Eating Disorders
in Children and Adolescents

Eating Disorders in Children and Adolescents

A CLINICAL HANDBOOK

edited by

Daniel Le Grange
James Lock

THE GUILFORD PRESS
New York   London

© 2011 The Guilford Press
A Division of Guilford Publications, Inc.
72 Spring Street, New York, NY 10012
www.guilford.com

Printed in the United States of America

This book is printed on acid-free paper.

Last digit is print number: 9   8   7   6   5   4   3   2   1

The authors have checked with sources believed to be reliable in their efforts to provide information that is complete and generally in accord with the standards of practice that are accepted at the time of publication. However, in view of the possibility of human error or changes in behavioral, mental health, or medical sciences, neither the authors, nor the editors and publisher, nor any other party who has been involved in the preparation or publication of this work warrants that the information contained herein is in every respect accurate or complete, and they are not responsible for any errors or omissions or the results obtained from the use of such information. Readers are encouraged to confirm the information contained in this book with other sources.

Library of Congress Cataloging-in-Publication Data

Eating disorders in children and adolescents : a clinical handbook / edited by Daniel Le Grange, James Lock.
    p. cm.
    Summary: "Eating disorders typically first appear during childhood and adolescence. Despite this early age of onset, edited volumes on eating disorders have not focused on this age cohort. One of the primary purposes of this book is to redress this imbalance and target the unique issues that pertain to the development, assessment, and treatment of eating disorders in children and adolescents, a period of heightened vulnerability to these disorders and to the potential damage they can cause."—Provided by publisher.
    Includes bibliographical references and index.
    ISBN 978-1-60918-491-9 (hardback)
    1. Eating disorders in children. 2. Eating disorders in adolescence. I. Le Grange, Daniel. II. Lock, James.
    RJ506.E18E293 2011
    618.92′8526—dc22
                                                                    2011002832

To my mother, who inspires me every day
with her "glass is half full" philosophy of life
—D. L. G.

To the teachers, mentors, patients, and families
who have taught me so much
—J. L.

About the Editors

Daniel Le Grange, PhD, is Professor in the Department of Psychiatry and Behavioral Neuroscience and Director of the Eating Disorders Program at the University of Chicago. He trained at the Institute of Psychiatry, University of London, and was a member of the team at the Maudsley Hospital in London that developed family-based treatment for anorexia nervosa. He is the author of numerous research publications and received a National Institute of Mental Health (NIMH) Early Career Development Award. Dr. Le Grange is currently principal investigator for studies on treatment of both bulimia nervosa and anorexia nervosa.

James Lock, MD, PhD, is a child psychiatrist and Professor of Child Psychiatry and Pediatrics in the Division of Child and Adolescent Psychiatry and Child Development, Department of Psychiatry and Behavioral Sciences, Stanford University. He is Director of the Eating Disorders Program in the Division of Child Psychiatry and Psychiatric Director of an inpatient eating disorders program for children and adolescents at Lucile Salter Packard Children's Hospital at Stanford. The author of numerous scientific publications on eating disorders in youth, Dr. Lock is a recipient of the Price Family Foundation Award for Research Excellence from the National Eating Disorders Association, an NIMH Early Career Development Award, and an NIMH Mid-Career Development Award.

Contributors

Roslyn Binford Hopf, PhD, private practice, Koenigstein im Taunus, Germany, and Department of Psychiatry and Behavioral Neuroscience, University of Chicago, Chicago, Illinois

Susan J. Bondy, PhD, Division of Epidemiology, Dalla Lana School of Public Health, University of Toronto, Toronto, Ontario, Canada

Kerri N. Boutelle, PhD, Departments of Pediatrics and Psychiatry, University of California, San Diego, La Jolla, California

Harriet Brown, Syracuse, New York

Melanie Brown, MA, Department of Psychology, Fairleigh Dickinson University, Teaneck, New Jersey

Rachel Bryant-Waugh, MSc, PhD, Department of Child and Adolescent Mental Health, Great Ormond Street Hospital, London, United Kingdom

Cynthia M. Bulik, PhD, Departments of Psychiatry and Nutrition, University of North Carolina at Chapel Hill, Chapel Hill, North Carolina

Mari Campbell, DClinPsy, Child and Adolescent Eating Disorders Team, South London and Maudsley NHS Foundation Trust, London, United Kingdom

Angela Celio Doyle, PhD, Department of Psychiatry and Behavioral Neuroscience, University of Chicago, Chicago, Illinois

Jennifer Couturier, MD, Pediatric Eating Disorders Program, McMaster Children's Hospital, Hamilton, Ontario, Canada

Katherine E. Craigen, BA, Department of Psychology, Fairleigh Dickinson University, Teaneck, New Jersey

Kamryn T. Eddy, PhD, Department of Psychiatry, Massachusetts General Hospital, Harvard Medical School, Boston, Massachusetts

Ivan Eisler, PhD, Section of Family Therapy, Institute of Psychiatry, Kings College London, London, United Kingdom

Pennie Fairbairn, MSc, Michael Rutter Centre for Children and Adolescents, South London and Maudsley NHS Foundation Trust, London, United Kingdom

Sheri M. Findlay, MD, Department of Pediatrics, McMaster Children's Hospital and McMaster University, Hamilton, Ontario, Canada

Kara Fitzpatrick, PhD, Department of Psychiatry and Behavioral Sciences, Stanford University School of Medicine, Stanford, California

Debra L. Franko, PhD, Department of Counseling and Applied Psychology, Northeastern University, Boston, Massachusetts

Michal Munk Goldstein, BA, Department of Psychology, Fairleigh Dickinson University, Teaneck, New Jersey

David B. Herzog, MD, Department of Psychiatry, Massachusetts General Hospital, Harvard Medical School, Boston, Massachusetts

Renee Rienecke Hoste, PhD, Department of Psychiatry and Behavioral Neuroscience, University of Chicago, Chicago, Illinois

Debra K. Katzman, MD, Division of Adolescent Medicine, The Hospital for Sick Children, Toronto, Ontario, Canada

Walter H. Kaye, MD, Department of Psychiatry, University of California, San Diego, La Jolla, California

Kelly L. Klump, PhD, Department of Psychology, Michigan State University, East Lansing, Michigan

Richard Kreipe, MD, Department of Pediatrics, Division of Adolescent Medicine, University of Rochester Medical Center, Rochester, New York

Daniel Le Grange, PhD, Department of Psychiatry and Behavioral Neuroscience, University of Chicago, Chicago, Illinois

James Lock, MD, PhD, Department of Psychiatry and Behavioral Sciences, Stanford University, Stanford, California

Katharine L. Loeb, PhD, Eating and Weight Disorders Program, Mount Sinai School of Medicine, New York, New York

Ann Moye, PhD, private practice, Bloomfield Hills, Michigan

Dianne Neumark-Sztainer, PhD, Division of Epidemiology and Community Health, School of Public Health, University of Minnesota, Minneapolis, Minnesota

Dasha Nicholls, MBBS, MD, Department of Child and Adolescent Mental Health, Great Ormond Street Hospital, London, United Kingdom

Mark L. Norris, PhD, Department of Pediatrics, Children's Hospital of Eastern Ontario, University of Ottawa, Ottawa, Ontario, Canada

Sheetal Patel, DPhil, School of Journalism and Mass Communication, University of North Carolina at Chapel Hill, Chapel Hill, North Carolina

Tara Peris, PhD, Semel Institute for Neuroscience and Human Behavior, David Geffen School of Medicine, University of California, Los Angeles, Los Angeles, California

Leora Pinhas, MD, Eating Disorders Program, Department of Psychiatry, The Hospital for Sick Children, University of Toronto, Toronto, Ontario, Canada

Sarah E. Racine, MA, Department of Psychology, Michigan State University, East Lansing, Michigan

Tammy L. Root, PhD, Department of Psychiatry, University of North Carolina at Chapel Hill, Chapel Hill, North Carolina

Ulrike Schmidt, PhD, Eating Disorders Outpatients Unit, Institute of Psychiatry, Kings College London, London, United Kingdom

Autumn Shafer, PhD, School of Journalism and Mass Communication, University of North Carolina at Chapel Hill, Chapel Hill, North Carolina

Mima Simic, PhD, Michael Rutter Centre for Children and Adolescents, South London and Maudsley NHS Foundation Trust, London, United Kingdom

Wendy Spettigue, MD, Regional Eating Disorders Program, Children's Hospital of Eastern Ontario, Ottawa, Ontario, Canada

Hans-Christoph Steinhausen, MD, PhD, Department of Child and Adolescent Psychiatry, Aalborg Psychiatric Hospital, Aarhus University Hospital, Aalborg, Denmark; Clinical Psychology and Epidemiology, Institute of Psychology, University of Basel, Basel, Switzerland; and Department of Child and Adolescent Psychiatry, University of Zurich, Zurich, Switzerland

Michael Strober, PhD, Semel Institute for Neuroscience and Human Behavior, David Geffen School of Medicine, University of California, Los Angeles, Los Angeles, California

Marian Tanofsky-Kraff, PhD, Department of Medical and Clinical Psychology, Uniformed Services University of the Health Sciences, Bethesda, Maryland

Mary Tantillo, PhD, PMHCNS-BC, University of Rochester School of Nursing, University of Rochester Medical Center, Rochester, New York

Nancy L. Zucker, PhD, Department of Psychiatry and Behavioral Sciences, Duke University Medical Center, Durham, North Carolina

Contents

INTRODUCTION

CHAPTER 1

Childhood and Adolescence

Looking at Eating Disorders When They Start

Daniel Le Grange

E ating disorders typically first appear during childhood and adolescence. Despite this early age of onset, edited volumes on eating disorders have not focused on this age cohort. One of the primary purposes of this book is to redress this imbalance and target the unique issues that pertain to the development, assessment, and treatment of eating disorders in children and adolescents, which is a period of heightened vulnerability to the these disorders, as well as the potential damage they can cause. An esteemed group of colleagues have come together in this volume to articulate the unique perspective that should be considered in examining the vexing issues of etiology, diagnosis, and assessment of eating disorders in children and adolescents. Similarly, physical growth and cognitive and psychological maturation are considered when existing treatment efforts across the eating disorders spectrum are discussed for this young patient population. We also visit the ongoing challenge to understand the origins of these disorders in the context of prevention efforts in school-age children and adolescents. Parents and families are central to understanding and treating children. Consequently, just prior to the concluding chapter of this book, a parent's perspective is offered by a mother, who worked with her husband to support their teenage daughter in her struggle with anorexia nervosa (AN).

This book covers seven broad areas, and I introduce each of these separately: Etiology and Neurobiology (Chapters 2–4), Epidemiology and Course (Chapters 5 and 6), Diagnosis and Classification (Chapters 7 and 8), Medical Issues and Assessment (Chapters 9 and 10), Treatment (Chapters 11–21), Prevention (Chapters 22 and 23), and A Parent's Perspective (Chapter 24). My colleague and coeditor, James Lock, provides the concluding chapter to this volume (Chapter 25), with closing remarks and a look at future directions for the field of child and adolescent eating disorders.

Part I. Etiology and Neurobiology

During childhood and adolescence, critical changes take place in neural development, physical growth, and psychological maturity. Malnutrition and related medical consequences brought on by an eating disorder may in fact result in more severe and potentially

3

greater long-term costs if these occur during childhood and adolescence. The neurobiology of eating disorders is a relatively new field of inquiry, and understanding the intricate relationships among the neurobiological, physiological, and sociocultural determinants of these disorders, especially in young patients, is proving to be elusive, but is especially relevant given that eating disorders most often have their onset during childhood or adolescence. In Chapter 2, "Neurobiology of Anorexia Nervosa," Kaye outlines what is currently known about these issues. Racine, Root, Klump, and Bulik highlight the findings of twin studies in Chapter 3, "Environmental and Genetic Risk Factors for Eating Disorders: A Developmental Perspective," and in Chapter 4, "The Role of Family Environment in Etiology: A Neuroscience Perspective," Strober and Peris tackle another perplexing issue.

Part II. Epidemiology and Course

A recent epidemiological study of the prevalence and correlates of eating disorders in a large (N = 10,123) representative sample of adolescents (ages 13–18) in the United States showed the lifetime prevalence of AN, bulimia nervosa (BN), and binge-eating disorder (BED) was, respectively, 0.3%, 0.9%, and 1.6% (Swanson, Crow, Le Grange, Swendsen, & Merikangas, in press). In this study, an eating disorder diagnosis appeared to be often associated with other psychiatric disorders, suicidality in particular, as well as role impairment at home, in school/work, in the family, and in social life (e.g., unable to go to school or work or to carry out normal activities because of problems with eating or weight). A majority of adolescents with an eating disorder sought some form of treatment, although only a minority received treatment specifically for their eating or weight problems. Notwithstanding, high levels of service utilization underscore the severity of eating disorders, but the largely unmet treatment needs in the adolescent population highlight that these disorders represent a true public health concern. Norris, Bondy, and Pinhas provide a detailed summary in Chapter 5, "Epidemiology of Eating Disorders in Children and Adolescents," and in Chapter 6, "Course and Outcome," Steinhausen gives an account of the natural course of and effects of treatments on eating disorders in children and adolescents.

Part III. Diagnosis and Classification

The text revision of the fourth edition of the *Diagnostic and Statistical Manual of Mental Disorders* (DSM-IV-TR; American Psychiatric Association, 2000) presents significant challenges in terms of both the rather broad definition of eating disorder not otherwise specified (EDNOS) and its lack of sensitivity and specificity in the diagnosis of children and adolescents (Loeb et al., in press). An international workgroup of experts on the diagnosis and treatment of children and adolescents with eating disorders hopes to engineer improvements in the upcoming DSM-5 (Workgroup for Classification of Eating Disorders in Children and Adolescents [WCEDCA], 2010). The WCEDCA advocates an approach to diagnosis that is developmentally tailored toward this age group and takes diagnostic fluidity into consideration. It proposes (1) the use of lower and more developmentally sensitive thresholds of symptom severity as diagnostic boundaries for children and adolescents, (2) consideration of behavioral indicators in the absence of self-reported psychological features of eating disorder symptoms, and (3) utilization of informants such as parents to ascertain symptom profiles. Authors from the WCEDCA address an often neglected subject in "Diagnosis and Classification of Disordered Eating in Childhood" (Bryant-Waugh & Nicholls, Chapter 7) and in "Diagnosis and Classification of Eating Disorders in Adolescence" (Eddy, Herzog, & Zucker, Chapter 8). Both these chapters bring to light the importance of EDNOS and how to address this broad diagnostic group in younger patients, especially with an eye toward DSM-5.

Part IV. Medical Issues and Assessment

In addition to addressing the diagnostic dilemmas confronting clinicians and researchers working with children and adolescents, the recommendations by WCEDCA (2010) should also facilitate more accurate and earlier identification of eating disorders in these age groups. However, improved classification of eating disorders alone is not sufficient to facilitate accurate assessment of the medical status and cardinal psychological features of eating disorders. Many medical issues concerning eating disorders are unique in children and adolescents, such as slowed physical development, pubertal delay or interruption, and peak bone mass reduction at a time when peak bone mass should be achieved (Rome & Ammerman, 2003). Some of these deficits can be reversed with treatment. However, what makes the onset of an eating disorder particularly critical for children and adolescents is that height, for instance, can be stunted, a condition that may not be reversible even if healthy weight is achieved outside the period of maximum growth during adolescence, as discussed in Chapter 9, "Medical Issues Unique to Children and Adolescents," by Katzman and Findlay. Similarly, several psychological features of an eating disorder may not be easily articulated by children or adolescents. For example, adult sufferers of AN may describe a disturbance in the way in which one's body weight or shape is experienced, or emphasize that self-evaluation is unduly influenced by body shape, or deny the seriousness of the current low body weight, all of which helps clinicians better understand their patients' psychological characterization. Incorporating parents or other corroborating adults in the formal assessment of an eating disorder in younger patients can become an indispensable part in this complex process of evaluation and establishing diagnosis. Loeb and her colleagues provide an expansive review of all assessment measures typically employed in eating disorders and specifically how best to engage the parents in this process in Chapter 10, "Assessment of Eating Disorders in Children and Adolescents." Recognizing these distinctive medical and psychological features and challenges is essential for any professional involved in a comprehensive assessment clinic, which, in turn, has implications for early intervention, long considered to confer significant prognostic advantage (Deter & Herzog, 1994; Ratnasuriya, Eisler, & Szmukler, 1991; Schoemaker, 1997).

Part V. Treatment of Eating Disorders

We can all probably agree that early treatment is essential, yet several challenges remain to better ascertain which children and adolescents are appropriate candidates for early intervention or for one treatment versus another, as discussed in Chapter 18, "Early Treatment for Eating Disorders," by Loeb and colleagues. Numerous factors or obstacles, such as a low base rate, lack of diagnostic clarity, or the egosyntonic nature of most eating disorders, continue to beset the field of inquiry into treatment development, testing, and implementation across the spectrum of eating disorders. Despite these challenges, or perhaps because of them, inpatient treatment, an indispensable intervention for many patients, remains all too frequently the only and repeated form of management for many young patients, but with unpredictable long-term results (Gowers et al., 2007). Tantillo and Kreipe appreciate this dilemma and address the issue in Chapter 11, "Improving Connections for Adolescents across High-Intensity Settings for the Treatment of Eating Disorders."

Many clinical researchers have often argued that inpatient treatment for adolescents should be avoided if possible, and that instead, parents should be called upon to help bring about recovery on an outpatient basis (Dare & Eisler, 1997). Treatment in a hospital setting not only removes the patient from his or her regular environment, but often is experienced by the adolescent as traumatizing and disempowers parents. Compelling data now show that treatment should encourage parents in their efforts to support their child in an attempt to overcome their offspring's starvation or binge eating and purging (Le Grange, Crosby, Rathouz, & Leventhal, 2007; Lock et al., 2010). Family-based treatment for AN is described in Chapter 12 (Lock), and for BN in Chapter 15 (Le Grange). Evaluations of different forms of parental involvement, such as multifamily treatment (Chapter 13, "Multifamily Therapy for Adolescent Anorexia Nervosa," by Fairbairn and colleagues), and parent groups (Chapter 19, "Parent Groups in the Treatment of Eating Disorders," by Zucker and colleagues) are discussed in regard to possible new strategies to help families overcome eating disorders. Other individual psychotherapies, such as those that are adolescent focused (Chapter 14, by Moye and colleagues), cognitive-behavioral therapy (Chapter 16, by Campbell and Schmidt), or supportive psychotherapy (Chapter 17, by Hoste and Celio Doyle), are being investigated and are helpful, although perhaps not to the same degree alone as when parents are involved in treatment. There is also an urgent need to better understand the etiology and treatment of overeating in children. Given the current high rates of obesity in children and adolescents (Ogden, Carroll, Curtin, Lamb, & Flegal, 2010), targeting aberrant eating patterns for overweight in this patient population is also imperative, as discussed in Chapter 20 by Boutelle and Tanofsky-Kraff.

The collective efforts of those in our field to find effective treatments for children and adolescents with eating disorders have generally shied away from the use of pharmacotherapy. Although there is little empirical support for the use of medication in children and adolescents with eating disorders, pharmacotherapy is nevertheless common in clinical practice, and Chapter 21, "Pharmacotherapy for Eating Disorders in Children and Adolescents," by Couturier and Spettigue provides a helpful review of this subject. As is the case with other treatments for eating disorders, much more systematic inquiry into the use of medications in eating disorders is needed.

Part VI. Prevention

Eating disorder prevention in children and adolescents is one of the least understood and least researched domains in the field of eating disorders. Without a clearer idea of the etiological factors involved in these disorders, designing effective prevention efforts is a formidable challenge. Yet several efforts at better understanding the prevention of eating disorders have been undertaken. Eating disorder prevention efforts involve the identification, reduction, or elimination of critical modifiable risk factors for these disorders and at the same time involve the promotion of factors that are protective against eating disorders. These efforts are typically aimed at several audiences: individual, family, group, institutional, community, or the larger society. Neumark-Sztainer addresses these issues in Chapter 22, "Prevention of Eating Disorders in Children and Adolescents." Over the past two decades, innovative approaches to prevention (and intervention), such as the use of the Internet, have grown exponentially and are now beginning to reach the vast majority of people in developed nations, as reviewed in Chapter 23 by Celio Doyle and colleagues. The Internet no doubt is an impressive platform to provide programs to prevent and treat eating and weight disorders in children and adolescents.

Part VII. The Role of Parents

In the end, parents and families are seen to play a central role throughout the preceding six parts of this book, as children and adolescents are obviously firmly ensconced within their families. Whether we attempt to better understand the gene–environment interaction, appreciate the prevalence of eating disorders and the impact of these disorders on families and on service delivery, figure out how best to engage parents in the treatment of their offspring, or embark on efforts to improve our understanding at preventing these disorders, the parents' perspective on the well-being of their children should not be sidelined. Harriet Brown underscores these thoughts in Chapter 24 by providing a look at many of the dilemmas highlighted in this book. Professionals ought to join with patients and families and together promote awareness, encourage treatment, support research, and decrease stigma as we take a collective step forward in the field (see Brown, 2010).

In order to provide a comprehensive and focused discussion of eating disorders in younger populations, this cadre of outstanding clinicians and researchers, all of whom are devoting most of their careers to the field of child and adolescent eating disorder have contributed their expertise to this handbook. This is by no means an exhaustive treatment of this topic area, to be sure, but instead it is a focused guide that is both comprehensive and scholarly and should be useful to clinicians and researchers alike.

References

American Psychiatric Association. (2000). *Diagnostic and statistical manual of mental disorders* (4th ed., text rev.). Washington, DC: Author.

Brown, H. (2010). *Brave girl eating: A family's struggle with anorexia.* New York: HarperCollins.

Dare, C., & Eisler, I. (1997). Family therapy for anorexia nervosa. In D. M. Garner & P. E. Garfinkel (Eds.), *Handbook of treatment for eating disorders* (2nd ed., pp. 307–324). New York: Guilford Press.

Deter, H. C., & Herzog, W. (1994). Anorexia nervosa in a long-term perspective: Results of the Heidelberg–Mannheim study. *Psychosomatic Medicine, 56,* 20–22.

Gowers, S., Clark, A., Roberts, C., Griffiths, A., Edwards, V., Bryan, C., et al. (2007). Clinical effectiveness of treatments for anorexia nervosa in adolescents. *British Journal of Psychiatry, 191*, 427–435.

Le Grange, D., Crosby, R. D., Rathouz, P. J., & Leventhal, B. L. (2007). A randomized controlled comparison of family-based treatment and supportive psychotherapy for adolescent bulimia nervosa. *Archives of General Psychiatry, 64*, 1049–1056.

Lock, J., Le Grange, D., Agras, S., Moye, A., Bryson, S., & Booil, J. (2010). Randomized clinical trial comparing family-based treatment to adolescent focused individual therapy for adolescents with anorexia nervosa. *Archives of General Psychiatry, 67*, 1025–1032.

Loeb, K., Le Grange, D., Hildebrandt, T., Greif, R., Lock, J., & Alfano, L. (in press). Eating disorders in youth: Elusive diagnoses? *International Journal of Eating Disorders.*

Ogden, C. L., Carroll, M. D., Curtin, L. R., Lamb, M. M., & Flegal, K. M. (2010). Prevalence of high body mass index in US children and adolescents, 2007–2008. *Journal of the American Medical Association, 303*, 242–249.

Ratnasuriya, R., Eisler, I., & Szmukler, G. I. (1991). Anorexia nervosa: Outcome and prognostic factors after 20 years. *British Journal of Psychiatry, 156*, 495–456.

Rome, E. S., & Ammerman, S. (2003). Medical complications of eating disorders: An update. *Journal of Adolescent Health, 33*, 418–426.

Schoemaker, C. (1997). Does early intervention improve the prognosis in anorexia nervosa?: A systematic review of the treatment-outcome literature. *International Journal of Eating Disorders, 21*, 1–15.

Swanson, S. A., Crow, S. J., Le Grange, D., Swendsen, J., & Merikangas, K. R. (in press). Prevalence and correlates of eating disorders in adolescents: Results from the National Comorbidity Survey replication adolescent supplement. *Archives of General Psychiatry.*

Workgroup for Classification of Eating Disorders in Children and Adolescents. (2010). Classification of eating disturbance in children and adolescents: Proposed changes for the DSM-V. *European Eating Disorders Review, 18*, 79–89.

■ PART I ■

ETIOLOGY AND NEUROBIOLOGY

CHAPTER 2

Neurobiology of Anorexia Nervosa

Walter H. Kaye

How is it possible for people with anorexia nervosa (AN) to consume a few hundred calories a day and maintain an extremely low weight for many years, when most people struggle to lose even a few pounds?

People with AN exhibit a highly rigid, ritualized, and inadequate intake of food and so become severely underweight. They tend to resemble each other in other ways too: They often become sick around the same time (early adolescence), show similar symptoms and behaviors, and are mostly females (American Psychiatric Association, 2000). They typically resist eating and engage in a powerful pursuit of weight loss, yet paradoxically are obsessed with food and eating rituals. Even when underweight, they tend to see themselves as fat and deny being underweight. They tend to resist treatment and lack insight about the seriousness of the medical consequences of AN.

These similarities support the possibility that underlying neurobiological contributions drive the behaviors seen in AN.

Two types of eating-related behaviors are seen in AN. People with restricting-type AN lose weight purely by dieting, without binge eating or purging. People with binge-eating/purging-type anorexia (AN-BN) restrict food intake to lose weight, but periodically engage in binge eating and/or purging, as do those with bulimia nervosa (BN). Considering that transitions between syndromes occur in many, it has been argued that AN and BN share some risk and liability factors (Lilenfeld et al., 1998; Walters & Kendler, 1995). This chapter focuses on restricting-type AN.

Eating Disorder or Brain Disorder?

Although we call AN an eating disorder, we do not know whether it reflects a primary disturbance of the brain systems that regulate appetite, or whether changes in appetite are caused by other factors, such as anxiety or obsessional preoccupation with weight gain. Starvation and weight loss have powerful effects on the brain and other organ systems, causing neurochemical disturbances that may exaggerate preexisting traits (Pollice, Kaye, Greeno, & Weltzin, 1997), adding symptoms that maintain or accelerate the disease process. For example, patients with AN exhibit reduced brain volume (Katzman et al., 1996), altered metabolism of brain regions known to modulate emotion and thought

(Kaye, Wagner, Frank, & Bailer, 2006), and a return to childhood levels of female hormones (Boyar et al., 1974). The fact that such disturbances tend to normalize after weight restoration suggests that they are a consequence of AN rather than a cause.

A number of regions in the brain help regulate intake of foods and weight. In the hypothalamus, for instance, chemicals such as insulin and leptin send messages about hunger and energy balance. With weight loss, the levels of these chemicals become abnormal, signaling that the body doesn't have enough fuel and that the person needs to eat. The evidence suggests that such changes are driven by starvation and serve to conserve energy or stimulate hunger and feeding (Schwartz, Woods, Porte, Seeley, & Baskin, 2000); they likely do not cause AN. But people with AN seem able to override or ignore signals from lower brain regions such as the hypothalamus. New studies point to the ways uniquely human higher brain regions (e.g., the frontal cortex and insula) are implicated in the ongoing starvation of AN. These higher brain regions play a crucial role in emotions, personality, and rewards, all of which are thought to be important in AN.

AN and Personality Traits

Genes play a major role in causing eating disorders (Berrettini, 2000; Bulik et al., 2006; Walters & Kendler, 1995), likely contributing to a range of personality traits that put people at risk for AN. People who develop AN tend to display certain characteristics in childhood, years before they become ill, including anxiety and depression, perfectionism, people-pleasing behaviors, a drive for thinness, and obsessiveness. These traits tend to persist after recovery.

In AN, as in other illnesses, we often talk about *trait* versus *state*. People are born with certain personality traits, such as perfectionism or a tendency toward anxiety, that last their whole lives. States are more situation specific—say, the kind of anxiety many New Yorkers felt right after 9/11. States can be affected by environment or circumstances; traits cannot.

Obsessive personality traits include an overconcern for symmetry and exactness (Kaye, 1997). For instance, people with AN may color-code the clothes in their closets; they may have specific spots for items in their rooms and get upset if things are moved. On the plus side, they tend to be achievement oriented and compliant and make exceptional students. A child who later develops AN is typically described as "the best little girl (boy) in the world." Such young people tend to be rule abiding, rigid, and anxious children who are high in harm avoidance, a personality trait characterized by a tendency to criticize and doubt past thoughts and behaviors, worry about the future, and struggle with uncertainty (Cloninger, Przybeck, Svrakic, & Wetzel, 1994). Studies show that these personality traits are heritable and are often seen in unaffected family members, independent of body weight (Bulik et al., 2007), suggesting that they are risk factors for the development of AN. Not everyone who develops AN has all these traits, of course. Some people have only one or a few. Others may not have any. Still, our experience is that most people who develop AN show at least some of these personality traits and temperament in childhood.

One reason we are not sure is that it is challenging to design the kind of long-term studies that can look for these traits, given the young age of potential subjects, the rarity of the disorder, and the need to follow subjects for many years. An alternative strategy is to study people who have recovered from AN, avoiding the confounding influences of malnutrition and weight loss. There is no single agreed-upon definition of recovery from AN; in our research we use a definition that includes stable and healthy body weight for months or years, with stable nutrition, the relative absence of dietary abnormalities, and normal menstruation.

The process of recovery in AN is poorly understood and, in most cases, protracted. But we do know that between 50 and 70% of affected individuals will eventually have complete or moderate resolution of the illness, though this may not occur until their mid-20s (Steinhausen, 2002; Strober, Freeman, & Morrell, 1997; Wagner et al., 2006). Studies describe temperament and character traits that persist after long-term recovery, including negative emotionality, harm avoidance and perfectionism, desire for thinness, and mild dietary preoccupation. Such persistent symptoms may be "scars" caused by chronic malnutrition. But the fact that such behaviors (Casper, 1990; Srinivasagam et al., 1995; Wagner et al., 2006) are similar to those described in children who go on to develop AN (Anderluh, Tchanturia, Rabe-Hesketh, & Treasure, 2003; Lilenfeld, Wonderlich, Riso, Crosby, & Mitchell, 2006; Stice, 2002) argues that they reflect underlying traits rather than consequences of AN.

Some of the common behaviors seen in both recovered and acute AN are often found together. Our research group has been exploring how these behaviors are coded in the brain. It would be an oversimplification to think these traits are somehow contained in neurotransmitters or brain regions; the human brain is far too complex. But such behaviors may be encoded in the neural pathways that modulate emotion, reward, and the human ability to think about consequences and the future.

Two neural pathways—the limbic and the cognitive—affect appetite, emotionality, and cognitive control and seem to be particularly relevant to behavior in AN. The *limbic* neurocircuit includes the amygdala, insula, ventral striatum, and ventral regions of the anterior cingulate cortex (ACC) and orbitofrontal cortex (OFC); it seems to help people identify the emotional significance of events and stimuli and respond appropriately (Phillips, Drevets, & Lane, 2003; Phillips, Drevets, & Rauch, 2003). The *cognitive* neurocircuit affects selective attention, planning, inhibition, and emotional self-control and includes the hippocampus, dorsal regions of the ACC, the dorsolateral prefrontal cortex (DLPFC), and the parietal cortex (Phillips, Drevets, Rauch, & Lane, 2003; Phillips, Drevets, & Rauch, 2003). Earlier brain-imaging studies have demonstrated that people recovered from AN show altered activity in frontal, ACC, and parietal regions (Gordon, Lask, Bryant-Waugh, Christie, & Timimi, 1997; Rastam et al., 2001; Uher et al., 2003)—elements in both the limbic and cognitive pathways.

Neurobiology and Appetite

Appetite is a complex phenomenon, a function of signals coming from nerves and hormones in the brain and the gut and from fat and sugar stores throughout the body (Figure 2.1). Higher brain structures may be particularly involved in the kind of disturbed eating that characterizes AN. Recent studies suggest that the motivation to eat (or not eat) is related to the palatability of food, the level of a person's energy stores, and the cognitive ability to control or restrain eating (Elman, Borsook, & Lukas, 2006; Kelley, 2004; Saper, Chou, & Elmquist, 2002).

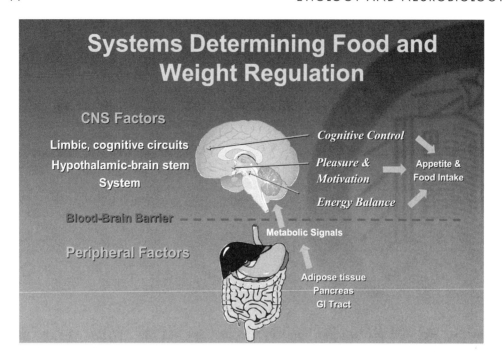

FIGURE 2.1. Overview of the many systems that contribute to food and weight regulation.

Appetite is clearly disturbed in AN. People with AN dislike high-fat foods (Drewnowski, Pierce, & Halmi, 1988; Fernstrom, Weltzin, Neuberger, Srinivasagam, & Kaye, 1994) and react differently to hunger and satiety cues than people without AN (Garfinkel, Moldofsky, & Garner, 1979; Santel, Baving, Krauel, Munte, & Rotte, 2006). For people with AN, eating less *reduces* anxiety, whereas eating makes them feel *more* anxious and/or depressed (Kaye et al., 2003; Strober, 1995; Vitousek & Manke, 1994). These responses to food are shared by most people with AN, supporting the possibility that they reflect some unusual function of the neural circuits involved in regulating eating behavior. They also tend to remain even after weight restoration.

In imaging studies, we often use a sweet-taste-perception (Figure 2.2) task to activate brain areas involved in regulating appetite. Receptors on the tongue respond to a sweet taste (Chandraskekar, Hoon, Ryba, & Zuker, 2006), then send a signal through the brain stem and lower brain regions to the primary taste center in the anterior insula (Faurion et al., 1999; Ogawa, 1994; Schoenfeld et al., 2004; Scott, Yaxley, Sienkiewicz, & Rolls, 1986; Yaxley, Rolls, & Sienkiewicz, 1990), an area deep in the brain near the frontal and temporal lobes, which is important in the perception and interpretation of physical sensations. The insula is the first area in the cortex to recognize when we have tasted something sweet, salty, or sour. Along with a related network including the amygdala, the ventral ACC, and the OFC, the insula helps determine whether we find a taste pleasant or unpleasant.

These regions of the brain seem to become more active when we are hungry and less active when we are full (Kringelbach, O'Doherty, Rolls, & Andrews, 2003; Morris & Dolan, 2001; Small, Zatorre, Dagher, Evans, & Jones-Gotman, 2001; Tataranni et al.,

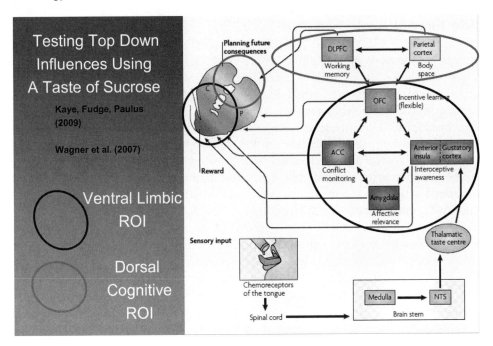

FIGURE 2.2. Pathways contributing to processing sweet taste. Receptors on the tongue detect a sweet taste. The signal is then transmitted through brain stem and thalamic taste centers to the primary taste cortex, which lies adjacent to and is densely interconnected with the anterior insula. The anterior insula is an integral part of a "ventral (limbic) neurocircuit" through its connections with the amygdala, the anterior cingulate cortex (ACC) and the orbitofrontal cortex (OFC), and the ventral striatum. Cortical structures involved in cognitive strategies (forming a dorsal neuro-circuit) send inputs to the dorsolateral striatum. The sensory aspects of taste are primarily an insula phenomenon, whereas higher cortical areas modulate pleasure, motivation, and cognitive aspects of taste. These aspects are then integrated, resulting in an "eat" or "do not eat" decision. Coding the awareness of pleasant sensation from the taste experience via the anterior insula may be altered in subjects with AN, tipping the balance of striatal processes away from normal, automatic reward responses mediated by the ventral striatum and toward a more "strategic" approach mediated by the dorsal striatum. From Kaye, Fudge, and Paulus (2009). Copyright 2009 by Walter H. Kaye. Reprinted by permission.

1999; Uher, Treasure, Heining, Brammer, & Campbell, 2006). When we are very hungry, food tastes better and we feel more motivated to eat. When we are full, food may still taste good, but it tends to be less rewarding. And even delicious food can become unpleasant: Eating a small piece of chocolate cake at dessert may be pleasing, but being forced to eat the whole cake may be a bad experience, thanks to a phenomenon called sensory-specific satiety, which explains why we grow "tired" of eating one food during a meal and switch to another.

The insula and related regions connect to a subcortical area, the ventral striatum, which is important in carrying out motivated behavior. Together, these regions help us sense the pleasurable, motivating value of food and how this value may change, depending on whether we are hungry or full.

Inside the AN Brain

Imaging studies show some intriguing differences between the brains of people who have had AN and the brains of healthy control subjects. Many of these differences may be seen in the insula. For instance, when people without AN are given sugar during a sweet-perception task, the more they say they enjoy the sugar, and the more activity they show in their insula, ACC, and striatum (Wagner et al., 2008), supporting the idea that these regions are important for sensing reward. People who are recovered from AN show less activity in these areas (Figure 2.3) when tasting sugar (Wagner et al., 2008).

When looking at pictures of food, both recovered and underweight people with AN show altered activity in the insula, the OFC, the mesial temporal and parietal cortices, and the ACC (Ellison et al., 1998; Gordon et al., 2001; Naruo et al., 2000; Nozoe et al., 1993; Uher et al., 2003, 2004). People recovered from AN showed less activity in the insula and other parts of the neural network, suggesting that the ability to perceive a palatable taste is fundamentally altered in AN, even after recovery, and that people with AN have a reduced incentive and/or motivation to approach food (Figure 2.4).

Overall, the results of these brain-imaging studies suggest that people with AN have lower-than-usual drive in a number of the systems that respond to hunger and appetite, which may explain how it is possible for them to pursue emaciation to the point of death. Normally, when people become hungry, neural networks around the brain become more active, making food taste more rewarding and driving the motivation to eat. People with

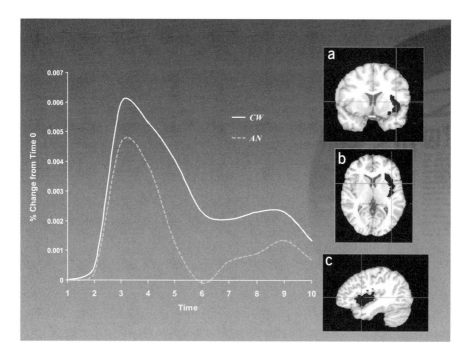

FIGURE 2.3. (a) Coronal, (b) axial, and (c) sagittal view of left insula. The graph shows the time course of BOLD signal as a mean of all 16 recovered restricting-type AN and 16 control women (CW) for taste-related (sucrose and water) response in the left insula. $p = .003$. From Wagner et al. (2008). Copyright 2008 by Angela Wagner. Reprinted by permission.

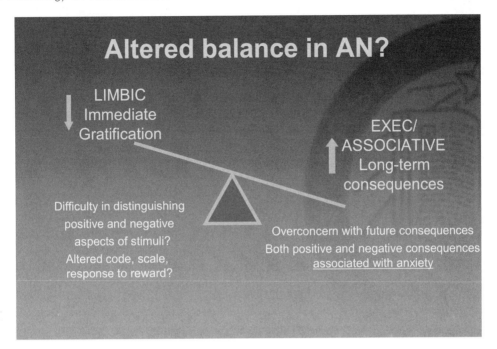

FIGURE 2.4. Data (Wagner et al., 2007) suggest that individuals who have recovered from AN have an imbalance between pathways that identify the emotional significance of environmental stimuli and pathways responsible for the performance of planning and effortful functions. People with AN do not live in the moment. They tend to have exaggerated and obsessive worry about the consequences of their behaviors, looking for rules when there are none, and they are unduly concerned about making mistakes. Individuals who have recovered from anorexia nervosa may be less able to precisely modulate affective response to stimuli and live in the here and now. They do appear to have increased traffic in neurocircuits concerned with planning and consequences.

AN may get mixed messages from various parts of the brain, which may explain why they often have obsessions with food and cooking yet do not have enough motivation to eat.

In addition to playing a role in taste, the insula is critically involved in *interoceptive processing* (Craig, 2009; Critchley, Wiens, Rotshtein, Ohman, & Dolan, 2004; Paulus & Stein, 2006), making us aware of physical sensations of pain, heat or cold, itch, tickle, muscle tension, air hunger, and other bodily processes (Craig, 2002). The insula is responsible for registering a change in any of these physiological processes and telling the body to do something about it; for instance, the insula becomes more active when a person is hungry, signaling the need to eat.

Some clinicians have theorized that altered interoceptive awareness may help trigger and reinforce AN (Bruch, 1962; Fassino, Piero, Gramaglia, & Abbate-Daga, 2004; Garner, Olmstead, & Polivy, 1983; Lilenfeld et al., 2006). Recent studies from our group suggest that people with AN may exhibit a generalized alteration of insula activity involving other interoceptive signals besides taste. This raises the question of whether altered insula function contributes to a fundamentally and physiologically altered sense of self in AN (Pollatos et al., 2008). Many of the most puzzling symptoms of AN, such as distorted body image, failure to appropriately respond to hunger, and diminished motivation to change, may be related to disturbed interoceptive awareness.

Reward Processing in AN

Many people with AN exercise compulsively and find little in life rewarding aside from the pursuit of weight loss (American Psychiatric Association, 2000). Like other traits, these too persist, in a more modest form, after recovery (Klump et al., 2004; Wagner et al., 2006). These particular traits all involve the neurotransmitter dopamine, which contributes to altered reward and affect, decision making, and executive control. There is considerable evidence that altered function of dopamine occurs in AN (Kaye, Fudge, & Paulus, 2009), possibly contributing to overexercise and decreased food intake (Frank et al., 2005).

Our group did a brain-imaging study in which we asked both healthy controls and people recovered from AN to perform a simple choice and feedback task (Wagner et al., 2007). The task was adapted from a well-characterized "guessing-game" protocol (Delgado, Nystrom, Fissel, Noll, & Fiez, 2000) known to activate the ventral striatum and ACC. In controls, the neural activity for winning money was very different from the activity for losing money. But in people recovered from AN, brain activity in the ACC and its ventral striatal target was similar whether they won or lost (Wagner et al., 2007). This suggests that people with AN may have trouble discriminating between positive and negative feedback and identifying the emotional significance of stimuli (Phillips, Drevets, Rauch, & Lane, 2003), which in turn may help explain why it is so tough to motivate them to go into treatment or to appreciate the consequences of their behaviors (Halmi et al., 2005).

Women who were recovered from AN also showed exaggerated activity in certain areas of the brain, specifically the DLPFC and the parietal cortex (Wagner et al., 2007). These regions are activated by tasks in which there is a perceived connection between action and outcome, *and* some uncertainty about whether the action will lead to the desired outcome (Tricomi, Delgado, & Fiez, 2004). Healthy control subjects were able to "live in the moment"; they realized they had to make a guess, they made a guess, and they moved on to the next task without undue concern. In contrast, people recovered from AN tended to worry about the consequences of their behaviors, looking for "rules" when there were none and feeling unduly concerned about making mistakes. A recent functional magnetic resonance imaging (fMRI) study, using a set-shifting task, showed similar findings in ill AN patients (Zastrow et al., 2009). Together these findings suggest that people with AN may be both unsure of how they feel in the moment and overconcerned about tasks involving planning and consequences (Figure 2.5).

One explanation for these findings may lie in the way neurocircuits overlap in the brain. For instance, the cortical regions included in the dorsal neurocircuit affect both cognitive and executive functions such as planning and sequencing, and at the same time overlap with ventral striatal areas (Chikama, McFarland, Armaral, & Haber, 1997; Fudge, Breitbart, Danish, & Pannoni, 2005) that modulate the approach to or avoidance of food. If the parts of this cognitive circuit that inhibit the drive to eat are overactive, that may let people with AN suppress and override signals about bodily needs such as hunger.

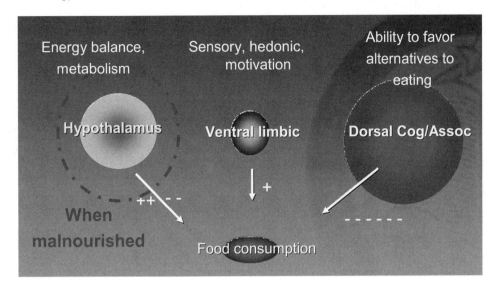

FIGURE 2.5. Multiple systems contribute to decisions about food consumption (Berthoud, 2006; Elman et al., 2006; Hinton et al., 2004; Kelley, 2004; Morton, Cummings, Baskin, Barsh, & Schwartz, 2006; Saper et al., 2002). We hypothesize that individuals with AN have a trait for altered ventral limbic system function, so thus have a diminished sensory-hedonic-motivational "drive" to consume food. In contrast, they have a trait for exaggerated dorsal cognitive function, so that they have enhanced inhibitory abilities and thus can "favor" alternatives to eating. These traits persist after recovery, but individuals with AN learn to compensate by choosing to eat the same amounts of the same foods every day, so that they are able to maintain their weight and have adequate nutrition. Thus hypothalamic systems, which are important for responding to deficits in energy balance, are normal. However, when malnourished and underweight, the hypothalamus senses a deficit in energy balance and responds with altered levels of neuropeptides and hormones that serve to drive appetite and conserve energy. We suspect that the puzzling appetitive behaviors that ill AN patients show (restricted eating, yet obsessed with food, afraid to eat but scared that they cannot stop, etc.) are due to these mixed signals.

Conclusions and Future Directions

Like other eating disorders, AN typically appears during adolescence, a time of profound biological, psychological, and sociocultural change. A considerable degree of flexibility is required to successfully manage the transition into adulthood (Connan, Campbell, Katzman, Lightman, & Treasure, 2003). Teenagers leave the security of their home environments and must learn to balance immediate and long-term needs and goals to achieve independence (Connan et al., 2003).

Neurobiology may offer some answers as to why AN typically develops during adolescence. AN is thought to be a disorder of complex etiology, in which genetic, biological, psychological, and sociocultural factors, and interactions between them, create susceptibility (Connan et al., 2003; Jacobi, Hayward, de Zwaan, Kraemer, & Agras, 2004; Lilenfeld et al., 2006; Stice, 2002). No single factor has been shown to be either necessary or sufficient for causing AN.

AN often begins with a restricted diet and weight loss during adolescence, which progresses to an out-of-control spiral. People who develop AN may cross a threshold where temperament interacts with stress and/or psychosocial factors, leading to an illness with impaired insight and a powerful, obsessive preoccupation with dieting and weight loss. Psychologically, the changes of adolescence may challenge the perfectionism, harm avoidance, and rigidity of those at risk for AN and thus fuel an underlying vulnerability. The biological changes of puberty may also help trigger the onset of AN (Klump, Burt, McGue, & Iacono, 2007). Those at risk for AN may feel overwhelmed by the difficulties of learning to interact flexibly and master complex and mixed cultural and societal messages—a set of tasks made more difficult for them because of their underlying neurobiology.

An interesting question about AN is why so many more females develop it than males. The answer may lie in the biological changes associated with adolescence, which differ between males and females. For example, menarche is associated (Connan et al., 2003) with a rapid change in body composition and the neuropeptides modulating metabolism. The rise in estrogen levels associated with puberty in females may affect the serotonin system (Rubinow, Schmidt, & Roca, 1998) or levels of neuropeptides (Torpy, Papanicolaou, & Chrousos, 1997) that influence feeding, emotionality, and other behaviors. The brain changes associated with puberty may exacerbate these processes; for example, orbital and dorsolateral prefrontal cortex regions develop greatly during and after puberty (Huttenlocher & Dabholkar, 1997), and increased activity in these cortical areas may trigger the excessive worry, perfectionism, and strategizing common to those with AN. Stress and/or cultural and societal pressures may also contribute by amplifying anxious and obsessional temperament. People at risk for AN find that restricting food intake makes them feel less anxious, and so they enter a vicious cycle in which eating exaggerates anxiety and food refusal reduces it—a fact that may account for the chronicity of the disorder.

It is important to remember that the temperament and personality traits that may create a vulnerability for developing AN are not all bad. Traits like attention to detail, concern about consequences, and a drive to accomplish and succeed can all be positive. It is tempting to speculate that the ability to plan ahead, control impulses, and avoid harm may have had highly adaptive value for ancestors who lived in environments where food supplies were constrained by long periods of cold weather (e.g., worry in July about food supplies in January). Thus, it is our clinical experience that many people who recover from AN go on to do well in life.

Acknowledgments

Funding for this work was provided by the National Institute of Mental Health (Grant Nos. MH046001, MH042984, MH076286, and MH086017), the Price Foundation, the Peterson Foundation, and the Hilda & Preston Davis/Joan Wisemer Foundations.

References

American Psychiatric Association. (2000). *Diagnostic and statistical manual of mental disorders* (4th ed., text rev.). Washington, DC: Author.

Anderluh, M. B., Tchanturia, K., Rabe-Hesketh, S., & Treasure, J. (2003). Childhood obsessive–compulsive personality traits in adult women with eating disorders:

Defining a broader eating disorder phenotype. *American Journal of Psychiatry, 160*(2), 242–247.

Berrettini, W. (2000). Genetics of psychiatric disease. *Annual Review of Medicine, 51*, 465–479.

Berthoud, H. R. (2006). Homeostatic and non-homeostatic pathways involved in the control of food intake and energy balance. *Obesity, 14*, 197S–200S.

Boyar, R. K., Finkelstein, J., Kapen, S., Weiner, H., Weitzman, E., & Hellman, L. (1974). Anorexia nervosa. Immaturity of the 24-hour luteinizing hormone secretory pattern. *New England Journal of Medicine, 291*(17), 861–865.

Bruch, H. (1962). Perceptual and conceptual disturbances in anorexia nervosa. *Psychosomatic Medicine, 24*, 187–194.

Bulik, C., Hebebrand, J., Keski-Rahkonen, A., Klump, K., Reichborn-Kjennerud, K. S., Mazzeo, S., et al. (2007). Genetic epidemiology, endophenotypes, and eating disorder classification. *International Journal of Eating Disorders, 40*(Suppl.), S52–S60.

Bulik, C., Sullivan, P. F., Tozzi, F., Furberg, H., Lichtenstein, P., & Pedersen, N. L. (2006). Prevalence, heritability and prospective risk factors for anorexia nervosa. *Archives of General Psychiatry, 63*(3), 305–312.

Casper, R. C. (1990). Personality features of women with good outcome from restricting anorexia nervosa. *Psychosomatic Medicine, 52*(2), 156–170.

Chandraskekar, J., Hoon, M., Ryba, N., & Zuker, C. (2006). The receptors and cells for mammalian taste. *Nature, 444*, 288–294.

Chikama, M., McFarland, N., Armaral, D., & Haber, S. (1997). Insular cortical projections to functional regions of the striatum correlate with cortical cytoarchitectonic organization in the primate. *Journal of Neuroscience, 17*(24), 9686–9705.

Cloninger, C., Przybeck, T., Svrakic, D., & Wetzel, R. (1994). *The Temperament and Character Inventory (TCI): A guide to its development and use.* St. Louis: Washington University School of Medicine.

Connan, F., Campbell, I., Katzman, M., Lightman, S., & Treasure, J. (2003). A neurodevelopmental model for anorexia nervosa. *Physiology and Behavior, 79*(1), 13–24.

Craig, A. (2009). How do you feel—now? The anterior insula and human awareness. *Nature Reviews Neuroscience, 10*(1), 59–70.

Craig, A. D. (2002). How do you feel? Interoception: The sense of the physiological condition of the body. *Nature Reviews Neuroscience, 3*(8), 655–666.

Critchley, H., Wiens, S., Rotshtein, P., Ohman, A., & Dolan, R. (2004). Neural systems supporting interoceptive awareness. *Nature Neuroscience, 7*, 189–195.

Delgado, M., Nystrom, L., Fissel, C., Noll, D., & Fiez, J. (2000). Tracking the hemodynamic responses to reward and punishment in the striatum. *Journal of Neurophysiology, 84*, 3072–3077.

Drewnowski, A., Pierce, B., & Halmi, K. (1988). Fat aversion in eating disorders. *Appetite, 10*, 119–131.

Ellison, Z., Foong, J., Howard, R., Bullmore, E., Williams, S., & Treasure, J. (1998). Functional anatomy of calorie fear in anorexia nervosa. *Lancet, 352*(9135), 1192.

Elman, I., Borsook, D., & Lukas, S. (2006). Food intake and reward mechanisms in patients with schizophrenia: Implications for metabolic disturbances and treatment with second-generation antipsychotic agents. *Neuropsychopharmacology, 31*(10), 2091–2120.

Fassino, S., Piero, A., Gramaglia, C., & Abbate-Daga, G. (2004). Clinical, psychopathological and personality correlates of interoceptive awareness in anorexia nervosa, bulimia nervosa and obesity. *Psychopathology, 37*(4), 168–174.

Faurion, A., Cerf, B., Van De Moortele, P. F., Lobel, E., Mac Leod, P., & Le Bihan, D. (1999). Human taste cortical areas studied with functional magnetic resonance imaging: Evidence of functional lateralization related to handedness. *Neuroscience Letters, 277*(3), 189–192.

Fernstrom, M. H., Weltzin, T. E., Neuberger, S., Srinivasagam, N., & Kaye, W. H. (1994). Twenty-four-hour food intake in patients with anorexia nervosa and in healthy control subjects. *Biological Psychiatry, 36*(10), 696–702.

Frank, G., Bailer, U. F., Henry, S., Drevets, W., Meltzer, C. C., Price, J. C., et al. (2005). Increased dopamine D2/D3 receptor binding after recovery from anorexia nervosa measured by positron emission tomography and [^{11}C]raclopride. *Biological Psychiatry, 58*(11), 908–912.

Fudge, J., Breitbart, M., Danish, M., & Pannoni, V. (2005). Insular and gustatory inputs to the caudal ventral striatum in primates. *Journal of Comparative Neurology, 490*(2), 101–118.

Garfinkel, P., Moldofsky, H., & Garner, D. M. (1979). The stability of perceptual disturbances in anorexia nervosa. *Psychological Medicine, 9*(4), 703–708.

Garner, D. M., Olmstead, M. P., & Polivy, J. (1983). Development and validation of a multidimensional eating disorder inventory for anorexia and bulimia nervosa. *International Journal of Eating Disorders, 2*, 15–34.

Gordon, C. M., Dougherty, D. D., Fischman, A. J., Emans, S. J., Grace, E., Lamm, R., et al. (2001). Neural substrates of anorexia nervosa: A behavioral challenge study with positron emission tomography. *Journal of Pediatrics, 139*(1), 51–57.

Gordon, I., Lask, B., Bryant-Waugh, R., Christie, D., & Timimi, S. (1997). Childhood-onset anorexia nervosa: Towards identifying a biological substrate. *International Journal of Eating Disorders, 22*(2), 159–165.

Halmi, K., Agras, W. S., Crow, S., Mitchell, J., Wilson, G., Bryson, S., et al. (2005). Predictors of treatment acceptance and completion in anorexia nervosa. *Archives of General Psychiatry, 62*, 776–781.

Hinton, E. C., Parkinson, J. A., Holland, A. J., Arana, F. S., Roberts, A. C., & Owen, A. M. (2004). Neural contributions to the motivational control of appetite in humans. *European Journal of Neuroscience, 20*, 1411–1418.

Huttenlocher, P., & Dabholkar, A. (1997). Regional differences in synaptogenesis in human cerebral cortex. *Journal of Comparative Neurology, 387*, 167–178.

Jacobi, C., Hayward, C., de Zwaan, M., Kraemer, H., & Agras, W. (2004). Coming to terms with risk factors for eating disorders: Application of risk terminology and suggestions for a general taxonomy. *Psychological Bulletin, 130*, 19–65.

Katzman, D. K., Lambe, E. K., Mikulis, D. J., Ridgley, J. N., Goldbloom, D. S., & Zipursky, R. B. (1996). Cerebral gray matter and white matter volume deficits in adolescent girls with anorexia nervosa. *Journal of Pediatrics, 129*, 794–803.

Kaye, W. (1997). Anorexia nervosa, obsessional behavior, and serotonin. *Psychopharmacology Bulletin, 33*(3), 335–344.

Kaye, W., Barbarich, N. C., Putnam, K., Gendall, K. A., Fernstrom, J., Fernstrom, M., et al. (2003). Anxiolytic effects of acute tryptophan depletion in anorexia nervosa. *International Journal of Eating Disorders, 33*(3), 257–267.

Kaye, W., Fudge, J., & Paulus, M. (2009). New insight into symptoms and neurocircuit function of anorexia nervosa. *Nature Reviews Neuroscience, 10*(8), 573–584.

Kaye, W., Wagner, A., Frank, G., & Bailer, U. (2006). Review of brain imaging in anorexia and bulimia nervosa. In J. Mitchell, S. Wonderlich, H. Steiger, & M. deZwaan (Eds.), *AED annual review of eating disorders*: Part 2 (pp. 113–130). Abingdon, UK: Radcliffe.

Kelley, A. E. (2004). Ventral striatal control of appetite motivation: Role in ingestive behavior and reward-related learning. *Neuroscience Biobehavioral Review, 27*, 765–776.

Klump, K., Burt, S., McGue, M., & Iacono, W. (2007). Changes in genetic and environmental influences on disordered eating across adolescence. A longitudinal twin study. *Archives of General Psychiatry, 64*(12), 1409–1415.

Klump, K., Strober, M., Johnson, C., Thornton, L., Bulik, C., Devlin, B., et al. (2004). Personality characteristics of women before and after recovery from an eating disorder. *Psychiatric Medicine, 34*(8), 1407–1418.

Kringelbach, M. L., O'Doherty, J., Rolls, E., & Andrews, C. (2003). Activation of the human orbitofrontal cortex to a liquid food stimulus is correlated with its subjective pleasantness. *Cerebral Cortex, 13*, 1064–1071.

Lilenfeld, L., Wonderlich, S., Riso, L. P., Crosby, R., & Mitchell, J. (2006). Eating disorders and personality: A methodological and empirical review. *Clinical Psychology Review, 26*(3), 299–320.

Lilenfeld, L. R., Kaye, W. H., Greeno, C. G., Merikangas, K. R., Plotnicov, K., Pollice, C., et al. (1998). A controlled family study of anorexia nervosa and bulimia nervosa: Psychiatric disorders in first-degree relatives and effects of proband comorbidity. *Archives of General Psychiatry, 55*(7), 603–610.

Morris, J. S., & Dolan, R. J. (2001). Involvement of human amygdala and orbitofrontal cortex in hunger-enhanced memory for food stimuli. *Journal of Neuroscience, 21*(14), 5304–5310.

Morton, G. J., Cummings, D. E., Baskin, D. G., Barsh, G. S., & Schwartz, M. W. (2006). Central nervous system control of food intake and body weight. *Nature, 443,* 289–295.

Naruo, T., Nakabeppu, Y., Sagiyama, K., Munemoto, T., Homan, N., Deguchi, D., et al. (2000). Characteristic regional cerebral blood flow patterns in anorexia nervosa patients with binge/purge behavior. *American Journal of Psychiatry, 157*(9), 1520–1522.

Nozoe, S., Naruo, T., Nakabeppu, Y., Soejima, Y., Nakajo, M., & Tanaka, H. (1993). Changes in regional cerebral blood flow in patients with anorexia nervosa detected through single photon emission tomography imaging. *Biological Psychiatry, 34*(8), 578–580.

Ogawa, H. (1994). Gustatory cortex of primates: Anatomy and physiology. *Neuroscience Research, 20*(1), 1–13.

Paulus, M., & Stein, M. B. (2006). An insular view of anxiety. *Biological Psychiatry, 60*(4), 383–387.

Phillips, M., Drevets, W., & Rauch, S. L. (2003). Neurobiology of emotion perception: II. Implications for major psychiatric disorders. *Biological Psychiatry, 54*(5), 515–528.

Phillips, M., Drevets, W. R., Rauch, S. L., & Lane, R. (2003). Neurobiology of emotion perception: I. The neural basis of normal emotion perception. *Biological Psychiatry, 54*(5), 504–514.

Pollatos, O., Kurz, A.-L., Albrecht, J., Schreder, T., Kleemann, A., Schopf, V., et al. (2008). Reduced perception of bodily signals in anorexia nervosa. *Eating Behavior, 9,* 381–388.

Pollice, C., Kaye, W. H., Greeno, C. G., & Weltzin, T. E. (1997). Relationship of depression, anxiety, and obsessionality to state of illness in anorexia nervosa. *International Journal of Eating Disorders, 21*(4), 367–376.

Rastam, M., Bjure, J., Vestergren, E., Uvebrant, P., Gillberg, I. C., Wentz, E., et al. (2001). Regional cerebral blood flow in weight-restored anorexia nervosa: A preliminary study. *Developmental Medicine and Child Neurology, 43*(4), 239–242.

Rolls, E. T. (20050. Taste, olfactory, and food texture processing in the brain, and the control of food intake. *Physiology and Behavior, 85,* 45–56.

Rubinow, D. R., Schmidt, P. J., & Roca, C. A. (1998). Estrogen-serotonin interactions: Implications for affective regulation. *Biological Psychiatry, 44*(9), 839–850.

Santel, S., Baving, L., Krauel, K., Munte, T., & Rotte, M. (2006). Hunger and satiety in anorexia nervosa: fMRI during cognitive processing of food pictures. *Brain Research, 1114,* 138–148.

Saper, C. B., Chou, T. C., & Elmquist, J. K. (2002). The need to feed: Homeostatic and hedonic control of eating. *Neuron, 36*(2), 199–211.

Schoenfeld, M., Neuer, G., Tempelmann, C., Schussler, K., Noesselt, T., Hopf, J., et al. (2004). Functional magnetic resonance tomography correlates of taste perception in the human primary taste cortex. *Neuroscience, 127*(2), 347–353.

Schwartz, M. W., Woods, S. C., Porte, D., Jr., Seeley, R. J., & Baskin, D. G. (2000). Central nervous system control of food intake. *Nature, 404,* 661–671.

Scott, T. R., Yaxley, S., Sienkiewicz, Z., & Rolls, E. (1986). Gustatory responses in the frontal opercular cortex of the alert cynomolgus monkey. *Journal of Neurophysiology, 56,* 876–890.

Small, D., Zatorre, R., Dagher, A., Evans, A., & Jones-Gotman, M. (2001). Changes in brain activity related to eating chocolate:

From pleasure to aversion. *Brain*, *124*(9), 1720–1733.

Srinivasagam, N. M., Kaye, W. H., Plotnicov, K. H., Greeno, C., Weltzin, T. E., & Rao, R. (1995). Persistent perfectionism, symmetry, and exactness after long-term recovery from anorexia nervosa. *American Journal of Psychiatry*, *152*(11), 1630–1634.

Steinhausen, H.-C. (2002). The outcome of anorexia nervosa in the 20th century. *American Journal of Psychiatry*, *159*(8), 1284–1293.

Stice, E. (2002). Risk and maintenance factors for eating pathology: A meta-analytic review. *Pychopharmacology Bulletin*, *128*, 825–848.

Strober, M. (1995). Family–genetic perspectives on anorexia nervosa and bulimia nervosa. In K. D. Brownell & C. G. Fairburn (Eds.), *Eating disorders and obesity: A comprehensive handbook* (pp. 212–218). New York: Guilford Press.

Strober, M., Freeman, R., & Morrell, W. (1997). The long-term course of severe anorexia nervosa in adolescents: Survival analysis of recovery, relapse, and outcome predictors over 10–15 years in a prospective study. *International Journal of Eating Disorders*, *22*(4), 339–360.

Tataranni, P. A., Gautier, J. F., Chen, K., Uecker, A., Bandy, D., Salbe, A. D., et al. (1999). Neuroanatomical correlates of hunger and satiation in humans using positron emission tomography. *Proceedings of the National Academy of Sciences of the United States of America*, *96*(8), 4569–4574.

Torpy, D., Papanicolaou, D., & Chrousos, G. (1997). Sexual dismorphism of the human stress response may be due to estradiol-mediated stimulation of hypothalamic corticotropin-releasing hormone synthesis. *Journal of Clinical Endocrinology and Metabolism*, *82*, 982.

Tricomi, E. M., Delgado, M. R., & Fiez, J. A. (2004). Modulation of caudate activity by action contingency. *Neuron*, *41*, 281–292.

Uher, R., Brammer, M., Murphy, T., Campbell, I., Ng, V., Williams, S., et al. (2003). Recovery and chronicity in anorexia nervosa: Brain activity associated with differential outcomes. *Biological Psychiatry*, *54*, 934–942.

Uher, R., Murphy, T., Brammer, M., Dalgleish, T., Phillips, M., Ng, V., et al. (2004). Medial prefrontal cortex activity associated with symptom provocation in eating disorders. *American Journal of Psychiatry*, *161*(7), 1238–1246.

Uher, R., Treasure, J., Heining, M., Brammer, M. C., & Campbell, I. C. (2006). Cerebral processing of food-related stimuli: Effects of fasting and gender. *Behavioral Brain Research*, *169*(1), 111–119.

Vitousek, K., & Manke, F. (1994). Personality variables and disorders in anorexia nervosa and bulimia nervosa. *Journal of Abnormal Psychology*, *103*(1), 137–147.

Wagner, A., Aizenstein, H., Frank, G. K., Figurski, J., May, J. C., Putnam, K., et al. (2008). Altered insula response to a taste stimulus in individuals recovered from restricting-type anorexia nervosa. *Neuropsychopharmacology*, *33*(3), 513–523.

Wagner, A., Aizenstein, H., Venkatraman, M., Fudge, J., May, J., Mazurkewicz, L., et al. (2007). Altered reward processing in women recovered from anorexia nervosa. *American Journal of Psychiatry*, *164*(12), 1842–1849.

Wagner, A., Barbarich, N., Frank, G., Bailer, U., Weissfeld, L., Henry, S., et al. (2006). Personality traits after recovery from eating disorders: Do subtypes differ? *International Journal of Eating Disorders*, *39*(4), 276–284.

Walters, E. E., & Kendler, K. S. (1995). Anorexia nervosa and anorexic-like syndromes in a population-based female twin sample. *American Journal of Psychiatry*, *152*(1), 64–71.

Yaxley, S., Rolls, E., & Sienkiewicz, Z. (1990). Gustatory responses of single neurons in the insula of the macaque monkey. *Journal of Neurophysiology*, *63*(689–700).

Zastrow, A., Kaiser, S., Stippich, C., Walthe, S., Herzog, W., Tchanturia, K., et al. (2009). Neural correlates of impaired cognitive-behavioral flexibility in anorexia nervosa. *American Journal of Psychiatry*, *166*(5), 608–616.

CHAPTER 3

Environmental and Genetic Risk Factors for Eating Disorders

A Developmental Perspective

Sarah E. Racine
Tammy L. Root
Kelly L. Klump
Cynthia M. Bulik

Over the past two decades it has become increasingly clear that early conceptualizations of eating disorders as primarily influenced by sociocultural factors are false. Behavioral genetic investigations have implicated genetic and environmental factors in the etiology of eating disorders (i.e., anorexia nervosa [AN], bulimia nervosa [BN], binge-eating disorder [BED]), as well as component eating attitudes and behaviors (e.g., weight preoccupation, binge eating). In addition, given that eating disorders typically have their onset in adolescence, developmental twin methods have been used to elucidate etiological influences that may contribute to critical periods for the emergence of eating disorders.

This chapter reviews twin studies to illustrate differences in genetic and environmental effects on disordered eating across development. We set the stage by first reviewing twin studies of eating disorders and disordered eating attitudes and behaviors in adulthood. We then focus on developmental twin studies to illustrate changes in environmental and genetic influences on disordered eating phenotypes across development. Finally, puberty is examined as a critical period for developmental shifts in the etiology of disordered eating and the potential role of ovarian hormones in these relationships is discussed.

Twin Study Method

Twin studies represent a natural experiment that allows us to quantify and separate the effects of genes and environment on the etiology of a disorder or trait. These studies capitalize on the fact that monozygotic (MZ; identical) twins share approximately 100% of their genome, whereas dizygotic (DZ; fraternal) twins share approximately 50% of their segregating genetic material. Thus, if members of MZ twin pairs are more frequently concordant for a disorder (both members of the twin pair display the disorder or trait) than members of DZ twin pairs, a genetic contribution is suggested. With the use of statistical modeling, the total variance in a phenotype within a given population can be partitioned into additive genetic (i.e., the additive effects of multiple genes), shared environmental (i.e., factors that make members of a twin pair similar to one another), and nonshared environmental influences (i.e., factors that make members of a twin pair different from one another (Plomin, DeFries, McClearn, & McGuffin, 2008).

Twin Studies of Disordered Eating

Previous family and twin studies have reported that AN (Bulik et al., 2006; Lilenfeld et al. 1998; Strober, Freeman, Lampert, Diamond, & Kaye, 2000; Walters & Kendler 1995) and BN (Bulik, Sullivan, & Kendler, 1998; Kendler et al., 1991) run in families, and that a substantial portion of this observed familiality is due to genetic factors. Twin studies have reported heritability estimates that range from 31 to 76% for AN (e.g., Bulik et al., 2006; Bulik, Slof-Op't Landt, van Furth, & Sullivan, 2007; Klump, Miller, Keel, McGue, & Iacono, 2001) and from 28 to 83% for BN (e.g., Bulik et al., 1998; Bulik,

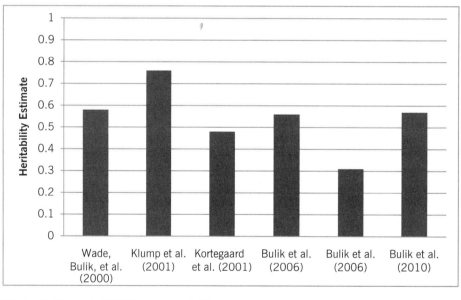

Wade, Bulik, et al. (2000)	0.58
Klump et al. (2001)	0.76
Kortegaard et al. (2001)	0.48
Bulik et al. (2006)	0.56
Bulik et al. (2006)	0.31
Bulik et al. (2010)	0.57

FIGURE 3.1. Heritability estimates for AN in adulthood. Twin studies of AN in adulthood indicate that it is significantly heritable, with heritability estimates ranging from 31 to 76%.

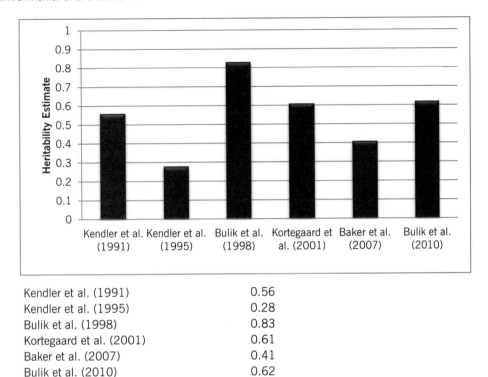

Kendler et al. (1991)	0.56
Kendler et al. (1995)	0.28
Bulik et al. (1998)	0.83
Kortegaard et al. (2001)	0.61
Baker et al. (2007)	0.41
Bulik et al. (2010)	0.62

FIGURE 3.2. Heritability estimates for BN in adulthood. Twin studies of BN in adulthood indicate that it is significantly heritable, with heritability estimates ranging from 28 to 83%.

Sullivan, Wade, & Kendler, 2000) in adulthood (see Figures 3.1 and 3.2). DSM-IV diagnostic criteria for AN have also been assessed at the individual-item level using an item-factor approach, and variability in the heritability of these items was detected (Mazzeo et al., 2009). The items with the lowest heritability estimates were amenorrhea (16%) and "did others tell you that your low weight was a hazard to your health? (9%)," whereas the highest heritability estimates were found for "weight loss of more than 15 pounds (34%)" and lowest lifetime body mass index (BMI) (33%).

Heritability estimates for disordered eating attitudes and behaviors (e.g., weight preoccupation, body dissatisfaction, dietary restraint, binge eating, compensatory behaviors) are similar to those for eating disorders and range from 34 to 65% (see Figure 3.3). This indicates that the symptoms that commonly precede the development of AN and BN are also highly heritable. The remaining variance in liability to eating disorders and disordered eating in adulthood is usually accounted for by unique, nonshared environmental influences. Nonshared environmental factors for disordered eating can include individual life experiences, peer group influences, and differential parental treatment (Klump, Wonderlich, Lehoux, Lilenfeld, & Bulik, 2002), but measurement error is also contained in the estimate of the nonshared environment. Only a few studies (e.g., Kendler et al., 1995; Reichborn-Kjennerud, Bulik, Tambs, & Harris, 2004) have reported that shared environmental influences significantly contribute to the variance in eating pathology in adulthood.

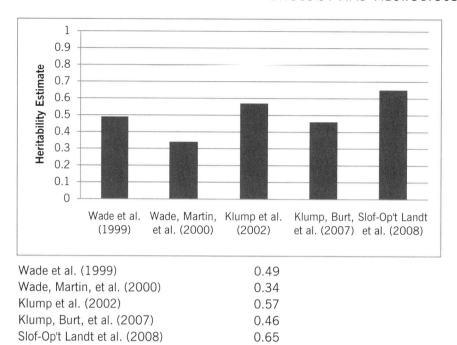

Wade et al. (1999)	0.49
Wade, Martin, et al. (2000)	0.34
Klump et al. (2002)	0.57
Klump, Burt, et al. (2007)	0.46
Slof-Op't Landt et al. (2008)	0.65

FIGURE 3.3. Heritability estimates for overall disordered eating in adulthood. Twin studies of overall disordered eating, measured continuously, in adulthood indicate that disordered eating is significantly heritable, with heritability estimates ranging from 34 to 65%.

Developmental Twin Studies of Disordered Eating

Eating disorder onset often occurs during adolescence, and studies examining genetic and environmental influences on disordered eating from a developmental perspective can provide valuable information regarding mechanisms of onset. Knowledge of critical periods for the development of disordered eating can also be useful in understanding how and when to intervene to reduce these potentially harmful outcomes.

The first study to empirically examine the developmental nature of the etiology of disordered eating was conducted by Klump, McGue, and Iacono (2000) using a large cross-sectional twin sample from the Minnesota Twin Family Study (MTFS). Etiological effects on disordered eating attitudes and behaviors were compared in 11- and 17-year-old female twins. Genetic and environmental influences on overall levels of disordered eating as well as weight preoccupation differed by age and were independent of BMI. Specifically, for the 11-year-old twins, the variance in disordered eating was predominantly due to shared and nonshared environmental effects, and genetic influences were nominal. However, the heritability of disordered eating was substantial in the 17-year-old twins, and the remaining variance was explained by unique environmental influences.

Extending these findings, Klump, Burt, McGue, and Iacono (2007) used longitudinal data to investigate developmental *changes* in genetic and environmental influences on disordered eating (i.e., body dissatisfaction, weight preoccupation, binge eating, and the use of compensatory behaviors) across MTFS female twins assessed at ages 11, 14, and 18. Results were consistent with the original study in that genetic effects became more pronounced as age increased. Genetic influences were minimal at age 11 (6%), increased substantially at age 14, and remained constant through age 18 (46%). This suggests that a critical period for the emergence of genetic influences on disordered eating occurs between ages 11 and 14.

Silberg and Bulik (2005) conducted a developmental study examining unique and common etiological influences on eating, depressive, and anxiety symptoms. With the use of longitudinal data from the Virginia Twin Study of Adolescent Behavioral Development, female twins were compared in childhood–young adolescence (8–13 years) and mid–late adolescence (14–17 years). Results suggested a common genetic factor underlying all internalizing symptoms in both age groups, and a unique genetic factor influencing only liability to disordered eating in the 8- to 13-year-old group. In regard to environmental influences, one shared environmental factor influenced risk for early depressive symptoms and early eating pathology, and another shared environmental factor was common to both early and late separation anxiety and later disordered eating. Findings are significant in suggesting both common and unique genetic and shared environmental effects on internalizing phenotypes across development.

Like Klump and colleagues (2000; Klump, Burt, et al., 2007; Klump, Perkins, et al., 2007), Silberg and Bulik (2005) found that genes accounted for more variance in eating disorder symptoms in the older (14–17 years) versus younger (8–13 years) twins. However, a unique set of genetic factors (that did not influence risk for other internalizing disorders) contributed to the variance in eating disorder symptoms in the younger group. This discrepancy may be due to differences in the measures used to assess disordered eating or to differences in age categorizations across the studies—that is, the preadolescent group in Silberg and Bulik (2005) included twins whose ages overlapped with both the 11- (10–12 years) and 14- (13–15 years) year-old groups in Klump, Burt, and colleagues (2007).

Collectively, the aforementioned studies suggest clear developmental differences in the etiological influences on disordered eating. Although the critical period for genetic influences on disordered eating differs slightly across studies, early adolescence appears to be a time during which genetic risk for disordered eating increases.

Puberty as a Critical Developmental Period

Puberty marks a time of significant biological and psychosocial change (Herman-Giddens et al., 1997) and has been associated with increased rates of disordered eating and eating disorders (Killen et al., 1992). An important line of research has examined puberty as a potential mechanism for age-related increases in the genetic influences on disordered eating. Indeed, pubertal development appears to moderate the heritability of disordered eating, independent of age (Culbert, Burt, McGue, Iacono, & Klump, 2009; Klump, McGue, & Iacono, 2003; Klump, Perkins, Burt, McGue, & Iacono, 2007). In the first study of its kind, Klump and colleagues reported minimal genetic effects on disordered eating in prepubertal 11-year-old twins, but substantial genetic effects (~50%) in 11-year-old twins who were in mid-to-late puberty (Klump et al., 2003). An important finding was that 11-year-old twins who had begun puberty closely resembled adult twins in the magnitude of genetic effects, such that the heritability of disordered eating could be constrained to be equal in 11-year-old pubertal and adult twins. Similar findings have been reported when puberty was examined as a continuous variable, as Klump, Perkins, and colleagues (2007) found that genetic influences on disordered eating increased linearly with increasing pubertal development.

Findings implicating puberty in the activation of genetic influences on disordered eating have now been replicated in an independent sample of twins from the Michigan State University Twin Registry (Culbert et al., 2009). Similar to the findings of Klump and colleagues (2003), genetic influences on disordered eating were nominal in prepubertal twins and increased substantially during midpuberty, after controlling for age and BMI. In addition, the study by Culbert and colleagues (2009) demonstrated that differences in the etiology of disordered eating depending on pubertal status may be missed if later markers of pubertal development are used. Rowe, Pickles, Simonoff, Bulik, and Silberg (2002) found that genetic effects on bulimic symptoms could be constrained to be equal across pre- and postmenarcheal female twins. These findings were thought to be inconsistent with puberty-related differences in the etiology of disordered eating reported by Klump and colleagues. Culbert and colleagues (2009) resolved this discrepancy by examining differences in genetic and environmental effects on disordered eating when categorizing twins using either midpuberty or menarche. When midpuberty was used, nominal genetic effects in prepubertal twins and substantial genetic influences in pubertal twins were observed. When menarcheal status was used, moderate and significant genetic effects were found for both groups. These findings highlight puberty as a critical period for developmental changes in the genetic and environmental influences on disordered eating.

Ovarian Hormones: Activation of Genetic Influences?

Given the importance of puberty in regard to genetic influences on disordered eating, researchers are beginning to explore which changes at puberty (e.g., ovarian hormones, body weight, mood, peer influences) may be responsible for these findings. One line of research has hypothesized that ovarian hormones may be specifically relevant for genetic effects on disordered eating over and above the effects of other physical and psychological variables. Preliminary findings suggest that estradiol moderates genetic influences on disordered eating in 10- to 15-year-old female twins (Klump, Keel, Sisk, & Burt, 2010). Genetic influences were significantly higher in twins with high versus low estradiol levels, and these effects could not be accounted for by age, BMI, or the physical changes of puberty. Estrogen's onset at puberty may partially account for the increase in genetic influences on disordered eating with increasing pubertal development. Moreover, data collected across the menstrual cycle has demonstrated phenotypic relationships between ovarian hormones and binge eating in both women with BN (Edler, Lipson, & Keel, 2007) and nonclinical samples of women (Klump, Keel, Culbert, & Edler, 2008). Thus, research suggests that ovarian hormones may be involved in both phenotypic and genetic relationships with disordered eating.

Conclusions

Clearly, the relative influence of genes and environment is not constant across the lifespan, with genetic factors becoming more prominent after puberty. This observation raises several questions. First, when eating disorders do emerge prior to puberty, it is unclear whether they are etiologically similar to eating disorders that develop during adolescence and adulthood. It is known that the presentation of eating disorders in children often differ from the prototypes that are included in the DSM (Bravender et al., 2010), although the extent to which this is due to fundamental differences in genetic and environmental factors is unknown. Second, from a treatment perspective, we have not yet addressed whether optimal intervention tailoring should consider the emergence of genetic factors for disordered eating during puberty. It is clear that family-based approaches confer advantage in the treatment of AN and BN in youth (Berkman et al., 2006). Moreover, treatment success is more likely with younger patients (Le Grange & Loeb, 2007). One possibility is that intervention can be more successful before the genetic activation of risk for disordered eating at puberty occurs. The activation of genetic factors around the time of puberty may render eating disorders more biologically entrenched—further complicating treatment. Although speculative, these considerations underscore the importance of early detection and treatment of eating disorders. The identification and reversal of early symptoms may prevent the emergence of more persistent presentations that are less amenable to intervention.

References

Baker, J. H., Mazzeo, S. E., & Kendler, K. S. (2007). Association between broadly defined bulimia nervosa and drug use disorders: Common genetic and environmental influences. *International Journal of Eating Disorders, 40*, 673–678.

Berkman, N., Bulik, C., Brownley, K., Lohr, K., Sedway, J., Rooks, A., et al. (2006). *Management of eating disorders* (Evidence Report/Technology Assessment No. 135; AHRQ Publication No. 06-E010). Rockville, MD: Agency for Healthcare Research and Policy. (Prepared by the RTI International–University of North Carolina Evidence-Based Practice Center under Contract No. 290-02-0016)

Bravender, T., Bryant-Waugh, R., Herzog, D., Katzman, D., Kreipe, R. D., Lask, B., et al. (2010). Classification of eating disturbance in children and adolescents: Proposed changes for the DSM-V. *European Eating Disorders Review, 18*, 79–89.

Bulik, C. M., Slof-Op't Landt, M. C., van Furth, E. F., & Sullivan, P. F. (2007). The genetics of anorexia nervosa. *Annuual Review of Nutrition, 27*, 263–275.

Bulik, C. M., Sullivan, P. F., & Kendler, K. S. (1998). Heritability of binge-eating and broadly defined bulimia nervosa. *Biological Psychiatry, 44*, 1210–1218.

Bulik, C. M., Sullivan, P. F., Tozzi, F., Furberg, H., Lichtenstein, P., & Pedersen, N. L. (2006). Prevalence, heritability, and prospective risk factors for anorexia nervosa. *Archives of General Psychiatry, 63*, 305–312.

Bulik, C. M., Sullivan, P. F., Wade, T. D., & Kendler, K. S. (2000). Twin studies of eating disorders: A review. *International Journal of Eating Disorders, 27*, 1–20.

Bulik, C. M., Thornton, L. M., Root, T. L., Pietsky, E. M., Lichenstein, P., & Pedersen, N. L. (2010). Understanding the relation between anorexia nervosa and bulimia nervosa in a Swedish national twin sample. *Biological Psychiatry, 67*, 71–77.

Culbert, K. M., Burt, S. A., McGue, M., Iacono, W. G., & Klump, K. L. (2009). Puberty and the genetic diathesis of disordered eating attitudes and behaviors. *Journal of Abnormal Psychology, 118,* 788–796.

Edler, C., Lipson, S. F., & Keel, P. K. (2007). Ovarian hormones and binge eating in bulimia nervosa. *Psychological Medicine, 37,* 131–141.

Fichter, M. M., & Noegel, R. (1990). Concordance for bulimia nervosa in twins. *International Journal of Eating Disorders, 9,* 255–263.

Herman-Giddens, M. E., Slora, E. J., Wasserman, R. C., Bourdony, C. J., Bhapkar, M. V., Koch, G. G., et al. (1997). Secondary sexual characteristics and menses in young girls seen in office practice: A study from the Pediatric Research in Office Settings network. *Pediatrics, 99,* 505–512.

Kendler, K. S., MacLean, C., Neale, M., Kessler, R., Heath, A., & Eaves, L. (1991). The genetic epidemiology of bulimia nervosa. *American Journal of Psychiatry, 148,* 1627–1637.

Kendler, K. S., Walters, E. E., Neale, M. C., Kessler, R. C., Heath, A. C., & Eaves, L. J. (1995). The structure of the genetic and environmental risk factors for six major psychiatric disorders in women: Phobia, generalized anxiety disorder, panic disorder, bulimia, major depression, and alcoholism. *Archives of General Psychiatry, 52,* 374–383.

Killen, J. D., Hayward, C., Litt, I., Hammer, L. D., Wilson, D. M., Miner, B., et al. (1992). Is puberty a risk factor for eating disorders? *American Journal of Disorders in Childhood, 146,* 323–325.

Klump, K. L., Burt, S. A., McGue, M., & Iacono, W. G. (2007). Changes in genetic and environmental influences on disordered eating across adolescence: A longitudinal twin study. *Archives of General Psychiatry, 64,* 1409–1415.

Klump, K. L., Keel, P. K., Culbert, K. M., & Edler, C. (2008). Ovarian hormones and binge eating: Exploring associations in community samples. *Psychological Medicine, 38,* 1749–1757.

Klump, K. L., Keel, P. K., Sisk, C., & Burt, S.

A. (2010). Preliminary evidence that estradiol moderates genetic influences on disordered eating attitudes and behaviors during puberty. *Psychological Medicine, 40,* 1745–1753.

Klump, K. L., McGue, M., & Iacono, W. G. (2000). Age differences in genetic and environmental influences on eating attitudes and behaviors in preadolescent and adolescent female twins. *Journal of Abnormal Psychology, 109,* 239–251.

Klump, K. L., McGue, M., & Iacono, W. G. (2003). Differential heritability of eating attitudes and behaviors in prepubertal versus pubertal twins. *International Journal of Eating Disorders, 33,* 287–292.

Klump, K. L., Miller, K. B., Keel, P. K., McGue, M., & Iacono, W. G. (2001). Genetic and environmental influences on anorexia nervosa syndromes in a population-based twin sample. *Psychological Medicine, 31,* 737–740.

Klump, K. L., Perkins, P. S., Burt, S. A., McGue, M., & Iacono, W. G. (2007). Puberty moderates genetic influences on disordered eating. *Psychological Medicine, 37,* 627–634.

Klump, K. L., Wonderlich, S., Lehoux, P., Lilenfeld, L. R., & Bulik, C. M. (2002). Does environment matter? A review of nonshared environment and eating disorders. *International Journal of Eating Disorders, 31,* 118–135.

Kortegaard, L. S., Hoerder, K., Joergensen, J., Gillberg, C., & Kyvik, K. O. (2001). A preliminary population-based twin study of self-reported eating disorder. *Psychological Medicine, 31,* 361–365.

Le Grange, D., & Loeb, K. L. (2007). Early identification and treatment of eating disorders: Prodrome to syndrome. *Early Intervention in Psychiatry, 1,* 27–39.

Lilenfeld, L. R., Kaye, W. H., Greeno, C. G., Merikangas, K. R., Plotnicov, K., Pollice, C., et al. (1998). A controlled family study of anorexia nervosa and bulimia nervosa: Psychiatric disorders in first-degree relatives and effects of proband comorbidity. *Archives of General Psychiatry, 55,* 603–610.

Mazzeo, S. E., Mitchell, K. S., Bulik, C. M., Reichborn-Kjennerud, T., Kendler, K. S., &

Neale, M. C. (2009). Assessing the heritability of anorexia nervosa symptoms using a marginal maximal likelihood approach. *Psychological Medicine, 39,* 463–473.

Plomin, R., DeFries, J. C., McClearn, G. E., & McGuffin, P. (2008). *Behavior genetics* (5th ed.). New York: Worth.

Reichborn-Kjennerud, T., Bulik, C. M., Tambs, K., & Harris, J. R. (2004). Genetic and environmental influences on binge eating in the absence of compensatory behaviors: A population-based twin study. *International Journal of Eating Disorders, 36,* 307–314.

Rowe, R., Pickles, A., Simonoff, E., Bulik, C. M., & Silberg, J. L. (2002). Bulimic symptoms in the Virginia Twin Study of Adolescent Behavioral Development: Correlates, comorbidity, and genetics. *Biological Psychiatry, 51,* 172–182.

Silberg, J. L., & Bulik, C. M. (2005). The developmental association between eating disorders symptoms and symptoms of depression and anxiety in juvenile twin girls. *Journal of Child Psychology and Psychiatry, 46,* 1317–1326.

Slof-Op't Landt, M. C. T., Bartels, M., Van Furth, E. F., Van Beijsterveldt, C. E. M., Meulenbelt, I., Slagboom, P. E., et al. (2008). Genetic influences on disordered eating behaviour are largely independent of body mass index. *Acta Psychiatrica Scandinavica, 117,* 348–356.

Strober, M., Freeman, R., Lampert, C., Diamond, J., & Kaye, W. (2000). Controlled family study of anorexia nervosa and bulimia nervosa: Evidence of shared liability and transmission of partial syndromes. *American Journal of Psychiatry, 157,* 393–401.

Wade, T. D., Bulik, C. M., Neale, M., & Kendler, K. S. (2000). Anorexia nervosa and major depression: Shared genetic and environmental risk factors. *American Journal of Psychiatry, 157,* 469–471.

Wade, T., Martin, N. G., Neale, M. C., Tiggemann, M., Treloar, S. A., Bucholz, K. K., et al. (1999). The structure of genetic and environmental risk factors for three measures of disordered eating. *Psychological Medicine, 29,* 925–934.

Wade, T., Martin, N. G., Tiggemann, M., Abraham, S., Treloar, S. A., & Heath, A. C. (2000). Genetic and environmental risk factors shared between disordered eating, psychological and family variables. *Personality and Individual Differences, 28,* 729–740.

Walters, E. E., & Kendler, K. S. (1995). Anorexia nervosa and anorexic-like syndromes in a population-based female twin sample. *American Journal of Psychiatry, 152,* 64–71.

CHAPTER 4

The Role of Family Environment in Etiology

A Neuroscience Perspective

Michael Strober
Tara Peris

Through the Lens of Modern Science: Prospects and Challenges

The aim of this chapter is to selectively review findings relevant to a subject of impassioned debate in our field: Is family life experience a relevant factor in explaining etiology? With mounting evidence that eating disorders are heritable (see Chapter 3) and that involving parents more directly in treatment can aid in restoring weight and controlling binge eating (see Chapters 12 and 16), the question is timely. It is also meaningful because as technical sophistication in biological research grows, knowledge about the intrinsic relationship between developing behavioral systems, their organizing biology, and the social milieu is advancing rapidly. What is enriching about the paradigms now being used to explore this transaction is the concern with mechanisms of change and the different platforms available for approaching its complexity and many subtleties. Indeed, it has never been questioned that the major disruptions of early life—poverty, social disadvantage, out-of-home placement—can wreak havoc on the psychological growth of children; there is much empirical study to support this. But the typical life history associated with eating disorders is rarely burdened with such conspicuous vulnerability. Even so, difficulties in personal adjustment are almost always present and they are not trivial, even when the reactions concern seemingly ordinary life changes. We discuss the nature of these reactions and implications they have for understanding the neural mechanisms involved and how family life may pertain. Indeed, from work undertaken in recent decades we understand better that the unfolding impact of environment on development often involves mechanisms that are more faintly detailed, but whose later effects on adaptation are strong. As Panksepp (1998) described in his treatise on affective consciousness, even primitive operating systems in the brain that activate in infancy can sometimes place constraints on the processing of life events that will resonate for a lifetime. This point is crucial to our discussion in another sense, which is the need for caution when contemplating the meaning of certain family patterns in a developmental progression that includes many entering and exiting events, genetically influenced tendencies, and more.

Human development, from the most primordial expression of the newborn's response to a mother's presence to the evolution of higher consciousness, includes a stunningly diverse array of transitions and acquisitions that depend on a complex and cumulative discourse between innate drives and experience. Whether it is reasonable to expect that we can decode all that is involved and draw conclusions about the strength of the individual elements in time and space is another matter. Ontogeny is not predictable and because the interchange of innate proclivities and experience is so fluid, effects that once seemed core elements are ultimately overshadowed by new ones whose influence is deemed irrefutable. Indeed, the challenge was once considered so daunting that some scholars boldly declared (Baldwin, 1960) that efforts to isolate with credible precision the respective roles of innate propensity and life's unpredictability in behavioral outcomes could never succeed, others scoffing that it was professional madness (MacFarlane, 1971).

The case history we now present anchors the discussion from a new angle. It frames the issues differently because decades after these admonitions there is much new data that bear on the issues and illustrate how old controversies can be recast. It is a poignant story, illustrating that life is swayed by many different influences—genetic propensities on one hand, outside pressures on the other—and the pathways cross in ways not easy to track. This is our focus, how modern neuroscience can shed new light on the interchange of biology and experience in eating disorders and in doing so aid our understanding of the personal struggles it creates.

> Jill is 13 years old. She is formal and correct in her manner, to the point of being stilted; because of this she is teased mercilessly by classmates. At 5 feet, 71 pounds she concedes she is too thin. A superior student, she has boundless passion for learning and reads incessantly, but as her choice in books expands she finds herself increasingly troubled by newly felt curiosities that are in conflict with her rigid tendencies and the core beliefs valued strongly by her family; the conflict troubles her. She says she is a constant worrier, that change makes her nervous, and that she is preoccupied by a nagging fear that something may happen to her parents. She hints that a deafening confusion pervades thoughts she has about herself and her family, which bring much guilt and shame. She sometimes wonders if rather than a whole person who makes sense of things in an orderly way, she is a patchwork of different people; such thoughts make her feel dishonest and untrustworthy. She stumbles through her words, hesitant to fully open up, often seeking reassurance that it is permissible to share these experiences and wondering if she is impolite, rude, or disobedient. She receives the reassurance with a nod but a moment later seems more distressed; that she is extraordinarily gifted is evident. As she describes what it is like to be the person she is, it is evident that an adult-like maturity sharpens her sense of how estranged she is from her surroundings—that she must shield all that defines her to avoid being mocked; it can be easily sensed how hopelessly lost she feels. She says she cannot understand why her weight loss makes her feel better but admits it is a discipline she can no longer control. She reluctantly concedes she is afraid and needs help.

Up to this point, there is likely to be broad agreement about the clinical presentation. Like that of so many people with anorexia nervosa (AN), Jill's development from early on bears the stamp of pervading anxiety about change and her parents' safety, inhibition of expression, compulsiveness of routine, difficulty with self-initiation and assertion, and a perfectionism that both she and her parents readily agree leaves her exhausted at day's end, physically and mentally. She routinely abides by her parents' wishes, is never cross, cares dutifully for her siblings, and is surely one of her teachers' most devoted and cherished students.

But as more of the case material unfolds, parsing issues of cause and effect becomes a more complicated interpretive challenge.

Jill's parents are devoutly religious, believing that sacrifice is among the holiest of virtues and that self-interest and appetitive arousals are vices to shun. These notions are similarly reflected in attitudes concerning meal quality and quantity—namely, that food should be consumed sparingly, that rich desserts are excesses to be enjoyed only on special occasions. An important fact is that neither parents nor extended family members have ever shown weight or shape concerns. Jill reveres her mother's iron will and discipline, attributes she believes she has herself but which can stand to be more finely honed. She loves her parents dearly and their concern for her is no less evident. But at one point, when asked if she ever took issue with anything her parents did or thought, her eyes flared—the look of someone venturing with apprehension into a strange place only to discover something repelling—saying never would she even contemplate such a thing. She can't explain why the question shakes her; when pressed further she frowned and slumped low in her chair, as if seeking retreat from a dialogue too unsettling. After several moments of silence she looked up, tears welling in her eyes.

Several weeks later Jill spoke of the challenge of having three younger siblings—each of whom she describes, in not so endearing terms, as "more annoying and obnoxious than the next"—and hearing day after day her parents saying how much they benefit from the support she gives them in managing household chores and keeping the children out of their hair. She is described admiringly as her "parents' apprentice," which, Jill says, is indeed an honor valued deeply; but it also triggers guilt as she reluctantly concedes a wish to have more free time. Still, there is only so much she can do to maintain even a semblance of order in the home. Most of the time, she says, the living space is uncomfortably loud and to an outsider would surely appear turned upside down. Because her own sensitivities require more order and stability than is needed by either her parents or any of her siblings, she often feels she is "going insane." Never does she doubt how strongly she is loved, but she does not know what physical affection is or how to express it herself; even the mere desire to know what it might feel like is viewed as a betrayal of family loyalty. She wonders, too, whether it is sinful that her dreams are full of so many desires and is in awe of children at school who seem carefree and spontaneous in their expressed emotion. She reveals, with much trepidation, that many times during the past year she would retreat to her room after dinner, hands draped over her ears in the hope that she might grab a moment of silence. And, finally, as if all this isn't stress enough, several months before the weight loss began, her father revealed that he is gravely ill, the prognosis uncertain. Her parents say it is best not to speak of this further.

Jill's parents agree that the narrative paints a fair picture of their daughter, themselves, and their family life. But in the months leading up to this consultation no agreement was reached on what explained Jill's starvation. Among the ideas put forward by the many practitioners whose advice the family sought were that Jill had turned away from her spiritual and religious values and was thus experiencing extreme guilt and self-punishment; because she felt undeserving of her family's love, she starved in penitence; she was rebelling against an oppressive and overcontrolling family structure; she was beginning to mourn her father's anticipated death; her family life had little relevance because it is now understood that AN is a disorder of unbalanced chemistry, no different from other psychiatric conditions. When asked about these various theories, Jill, shaking her head, whispered, "I don't think so; I think what's going on is more complicated." Indeed, an additional element of the history implies that this is so: Jill has an older sister who, by everyone's description, is exuberant and free-spirited. Although her parents say she is sometimes a thorn in their side because their values clash, she is at ease with her full-figured frame and well adjusted in every way. When this sister's opinion was sought on all the family has been through, she said unhesitatingly, "Jill and I are just different, way different. She is sensitive to everything that goes on, I'm not. I think my family is great but I just ignore a lot of what they say. Jill takes it all in; she can't ignore anything. She's exactly like our dad." (She has already told us that, like Jill, he is a man who from childhood has been nervous and rigid in his ways.)

The case, layered in complexities arguably greater than those we see in most other families, was, in fact, selected for this reason—because it highlights so vividly the questions that pervade our field: What individual elements in this complex history are most relevant? Where do we place the connecting lines that link innate behavioral traits with life events and family attitudes that seem relevant too, and exactly how does the bridge build over time? Do we give precedence to biology within the culture of Jill's family life, or is it the other way around? Do her symptoms evolve from a defective anatomy—a processing of visual information, affect experience, and appetitive motivation come undone—or is it life experience and learned attitudes that have skewed a young child's mind to such a degree that puberty and the nutrients that fuel it are now shunned? No matter how the case is approached—whether seen through a clinician's lens or a model builder's theoretical calculus—the clash of opinions is bound to be sharp, and perspective taking to find common ground will not be so easy. Yet overshadowing the debate remains a more heartfelt and difficult struggle: patient and loved ones trying to make sense of it all—too often a private, bewildering anguish mired in contradictory formulations, some with too little detail to even ponder, others accusatory in tone. This is why the challenge of bringing sense to *non-sense* is worthy.

As noted, there is at least one area of common ground—the contributory role of temperament, the pattern of behavior that appears regularly in advance of weight loss. In AN, it is composed of rigidity, sensitivity to negative consequences, reticence and discomfort in the presence of novelty and ambiguity, chronic worry, low appetitive motivation, and fearfulness; some of the same features are seen in advance of bulimia nervosa (BN) as well. The reason that temperament has been implicated as a possible clue to at least certain biological underpinnings from which the illness emerges, especially in AN (see Bulik, Sullivan, Fear, & Joyce, 1997; Bulik et al., 2006; Kaye, Bulik, Thornton, Barbarich, and the Price Foundation Collaborative Group, 2004; Keel, Klump, Miller, McGue, & Iacono, 2005; Strober, 2010; Strober, Freeman, Lampert, & Diamond, 2007), is that (1) these traits are moderately heritable and confer risk for later anxiety disorder and depression, (2) anxiety disorders especially are common precursors to AN and are also seen in family members (as are traits of perfectionism and compulsive personality),

(3) the risk of anxiety disorder is elevated in the non-eating-disordered identical co-twins of persons with eating disorders, thus suggesting a common genetic diathesis, and (4) the phenomenology of anxiety—hypervigilance, biased attention to negatively valenced environmental cues, avoidance when threat is perceived—mirrors well the exaggerated fear and avoidance of weight and shape changes associated with eating disorders.

We are not arguing that the vulnerabilities underlying anxiety and eating disorders are identical; rather that their commonalities—similarity in symptom structure, ubiquity of anxious phenotypes prior to their onset, significant familial aggregation—argue persuasively for an association. It is for this reason that a consideration of what is known about the role of genetic variation, developmental stress, and moderators of outcome in anxiety phenotypes may helpfully inform the dialogue about causal processes in eating disorders. Thus we discuss, in broad terms, several levels of observation: the genetics and neurobiology of stress and anxiety proneness; how chronic stress, including disruptions in the emotional environment, alters brain development in regions that normally regulate vigilance, sensory processing, emotional learning, and motivational behavior; how early life circumstances can buffer the expression of genes that predispose a person to anxiety and stress; and family processes that are associated with childhood anxiety.

Admittedly, generalizing this literature rests heavily on conjecture, as the study of stress and emotion-regulating circuitry in eating disorders is in its infancy. However, the extent of relevant animal and human translational research is now so vast that a potential to deepen understanding of how the interchange of biology and social environment may play out in eating disorders cannot be ignored. Consider just two findings in the neuroscience literature that lend support, which we explore in more detail:

1. The anxious temperament associated with AN has been connected to excitability of the limbic forebrain, especially in the amygdala, a region implicated not only in anxiety, fear, and vigilance for threat (LeDoux, 2000), but also in the regulation of energy balance and weight in the face of chronic stress (Soloman, Jones, Packard, & Herman, 2009).

2. Stress exposure during developmentally sensitive periods has been implicated in tissue-damaging levels of glucocorticoids as well as alterations in gene expression that have lasting consequences for stress reactivity, hypervigilance, and high arousal to novelty (Heim & Nemeroff, 2001; Shin & Liberzon, 2010)—features indisputably central to the psychology of AN. Conversely, learning to cope better with stress early in development appears to increase surface expression of prefrontal brain cortices that effectively regulate limbic arousal to novelty and support the retention of fear extinction (Katz et al., 2009).

That these findings are possibly germane to understanding how neural processes can mechanistically shape symptom phenomena in eating disorders and increase risk of long-term chronicity is difficult to argue, and we offer here some speculative ideas. Clearly, an exclusively psychological theory of eating disorders is difficult to argue against the backdrop of today's science. But there are some caveats. First, it is surely the case that multiple causal pathways are involved (see Berridge, 2009; Steinglass & Walsh, 2006), including circuitry and transmitter chemistry that regulate reward, habit patterns, and appetitive motivation; and, obviously, more than anxiety proneness is involved as the large majority of anxiety-prone people never develop disordered eating. Second, clinical experience shows that for every family affected by an eating disorder where there are parallels to our case, there are others that are dramatically different. This is why understanding the normally occurring variation in family environments within a neuroscience perspective and how it informs clinical work is important too. We selected this particular case vignette because it highlights so vividly the range of issues we believe essential to explore.

In this regard, a conceptual principle on which we all agree is that eating disorders are no less complex than other psychiatric phenotypes—single disciplinary approaches are bound to be insufficient; complex explanatory models are needed if the search for more effective therapies is to succeed. Regarding Jill's history, we expect the idea of an integrative approach to be widely embraced; indeed, nearly three decades after Garfinkel and Garner's (1982) seminal text on the multidimensional nature of AN even the acknowledgment of its importance seems gratuitous.

However, for Jill's family there was no shortage of opinions on "the true heart of the problem"—whether precedence should be accorded biological determinism or influences more social in nature—each championed with conviction. Strong though it may be, cross-discipline agreement on complexity does not set aside this altogether more complicated debate, not that we would expect it to. Many of us have trained in programs firmly rooted in one particular tradition or another, and there is an inevitable hold that training and well-honed technical skills have on how we contemplate clinical material. What is curious, however, is that the boundary between biology and social influence is less decisively debated in other areas of psychopathology. Take, for example, schizophrenia, anxiety, depression, posttraumatic stress; in each case contemporary models emphasize how vulnerability and pathogenesis depend not solely on genetic risk but rather on complex interactions between innate susceptibility, chronic life stress, and molecular adaptations that over time impact neural and behavioral plasticity. And, analogously, it is also argued that depending on how individual genes and environmental effects shuffle along these pathways, the long-term prospect is better for some than for others.

So although it is true that research on causal mechanisms in eating disorders has moved closer to accepting as "truth" the importance of genetic and biological vulnerability (see Klump, Bulik, Kaye, Treasure, & Tyson, 2009; Racine, Root, Klump, & Bulik, Chapter 3, this volume), the nod toward biology raises an important question: Does this mean that environment, including aspects of family life, is no longer relevant, either theoretically or clinically (see Le Grange, Lock, Loeb, & Nicholls, 2010)? But how could this be if the research disciplines advocating loudest for studying environmental effects in complex behavior are molecular biology and genetics (Meaney, 2010)? And if we accept the call of contemporary neuroscience that family environment is relevant, how do we avoid fostering the misleading impression that such influences are *causative*, or singularly crucial, when neither of these two ideas is supported by theory or empirical evidence (Klump et al., 2009; Le Grange et al., 2010)?

Allegiance to discipline being what it is, debate will continue as to which level of discourse is the more relevant one, although psychopathologists in other fields insist, as they have for decades (Neufeld, 1982), that such a debate is counterintuitive and unhelpful. Indeed, an immediate reason for setting the debate aside is that disciplines that once labored in isolation—from developmental psychology and clinical psychology, to epidemiology, quantitative genetics, and molecular neuroscience—now work in collaborations that have dramatically reshaped ideas about the nature of complex interactions that promote healthy and unhealthy development, and how syndromes long considered separate may, in fact, relate. Hence, it is not a contradiction that modern neuroscience discredits the idea that faulty learning or a "harmful" family is the root of abnormal behavior as strongly as it argues that effects of genes and biology are not absolute—that to understand behavior and its evolution is to understand the interdependency of biology and experience; our case history illustrates this well.

So if complexity in psychopathology is the rule, then translational neuroscience—the new science of mind and behavior—may help to better explain how interchanges between biology, stress, and family environment are similarly relevant to eating disorders. But in this regard it is also important to be precise as to what we are *not* saying. We are not asserting that a causal explanation of eating disorders in familial terms is valid, or that family factors in vulnerability or illness course are more influential than nonfamilial ones. We believe strongly, in line with recent reviews (Klump et al., 2009; Le Grange et al., 2010) and consistent with the detailed analysis of risk factor studies presented by Jacobi, Hayward, de Zwaan, Kraemer, and Agras (2004), that no substantive evidence supports the idea that eating disorders are "family caused." What is plausible, however, is that familial effects have potential theoretical and clinical relevance.

For ease of discussion, and given limitations of space and scope, we focus more on AN, but refer to binge eating where research argues empirically, or intuitively, for the bridge. Beyond these constraints, the editors imposed no restrictions on the content of this chapter, asking only that we think broadly and speculate freely.

The generalizations on which our discussion is based are drawn from a number of comprehensive reviews (for each set, readers are directed to these articles for specific, individual source material). There is overlap among them—and along with this some redundancy in the discussion—but taken as a whole the following generalizations validly support the premise that the interchange of biology and experience is no less relevant to eating disorders than to other complex psychological disorders.

The Primacy of Genetic Effects

Much of the variation in behavioral tendencies—how we react to stress and novelty, personality structure, neural function, and proneness to psychological illness—can be attributed to additive genetic factors (Faraone, Tsuang, & Tsuang, 1999). Our case illustrates what many parents of multisibling families know all too well: their affected child stood out from the very beginning. Jill certainly knew this, and as her capacity for self-contemplation grew, so did the intuition that her nervousness, disdain of change, and extreme discipline felt more like destiny than a matter of choice. However, in contemporary models of illness gene effects are not invariant, they often require a particular environment to activate the vulnerability they confer, and absent a dominant locus that is fully penetrant many different genes of small individual effect shape a continuum of behavioral risk. In effect, this means that in complex inheritance risk genes are not distinctively causal, as long-term outcomes are determined by multiple other sources of vulnerability and protective influences linked together over time in both early-acting and late-acting interactive causal chains (Rutter, 1988). In short, we no longer question the role of genes in abnormal behavior, but hold that genomic effects are not predictable nor do they "program" illness per se.

Gene–Environment Interaction

Relevant here is Plomin's (1986) reminder, "There can be no behavior without both genes and environment" (p. 92). This elegantly simple truth is reflected in another crucial dictum of behavior genetics: that variation in behavior across the lifespan expresses not simply the effects of either one but rather the joint effects of both—an interaction between genotype and environment. Gene effects and environments are also correlated wherein each bears witness to either the child's or parents' genetic propensities. These correlations operate in several ways. As genes and family environment are shared—their effects are perfectly confounded—a trait passed from one or both parents can similarly determine the environment they create for the child; here the correlation between genotype and environment is a passive one (Jill's mother, like Jill, is highly disciplined, goal oriented, and affectively restrained. Similarly, Jill and her father are compulsive in their routines, nervous, and fearful). It is also plausible that experiences in both home and nonfamily settings unfold partly in response to (sometimes preferentially so) a child's genetically formed characteristics—in this case a correlation that is reactive (it was Jill, not her "less dependable," free-spirited sister who was relied upon by parents to assist with household chores, in the same way that Jill was often engaged by her homeroom teacher to assist in the classroom). And third, however inhibited or reticent a child may be, the child is hardly passive in his or her interactions with the environment; to the contrary, the child actively seeks out or evokes—obviously, some children more than others—environments that mirror his or her genetic traits (Jill would routinely shun personal interests to lend parents a helping hand, feeling it was not only a duty but a moral imperative). Overall, the single strongest effect a family environment exerts on its members is to accentuate the underlying differences between them.

Variation in the Effects of Stress

It is well accepted that chronic stress can be a starting point for psychopathological outcomes (Barrett, Rose, & Klerman, 1979; Neufeld, 1982). The following discussion considers the fact that environmental effects sometimes endure because stress can mechanistically retune brain morphology and signal a programming of genes in regions vital to emotional memory and motivational action. What results from this interchange is a series of molecular events that encode information about the prevailing environment, which in turn become a link in the causal chain that eventuates in either adaptive or maladaptive outcomes. But in the same way that gene effects are not invariant, much the same can be said of stressful environments; for some the exposure proves disabling, whereas others are resilient. And there is another especially relevant point here: not all stress during development is inherently pathogenic, and a parent's instinct to protect a child from exposure to adversity is not without significant risk. This is because mild stress exposures often promote a child's later resilience. Thus, as we come to see more clearly that complex behavior does not begin and end with genes or stress, but rather with gene–environment interplays that set in motion longlasting causal chains, we had better appreciate not only why there is significant gloss to human development but also why modeling causal factors is not straightforward. Place a genotype associated with greater anxiety risk and stress responsiveness in a rearing environment that offers stability, security, and strong social bonding, and later problem behaviors may be few (Meaney, 2010).

Given that support for these generalizations is strong, they merit consideration as the prism through which what is known about family environments in AN and BN should pass for interpretation. So in considering the next section of this chapter, it is to be remembered that gene effects are at a distance from symptom development, that they cannot be divorced from the social context in which they are expressed, and that risk of later adversity cannot be inferred without reference to genotype—consider one element in isolation, and knowledge of causal mechanisms is bound to be insufficient. These generalizations and their caveats must surely apply in contemplating the possible relevance of family life to a more complete knowledge of eating disorders.

Family Experience in Eating Disorders: A Brief Summary

The topic of family experience has hardly been ignored as a field of inquiry (for background, see Jacobi et al., 2004; Steiger & Stotland, 1995; Strober, 1992) in the nearly 150 years since Gull's (1874) admonition that parents cannot offer the "moral conditions" required for proper treatment of AN. Whether or not the insights gained since Gull can be considered substantive knowledge has been debated, as most of this research compares cases of ill persons and non-ill control persons without establishing cleanly whether the differences shown are precursors or consequences of illness (Jacobi et al., 2004). For this reason it is doubtful that any of these findings usefully point in the direction of contributing vulnerability, and it is equally just to say that evidence for a distinct family transactional style in eating disorders is lacking (Le Grange et al., 2010).

Still, it would be premature to dismiss outright the entirety of this literature in light of what neuroscience has revealed about environmental effects. Moreover, there are several rigorously designed and expertly conducted community and cohort risk factor studies of eating disorders (Fairburn, Cooper, Doll, & Welch, 1999; Fairburn, Welch, Doll, Davies, & O'Connor, 1997; Pike et al., 2008) and the findings are intriguing. The following is a concise summary of this literature, drawn from the review articles cited above; again, readers interested in specific articles that support the generalizations are referred to these resources.

Descriptive and Observational Accounts

What emerges from the studies of descriptive and observational accounts is a rather long list of parent maladies, most derived from anecdotal impressions of unknown reliability, some from psychometric instruments. They include obsessionality, hostility, passivity, rigidity, introversion, demandingness, social maladjustment, and impulsivity. In similar fashion, family interactions have been described impressionistically as showing maternal insecurity coupled with paternal detachment as well as submissiveness and emotional reserve, consistent with the idea that family environments in cases of eating disorders express a global transactional pattern marked by constraining rules that impair the normal process of psychological separation and autonomous functioning, that encourage sustained dependencies and solicitations of protection, and that promote enmeshment, conflict avoidance, and high levels of negative expressed emotion.

The caveats are several. First and most significant, given that these findings are largely cross-sectional, the characteristics portrayed are correlates rather than indicators of risk or causal mechanisms (see Jacobi et al., 2004). Second, they are subject to a variety of reporting and observer biases and some may be influenced by the type, time course, and intensity of treatments received. Third, it remains in question as to what degree the findings reflect severity biases common to clinic cases (although findings, still sparse, in nonclinic samples tend to largely parallel these reports; see Steiger & Stotland, 1995). And fourth, they are muddled and confounded by diagnostic heterogeneity within eating disorders.

Patterns of Heterogeneity

Limitations of method aside, the characteristics described are not universal, as many families show no obvious dysfunction by clinical observation or when compared with non-ill control families in which childhood and family background characteristics are carefully assessed retrospectively (see, e.g., Crisp, Hsu, Harding, & Hartshorn, 1980; Webster & Palmer, 2000). Second, and most striking, are differences by clinical subtype of illness. Here it has been observed quite consistently that families with the binge-eating form of AN and those with BN differ from families with classic, restricting-type AN; specifically, they are more likely to exhibit lower expressed warmth, less affection, less mutuality of support, greater family discord and adversity, less general cohesion, and more belittling attitudes and negative expressed emotion (Steiger & Stotland, 1995; Strober, 1992).

Risk Factor Studies

The importance of risk factor studies is that they carefully establish the antecedence of putative measures of risk and compare their occurrence in matched samples of cases and controls. The major findings (Fairburn et al., 1997, 1999; Pike et al., 2008) are that many of the risk factors shown to be more common in persons with eating disorders as compared with healthy persons (controls) similarly distinguish cases of non-eating-disorder psychopathology (mainly depression and anxiety diagnoses); but intriguingly, some are specific to AN, others to BN. Factors shown to separate persons with eating disorders from healthy persons (controls) include family discord, emotional over- and underinvolvement, low affection, high expectations and demands, and parental health problems. In both the Fairburn and colleagues (1999) and Pike and colleagues (2008) studies, high parental expectations/demands and underinvolvement also distinguished AN from non-eating-disorder psychopathology, arguing for specificity. This particular finding may bear some relationship to the significant association of AN with higher social class reported in a Swedish population cohort study (Lindberg & Hjern, 2003), but negative findings concerning social class have also been reported (see Lindberg & Hjern, 2003).

Strongly in line with findings concerning heterogeneity, the risk factor data discussed earlier similarly show that BN and AN with binge-eating history are characterized by even greater exposure to parental depression and substance abuse, parent underinvolvement and high demands, and early life disruptions than that found in psychiatric controls, again suggesting a degree of specificity. It is therefore conceivable that the overall level of antecedent life stress—in the form of certain parenting problems and family dysfunction—is differentially associated with binge-eating subforms of eating disorder. But it is also plausible that these associations are mediated partly by personality and impulse-related complications linked to the parental psychiatric disorders reported, and that the high novelty seeking often seen in persons with binge eating and purging may similarly share this genetic diathesis. Also needing consideration in this regard is the potentially overlapping environmental effect of disturbances in rearing, attachment, and other aspects of parenting behavior that are well-documented consequences of parental depression (Weissman & Paykel, 1974). In short, eating disorders share antecedent vulnerabilities in common with disorders whose major distinguishing features involve disturbances of emotion.

Predictors of Illness Outcome

The relationship of family environment to illness course and outcome has received attention, but interpretation of existing data is problematic (Steinhausen, 2002; Steinhausen & Weber, 2009; see also Steinhausen, Chapter 6, this volume). There is some evidence that a negative parent–child relationship predicts poorer short-term outcome and early dropout from treatment in AN; conversely, there is far stronger evidence that a positive relationship is a favorable prognostic indicator. Regarding BN, with the exception of one strong finding (Fallon, Sadik, Saoud, & Garfinkel, 1994) linking negative outcome to severe family maladjustment, reliable family predictors for this condition have not been shown, although rigorously executed studies are few (Steinhausen & Weber, 2009). Notably, the same broad features of family environment associated with binge eating—high parental criticism and poor bonding—have been shown in two prospective studies (Strober, Morrell, & Freeman, 1997; Tozzi et al., 2005) to predict the eventual progression of restricting AN to BN.

In summary, although early theories of a psychosomatic family foundation for eating disorders (Minuchin, Rosman, & Baker, 1978; Palazzoli, 1978) had heuristic merit, no empirical finding supports their validity as a model of causation. Moreover, because of the many conceptual hurdles faced in investigating family environment and the wide differences in the methods that have been applied, it is unsurprising that the findings reported are neither easy to interpret nor to reconcile. What the evidence reviewed does show are broad trends that line up with basic knowledge of familial precursors of affective psychopathology: that problem parenting and family dysfunction are seen, but not always. In addition, there is at least some evidence to posit more eating-disorder-specific influences in the family domain—namely, high parental expectations and lack of affectionate care. However, specificity is not equivalent to universality, and problems of interpretation remain. Indeed, one can reasonably offer two parsimonious models for explaining the relationship: (1) that a parental effect creates an evolving family climate that acts independently on, and interactively with, the child's underlying genetic traits and (2) that high parental demands, on one hand, and certain temperamental precursors of eating disorder, on the other—namely, perfectionism, neuroticism, rigid obedience, and goal directedness—are related phenotypes that share a common genetic determination (note previously discussed evidence of familial transmission of compulsive personality in AN (Strober et al., 2007). So whether these studies are seen as evidence of an essentially environmental effect or another example of a complex interactive chain may well depend on one's theoretical point of view. Regardless, they are meaningful phenomena that illustrate how much remains to be learned about how the nexus of intrinsic individuality and family environment shapes risk.

These issues circle back to a crucial question: How is it possible to apportion these influences when members of the same family are not affected equally by stress, environmental and genetic effects interact, genetic characteristics of parent and child are partly shared and themselves have correlative associations with family environment, and the relationship between family environment and illness outcome may conceivably reflect a biological confound? The challenge is daunting but it should not deter study of how environmental pressures may be operating in the causal chain.

In the next sections we consider some of the advances in developmental neuroscience that may benefit this analysis. We first consider the existing literature on family processes in childhood anxiety to see if what has been documented here complements the observations reviewed earlier. Indeed, the findings show a clear parallel in how common it is for negative, escalating chain reactions to unfold in families that transmit anxiety and stress.

The Familial Context of Childhood Anxiety

There is a considerable recent literature on the role of inheritance, parent psychopathology, and family environment in child anxiety (Ginsburg, Siqueland, Masia-Warner, & Hedtke, 2004). As in the case of eating disorders, pharmacological and psychosocial treatments have proliferated over the past decade (Barrett, Farrell, Pina, Peris, & Piacentini, 2008), but for many youth the response is incomplete and impairment lingers. Another parallel lies in efforts to improve treatment response by alleviating maladaptive family interactions that constrain treatment adherence and therapeutic gains. Such work is based on evidence that parental accommodation and critical attitudes are common features of the family environment for both adults and children with anxiety—obsessive–compulsive disorder especially—and when present they increase the risk of poor treatment outcome and later relapse (Amir, Freshman, & Foa, 2000; Chambless & Steketee, 1999; Leonard et al., 1993), similar to findings in eating disorders.

At the core of these treatments is direct, active engagement of parents as coaches or co-therapists (Freeman et al., 2003; Scahill et al., 1997). And here, too, what has been observed is not unlike the results we see in our field (see Lock, Chapter 12, and Campbell & Schmidt, Chapter 16, this volume) – namely, symptom change can be impressive but for many youths illness persists (Barrett, Farrell, Dadds, & Boulter, 2005). Also attesting to how difficult it can be to alter the family climate, these interventions have thus far shown limited benefit in reducing parental distress and accommodation to the child's persisting difficulties. What remains unknown is whether resistance to change in this domain is the result of greater parental vulnerability, which in turn transmits a more severe anxiety phenotype to offspring—a common genetic influence—or conversely, the understandable frustration of parents attempting to reign in, unsuccessfully, the putatively greater intractability of early-onset anxiety disorder. Although work addressing the question is limited, there is some evidence that level of vulnerability may be at play in that baseline symptom severity in the child with obsessive–compulsive disorder has been shown to predict poorer treatment outcome (Barrett et al., 2005; Piacentini, Bergman, Jacobs, McCracken, & Kretchman, 2002).

The parallel to what occurs in families of persons with eating disorders is evident. Parents of anxious and eating-disordered youth alike face challenges under the best of circumstances, but the struggle is infinitely greater if their own predisposition to nervousness enters the mix. And should that happen, anxiety will pervade the home to an even greater extent, the waves of emotional arousal becoming so constant that disruptions, accommodations, and hostile attitudes seem normative; the unfortunate consequence of this pattern is poorer treatment response and higher rates of relapse (Peris et al., 2008; Piacentini, Bergman, Keller, & McCracken, 2003; Renshaw, Steketee, & Chambliss, 2005). What this stress expresses and how emotional environments can impact biological pathways that influence developmental outcomes are now considered.

Stress, Anxiety, and the Environment

The material in this section is drawn from recent comprehensive, integrative reviews (Aggleton, 2000; Caspi, Hariri, Holmes, Uher, & Moffitt, 2010; Gross & Hen, 2004a, 2004b; Gunnar, 2003; Heim & Nemeroff, 2001; Kappelar & Meaney, 2010; Leonardo & Hen, 2008; LeDoux, 2000; Meaney, 2010; Panksepp, 1998; Shin & Liberzon, 2010) that highlight the physiology, molecular chemistry, and neurocircuitry of stress and anxiety and the role of environment in shaping plasticity within these systems. The main insight gained from this literature is that genetic vulnerability and early emotional environment are neither independent of each other nor mutually exclusive and that differences within each of these domains matters greatly in how people adapt.

Regulatory aspects of neural operating systems that mediate adaptation to environmental demands have been evolutionarily conserved within a widely distributed circuitry, of which prefrontal cortices, extended amygdala, and hippocampus are key regions. The cascades involved are evident early in life, as are individual differences in their intensity and long-term effects, underlining the fact that a capacity for detecting and then reacting automatically to adverse environments is present from early in development. Consistent with the imperative of natural selection, when threats to survival are obvious individual differences in corticolimbic stress/anxiety reaction patterns are essentially negligible; all organisms are capable of mobilizing basic resources when faced with events that threaten survival. But as evolutionary pressures became more diverse so did the evolving genome, giving rise to variations that expressed reaction patterns better suited to life's emerging vicissitudes, promoting adaptations that were a logical fit to the unique environmental pressures faced. Bearing on this point are two fundamental "truths" in modern developmental psychopathology that explain why it is difficult to contemplate the eventual course of any single life history. First, genetic variation in stress and anxiety proneness is substantial, yet the expression of risk genes is highly context dependent. Second, and arguably more intriguing, is evidence that although stress during sensitive periods of early development—unstable attachments, unpredictable parental care, and disorganization in the rearing environment—programs the brain in a way that produces later stress and anxiety-prone behavior, offspring of the following generation—that is, offspring of these high-stress/anxious parents—also tend to exhibit anxious traits even when trauma in their own history is absent (Frank et al., 2010). How this cross-generation transmission of stress susceptibility comes about remains little understood (we return to the question in a following section). What we can assume is that assimilations between genotype, environment, and biology create wide, not easy to predict, individual differences in how environmental signals are appraised and processed, and that these effects can be transmitted over generations. Simply put, this is why the adjustments of children facing a common set of family or outside environmental challenges rarely follow a predictable behavioral or biological ontogeny.

By and large, individual differences in stress reaction and vigilance regulation are stable over time, the substrates involved have intrinsically subtle properties, and there are sexual dimorphisms that differentiate at a remarkably early age. Two trends in this latter regard are pertinent: First, as compared with infant boys, girls exhibit more spontaneously expressed socioemotional behavior, they are more sensitive to the hedonics of taste, they react more strongly to auditory and tactile stimulation, and they ultimately show greater anxiety sensitivity (see Korner, 1969, 1973). Second, not only do persons with high trait anxiety show greater amygdala activation as compared with persons low in anxiety when processing stimuli that convey emotional threat, the contrast is observed even when the stimulus is presented outside conscious awareness (Etkin et al., 2004), supporting the idea that predisposition to anxiety promotes a vigilance for threat in the environment that is unconscious. What can be inferred from these observations is that from early in life girls show a distinctively different emotional resonance with their rearing environment, which coincides with expression of genetic differences in stress and anxiety proneness. These differences parsimoniously explain why females are more likely than males to imbue environmental signals with greater affective valence, a speculation that also fits well with emerging evidence of structural differences between the sexes in subcortical areas that mediate fear and anxiety (see Gorski, 2000).

At a theoretical level, the relevance of these findings to eating disorders is persuasive. Elsewhere (Strober, 2010), one of us (M. S.) offered the heuristic idea that in a child prone to anxiety, averse to novelty, and compulsively rigid in his or her habits, feelings of shame and ineffectiveness are bound to rise with puberty's approach, and for these reasons the coincidence of startling body change and developmental challenge signals impending "threat," which in turn greatly increases the child's level of vigilance. In this scenario not only is the body linguistically tagged with negative emotional connotations, but, given what is known about how emotion-regulating circuitry mediates threat appraisal and how innate differences affect the neurosymbolic intensity of vigilance (Panksepp, 19980, a reasonable further speculation is that biological mechanisms come into play. And this may be an insight into how it is that one child insists loudly and absolutely that he or she does indeed "see" a looming presence—an unwelcome new body running wild—that is imperceptible to another.

Turning back to the role of environment, in one sense its importance to emotional development is all too obvious. Verbal instruction and observational learning are influential in shaping the content of mental life—our perceptions, thought patterns, attitudes, and motivations—and family experience is an inarguably powerful medium. Until we learned how gene–environment interactions give shape to variations in learning, it was naturally assumed that environment's role was more or less deterministic. Today, the concepts invoked to explain emotional learning are vastly different, with the mechanisms involved complexly intertwined in a dynamic chain of gene–environment signaling designed to support the greatest possible flexibility in adaptation; but should stress be chronically high during early development, the plasticity of learning and adaptation is constrained and outcomes are less favorable. Illustrating the point are a number of solidly established findings (Cahill et al., 1996; Frank et al., 2010; Goldin, McRae, Ramel, & Gross, 2008; LeDoux, 2000; Phelps et al., 2001; Reeb-Sutherland et al., 2009; Shin & Liberzon, 2010):

1. The amygdala activates not only when exposed to unconditionally aversive stimuli but also to stimuli given emotional meaning through simple conditioning—that is, certain fears are innately driven whereas others are learned, yet both register in the same neural structure.
2. The strength of amygdala activation during learning correlates with later capacity to retrieve these cues from memory—that is, we are more likely to retain memories when they are attached to powerful emotion; this is why strong fears may be especially difficult to extinguish.
3. Prompting an experimental subject to reappraise the meaning of a stimulus presentation or suggesting a new context for its interpretation activates prefrontal regions of the brain that, as mentioned earlier, normally modulate, one might say "tame," limbic system arousal—that is, brain substrates that support anxiety expression are malleable, at least for some.
4. When anxiety is extreme and limbic structures are hyperexcitable, threat signaling is not effectively regulated by this top-down control—that is, highly anxious persons experience far greater challenge when evaluating the environment for threat and thus overgeneralize their fears.

These points fit well with two other observations on how stress, genetic variation, and the environmental milieu interface adaptively during early development:

1. Components within the limbic circuitry that mediate the reaction to stress overlap with those mediating the response to novelty, anxiety, and fear in ways complementary and synergistic. This is intuitive, inasmuch as stress, apprehension, and vigilance operate together to facilitate survival; if innate anxiety is high, an indiscriminant hypervigilance will linger.
2. Depending on genotype and the milieu's emotional ambience, biological adaptations during development can differ sharply, but each adaptive phenotype is, in effect, preparing the organism to anticipate similar future emotional demands. When the rearing milieu is one of security and high emotional care, and assuming a relative absence of genes that confer high trait anxiety, offspring who experience stress of mild intensity during sensitive periods show enhanced learning and greater ease in exploring novel environments. But should early life stress be intense and chronic, hormonal and chemical cascades enhance anxiety, facilitate the conditioning of fear to environmental events, promote withdrawal and social defeat, and strengthen the resistance of negative emotional memories to extinction, all of which strengthen the impulse to retreat when future challenges arise. On one hand, this makes logical sense—it is functionally relevant for fear to remain prepotent if early life experience was marked by repeated threat—however, on the other hand, the social and psychological disadvantages that follow from chronic hypervigilance are great.

The point here is that although differences in the phenotypes are sharp—one is marked by constant avoidance and suffering, the other by resilience and relatively greater protection from ill health—each is functional in its own right from the standpoint of early adaptive demands. Panksepp's (1998) hypothesis that these very same adaptive mechanisms play a role in shaping the foundation of higher-order affective consciousness that ultimately defines "the self" is relevant here as it offers a rational explanation of how AN can serve an adaptive purpose—"managing" the agonizing, unwelcome novelties of development from which it emerges—yet leaving in its path a life painfully constrained by avoidance, doubt, and self-deprivation.

So how then, in specific terms, does environment enter into this causal chain? There are several convergent findings.

Adverse Effects of Stress on Brain Morphology and Function

Historical precedents for linking stress to psychopathology involved the study of how loss of primary attachments correlated with later maladaptive emotional functioning. What is known today is that part of the causal chain involves disruptions in the evolving structure and function of the brain's emotional circuitry. The basis for this new model concept is evidence from clinical and translational research that chronic environmental stress (1) alters the expression of brain receptors, which in turn influences anxiety and appetitive behaviors, (2) activates transcription factors critical to a broad range of adaptive functions, and (3) impacts cellular morphology in regions implicated in anxiety and fear—specifically, reducing dendrite growth in the hippocampus, a region implicated in the contextual modulation of anxiety/fear, while increasing dendrite branching in the amygdala, the major locus of fear conditioning. This neural signature of stress has been advanced as a plausible model of pathological anxiety, greater ease of fear development, and symptom persistence due to impairments in habituation and extinction learning.

Associations between Early Adversity and Pathological Outcomes

In humans, as the number of individual exposures to traumatic life events increases, there is correspondingly greater risk of later depression and poor stress regulation. Strongly compatible with this observation are the results of studies in rodents and primates showing that when mothers are taken from their pups during early infancy or when they must forage for food supplies under conditions of unexpectedly high environmental uncertainty, their offspring develop greater propensity for later anxiety, they are more submissive, and their hormonal secretions upon reexposure to stress are sharply increased.

An analogous line of research has investigated the prospective effect on offspring of exposure to naturally occurring variations in the quality of maternal care. Similar to the effects generated by maternal separation, rodent offspring of mothers who normally display low licking and grooming behaviors (a model of low emotional care) are more likely to develop anxiety phenotypes and to secrete more glucocorticoids when later stressed, as compared with pups reared by mothers displaying high licking and grooming. An important point is that experiments that use cross-fostering show that this particular outcome is highly regulated by environmental signals. The basis for this conclusion is that when offspring of low-grooming mothers are fostered by those high in displays of grooming behavior, the risk of later anxiety and fear is low. Analogously, females fostered by high-grooming mothers similarly develop a high-grooming phenotype and in turn give birth to offspring low in anxiety; but it is important to note that this occurs even if they are birthed by low-grooming mothers. However, the environmental effect is not seen in the reverse pattern of cross-fostering. Specifically, offspring of high-grooming mothers are resilient to the negative effect of rearing by low-grooming foster mothers (who also exhibit naturally higher levels of anxiety), a trajectory indicating transmission of genes by high-grooming biological mothers that protect against the anxiogenic effect of low maternal care during infancy. In short, disrupting the normal course of rearing and social attachments, a model of chronic stress, can pose significant risk to maturing biological systems, but certain genotypes buffer the potential adverse effect.

The Interaction of Genes and Environment

We noted that the evolving capacity to adapt flexibly to anxiety-generating encounters with novel environments was essential to fitness. This is surely why the number of genes with regulatory functions in emotion and motivation circuitry is large; the best studied are those involved in serotonergic (5-HT) neurotransmission. We know from murine and rodent studies in which specific genes are removed or mutated to observe their effects on anxiety phenotypes that the 5-HT system plays a central role in priming locomotor and emotion-mediating circuits during sensitive periods of postnatal development. Thus it is unsurprising from the standpoint of evolutionary fitness that the course of anatomical, chemical, and molecular changes that characterize 5-HT effects match up in time with the animal's strengthening capacity for free-ranging exploration of a novel environment. Although legitimate questions remain about whether these findings generalize to the underpinnings of anxiety in humans, homologies across species in the biological foundations of emotional behavior are sufficiently impressive to justify their consideration in the study of human gene–environment interaction.

To date, the largest body of primate and human research modeling gene–environment interaction in stress and anxiety reactions involves study of polymorphic variations in the promoter region of the 5-HT transporter—the major variants being a short (*s*) allele associated with reduced transcriptional efficiency and lower reuptake of serotonin, and a long (*l*) allele whose transcription efficiency is greater. As the Caspi and colleagues (2010) review of this literature shows, there are strong consistencies across diverse research designs and methodologies. There are two major, complementary finds:

1. Inheriting at least one copy of the low 5-HT transporter expressing *s* allele confers greater negative emotionality and stress reactivity. The number of *s* allele-dependent effects is large, but unity among the neural and behavioral phenotypes expressed is striking: neuroticism, elevated anxiety-like behavior in infancy, easier acquisition of conditioned fear, increased auditory startle, affective lability, stress secretory activity, increased activation of the amygdala to emotionally threatening stimuli, disruption in frontal–limbic modulating circuitry, and attentional bias toward negatively valenced environmental stimuli. Given how widespread the features of *s* allele inheritance are, it seems clear that this variant measurably shifts the brain's processing of novelty and negatively valenced emotional stimuli toward greater intensity and more distressing arousal.

2. However, neither the action of genes nor the effects of environmental adversity alone adequately explains behavioral outcomes. Support for this generalization is strong, with convergent evidence in primates and humans showing (a) that effects of the *s* allele genotype are moderated by quality of the rearing environment and (b) that depressiono-genic effects of stress are moderated by inheritance of the short allele. Specific examples

of these interactions are that home-reared monkeys express developmentally normal levels of 5-HT metabolism whether or not they carry an *s* allele genotype, whereas deleterious effects of maternal separation and peer rearing on later socioemotional adjustment and neuroendocrine stress activity occur only in offspring with an *s* allele genotype. Precisely the same interaction is seen in the nearly three dozen human studies reviewed in Caspi and colleagues (2010): susceptibility to the potentially deleterious effects of environmental stress depends, at least in this one sense, on which of the two 5-HT promoter region variants one has.

A final piece of research dramatically illustrates how exquisitely sensitive emergent biological processes are to the environment's emotional ambience. Work by Kent Berridge and colleagues (Reynolds & Berridge, 2008) has shown that chemical signaling from prefrontal and subcortical inputs to the nucleus acumbens—a region linked closely to motivational processes—will activate either appetitive (feeding/drinking) or defensive (fear and withdrawal) behavior, depending on where the signal occurs along a keyboard-like gradient in the medial shell region of the acumbens. Under normal circumstances signaling the rostral region of the shell promotes stronger appetitive motivation, whereas behavior becomes steadily defensive in character as the locus of signaling moves in a caudal direction. But the position of these motivation-generating zones is not fixed; instead, the shell's anatomy exhibits remarkably significant plasticity, radiating in one direction or the other, depending on the environment's prevailing emotional tone. Specifically, when rats are exposed to a naturally preferred, safe environment, fear-generating zones retract whereas zones that instantiate appetitive behavior expand into the caudal space, soon occupying roughly 90% of the region. And the converse is true: change the exposure to an environment that is distressingly unfamiliar, and zones that normatively generate fear and other defensive actions shift rostrally, now making up most of this rostrocaudal gradient. The implication of this plasticity for understanding how environment affects behavior is profound, and its application to the study of pathological outcomes is clear. Rather than a structure fixed in time and space, neuronal architecture in this motivation circuit is fully reversible when signaled affectively, an adaptive plasticity that keys behavior to its ever-changing environment. This has intriguing clinical ramifications, which in turn invite many questions: What occurs over time if the signaling valence is relatively constant during early life? We can easily see how the question pertains to AN inasmuch as the fearful anticipation of change begins early in development and shadows the perception of daily life up to the time symptoms emerge. Is it conceivable that in such a developmental trajectory the circuit's flexibility to retune is genetically constrained? Or is there a point where motivational anatomy in the brain's reward center adapts unalterably to a milieu whose ambience is continuously experienced as fearful by an innately anxious child? Likewise, as fear-generating zones fill the signaling space, do appetitive arousal and hedonic drive become so dulled that chronicity of illness is inevitable? And are low emotional care and chronic family stress during early development factors in this biological adaptation?

In short, stress during early rearing, emotional ambience of the surrounding milieu, and inheritance of specific genotypes all play intricately coordinated roles in shaping behavioral plasticity over time and influencing what capacities for later adaptation are, or are not, accessible to the developing child—which brings us to a final area of study.

Epigenetic Programming of Environmental Effects

It is becoming increasingly well understood (see Kappeler & Meaney, 2010; Meaney, 2010) how these environment events molecularly program and physically imprint the genome to sustain plasticity changes well beyond the time of a child's exposure to early challenges. As previously discussed, the amount of licking and grooming lactating rodents display with their offspring is a fairly stable phenotype unless grooming is curtailed by stress in the environment. Regarding the biological mechanisms involved, this research shows that adult offspring who received high levels of grooming (i.e., greater emotional care) differentially express genes in brain regions—the hippocampus in particular—that coordinate hormonal feedback essential for the effective operation of stress and emotion circuitry. Although a detailed description of the entire cascade of events is beyond the scope of this chapter—for background, see the Kappelar and Meaney (2010) and Meaney (2010) reviews—it suffices our purpose to summarize the main findings succinctly.

In brief, as we previously discussed, offspring who receive high licking and grooming in their infancy (i.e., reliable emotional care) enter adulthood displaying less startle and fear in response to novel environments they encounter as adults; the reverse continuity is seen too—namely, distinctly higher level of stress and fear upon confronting novelty among adult offspring reared in infancy by mothers with low licking and grooming. At least one of the critical mediating factors involved is release of corticotrophin releasing factor (CRF), whose expression and triggering of norepinephrine release in corticolimbic regions is linked to increased fear along with suppression of appetitive motivation. What is clear from the work of Meaney and colleagues is that offspring of high-grooming mothers exhibit lower levels of CRF in fear-generating limbic structures as compared with offspring reared by low-grooming mothers. But there are further differences, all of which support a more effective modulation of stress and fear. Key among these are (1) increased receptor expression for the brain's principal source of neural inhibition (gamma-aminobutyric acid [GABA]) and (2) increased hippocampal glucocorticoid receptor expression that results in enhanced negative feedback sensitivity to circulating stress hormones—in essence, a neural signature for better stress regulation and greater anxiety resilience.

Perhaps the most critical aspect of the story concerns the mechanisms by which these cellular effects of maternal care are carried forward in time—how they generate a script of sorts that physically imprints the genome through dynamic remodeling of DNA's chemical and structural environment. These changes involve chromatin structure and methylation, which in turn influence gene transcription—modifications that are the essence of epigenesis. And because the processes by which such epigenetic tags mediate gene expression and behavioral plasticity are malleable and thus potentially reversible, they are deemed the cornerstone of how gene–environment interaction operates (Meaney, 2010) and arguably the most important of the fresh new insights into how and why early environment is a crucial link between the genome and long-term health.

The crucial point about epigenesis is that it shows the genome to be sensitively and dynamically regulated by signals from the prevailing emotional environment that leave physical imprints, later activated by new adaptive pressures. It seems irrefutable that we would do well to consider how the new science of epigenetics, along with growing knowledge of how stress impacts development, brings fresh ideas for how genes, biology, and environment interact in the emergence of eating disorders.

Clinical Implications and Caveats

The general aim of this review was to illustrate the value of merging perspectives in the approach to causal study. We made much of the fact that multiple lines of evidence from animal and human study show how each domain of inquiry—biology and environment— is important to understanding how behavioral adaptations are shaped, and that by taking both into account the complex interplay is better grasped. The complexity involved is not discounted and there is much to understand about how all of this applies to the development of eating disorders; but their application is, without question, plausible.

First, this work convincingly shows that there are environmental factors that strongly affect the development of neural circuits involved in the mediation of stress, anxiety, fear, and appetitive arousal, the relevance of which to eating disorders is indisputable. Furthermore, the relationship is not one-sided, in that genetic sensitization of these circuits is also well documented, explaining why certain life histories become ever more complicated over time. Thus, as new light is shed on biological mechanisms that play a role in symptom development, we are also learning about the importance of environment in their epigenetic programming and how early family emotional stability may be protective.

What is new in the story of early adversity and later life problems is how the chain forms and evolves—and, analogously, why maladaptive outcomes following stress are not always seen and why illness can emerge even when life adversity is absent. Whether our attention turns first and foremost to a gene's composition or to the environment's emotional tone, today's science tells us that generalizations about complex behaviors will suffer unless a wide scope of knowledge is used for modeling the arc of long-term development and for explaining why life histories diverge so dramatically and unexpectedly from what is adaptive.

Our premise in considering this material is that it has wide application to eating disorders. Even though empirical data are scant, the premise is not unreasonable, given that high stress, anxiety syndromes, and rigidly formed habits are unusually common in both the premorbid and morbid state and strains in a family's emotional environment prior to onset are also seen. At the same time these odd and implacable conditions emerge in families lacking adaptive problems with other children who are exuberant and carefree. This is why it is not surprising that stress and anguish in functionally well families is typically transient—not psychopathology but rather the expected reaction of parents who come to realize that their child's intention to lose even more weight is deadly serious, an act that defies all logic; as symptoms remit so does family turmoil. Clearly, the mechanisms that give rise to eating disorders are not random but rather favor some over others because of innate vulnerabilities still unknown. This is why the idea that genes coding for systems that affect appetitive motivation, high stress reactivity, rigid habits, and excitement of anxiety and fear play a role is plausible.

Equally critical to consider is how adversity, family tensions, and the emotional environment factor in the trajectory, an equally plausible idea in light of what new paradigms have revealed. Modern psychology and neuroscience leave no doubt that genes bias the emergent structure of mind and experience, but how this plays out during early development cannot be grasped without knowing how environmental signals may influence behavioral plasticity; and because gene–environment interaction is nearly ubiquitous and entails an essentially dynamic process, it is not variation in genomic sequence that causes people to differ dramatically as much as the epigenetic remodeling of DNA by environmental signals that affect gene transcription.

We highlighted literature on stress and anxiety because these phenotypes appear so often in patients and families, no doubt the result of hereditary influence, and there is no longer any argument that biology is undisputedly important to the genesis of eating disorders. But an informed understanding of "how" requires taking note of evidence showing that emotion circuitry is altered by early adversity and unreliable rearing, that stressful environments impair later adjustment, and that poorer outcomes are arguably more likely when the loading of anxiety-promoting genes is greater. However, this literature also points out that persons who inherit risk-conferring genes but who are reared in low-stress, high-nurturing homes show resilience in the face of novelty and stress. Thus, no logical reason can be offered for dismissing the relevance of these findings to a more complete understanding of how eating disorders emerge and what shapes their long-term trajectory.

Consider again the findings from risk factor studies (Fairburn et al., 1997, 1999; Pike et al., 2008). They show that the same types of maladaptive early stress and parenting behavior linked to later anxiety and stress reactivity appear in a certain proportion of families with eating-disordered offspring in advance of symptom onset. When considered in connection with outcome studies in AN that show a relationship between positive parent–child relationships and better prognosis, a reasonable speculation is that this trajectory reflects the same type of protective gene–environment interaction and epigenetic modeling by the environmental signaling described in animal and human studies. And equally plausible is the converse: that when children genetically predisposed to anxiety then face ongoing developmental adversity, neural systems that affect emotion and appetitive behavior become constrained and even more so if stress mounts cumulatively. In such cases, it can be reasoned that outcomes will be less favorable, but this remains only an intuitive idea that needs empirical study.

A recent illustration (Hancock & Grant, 2009) of how this interaction may hypothetically predispose to greater severity in AN involves the use of the activity-based anorexia (ABA) paradigm in which rats receive a pairing of limited daily access to food with unlimited access to an activity wheel. Exposed to such a combination, rats reduce feeding, lose weight rapidly, and increase their running steadily to the point of exhaustion and death. Hancock and Grant (2009) studied effects of the ABA paradigm in two groups of rats—one separated from the birth cage for short periods, the second for a more prolonged period, thereby modeling maternal separation and its long-term adverse changes in neural development as discussed earlier. The results were striking in two respects: (1) maternally separated rats consumed less food, and (2) they had a steeper weight decline, with these effects more pronounced in females. In a complementary study, Carrera, Gutierrez, and Boakes (2006) showed that there was less ABA-induced weight loss in rats who received brief periods of handling prior to testing, a manipulation that increases maternal care behaviors such as licking and grooming when the rat is returned to the home cage. The relevance of these reports to this chapter's premise is immediately apparent.

Another direct clinical application concerns binge eating. Cycles of caloric restriction and refeeding, followed later by exposure to stress, has been advanced as an ecologically valid model of binge eating (Boggiano et al., 2005). Although evidence shows that genes play a role in human susceptibility to this pattern (see Chapter 3), the generally greater family stress—deprivations, parent–child conflict, rancor, negative comments about weight and shape, and familial obesity—differentially associated with binge eating, including crossing over from AN to BN, suggests another possible example of how genetic risk and family environment are mutually or interactively involved. Exactly how is not well understood, but the following hypothesized chain of events is not far-fetched: a transmission (be it genetic or nongenetic) of negative attitudes and pressures in a fractured, antagonistic family setting can result in unstable food consumption; in time, food assumes hedonic, emotion-soothing properties; dieting pressures naturally quicken in adolescence; and given genetic differences in brain systems that influence hedonic and motivational aspects of feeding, emergent stress triggers loss-of-control feeding in susceptible individuals. Recent theoretical and empirical study (see Berridge, Ho, Richard, & DiFeliceantonio, 2010; Dallman, 2010) of how overconsumption can result from an adaptive synergy between chronic stress and neural circuits that influence appetitive motivation is relevant. Dallman (2010) has proposed that as stress increasingly biases cognition toward emotional activity and previously formed habits, the consumption of palatable foods is adaptively reinforced via reduction in hormones secreted during stress—a form of hedonic self-medication. Berridge and colleagues (2010) offer an alternative though a complementary idea, that stress activation of mesolimbic dopaminergic reward pathways is also in play, directly amplifying the incentive salience (or "wanting") of reward cues in the environment and thus increasing palatable feeding—a model of "cue-triggered bursts of binge eating"—which may help explain why binge eating can arise in response to emotions of intense pleasure or positive excitement. But, again, the issue of susceptibility is crucial inasmuch as this final outcome can be seen in only a small minority of youth coming from such a background.

We end this chapter on some notes of caution. The mechanisms by which eating disorders emerge from the actions of genes and environment are still a mystery. Our intent in discussing the role of family was not to enumerate a set of putative causes, but rather to offer generative ideas that have applicability to new research and to clinical ideas that offer a more carefully nuanced approach to patient care. That there is a basis for assuming the ideas discussed have applicability is clear—family stress and problems in emotional care are in the history of some of our patients, and to assume they are inconsequential, when an impressively large body of evidence shows that early life stress and parental behavior play a role in remodeling gene expression with sometimes lasting influence on adaptive phenotypes, is unhelpful.

Also meriting consideration is that developmental outcomes in children raised in highly stressed environments are not predicatively negative, perhaps depending on the *level of stress* encountered and inheritance of protective genes. Consider Jill's sister, whose development and self-esteem thus far have been problem free. So again, not only is it crucial to address the role of environmental signals, it is also important to consider genes that bias psychological development. Evidence of the subtleties involved was cited in Meaney's (2010) review, which noted that when offspring of rodent mothers with low licking and grooming encountered stress of *mild* intensity, synaptic plasticity and learning were enhanced, suggesting an adaptive demand signaled by limited parental availability. In one sense most parents already intuitively understand the importance of genetics perfectly well. They know clearly who among their children will rise fearlessly to a challenge and who will retreat in fear, submission, and self-castigation; they often understand as well that how children stand up to life's perturbations and good fortunes bears the stamp of heredity.

Of course, generalizations at this time concerning environmental effects can be risky, as the effects are not always reliably inferred. For most children the normal, everyday roll call of life's routine—homework, a family move, a new social group, a change of teacher, a shift in vacation plans—is a tedium well tolerated. But for those nervous and stress prone, it is neither ordinary nor welcome; rather, the humdrum is intensive, drastic, and emotional, posing a risk to psychological well-being in ways difficult for parents, siblings, and friends to easily comprehend. Indeed, Jill eventually confided to her family that she hardly ever felt her life had balance and for this reason she thought of herself in shameful terms—an absurdly nervous person, almost farcical in the eyes of others. So in one sense it is not unexpected that annoyance, frustration, and accommodation—themes also common in families of anxious children—eventually become a larger systemic "demand" for more sustained emotional adjustment and coping. The point here is that we can see how a narrow view of etiology runs the risk of falsely interpreting family life events as pathogenic.

A further potential level of complexity needs consideration—namely, children with extreme traits instigate stress on their own as nervousness, rigid perfectionism, and high novelty, each creating his or her own cumulative burdens. How, then, to sort through all of these elements in modeling the causal chain—how to determine where and exactly when the multiple types of gene–environment correlation come into play, at the same time imputing not only the significance of high parent demands (when they are present) but also the effects of stress the child creates innately on his or her own—is certain to challenge the wizardry of any biostatistician.

But the importance of attempting this in some way, if only at the level of conjecture, is what the new science encourages. Repeating yet again a point made several times, if there is a single guiding maxim in contemporary psychopathology it is that causal models of complex phenotypes cannot be drawn from any single domain of study, however well elaborated the analysis may seem. Given what has been learned in recent years—the natural variation in how human beings respond to environmental demands, how stressful events and parental behavior influence gene expression and later adaptations, how these processes lead to vulnerability or resilience, how genes and environmental factors impinge on the many brain pathways that shape affective, cognitive, and appetitive actions, and how this nexus of biology, temperament, and experience ultimately affects how we contemplate our transaction with the social world—the need for balance and integration in our approach to clinical material has never been more evident, yet never so complicated. If there is perhaps one single organizing concept that rises to the top for understanding and clinical application it is how variation in the interchange of genes and environment signal the brain in ways that facilitate, for better or worse, later adaptation to similar environmental demands.

So there is a conundrum. Beyond the question of how to best approach the modeling of such data (Rutter, 1988) is the challenge of how to reliably gauge the individual importance and precedence of any one component of vulnerability when facing patient and family in the clinical setting. A dismissive attitude toward the idea that family effects matter is too implausible a position to defend, but assuming it is central is incorrect too; addressing it when it does seem important requires much thought and sensitivity.

This is obvious, given psychiatry's history of ill-conceived ideas: that malignant parenting coax even the most extreme forms of psychiatric and neurodevelopmental disease; that specific psychosexual conflicts lead to particular types of psychosomatic syndromes;

that mental disorders would ultimately be related predictably and precisely to specific abnormalities of brain structure and function; that it was only a matter of time before the study of psychopathology would prove no different than physics—a matter of illuminating cause and effect. We know now that all of this is false.

In summary, what is true is that the effects of genes are not easy to infer, that brain function cannot be understood without taking account of the environment, and that effects of parenting, family life, and social experience cannot be understood without taking account of heredity. In facing the challenge such complexity poses to our field, the perspectives gained from modern neuroscience may help.

References

Aggleton, J. P. (2000). *The amygdala: A functional analysis.* New York: Oxford University Press.

Amir, N., Freshman, M., & Foa, E. B. (2000). Family distress and involvement in relatives of obsessive–compulsive disorder patients. *Journal of Anxiety Disorders, 14,* 209–217.

Baldwin, A. L. (1960). The study of child behavior and development. In P. H. Mussen (Ed.), *Handbook of research methods in child development* (pp. 3–35). New York: Wiley.

Barrett, J. E., Rose, R. M., & Klerman, G. L. (Eds.). (1979). *Stress and mental disorder.* New York: Raven Press.

Barrett, P., Farrell, L., Pina, A., Peris, T. S., & Piacentini, J. (2008). Evidence-based treatments for child and adolescent OCD. *Journal of Clinical Child and Adolescent Psychology, 37,* 137–155.

Barrett, P. M., Farrell, L. J., Dadds, M., & Boulter, N. (2005). Cognitive-behavioral family treatment of childhood obsessive–compulsive disorder: Long-term follow-up and predictors of outcome. *Journal of the American Academy of Child and Adolescent Psychiatry, 44,* 1005–1014.

Berridge, K. C. (2009). "Liking" and "wanting" food rewards: Brain substrates and roles in eating disorders. *Physiology and Behavior, 97,* 537–550.

Berridge, K. C., Ho, C.-Y., Richard, J. M., & DiFeliceantonio, A. G. (2010). The tempted brain eats: Pleasure and desire circuits in obesity and eating disorders. *Brain Research, 1350,* 43–64.

Boggiano, M. M., Chandler, P. C., Viana, J. B., Oswald, K. D., Maldanado, C. R., & Wauford, P. K. (2005). Combined dieting and stress evoke exaggerated response to opioids in binge eating rats. *Behavioral Neuroscience, 119,* 1207–1214.

Bulik, C. M., Sullivan, P. F., Fear, J. L., & Joyce, P. R. (1997). Eating disorders and antecedent anxiety disorders: A controlled study. *Acta Psychiatrica Scandanavica, 96,* 101–107.

Bulik, C. M., Sullivan, P. F., Tozzi, F., Furberg, H., Lichtenstein, P., & Pedersen, N. L. (2006). Prevalence, heritability, and prospective risk factors. *Archives of General Psychiatry, 63,* 305–312.

Cahill, L., Haier, R. J., Fallon, J., Alkire, M. T., Tang, G., Keator, D., et al. (1996). Amygdala activity at encoding correlated with long-term, free recall of emotional information. *Proceedings of the National Academy of Science, 93,* 8016–8021.

Carrera, D., Gutierrez, E., & Boakes, R. A. (2006). Early handling reduces vulnerability of rats to activity-based anorexia. *Developmental Psychobiology, 10,* 520–527.

Caspi, A., Hariri, A. R., Holmes, A., Uher, R., & Moffitt, T. E. (2010). Genetic sensitivity to the environment: The case of the serotonin transporter gene and its implications for studying complex diseases and traits. *American Journal of Psychiatry, 167,* 509–527.

Chambless, D. L., & Steketee, G. (1999). Expressed emotion and behavior therapy outcome: A prospective study with obsessive–compulsive and agoraphobic outpatients. *Journal of Counseling and Clinical Psychology, 67,* 658–665.

Crisp, A. H., Hsu, L. K. G., Harding, B., & Hartshorn, J. (1980). Clinical features of anorexia nervosa: A study of consecutive series of 102 female patients. *Journal of Psychosomatic Research, 24,* 179–191.

Dallman, M. F. (2010). Stress-induced obesity and emotional nervous system. *Trends in Endocrinology and Metabolism, 21,* 159–165.

Etkin, A., Klemenhagen, K. C., Dudman, J. T., Rogan, M. T., Ren, R., Kandel, E. R., et al. (2004). Individual differences in trait anxiety predict the response of the basolateral amygdala to unconsciously processed fearful faces. *Neuron, 44,* 1043–1055.

Fairburn, C. G., Cooper, Z., Doll, H. A., & Welch, S. L. (1999). Risk factors for anorexia nervosa: Three integrated studies. *Archives of General Psychiatry, 56,* 468–476.

Fairburn, C. G., Welch, S. L., Doll, H. A., Davies, B. A., & O'Connor, M. E. (1997). Risk factors for bulimia nervosa: A community-based case-control study. *Archives of General Psychiatry, 54,* 509–517.

Fallon, B. A., Sadik, C., Saoud, J. B., & Garfinkel, R. S. (1994). Child abuse, family environment, and outcome in bulimia nervosa. *Journal of Clinical Psychiatry, 55,* 424–428.

Faraone, S. V., Tsuang, M. T., & Tsuang, D. W. (1999). *Genetics of mental disorders: What practitioners and students need to know.* New York: Guilford Press.

Frank, T. B., Russig, H., Weiss, I. C., Graff, J., Linder, N., Michalon, A., et al. (2010). Epigenetic transmission of the impact of early stress across generations. *Biological Psychiatry, 68,* 408–415.

Freeman, J. B., Garcia, A. M., Fucci, C., Karitani, M., Miller, L., & Leonard, H. (2003). Family-based treatment of early onset obsessive–compulsive disorder [Special issue: Obsessive–Compulsive Disorder]. *Journal of Child and Adolescent Psychopharmacology, 13*(Suppl.), S71–S80.

Garfinkel, P. E., & Garner, D. M. (1982). *Anorexia nervosa: A multidimensional perspective.* New York: Brunner Mazel.

Ginsburg, G. S., Siqueland, L., Masia-Warner, C., & Hedtke, K. A. (2004). Anxiety disorders in children: Family matters. *Cognitive and Behavioral Practice, 11,* 28–43.

Goldin, P. R., McRae, K., Ramel, W., & Gross, J. (2008). The neural bases of emotion regulation, reappraisal, and suppression. *Biological Psychiatry, 15,* 577–586.

Gorski, A. R. (2000). Sexual differentiation of the nervous system. In E. R. Kandel, J. H. Schwartz, & T. M. Jessell (Eds.), *Principles of neuroscience* (pp. 1131–1148). New York: McGraw-Hill.

Gross, C., & Hen, R. (2004a). The developmental origins of anxiety. *Nature Reviews, 5,* 545–552.

Gross, C., & Hen, R. (2004b). Genetic and environmental factors interact to influence anxiety. *Neurotoxicty Research, 6,* 493–501.

Gull, W. W. (1874). Anorexia nervosa (apepsia/hysterica, anorexia hysterica). *Transactions of the Clinical Society of London, 7,* 22–28.

Gunnar, M. R. (2003). Integrating neuroscience and psychological approaches in the study of early experience. *Annals of the New York Academy of Science, 1008,* 238–247.

Hancock, S., & Grant, V. (2009). Early maternal separation increases symptoms of activity-based anorexia. *Journal of Experimental Psychology, 35,* 394–406.

Heim, C., & Nemeroff, C. B. (2001). The role of childhood trauma in the neurobiology of mood and anxiety disorders. *Biological Psychiatry, 49,* 1023–1039.

Jacobi, C., Hayward, C., de Zwaan, M., Kraemer, H. C., & Agras, W. S. (2004). Coming to terms with risk factors for eating disorders: Application of risk terminology and suggestions for a general taxonomy. *Psychological Bulletin, 130,* 19–65.

Kappeler, L., & Meaney, M. J. (2010). Epigenetics and parental effects. *Bioassays, 32,* 818–827.

Katz, M., Liu, C., Parker, K. J., Ottet, M. C., Epps, A., Buckmaster, E. L., et al. (2009). Prefrontal plasticity and stress inoculation-induced resilience. *Developmental Neuroscience, 31,* 293–299.

Kaye, W. H., Bulik, C. M., Thornton, L., Barbarich, N., M., & the Price Foundation Collaborative Group. (2004). Comorbidity of anxiety disorder with anorexia and bulimia nervosa. *American Journal of Psychiatry, 161,* 2215–2212.

Keel, P. K., Klump, K. L., Miller, K. B., McGue, M., & Iacono, W. G. (2005). Shared transmission of eating disorders and anxiety disorders. *International Journal of Eating Disorders, 38,* 99–105.

Klump, K. L., Bulik, C. M., Kaye, W. H., Treasure, J., & Tyson, E. (2009). Academy for Eating Disorders Position Paper: Eating disorders are serious mental illnesses. *International Journal of Eating Disorders, 42,* 97–103.

Korner, A. (1969). Neonatal startles, smiles, erections, and reflex sucks as related to state, sex, and individuality. *Child Development, 40,* 1039–1053.

Korner, A. (1973). Sex differences in newborns with special reference to differences in the organization of oral behavior. *Journal of Child Psychology and Psychiatry, 14,* 19–29.

LeDoux, J. E. (2000). Emotion circuits in the brain. *Annual Review of Neuroscience, 23,* 155–164.

Le Grange, D., Lock, J., Loeb, K., & Nicholls, D. (2010). Academy for Eating Disorders Position Paper: The role of the family in eating disorders. *International Journal of Eating Disorders, 42,* 97–103.

Leonard, H. L., Swedo, S. E., Lenane, M. C., Rettew, D. C., Hamburger, S. D., & Bartko, J. J. (1993). A 2- to 7-year follow-up of 54 obsessive–compulsive children and adolescents. *Archives of General Psychiatry, 50,* 429–439.

Leonardo, E. D., & Hen, R. (2008). Anxiety as a developmental disorder. *Neuropsychopharmacology, 33,* 134–140.

Lindberg, L., & Hjern, A. (2003). Risk factors for anorexia nervosa: A national cohort study. *International Journal of Eating Disorders, 34,* 397–408.

MacFarlane, J. W. (1971). The Berkely studies: Problems and merits of the longitudinal approach. In M. C. Jones, N. Bayley, J. W. MacFarlane, & M. P. Honzig (Eds.), *The course of human development* (pp. 3–9). Waltham, MA: Xerox College.

Meaney, M. (2010). Epigenetics and the biological definition of gene × environmental interactions. *Child Development, 81,* 41–79.

Minuchin, S., Rosman, B. L., & Baker, L. (1978). *Psychosomatic families: Anorexia nervosa in context.* Cambridge, MA: Harvard University Press.

Neufeld, R. W. J. (Ed.). (1982). *Psychological stress and psychopathology.* New York: McGraw-Hill.

Palazzoli, M. S. (1978). *Self-starvation: From individual to family therapy in the treatment of anorexia nervosa.* New York: Aronson.

Panksepp, J. (1998). *Affective neuroscience: The foundations of human and animal emotions.* New York: Oxford University Press.

Peris, T. S., Bergman, R. L., Langley, A., Chang, S., McCracken, J. T., & Piacentini, J. (2008). Correlates of accommodation of pediatric obsessive–compulsive disorder: Parent, child, and family characteristics. *Journal of the American Academy of Child and Adolescent Psychiatry, 47*(10), 1173–1181.

Phelps, E. A., O' Connor, K. J., Gatenby, J. C., Gore, J. C., Grillon, C., & Davis, M. (2001). Activation of the left amygdala to a cognitive representation of fear. *Nature Neuroscience, 4,* 437–441.

Piacentini, J., Bergman, R. L., Jacobs, C., McCracken, J., & Kretchman, J. (2002). Cognitive-behavior therapy for childhood obsessive–compulsive disorder: Efficacy and predictors of treatment response. *Journal of Anxiety Disorders, 16,* 207–219.

Piacentini, J., Bergman, R. L., Keller, M., & McCracken, J. (2003). Functional impairment in children and adolescents with obsessive–compulsive disorder. *Journal of Child and Adolescent Psychopharmacology, 13,* 61–69.

Pike, K. M., Hilbert, A., Wilfley, D. E., Fairburn, C. G., Dohm, F.-A., Walsh, B. T., et al. (2008). Toward an understanding of risk factors for anorexia nervosa: A case-control study. *Psychological Medicine, 38,* 1443–1453.

Plomin, R. (1986). *Development, genetics, and psychology.* Hilldale, NJ: Erlbaum.

Reeb-Sutherland, B. C., Vanderwert, R. E., Dednan, K. A., Marshall, P. J., Perez-Edgar, K., Chronis-Tuscano, A. P., et al. (2009). Attention to novelty in behaviorally inhibited children moderates risk for anxiety. *Journal of Child Psychology and Psychiatry, 50,* 1365–1372.

Renshaw, K. D., Steketee, G., & Chambless, D. L. (2005). Involving family members in the treatment of OCD. *Cognitive Behavior Therapy, 34,* 164–175.

Reynolds, S. M., & Berridge, K. C. (2008). Emotional environments retune the valence of appetitive versus fearful functions in nucleus accumbens. *Nature Neuroscience, 11,* 423–425.

Rutter, M. (1988). Longitudinal data in the study of causal processes: Some uses and some pitfalls. In M. Rutter (Ed.), *Studies of psychosocial risk* (pp. 1–28). Cambridge, UK: Cambridge University Press.

Scahill, L., Riddle, M. A., McSwiggin-Hardin, M., Ort, S. I., King, R. A., & Goodman, W. K. (1997). Children's Yale–Brown Obsessive Compulsive Scale: Reliability and validity. *Journal of the American Academy of Child and Adolescent Psychiatry, 36,* 844–852.

Shin, L. M., & Liberzon, I. (2010). The neurocircuitry of fear, stress, and anxiety disorders. *Neuropsychopharmacology, 35,* 169–191.

Soloman, M. B., Jones, K., Packard, B. A., & Herman, J. P. (2009). The medial amygdala modulates body weight but not neuroendocrine responses to chronic stress. *Journal of Neuroendocrinology, 22,* 13–23.

Steinglass, J., & Walsh, B. T. (2006). Habit learning and anorexia nervosa: A cognitive neuroscience perspective. *International Journal of Eating Disorders, 38,* 267–275.

Steiger, H., & Stotland, S. (1995). Individual and family factors in adolescents with eating symptoms and syndromes. In H.-C. Steinhausen (Ed.), *Eating disorders in adolescents* (pp. 49–68). Berlin: Water de Gruyter.

Steinhausen, H.-C. (2002). The outcome of anorexia nervosa in the 20th century. *American Journal of Psychiatry, 159,* 1284–1293.

Steinhausen, H.-C., & Weber, S. (2009). The outcome of bulimia nervosa: Findings from one-quarter century of research. *American Journal of Psychiatry, 166,* 1331–1341.

Strober, M. (1992). Family factors in adolescent eating disorders. In P. J. Cooper & A. Stein (Eds.), *Feeding problems and eating disorders in children and adolescents* (pp. 139–146). Chur, Switzerland: Harwood Academic Press.

Strober, M. (2010). The chronically ill patient with anorexia nervosa: Development, phenomenology, and therapeutic considerations. In C. M. Grilo & J. E. Mitchell (Eds.), *The treatment of eating disorders: A clinical handbook* (pp. 225–238). New York: Guilford Press.

Strober, M., Freeman, R., Lampert, C., & Diamond, J. (2007). The association of anxiety disorders and obsessive compulsive personality disorder with anorexia nervosa. *International Journal of Eating Disorders, 40,* S546–S551.

Strober, M., Morrell, W., & Freeman, R. (1997). The long-term course of severe anorexia nervosa in adolescents: Survival analysis recovery, relapse, and outcome predictors over 10–15 years in a prospective study. *International Journal of Eating Disorders, 22,* 339–360.

Tozzi, F., Thornton, L., M., Klump, K. L., Fichter, M., M., Halmi, K. A., Kaplan, A. S., et al. (2005). Symptom fluctuation in eating disorders: Correlates of diagnostic crossover. *American Journal of Psychiatry, 162,* 732–740.

Webster, J. J., & Palmer, R. L. (2000). The childhood and family background of women with clinical eating disorders: A comparison with women with major depression and women without psychiatric disorder. *Psychological Medicine, 30,* 53–60.

Weissman, M. M., & Paykel, E. S. (1974). *The depressed woman: A study of social relationships.* Chicago: University of Chicago Press.

■ PART II ■
EPIDEMIOLOGY AND COURSE

CHAPTER 5

Epidemiology of Eating Disorders in Children and Adolescents

Mark L. Norris
Susan J. Bondy
Leora Pinhas

The documentation of the incidence and prevalence of eating disorders is vital for health care workers, policymakers, educators, and administrators. It assists in the understanding of these illnesses both as they currently appear and how they may evolve in the future. Valid and reliable data allow for better decisions related to the necessities of prevention programs, screening interventions, and treatment options. Good epidemiological data can result in improved advocacy as well as planning for resource allocation and treatment by policymakers and health care providers (Garfinkel, 2002).

The Meaning of Incidence and Prevalence in Eating Disorders

Incidence and prevalence statistics are related measures that describe important aspects of the burden of disease in a given population (Last & International Epidemiological Association, 2001; Rothman, Greenland, & Lash, 2008). The incidence of disease is typically defined as the number of new cases in a population over a specified time interval, often 1 year (Last & International Epidemiological Association, 2001; Rothman et al., 2008). "Disease prevalence" refers to the total number of people with the disease, which includes new, continuing, and recurring events in the population. Prevalence estimates may describe one moment in time, point prevalence, or an annual rate. High prevalence of disease may be driven either by a high incidence of new cases or by a long duration of the disorder (Last & International Epidemiological Association, 2001; Rothman et al., 2008). Both rates may variously be reported as a percentage or per 10,000 or 100,000 population. Both incidence and prevalence may also be estimated in terms of the lifetime rate or risk (Last & International Epidemiological Association, 2001; Rothman et al., 2008).

It is important to understand the challenges associated with epidemiological research in eating disorders to appreciate why such seemingly simple questions are difficult to answer. This chapter summarizes and presents, where possible, the existing available epidemiological literature for children and adolescents. However, given the paucity of data available and the gaps that remain, studies that have included young adult data are also cited in an effort to be as informative as possible.

Overview of the Limitations in the Epidemiological Data on Eating Disorders

The number of studies in eating disorders has increased greatly in the last 30 years. However, the epidemiology of eating disorders remains underdeveloped. This is especially true in the epidemiology of child and adolescent eating disorders, in which studies are fewer in number and often limited in scope. This is regardless of the fact that the same literature reports the age of onset to be between 10 and 20 years for the vast majority of subjects (Preti et al., 2009).

Published epidemiological studies of eating disorders typically draw upon and report data from several types of health-related data sources: cross-sectional or longitudinal disease-specific case registries, cross-sectional mental health surveys, and ongoing registries of defined populations, including in this population, school systems and one registry of twin births (Milos, Spindler, Buddeberg, & Crameri, 2003). All of these methods have relative strengths and weaknesses. However, none of them have been used consistently across various populations in different countries across time, thus making comparisons difficult. The paucity of studies that have been published, often at sporadic intervals, makes it very difficult to assess differences in incidence or prevalence rates in different countries/populations or the stability or change in rates over time.

A common tool to estimate the incidence and prevalence of a variety of mental disorders has been the use of large cross-sectional surveys in the community, which interview participants for specific diagnoses. In studying rare disorders, these studies require very large samples to generate precise estimates of prevalence or incidence. Although more cost-effective methods have been developed—including the use of self-report measures rather than interviews to identify symptoms or diagnoses—when possible, the well-established two-stage approach to case detection (Hoek & van Hoeken, 2003) is preferred. In the first stage, large representative samples of respondents are screened for the presence of eating disorder symptoms using validated self-report questionnaires. These measures can often identify people potentially "at risk" for an eating disorder. Each individual identified as being at risk then undergoes a diagnostic interview, to exclude false-positive cases (Hoek, 2006; Hoek & van Hoeken, 2003; Williams, Tarnopolsky, & Hand, 1980). Studies that apply diagnostic case definitions can be expected to produce somewhat lower overall prevalence or incidence estimates relative to studies that rely on self-administered measures, which tend to be less specific and may overestimate the proportion of the population with the disorder (Fairburn & Beglin, 1990).

Studies based on representative population samples (e.g., surveys and population registries) tend to yield more valid estimates of rates in the population, relative to mechanisms such as clinical case series. However, because the ability of a study to estimate incidence and prevalence is dependent on the number of cases detected, many population-based mental health surveys have either not attempted to estimate the occurrence of eating disorders or have been unable to report estimates with satisfactory margins of error.

Some population-based studies fail to identify any prevalent adolescent cases of either anorexia nervosa (AN) or bulimia nervosa (BN) (Colton, Olmsted, & Rodin, 2007; de Azevedo & Ferreira, 1992; Isomaa, Isomaa, Marttunen, Kaltiala-Heino, & Björkqvist, 2009; Sancho, Arija, Asorey, & Canals, 2007). Because diagnoses of eating disorders are relatively infrequent, even small variations in the number of detected cases have the potential to strongly influence calculations of incidence, prevalence, and mortality rates (Fombonne, 1995; Pagsberg & Wang, 1994). As a result, much of the data in this field have come from clinical case registries instead.

In contrast to community surveys, eating disorder case series and registries of diagnosed eating disorder cases rely on clinical presentation and detection to identify cases in the population. These designs have distinct challenges with respect to error and bias in the measures used to define cases. There are also important potential sources of selection bias related to the probability that an individual in the population with the disorder will be properly identified as a case. The effects of secrecy and shame related to having an eating disorder can result in avoidance of help seeking and therefore lead to an underestimate of rates of disease when a clinical cohort is utilized for epidemiological study. In fact, the adult literature suggests that the proportion of subjects with a lifetime diagnosis of eating disorder who request general medical treatment for emotional problems is quite low: 33–48% among those with BN, 35–50% among those with AN, less than 30% among those with any other eating disorder (Keski-Rahkonen et al., 2007, 2009; Preti et al., 2009). Differences and changes in availability of care across regions and over time can adversely affect the comparability of estimates and result in high variability of estimates across data sources.

Clinical case detection relies on validated and standardized diagnostic criteria, but inconsistencies may arise across evaluators or settings and may not be valid across all settings and case populations. The incomplete understanding of the role of transcultural reliability, and the limitations of the current standardized diagnostic criteria (Hoek, 2006; Lahortiga-Ramos et al., 2005; Nicholls, Chater, & Lask, 2000), can also be problematic.

Studies relying on longitudinal population-based registries are designed to follow and evaluate a representative population over the time course in which an eating disorder occurs. An example of a population-based registry is a birth cohort of twins (Keski-Rahkonen et al., 2007, 2009) who undergo assessment every 2 years. Others are based on school-age populations, with planned follow-up contacts. These designs are believed to provide greater representativeness, as case identification is less influenced by health services use patterns and impediments to access of care. Relative to cross-sectional surveys, which may ask about symptoms over an entire lifetime, population-based registry studies may suffer less from recall error and bias as well. General population registries are valuable designs, but they exist in only some locations, tend to be limited in geographical area of coverage, and often describe study populations of modest size either because they are designed to describe a population of finite size (e.g., a localized school system or twins) or because of the high costs associated with active tracking of individuals over time.

Regardless of the sampling method, measurement error and bias in diagnostic practices are important considerations in prevalence and incidence studies. Beyond the possibility of errors introduced by the evaluator, eating disorders present inherent problems in the development and uniform application of valid case definitions. Challenges related to case definition, used for case ascertainment, include the gradual onset of illness, the chronic nature of eating disorders, and the fluidity of symptom profiles (subjects can exhibit tremendous heterogeneity, and symptom expression can evolve over a period of time within one individual). As a result, many subjects at some point in their course of illness fall under the umbrella of eating disorder not otherwise specified (EDNOS), which is the most common eating disorder diagnosis reported in specialized treatment settings (Peebles, Wilson, & Lock, 2006). In an attempt to keep our review as "clean" as possible, we have purposefully limited data on EDNOS to those defined by the DSM (American Psychiatric Association, 2000) and, for the most part, omitted studies or portions therein that report on "partial" AN or BN, as these cases are not easily placed in recognizable or necessarily valid diagnostic categories.

Despite these methodological and sampling difficulties, certain patterns have emerged over time and seem to recur in multiple studies. Incidence and prevalence rates of BN typically outnumber those seen in AN in adults and adolescents, but not necessarily in children, and rates of eating disorders tend to be highest in female adolescents ages 14–16 years (Joergensen, 1992; Lucas, Beard, O'Fallon, & Kurland, 1991; Nielsen, 1990).

Early-Onset Eating Disorders

Although several major epidemiological reviews of eating disorders have been published in peer-reviewed journals, not one review has focused solely on eating pathology, diagnosis, and epidemiology in children and adolescents (Fairburn & Beglin, 1990; Fombonne, 1995; Hoek, 2006; Hoek & van Hoeken, 2003; Hsu, 1996; Szmukler, 1985). There are a number of factors that have likely plagued the epidemiological study of early-onset eating disorders (EOED). First, such diagnoses are extremely uncommon in children. For example, data from a clinical registry database published in 1996 reported an incidence of AN in children ages 0–9 years of 0.3 per 100,000 (Turnbull, Ward, Treasure, Jick, & Derby, 1996). Other studies, regardless of methodology, have found few, if any, cases in children (Currin, Schmidt, Treasure, & Jick, 2005; Lucas et al., 1991; Pagsberg & Wang, 1994; van Son, van Hoeken, Bartelds, van Furth, & Hoek, 2006b). However, a recent prospective study in Australia documented an incidence of 1.4 per 100,000 children ages 5–13 years. These were children hospitalized for renourishment and/or treatment related to eating disorders (Madden, Morris, Zurynski, Kohn, & Elliot, 2009). This suggests the need for further prospective studies in the area and defined services to meet these children's needs. Unfortunately, as a result of the low overall rates of diagnosis, many studies tend to focus on adolescents and often exclude children below the age of 13 altogether.

From a diagnostic standpoint, it has become obvious in recent years that, even within child and adolescent cohorts, the clinical features of presentation among youth can differ significantly, depending on age (Bravender et al., 2007, 2010; Nicholls & Bryant-Waugh, 2009; Peebles et al., 2006). Although the study by Madden and colleagues (2009) showed clearly that a significant number of children with restrictive EOEDs had similar psychological symptoms as compared with adults with AN, it also highlighted the significant minority of patients that could not be easily classified because of the challenges associated with current classification systems in this population and the potential for misdiagnosis or missed diagnoses (Madden et al., 2009). A study by Nicholls and colleagues in 2000 found that adult criteria were of little value in the classification of the eating difficulties of children, but that Great Ormond Street criteria, which were developed specifically for this cohort, had greater reliability. It is unclear as to what extent clinical programs that are often used to create registry-based epidemiology data utilize current diagnostic criteria to assess young children and how this affects eating disorder identification. A recent article published by an international workgroup of experts in child and adolescent eating disorders recommended that revisions to DSM-IV-R should incorporate changes that allow greater sensitivity to the expression of the spectrum of disordered eating in children and adolescents (Bravender et al., 2010).

Anorexia Nervosa

Incidence

Incidence rates of AN vary, depending on the methods used and population studied, making an overall estimate of incidence in the adolescent age group difficult. A comprehensive review completed by Hoek and van Hoeken in 2003 reported rates ranging from 0.10 per 100,000 persons per year to 12.0 per 100,000 across all ages, with the two studies cited at the extremes of this range coming from different continents using clinical registries completed a half-century apart (Lucas, Crowson, O'Fallon, & Melton, 1999; Theander, 1970). Females are diagnosed more often than males, and those of ages 15–19 years seem to be at greatest risk (Hoek & van Hoeken, 2003; Lucas et al., 1999; Theander, 1970). As noted in Table 5.1, studies reported rates over a variety of age ranges (0–9 years, 10–14 years, 10–19 years, 10–24 years, 12–18 years, 15–19 years, 15–24 years) and calculated rates using data from clinical registries, cross-sectional population surveys, and longitudinal cohort studies, in various settings, including primary care clinics, hospital admissions, community samples, or prospective cohorts of at-risk populations. Even across similar ages, there is variability. Studies by Neilsen, Keski-Rahkonen, and Lucas each provided incidence determinations for youth 15–19 years old, ranging from a low of 9.92/100,000 (case registry of hospital admissions) to 69.4 per 100,000 (registry of all clinical case records) to a high of 270 per 100,000 (longitudinal representative population study with a twin birth cohort) (Keski-Rahkonen et al., 2007). Longitudinal representative population-based studies theoretically provide the most valid results (Keski-Rahkonen et al., 2007; Lucas et al., 1991; Nielsen, 1990). Interestingly, longitudinal representative population-based studies also provide some insight into how frequently patients with AN seek medical care. Keski-Rahkonen and colleagues (2007) found that only half of the subjects with AN sought treatment for their eating disorders.

One of the earliest studies with one of the longest follow-up periods was that completed by Lucas and colleagues (1991). The study employed a case registry that used an extensive case-finding methodology to identify rates of AN in a community where treatment was provided by one regional health care institution. It was also one of the first to clearly delineate and report incidence rates among multiple-age groups and between the sexes. The authors concluded that AN was the third most common chronic illness in adolescent females (Lucas et al., 1991). The study reported incidence rates of 25.7 per 100,000 for adolescents ages 10–14 years, and 69.4 per 100,000 in female teenagers ages 15–19 years during the years 1935–1984, but reported no cases in those under 10 years of age. A later follow-up inquiry, extending the time frame of the study to 1989, indicated an increased incidence of AN in adolescent females ages 15–19 years, to 73.9 cases per 100,000 (Lucas et al., 1999). An epidemiological study of eating disorders in primary care settings in the United Kingdom, similarly utilizing a case registry, reported incidence

TABLE 5.1. Incidence Rates of AN in Adolescents

Study authors	Country	Source	Ages	Incidence/100,000 (SD)		
				Females	Males	Total
Nielsen (1990)	Denmark	Case register admissions	10–14 15–19	1973–1987: 4.16 1973–1987: 9.92	1973–1987: 0.85	
Turnbull et al. (1996)	UK	Case register	0–9 10–19	1993: 0.7 (0–1.9) 1993: 34.1 (24.5–43.6)	1993: 0 1993: 1.3 (0–3.2)	1993: 0.3 (0–0.9) 1993: 17.5 (12.7–22.3)
Currin et al. (2005)	UK	Case register	0–9 10–19	1998–1993: 0 1998–1993: 34.6 (22–47.1)	1998–1993: 0 1998–1993: 2.3 (0–5.4)	1998–1993: 0 1998–1993: 18 (11.7–24.4)
van Son et al. (2006a)	Netherlands	Case register	5–9 10–14 15–19	1985–1989: 0 1995–1999: 4.5 1985–1989: 8.6 1995–1999: 18.4 1985–1989: 56.4 1995–1999: 109.2		
Moller-Madsen (1996)	Denmark	Case register	15–24	1970: 3.37 1989: 8.97		1970: 1.64 1989: 4.62
Joergensen (1992)	Denmark	Case register	10–14 15–19	1977–1986: 9.2 1977–1986: 11.9		
Pagsberg & Wang (1994)	Denmark	Case register, records	10–24	1970–1984: 11.9 1985–1989: 57.1		
Lucas et al. (1991)	US	Case records	0–9 10–14 15–19	1935–1984: 0 1935–1984: 25.7 1935–1984: 69.4	1935–1984: 0 1935–1984: 3.7 1935–1984: 7.3	1935–1984: 0 1935–1984: 14.6 1935–1984: 43.5
Hoek et al. (2005)	Netherlands	Case records	15–24	1995–1998: 17.5		
Mitrany et al. (1995)	Israel	Case records	12–18	1989–1993: 29		

(cont.)

TABLE 5.1. *(cont.)*

Study authors	Country	Source	Ages	Incidence/100,000 (*SD*)		
				Females	Males	Total
Milos et al. (2003)	Switzerland	Case records	12–25	1956–1958: 3.99 1993–1995: 19.72		
Keski-Rahkonen et al. (2007)	Finland	Cohort twin study	15–19	1990–1998: 270 (180–360)		
Raevuori et al. (2009)	Finland	Cohort twin study	10–24		1997–2006: 15.7 (6.6–37.8)	
Lahortiga-Ramos et al. (2005)	Spain	Cohort study	13–22	Year not specified: 200		Year not specified: 3,200

rates of 0.7 per 100,000 female children ages 0–9 years and 34.1 per 100,000 in females ages 10–19 years. In both studies, only patients who sought medical treatment could be counted, thus underestimating the true incidence in the community (Keski-Rahkonen et al., 2007; Preti et al., 2009).

In addition to the longitudinal representative population study published by Keski-Rahoken and colleagues (2007), which reported an incidence rate of 270 per 100,000 person-years in females ages 15–19 years, two other recent European studies offer useful information. An incidence study of Spanish adolescents ages 13–22 years used the preferred two-step methodological sampling in a longitudinal representative population-based inquiry and documented an incidence rate of 200 new cases/100,000/year for AN in females (Lahortiga-Ramos et al., 2005). In this study, there were no significant differences in the incidence values across age groups. A recent case registry study from the Netherlands (van Son, van Hoeken, Bartelds, van Furth, & Hoek, 2006a), however, described a significant increase (94%) in the incidence rate among 15- to 19-year-old females in the years 1995–1999 of 109.2 per 100,000 female-years as compared with 56.4 per 100,000 female-years in 1985–1989. The rates reported here are about half of those reported in the population-based longitudinal studies; this is in keeping with the data reporting that only about half of the patients with AN come to clinical attention (Keski-Rahkonen et al., 2007). This study also reported that the age-specific incidence was highest in the 15- to 19-year-age group across both study points (van Son et al., 2006a).

The only longitudinal representative population cohort study to report on males was based on a twin birth cohort in Finland and reported an incidence rate in males ages 10–22 years of 15.7/100,000 person-years (Raevuori et al., 2009). Clinical registries report incidence rates ranging from 0.85/100, 000 person-years in males ages 10–14 years, between 1973 and 1987 in Denmark (Nielsen, 1990), to 3.7/100,000 person-years in males ages 10–14 years and 7.3/100,000 person-years in males ages 15–19 years in Rochester, Minnesota, between 1935 and 1984 (Lucas et al., 1991), to 2.3/100,000 in males ages 10–19 years in the United Kingdom in 2000 (Currin et al., 2005). Few studies have ever reported separately on children under 10 years of age. In AN, based on only one clinical case registry from the United Kingdom, the reported incidence in females under 10 years of age has been reported as 0.4/100,000 person-years (Lucas et al., 1991; Turnbull et al., 1996) and among males under 10 years of age as 0.3/100 000 person-years (Turnbull et al., 1996).

Prevalence

In general, regardless of the methodology, prevalence rates of AN in adolescents tend to be lower than those for BN or EDNOS. Once again, longitudinal representative population-based studies employing a two-step methodology provide the most valid data available, but results vary depending on the country and the age range studied. Marchi and Cohen (1990) followed a representative American population-based sample of children ages 1–10 years for 10 years and reported AN prevalence rates in children 9–18 years of age to be 1.7% for females. Similarly, a 3-year study in Finnish adolescent females with a somewhat older mean age of 15.4 years documented a point prevalence of 0.7%, with a lifetime prevalence of 1.8–2.6%. In contrast, a Spanish study of 13-year-old females, completed over a 2-year period, documented a point prevalence of only 0.17% (Rodriguez-Cano, Beato-Fernandez, & Belmonte-Llario, 2005). Isomaa and colleagues (2009), reported prevalence rates in adolescent Finnish females, ages 15 years at the beginning of the study, in their two-step, 3-year follow-up study, of 1.8%. Longitudinal studies have provided additional estimations of prevalence right into the third decade of life. Stice, Marti, Shaw, and Jaconis (2009) completed diagnostic interviews of a culturally diverse community sample of 496 adolescent females over an 8-year period, with a mean start age of 13 years, and documented lifetime prevalence by the age of 20 years to be 0.6%.

Cross-sectional representative population-based surveys report prevalence rates for AN ranging from 0.7% in Norwegian females ages 14–15 years (Kjelsas, Bjornstrom, & Götestam, 2004), to 0.9% for females ages 15–19 years in Iran (Nobakht & Dezhkam, 2000). Clinical case registry studies have also demonstrated similar variability in lifetime prevalence rates of AN across varying time frames (with respect to calendar year and the ages of the populations studied) and varying clinical settings. Studies of inpatients and outpatients in Rochester, Minnesota (Lucas et al., 1991) produced prevalence rates of 480/100,000 person-years (0.48%) for females ages 15–19 years in 1985. In Denmark, between 1977 and 1986, prevalence ranged from 70/100,000 person-years in females ages 10–14 years (0.07%) to 120/100,000 person-years (0.12%) in females ages 15–19 years (Joergensen, 1992).

There is little information on the prevalence of AN in adolescent males or in children. Marchi and Cohen (1990) reported the AN prevalence rate of 0.3% for males ages 9–18 years. There were only two studies identified that reported prevalence rates for adolescent males separately. Using a sample of 953 Norwegian males ages 14–15 years who completed a self-report questionnaire, Kjelsas and colleagues (2004) provided a period prevalence rate of 0.2%. In a cross-sectional two-step study of Swedish grade 8 students, Rastam and colleagues found somewhat lower rates (0.09%) in the reported lifetime prevalence rates in adolescents 15 years of age. Although we were unable to identify any study that focused on prevalence rates in children under the age of 12 years, Kuboki and colleagues reported a rate of 17.5/100,000 person years in a cohort of inpatient and outpatient females under 14 years of age (Kuboki, Nomura, Ide, Suematsu, & Araki, 1996).

Bulimia Nervosa

Incidence

BN is characterized by long-standing urges and symptoms and gradual recovery and is most common in older adolescents and young adults (Anderluh, Tchanturia, Rabe-Hesketh, Collier, & Treasure, 2009; Keski-Rahkonen et al., 2009). In contrast, binge–purge behavior in those ages 12 years and younger appears to be extremely uncommon. In general, there are few overall studies available that have examined incidence rates of BN in adolescents and next to no studies with a focus on BN in children less than 12 years of age. Adolescent studies that have reported incidence rates for BN are summarized and presented in Table 5.2.

TABLE 5.2. Prevalence Rates of AN in Adolescents

Study authors	Country	Source	Ages	Prevalence	
				Females	Males
Nielsen (1990)	Denmark	Case register admissions	10–14 15–19	1973–1987: 14.5 1973–1987: 34.7	
Pelaez Fernandez et al. (2007)	Spain	Cohort	12–21	2001–2002: 0.33	2001–2002: 0
Rastam, Gillberg, & Garton (1989)	Sweden	Cohort	14–15	1985: 0.7	1985: 0.09
Tseng et al. (2007)	Taiwan	Cohort	15.9 (mean)	2003: 0.1	
de Azevedo & Ferreira (1992)	Portugal	Cohort	15–17	1987: 0	1987: 0
Pagsberg & Wang (1994)	Denmark	Case register, records	10–24	1989: 222	
Lucas et al. (1991)	US	Case records	15–19	1930–1980: 480.3	
Machado, Machado, Gonçalves, & Hoek (2007)	Portugal	Cohort	12–23	Year not specified: 0.39	
Ackard, Fulkerson, & Neumark-Sztainer (2007)	US	Cohort: self-report survey only	14.9 (mean)	1998–1999: 0.04	0
Fichter, Quadflieg, & Gnutzmann (1998)	Greece	Cohort	12–21	1998: 0.59	1998: 0
Steinhausen (1997)	Switzerland	Cohort study	14–17	1994–95: 0.7	1994–95: 0
Kjelsas et al. (2004)	Norway	Cohort study	14–15	1991: 0.6%	1991: 0.2%
Isomaa et al. (2009)	Finland	Cohort study	15	2004: lifetime prevalence: 1.8% point prevalence: 0.7%	0%

Like those found in studies of AN, incidence rates identified for BN vary tremendously by both age and gender. Recent data suggest that only about one-third of subjects with BN report for treatment (Keski-Rahkonen et al., 2009), highlighting the fact that clinical registries likely underestimate the incidence of BN. Therefore it is not surprising that the longitudinal representative population-based cohort studies (Keski-Rahkonen et al., 2009; Lahortiga-Ramos et al., 2005) report incidence rates for BN that are far higher than those of more clinically based studies. Unfortunately, regardless of methodology, studies have had limited ability to report rates for specific age ranges. Studies that provide adolescent-specific data are cited in Table 5.3. The longitudinal representative population-based studies report the incidence rate of BN in females in Finland ages 16–20 years as 300/100,000 person-years and as 150/100,000 person-years for the broader age range of 10–24 years (Keski-Rahkonen et al., 2009). Similarly, in Spain the incidence of BN in females ages 12–22 years was reported as 200/100,000 person-years (Lahortiga-Ramos et al., 2005).

TABLE 5.3. Incidence Rates of BN in Adolescents

Study authors	Country	Source	Ages	Incidence (95% CI)		
				Females	Males	Total
Turnbull et al. (1996)	UK	Case register	0–9 10–19	1993: 0 1993: 41 (30.6–51.5)	1993: 0 1993: 0.7 (0–2)	1993: 0 1993: 20.5 (15.3–25.7)
Pagsberg & Wang (1994)	Denmark	Case register, records	10–24	1970–1984: 5.3 1985–1989: 17.6		
Joergensen (1992)	Denmark	Case register	10–14 15–19	1977–1986: 3.3 1977–1986: 3		
van Son et al. (2006a)	Netherlands	Case register	10–14 15–19	1985–1989: 4.3 (0.1–24) 1995–1999: 0 1985–1989: 29.8(13.7–56.7) 1995–1999: 41(18.7–77.8)		
Currin et al. (2005)	UK	Case register	0–9 10–19	2000: 0 2000: 35.8 (23–48.6)	2000: 0 2000: 3.4 (0–7.3)	2000: 19.2 (12.6–25.7)
Soundy et al. (1995)	US	Case register, records	0–9 10–14 15–19	1980–1990: 0 1980–1990: 13 1980–1990: 125.1	1980–1990: 0 1980–1990: 0 1980–1990: 0	1980–1990: 0 1980–1990: 6.3 1980–1990: 66.6
Lahortiga-Ramos et al. (2005)	Spain	Cohort study	13–22	Year not specified: 200		
Keski-Rahkonen et al. (2009)	Finland	Cohort study	15–19	1990–1998: 210		

In Pagsberg and Wang's (1994) study using a Danish case registry, the average annual incidence rates were relatively constant from 1970 to 1984 but increased fourfold during the last 4 years of the study (1985–1989). The highest incidence rate was recorded in the final year of the study, leaving the possibility of further increases had data collection continued. Turnbull and colleagues' (1996) clinical registry study also demonstrated a rise in incidence rates calculated in primary care settings in the early 1990s in all females ages 10–39 years. The estimated highest overall incidence rates were 30.5 per 100,000 in females ages 20–39 years, followed by a rate of 24.2 per 100,000 in females ages 10–19 years. In contrast, van Son's clinical registry study reported that rates remained stable between the calendar years of 1985–1989 and 1995–1999 (van Son et al., 2006a). Rising rates in a clinical registry may reflect changes in incidence and prevalence, but they may also simply reflect increased availability of treatment interventions or improved screening and identification of patients rather than true changes in rates.

The peak age of incidence of BN remains unclear. Studies are limited in the manner in which data are presented (i.e., different age groups represented), although the majority of studies report peak ages between 16 and 20 years. For example, a review of case records completed over a 5-year period (1989–1993) in Israel found the median age of patients with BN to be 16 years (Mitrany, Lubin, Chetrit, & Modan, 1995). Keski-Rahkonen and colleagues (2009), using data collected from a longitudinal representative population-based cohort study, reported that the incidence of BN peaked between 16 and 20 years. Other studies, including the case registry data from the Rochester Epidemiology Project (Soundy, Lucas, Suman, & Melton, 1995), reported 35% of incident cases of BN also fell within the 15- to 19-year age group. Finally, Stice and colleagues' (2009) study of a community sample of adolescents revealed the peak age of onset for BN to be between 17 and 18 years. In contrast, Turnbull and colleagues' (1996) clinical registry study, reported on cases identified in the early 1990s, produced its highest incidence rates outside the adolescent age period. It should be noted, however, that this study reported cohorts from 0 to 9

TABLE 5.4. Prevalence Rates of BN in Adolescents

Study authors	Country	Source	Ages	Prevalence	
				Females	Males
Tseng et al. (2007)	Taiwan	Cohort	15.9 (mean)	2003: 1.0	
Pelaez Fernandez et al. (2007)	Spain	Cohort	12–21	2001–2002: 2.29	2001–2002: 0.16
Ackard et al. (2007)	US	Cohort: self-report survey only	14.9 (mean)	1998–1999: 0.3	1998–1999: 0.2
Fichter et al. (1998)	Greece	Cohort	12–21	1998: 1.18	1998: 0.68
Steinhausen (1997)	Switzerland	Cohort	14–17	1994–1995: 0.5	1994–1995: 0
Machado et al. (2007)	Portugal	Cohort	12–23	Year not specified: 0.3	
de Azevedo & Ferreira (1992)	Portugal	Cohort	15–17	1987: 0.16	1987: 0

years (incidence 0), 10 to 19 years (incidence 41/100,000), 20 to 39 years (56.7/100,000), and 40+ years (3.2/100,000). Van Son and colleagues (2006a) also documented highest incidence rates among 25- to 29-year-old subjects to occur during the first time period of their registry study (1985–1989). However, they noted a downward shift in age in the years 1995–1999, in which the highest rates were found in females ages 15–19 years and 20–24 years.

There are several studies that document the incidence of BN in males. From clinical registry data in the United Kingdom in 2000, the incident rate was reported as 3.4/100,000 in males ages 10–19 years (Currin et al., 2005). In Rochester, Minnesota, between 1980 and 1990, it was 6.3/100,000 in males ages 10–14 years and 66.6/100,000 in males ages 15–19 years (Soundy et al., 1995). Given the wide range of rates and the small number of studies, it is hard to draw any conclusions. Only three studies included children less than 10 years of age. These studies relied on case registries and were retrospective in nature. There were no identified cases of BN in these studies. Madden's study of patients with early-onset eating disorders in Australia found that 11% of the total sample studied, ages 5–13 years, engaged in self-induced vomiting, although no patient met the full criteria for BN. The study was limited methodologically, as it was focused on restricting eating disorders and was not designed to identify BN (Madden et al., 2009).

Prevalence

Despite the fact that prevalence rates of BN tend to be higher than those of AN in adolescents in the majority of epidemiological studies, there are fewer studies targeting BN. This is especially true for young adolescents. Point prevalence rates as low as 0.14% have been documented in a young population-based longitudinal cohort of Spanish children with a mean age of 11.4 years (Pelaez Fernandez, Labrador, & Raich, 2007). Lifetime prevalences have been documented to be as high as 3.2% for adolescent females ages 15–18 years in a case registry-based study in Iran (Nobakht & Dezhkam, 2000).

The majority of studies that have reported data for AN also provide estimates on rates of BN. Studies focusing on young adolescents are less conclusive and have at times found BN to be less prevalent than AN. The population-based longitudinal cohort study published by Isomaa and colleagues (2009) found that the point prevalence for BN (0.4%) was lower than that observed for AN (0.7%), although 3-year prevalence rates were equal at 0.9% among Finnish adolescents with a mean start age of 15.4 years. This is not always the case, however. A Spanish two-step study, of 2 years' duration, involving subjects with a mean starting age of 13 years found a higher point prevalence for BN (1.38%) as compared with AN (0.17%) (Rodriguez-Cano et al., 2005).

Again, longitudinal population-based cohort studies that follow subjects through adolescence tend also to report higher lifetime prevalence rates of BN as compared with AN. An 8-year longitudinal study of an American community sample of adolescent females reported a lifetime prevalence for BN, by the age of 20 years, of 1.6% (as compared with 0.6% for AN), and a 10-year longitudinal study reported rates for females ages 9–18 years of 2.8% (Marchi & Cohen, 1990).

Representative cross-sectional population surveys reported a lifetime prevalence rate of BN in females, ranging from 1.2% in Norwegians ages 14–15 years (Kjelsas et al., 2004) to 3.2% for older adolescents, ages 15–18 years, in Iran (Nobakht & Dezhkam, 2000). Case registry-based data from 1977 to 1986, reported prevalence rates of BN in females in Denmark as 70/100,000 in females ages 15–19 years and 40/100,000 in females ages 10–14 years (Nicholls et al., 2000), and that the prevalence rate, among subjects ages 10–24 years, went from 25 to 89/100,000 between 1970 and 1989 (Pagsberg & Wang, 1994).

As is the case for most of the literature pertaining to eating disorders, data on males or children with BN are extremely sparse. There are three longitudinal population-based cohorts that do report on males. Sancho and colleagues' (2007) study of Spanish youth, with a mean age of 11.4 years, found higher rates of BN in males as compared with females, with a point prevalence of BN of 0.14% in females and 0.3% in males. An American study reported prevalence rates of 0.3% in males among subjects between 9 and 18 years of age at the end of 10-year follow up, (Marchi & Cohen, 1990). A second American study analyzed National Health and Nutrition Examination Survey data over a 4-year period. This study focused on children between the ages of 8 and 15 years and reported a 12-month prevalence of 0.1% of BN for both males and females. Finally, there is one case registry study of Iranian youth that documented prevalence rates of 0.4% in 14- to 15-year-old males (Nobakht & Dezhkam, 2000).

Eating Disorder Not Otherwise Specified

Incidence

There are very few studies reporting on EDNOS. The rate of EDNOS has been reported in two representative population-based registries. In Spain the incidence rate in females between the ages of 12 and 22 years was 2,800/100,000 person-years (Lahortiga-Ramos et al., 2005). This is similar to a study from Finland reporting on the incidence of all eating disorders, in which the vast majority of cases identified were EDNOS. This study reported an incidence rate of 1641/100,000 person-years in females ages 15–18 years (Isomaa et al., 2009). There have been no well-designed population-based studies that have reported on EDNOS in adolescent males nor any eating disorders in children, although American survey data are anticipated within the next few years that may present such estimates for adolescents (Kessler, 2000; Kessler et al., 2009).

Prevalence

Despite the fact that the diagnosis of EDNOS diagnosis is often the most prevalent among the eating disorders, as a category, it is often omitted in large epidemiological surveys of eating disorders. This may be related to the overwhelming variability and heterogeneity present within the category and the challenges that it creates for researchers. As a result, there is more variance in reported rates of EDNOS among studies than that witnessed for AN or BN, although the majority of the studies are of representative population-based cohorts with longitudinal follow-up. In Spain in a two-step, 2-year representative cohort study in which the starting age of the subjects was 13 years, the point prevalence of EDNOS in females was 4.86% and in males it was 0.6% (Rodriguez-Cano et al., 2005). The one cross-sectional representative population survey reported rates of 14.6% for females and 5% for males ages 14–15 years (Kjelsas et al., 2004). The lifetime rates of EDNOS have varied. In an American study, with a 10-year follow-up, the rate was reported to be 1.84% in females between the ages of 9 and 18 years. Yet in a second

8-year longitudinal study of an American community sample of adolescent females, 12% of the subjects experienced some form of EDNOS (defined as subthreshold AN, subthreshold BN, purging disorder, or binge-eating disorder [BED]) by the age of 20 years (Marchi & Cohen, 1990; Stice et al., 2009). In a Spanish cohort of children between the ages of 9.4 and 13.5 years, the point prevalence of EDNOS was 1.84–3.23% in males and 3.63–5.67% in females (Sancho et al., 2007).

Eating Disorders in Medically Ill Persons

Adolescents with chronic medical conditions have been reported to have higher rates of body dissatisfaction and to engage in more high-risk weight loss practices. This has been observed across a variety of conditions, regardless of whether the medical condition is nutrition related (such as diabetes) (Neumark-Sztainer, Story, Resnick, Garwick, & Blum, 1995). Although there is little data on eating disorders in specific medical conditions, there is one study reporting on adolescents with chronic medical conditions between the ages of 16 and 20 years that found that youth with chronic illness are at increased risk of developing an eating disorder (Suris, Michaud, Akre, & Sawyer, 2008). There has been some attention focused on cystic fibrosis, with most of the studies concluding that patients are not at increased risk (Duff, Wolfe, Dickson, Conway, & Brownlee, 2003; Raymond et al., 2000; Shearer & Bryon, 2004), and idiopathic scoliosis, in which the findings suggest higher prevalence rates of eating disorders. However, only type I diabetes has been studied in any depth.

In a clinical case series of 101 female subjects with type I diabetes ages 9–13 years, Colton, Olmstead, Daneman, Rydall, and Rodin (2004) reported that those who had type I diabetes had higher point prevalence rates of disordered eating, but not higher rates of eating disorders than those without diabetes. This was also the finding in a pediatric sample of 97 cases (Powers, Malone, Coovert, & Schulman, 1990) and in a study of 193 subjects between the ages of 8 and 18 years (Iafusco et al., 2004). In contrast, a recent study of 192 females ages 11–19 years found that eating disorders were significantly more common in the patients with diabetes than in the control group, with 27.5% of the group classified as having BN or BED (Smith, Latchford, Hall, & Dickson, 2008). The largest and therefore better-powered study, with 3,000 adults, found that diabetes was associated with an increased likelihood of eating disorders with an odds ratio of 2.3 after adjusting for differences in demographic characteristics and comorbid mental disorders. This effect was specific to diabetes and eating disorders were the only mental health disorders associated with a significantly increased risk of diabetes (Goodwin, Hoven, & Spitzer, 2003).

Although there are conflicting reports that eating disorder rates are more common in patients with diabetes, when the two disorders co-occur mortality is significantly elevated. In a 10-year follow-up of 510 patients with diabetes and 658 patients with AN, the mortality rate for type I diabetes was 2.2/1,000; for AN, it was 7.3/1,000; and for concurrent cases it was 34.6/1,000. The standardized mortality ratio for type I diabetes was 4.06; for AN, it was 8.86; and for concurrent cases it was 14.5 (Nielsen, Emborg, & Molbak, 2002).

The data on the association of eating disorders and idiopathic scoliosis is less well studied. However, a recent study of 207 females between the ages of 12 and 19 years who had been in treatment for a minimum of 3 years reported statistically significantly higher point prevalence rates of AN, BN, and EDNOS in patients with idiopathic scoliosis. The prevalence rate of AN was 9.2%; of BN, 7.7 %; and of EDNOS, 5.3% (Alborghetti, Scimeca, Costanzo, & Boca, 2008). Earlier studies reported on differences in weight, although not specifically reporting on eating disorders. A clinic registry study of 44 patients between the ages of 13 and 19 years produced a statistically significant increased prevalence of low weight in patients with idiopathic scoliosis, in which 25% of patients had weights or body mass indexes (BMIs) that would meet the weight criterion for AN (Smith, Latchford, Hall, Millner, & Dickson, 2002; Smith et al., 2008).

The Utilization of Health Services and Hospitalizations

The examination of health service utilization and hospitalizations can aid in increasing the appreciation of the effect that the prevalence of eating disorders has on both the individual and his or her community. A handful of American studies reporting hospitalizations and health services utilization and costs have been published in the last 10 years. Health services studies in adults report that the use of health services among those with an eating disorder was significantly elevated in all service sectors as compared with matched controls without eating disorders. Contrary to expectations, health care utilization was found to be similarly high across the spectrum of eating disorders (Striegel-Moore et al., 2008) and non-eating-disorder psychiatric conditions (Striegel-Moore, 2005).

The Cost of Eating Disorders

European and American data provide information on the actual cost of eating disorders. A cost-of-illness analysis from Germany reports the annual cost per patient with AN is approximately 5,300 euros and for BN it is 1,300 euros. The hospitalization cost of 12,800 euros per patient with AN, or 11,700 euros per patient with BN, is markedly higher than the average hospitalization cost of 3,600 euros (Krauth, Buser, & Vogel, 2002).

In 1995, in New York State, for patients between the ages of 9 and 17 years, with a mean length of stay of 18 days, the cost of treatment of an eating disorder ranged from $341.78 to $148,471.00, with a median of $3,817 and a mean of $10,019. It is important to note that in this study, the length of stay was influenced only by the availability of insurance and payer status (Robergeau, Joseph, & Silber, 2006) and that in other countries; length of stay was typically longer. For example, in Switzerland the mean length of stay has been reported at 59 days (Warnke & Rossler, 2008). More recently, in the United States the estimated cost per patient per year of treatment was $33,105 for adolescents with AN, and this cost factored in both inpatient and outpatient care (Lock, Couturier, & Agras, 2008).

In the Canadian province of British Columbia, the cost to government of long-term disability secondary to having an eating disorder ranged from $2.5 million to $101 million, which was 30 times the amount spent on treatment of eating disorders (Su & Birmingham, 2003). In the United Kingdom, the health care cost of AN was estimated to be £4.2 million in 1990, whereas in Australia the health care cost of eating disorders was Aus$22 million for the year 1993/1994 (Simon, Schmidt, & Pilling, 2005).

Health Services Utilization in Children and Adolescents

Health services utilization data for children and adolescents with eating disorders are available in North America. In 2006 in the United States, 21.3% of youth between the ages of 12 and 17 years received mental health treatment for emotional distress, with 8.6% of these adolescents seeking mental health treatment for an eating disorder in the previous year. It is important to remember when interpreting these data, that because most children with significant emotional distress do not receive treatment, this is likely an underestimate of need (Knopf, Park, & Paul Mulye, 2008). A study employing the Pediatric Health Information System database identified 1,713 admissions between 2000 and 2004, representing 1,262 unique patients. Just over half of the patients were treated in an inpatient psychiatric unit. Patients admitted to a psychiatric unit were more likely to be older, to have a comorbid psychiatric disorder, and to have a longer length of stay. Females constituted 92% of the admissions and the mean age at discharge was 15.3 years. AN was the most common discharge diagnosis, found in 71% of the cases, with the rest being evenly split between BN and EDNOS. The mean length of stay was 15.7 days overall, with a range of 1–260 days. The longest mean length of stay was found in patients with AN. Interestingly, 1–2% of patients admitted had a comorbid diagnosis of diabetes (Calderon, Vander Stoep, Collett, Garrison, & Toth, 2007). In Canada the number of hospitalizations for an eating disorder was highest in females between the ages of 15 and 19 years, with 65 hospitalizations per 100,000 person-years, followed by females between the ages of 10 and 14 years, with a hospitalization rate of 22/100 (Government of Canada, 2006).

Using a large nationwide database of private health insurance claims, one American study explored changes in the patterns of inpatient psychiatric diagnoses in children and adolescents between 1995 and 2000. It found a sample of 5,346 children under the age of 18 years who received psychiatric inpatient treatment out of a total of 1,723,681 insured children. There was a dramatic and statistically significant increase in eating disorders in female adolescents (ages 13–18 years), in which the proportion grew from 2.3% in 1995 to 5.1% of all psychiatric admissions in 2000 (Harpaz-Rotem, Leslie, Martin, & Rosenheck, 2005). These results are similar to more recent American data from the Health Care Costs and Utilization Project (HCUP) that compared estimates of hospitalizations from 1999–2000 to 2005–2006. There were a number of statistically significant findings related to the diagnosis of eating disorders. There was a rise of 18% in hospital admissions over the study period, with 28,155 eating disorder–related stays in 2005–2006 with a total cost of $271 million (a 61% rise in cost). The average cost per stay in 2005–2006 was $9,628. There was no change in the mean length of stay of about 8 days. The inpatient death rate related to hospitalization was also unchanged at 0.6%. In 2005–2006, 4% of admissions were of children under the age of 12 years, and this represented an increase of 119% from 1999–2000. Twenty-three percent of admissions occurred in patients ages 12–19 years, representing a nonstatistically significant increase of 18%.

Are the Rates of Eating Disorders on the Rise?

A number of authors have attempted to determine whether the rates of eating disorders are on the rise—in recent years by replicating and undertaking reviews of studies previously completed as well as reviewing different data sets drawn from different time intervals (Fombonne, 1995; Hoek & van Hoeken, 2003; Pawluck & Gorey, 1998; Wakeling, 1996). Although these reviews were based on many similar sets of studies, authors have been unable to agree on whether a true increase has occurred. Despite the fact that we were unable to find a recent review on this topic, it appears that there are simply too many differences in methodologies and populations to make any meaningful interpretations valid or reliable (Fombonne, 1995; Lucas et al., 1999).

Some authors have attempted to use studies with long sampling periods as a way to address this question. These studies have, in general, demonstrated increases in rates of AN in specific age cohorts (Lucas et al., 1999; Pagsberg & Wang, 1994; Willi, Giacometti, & Limacher, 1990; Willi & Grossmann, 1983). Pagsberg and Wang (1994) reported incidence rates over a 20-year period using a clinical case registry in Denmark and suggested that rates increased in females ages 10–24 years over the last quarter of the study time frame, ranging from 7.8 per 100,000 for the years 1970–1974 to 57.1 per 100,000 for the period 1985–1989. Another Danish study, completed using the same case registry, attempted to build upon the rates previously reported by correcting for previous biases and examining rates in children ages 0–9 years and youth ages 10–19 years. The study authors found that rates per 100,000 in males were stable over the period of study (1970–1993) but showed a clear and significant increase in overall rates of diagnosis in hospitalized females over the 24-year period and a clearest increase in females ages 10–19 years (Munk-Jorgensen, Moller-Madsen, Nielsen, & Nystrup, 1995). Consistent with other studies, the rate for males was found to be only a minor fraction one-tenth of the rate for females (Munk-Jorgensen et al., 1995). The authors suggested in their discussion that although the results were clear, the increases could not definitively be accounted for by an actual rise in the population. Instead, because of the nature of their study and the fact that all cases were drawn from a clinical registry, their results could reflect an increased tendency for diagnoses to cross the nosocomial threshold or to have been the effect of increased attention from health care providers and/or services (Munk-Jorgensen et al., 1995).

Other studies have reported increases at various time intervals and in multiple countries from the 1930s through the 1980s (Jones, Fox, Babigian, & Hutton, 1980; Kendell, Hall, Hailey, & Babigian, 1973; Lucas, Beard, O'Fallon, & Kurland, 1988; Lucas et al., 1991; Szmukler & Russell, 1986; Theander, 1970; Willi et al., 1990; Willi & Grossmann, 1983). The study by Lucas and colleagues (1991) of a community-based epidemiological resource, which spanned a 50-year period, deserves special mention. Although it was based on an analysis of medical records, this study avoided many of the more common flaws seen in similar reviews relating to diagnostics, service availability, and the reporting of crude rates as opposed to age-specific rates (Fombonne, 1995). The study failed to show any increase in incidence rates in females over 20 years of age or in males but did show a very clear and distinct linear rise in females ages 15–24 years (Lucas et al., 1991). Fombonne (1995) has argued that the statistical trend was largely driven by an increase only in the last data point reported, which accounted for 23% of cases. However, in a follow-up study involving the same clinical resource, Lucas and colleagues (1999) showed that the trend of increasing rates of AN had continued over another 5-year period, between 1985 and 1989. A rise in the incidence was also noted among 10- to 14-year-old females over the four decades following 1950, the first year chosen for analysis (Lucas et al., 1999). Of interest, the authors of two reviews that focused on the question of changing rates (Hoek & van Hoeken, 2003; Wakeling, 1996) also concluded that there had been a substantial increase in the incidence of AN among females 15 to 24 years of age.

More recently, large population-based surveys and clinical registry studies have demonstrated cohort effects in which age-specific prevalence rates have been associated with birth year, indicating real changes over time (Last & International Epidemiological Association, 2001; Rothman et al., 2008). The largest study to report a cohort effect was a cross-sectional population representative study of adults with a total sample size of 21,425 subjects across six European countries. This study reported a consistent inverse association between cohort (age at interview) and lifetime risk: a younger cohort had significantly higher odds of receiving a diagnosis of eating disorder (AN, BN, or EDNOS) than the older cohort, indicating that the prevalence rates of eating disorders across diagnoses increased with each new generation of subjects, irrespective of gender (Preti et al., 2009). This finding was also reported in an American national representative face-to-face household survey, the National Comorbidity Replication Study. This study had a large but more limited sample size of 9,282 subjects and did not identify any subjects who had a prevalent diagnosis of AN in the previous year. Although the same pattern, as described in the previous study, was found across the diagnostic categories of eating disorders in both men and women, only BN, binge eating, and EDNOS had statistically significantly elevated odds ratios in the younger generations of subjects. The failure to find a statistically significant cohort effect for AN was likely due to the limited number of subjects with a history of AN identified in this study (Hudson, Hiripi, Pope, & Kessler, 2007). Similarly, in Italy a clinical registry of 2,459 females between the ages of 12 and 66 years reported a decrease in age of onset with increasing birth year, indicating that younger generations of young women are developing their eating disorders at an earlier age (Favaro, Caregaro, Tenconi, Bosello, & Santonastaso, 2009).

Regardless of whether the incidence and prevalence of eating disorders has changed in the general population, there is evidence supporting the impression that the rates of eating disorders have increased in adolescents in successive generations and that age of onset is younger than in previous generations (Favaro et al., 2009; Hudson et al., 2007; Preti et al., 2009). Multiple studies have also demonstrated a clear increase in the incidence of registered cases, and as a result the demand for services is now higher (Hoek & van Hoeken, 2003). This is quite relevant, as health care providers, funding agencies, and governments will need to work together to ensure that services are effective, not only in the detection of disease, but also in its assessment and timely treatment.

Does Age Affect Outcome in Eating Disorders?

Recovery

The literature describing the outcomes of eating disorders consists of follow-up (cohort) studies of children and adolescents drawn from a variety of patient populations, including clinical case series or representative population-based surveys or registries. Follow-up studies are even fewer in number than studies reporting on incidence or prevalence in children and adolescents. They also report on populations that are limited in sample size. To date, there is little to no information on BN or EDNOS and there are no population-based outcome studies in children, specifically. Therefore the relevant outcome data for children and adolescents are largely restricted to AN.

A number of clinical cohort studies examining long-term outcomes consider age as it relates to outcome. In the United States, Strober and colleagues reported on the 10–15-year follow-up of 95 patients (85 were female) admitted to a specialty program between 1980 and 1985. There was no difference in outcome based on age (Strober, Freeman, & Morrell, 1997). In Norway a female cohort of 51 adolescents, who began treatment for AN at a mean age of 14.9 years (range 8.2–16.8 years), was followed for a mean of 8.8 years. Age at treatment start did not predict outcome (Halvorsen, Andersen, & Heyerdahl, 2004). In Sweden 68 adolescent females with a median age of 15 years at admission were followed up for 16 years. Age of onset of symptoms, once again, did not affect outcome (Nilsson & Hagglof, 2005). There are two 1-year follow-up studies following inpatient admission for AN. In the United States, with a sample of 41 adolescents, higher discharge weight, but not age, predicted a greater likelihood of maintenance of weight (Lock & Litt, 2003). In Germany a 1-year follow-up of 55 females with a mean age of 15.8 years (age ranging from 12 to 18 years) admitted for inpatient stay for an average of 12 weeks of treatment, again found that age did not predict recovery or outcome (Salbach-Andrae et al., 2009). Finally, Steinhausen, Boyadjieva, Grigoroiu-Serbanescu, and Neumarker (2003) published a series of papers on a sizable cohort of adolescent patients ($N = 242$) admitted to the hospital for eating disorders across five European sites. The subjects were mostly female (more than 90%) and diagnosed with AN. At 8-year follow-up, lower age at first admission predicted a normal BMI (Steinhausen, 2009). The larger sample size of this last study may explain the statistically significant findings.

In a study that followed 75 adult and adolescent subjects, Casper and Jabine (1996) separated subjects by age at onset into early adolescence (11–15 years), late adolescence (16–18 years) and adult (19–27 years). As compared with adults, the two adolescent groups had higher BMI and better adjustment, but age at onset did not predict outcome from AN (Casper & Jabine, 1996). Similarly, Saccomani, Savoini, Cirrincione, Vercellino, and Ravera (1998) reported no prognostic value in age of onset in a study of 81 individuals between the ages of 9 and 21 years treated for AN in Italy. A study with one of the longest follow-ups of admitted patients with AN reported no differences in outcomes among the groups, with 76% of patients recovered at 24-year follow-up (Theander, 1985).

Steinhausen (1997, 2002) addressed age of onset in two review papers. In the first he compared 941 adolescent subjects with AN to 31 adult subjects with AN. There was a somewhat better global outcome for the adolescent patients in terms of recovery, improvement, and chronicity, but there was no consensus on the prognostic value of age at onset. Only in some studies did age confer a significant prognostic benefit (Steinhausen, 1997). In a more recent study with an expanded literature review (Steinhausen, 2002), the outcome in AN, in the adolescent-onset group, had a lower mortality rate and more favorable outcome as measured by rates in recovery, improvement, and chronicity.

There is very little literature on outcomes in children, most commonly defined as under the age of 13 or 14 years. In a 2-year follow-up of 30 subjects under the age of 14 years, 60% had a good outcome. Approximately half of the subjects were prepubertal in this study. Only a young age at referral, and not at illness onset, predicted a worse prognosis (Bryant-Waugh, Knibbs, Fosson, Kaminski, & Lask, 1988). Walford and McCune (1991) published a 3-year follow-up study of 15 children who had AN at the age of 13 years or younger and who were treated on an inpatient unit between 1976 and 1986. They reported a poorer outcome in patients under the age of 11 years at the onset of illness. Just over half of the patients were prepubertal at age of onset (Walford & McCune, 1991).

It appears that there is some evidence that adolescents have a better outcome as compared with adults; however, childhood onset may associated with a worse prognosis than adolescent onset. Caution must be exercised in considering these patterns, as the absence of more comprehensive data limits the reliability of these conclusions.

Mortality

Long-term follow-ups of clinical patients are the most common source of mortality data, but they provide no information on subjects who do not come to clinical attention. Conversely, population-based reviews of death certificates, where an eating disorder is listed as being related to the death, do address this gap, but are likely to miss some deaths resulting from an eating disorder as physicians may have no knowledge of the subject's medical history when completing the death certificate (Muir & Palmer, 2004). This limitation typically results in an underestimate of mortality rates. Mortality associated with any illness in children and adolescents requires consideration both as it relates to premature mortality in childhood or adolescence and as it relates to excess long-term mortality in later years. Not surprisingly, the data in both these situations are most commonly nonexistent for eating disorders. Studies on mortality that report standardized mortality ratios (SMRs) often present a single SMR that encompasses children and/or adolescents along with adults (Papadopoulos, Ekbom, Brandt, & Ekselius, 2009; Sullivan, 1995).

For all ages, in AN, an SMR of 6.2 in Sweden, 9.1 in Denmark, and 9.7 in Italy, have been reported in both sexes (Moller-Madsen, Nystrup, & Nielsen, 1996; Papadopoulos et al., 2009; Signorini et al., 2007), and patients were at increased risk of death resulting from cancer (SMR = 1.9), from endocrine (SMR = 7.9), cardiovascular (SMR =2.3), respiratory (SMR = 11.5), gastrointestinal (SMR = 5.4), urogenital (SMR = 10.8), and autoimmune (SMR = 8.8) difficulties, and psychoactive substance use (SMR = 18.9). The risk of death from suicide (SMR = 13.6) or undefined causes (SMR = 10.9) was also elevated (Papadopoulos et al., 2009). For BN, the death risk was nine times than expected (Harris & Barraclough, 1997). Causes of death are less well reported for BN; they include suicide, motor vehicle accidents, malnutrition (Keel & Mitchell, 1997), acute gastric dilation (Watanabe et al., 2008) and pancreatitis (Birmingham & Boone, 2004). EDNOS, despite being the most common eating disorder diagnosis, is rarely studied. Statistically significant elevated SMRs for EDNOS of 1.81 and 2.47 were reported recently (Button, Chadalavada, & Palmer, 2010; Crow et al., 2009; Moller-Madsen et al., 1996; Papadopoulos et al., 2009).

Clinical case registries either link a clinical database of patients with a national death registry to identify patients who have died, or they recontact patients at planned intervals to gather information directly. The only study providing an SMR specific to the age groups of interest reports an SMR of 6.6 in females between the ages of 15 and 19 years with AN admitted to a hospital and no reported deaths in females under the age of 15 years (Moller-Madsen et al., 1996). Although there are no age-specific reports of SMR for males, children, or adolescents with BN or EDNOS reported in the literature, one study does report the relative risk (RR) of death in older children and adolescents with eating disorders identified from a national clinical psychiatric admission registry and then linked to a death registry. These subjects were then compared with the age-matched general population. The RR of death in patients with any eating disorder, between the ages of 10 and 14 years, was 12; for adolescents ages 15–19 years, it was 10. Follow-up was a mean of 10 years. Patients who were not part of the clinical registry but had an eating disorder listed as a cause of death on their death certificates were also included (Emborg, 1999). Finally, there is one survival analysis of patients with AN reporting that females developing chronic AN between the ages of 10 and 15 years will see a 25-year reduction in lifespan (Harbottle, Birmingham, & Sayani, 2008; Papadopoulos et al., 2009).

Nielsen and colleagues (1998) reviewed and compared mortality rates across the age span, reported in eight studies. Based on five studies, the SMR in patients under 15 years of age (3.1) did not differ from the SMR in youth ages 15 to 19 years (3.2). However, as compared with subjects over the age of 20 years, subjects under the age of 20 years had lower SMRs (Nielsen et al., 1998). A handful of studies support the hypothesis that early-onset eating disorders do appear to be less fatal than those of later onset, but do not provide actual rates (Millar et al., 2005; Papadopoulos et al., 2009; Tanaka, Kiriike, Nagata, & Riku, 2001). Overall, younger age does seem to be associated with lower mortality, but given the limited number of studies, no conclusion can be drawn with any confidence.

Conclusions

This review highlights some of the methodological difficulties encountered in determining the incidence and prevalence of eating disorders in children and adolescents. Although research in the area has not been uniform over time, the information that is available has been helpful in beginning to shape our understanding of the epidemiological basis of these disorders. As our understanding of eating disorders has improved, so too has the recognition that a consistent methodological shift in studies of this nature is required. Moving forward, it will be crucial that investigators devise strategies that maximize patient and case identification (understanding that the use of strict categories, although helpful, limits our true understanding of the severity of all types of eating pathology present in populations) and as well come together to devise standardized means to capture and report data. Not only can this allow for improved comparisons across samples, but it can also help build on our ability to understand which trends are generalizable and which are not. At present, the epidemiological data on children with eating disorders remain inconsistent and inadequate.

References

Ackard, D. M., Fulkerson, J. A., & Neumark-Sztainer, D. (2007). Prevalence and utility of DSM-IV eating disorder diagnostic criteria among youth. *International Journal of Eating Disorders, 40*(5), 409–417

Alborghetti, A., Scimeca, G., Costanzo, G., & Boca, S. (2008). The prevalence of eating disorders in adolescents with idiopathic scoliosis. *Brunner-Mazel Eating Disorders Monograph Series, 16*(1), 85–93.

American Psychiatric Association. (2004).

Diagnostic and statistical manual of mental disorders (4th ed., text rev.). Washington, DC: Author.

Anderluh, M., Tchanturia, K., Rabe-Hesketh, S., Collier, D., & Treasure, J. (2009). Lifetime course of eating disorders: Design and validity testing of a new strategy to define the eating disorders phenotype. *Psychological Medicine, 39*(1), 105–114.

Birmingham, C. L., & Boone, S. (2004). Pancreatitis causing death in bulimia nervosa.

International Journal of Eating Disorders, 36(2), 234–237.

Bravender, T., Bryant-Waugh, R., Herzog, D., Katzman, D., Kreipe, R. D., Lask, B., et al. (2007). Classification of child and adolescent eating disturbances. Workgroup for Classification of Eating Disorders in Children and Adolescents (WCEDCA). *International Journal of Eating Disorders, 40*(Suppl.), S117–S122.

Bravender, T., Bryant-Waugh, R., Herzog, D., Katzman, D., Kreipe, R. D., Lask, B., et al. (2010). Classification of eating disturbance in children and adolescents: Proposed changes for the DSM-V. *European Eating Disorders Review, 18*(2), 79–89.

Bryant-Waugh, R., Knibbs, J., Fosson, A., Kaminski, Z., & Lask, B. (1988). Long term follow up of patients with early onset anorexia nervosa. *Archives of Disease in Childhood, 63*(1), 5–9.

Button, E. J., Chadalavada, B., & Palmer, R. L. (2010). Mortality and predictors of death in a cohort of patients presenting to an eating disorders service. *International Journal of Eating Disorders, 43*(5), 387–392.

Calderon, R., Vander Stoep, A., Collett, B., Garrison, M. M., & Toth, K. (2007). Inpatients with eating disorders: Demographic, diagnostic, and service characteristics from a nationwide pediatric sample. *International Journal of Eating Disorders, 40*(7), 622–628.

Casper, R. C., & Jabine, L. N. (1996). An eight-year follow-up: Outcome from adolescent compared to adult onset anorexia nervosa. *Journal of Youth and Adolescence, 25*(4), 499–517.

Colton, P. A., Olmsted, M. P., Daneman, D., Rydall, A., & Rodin, G. (2004). Disturbed eating behavior and eating disorders in preteen and early teenage girls with type 1 diabetes. A case controlled study. *Diabetes Care, 27*(7), 1654–1659.

Colton, P. A., Olmsted, M. P., & Rodin, G. M. (2007). Eating disturbances in a school population of preteen girls: Assessment and screening. *International Journal of Eating Disorders, 40*(5), 435–440.

Crow, S. J., Peterson, C. B., Swanson, S. A., Raymond, N. C., Specker, S., Eckert, E. D., et al. (2009). Increased mortality in bulimia nervosa and other eating disorders. *American Journal of Psychiatry, 166*(12), 1342–1346.

Currin, L., Schmidt, U., Treasure, J., & Jick, H. (2005). Time trends in eating disorder incidence. *British Journal of Psychiatry, 186*, 132–135.

de Azevedo, M. H., & Ferreira, C. P. (1992). Anorexia nervosa and bulimia: A prevalence study. *Acta Psychiatrica Scandinavica, 86*(6), 432–436.

Duff, A. J., Wolfe, S. P., Dickson, C., Conway, S. P., & Brownlee, K. G. (2003). Feeding behavior problems in children with cystic fibrosis in the UK: Prevalence and comparison with healthy controls. *Journal of Pediatric Gastroenterology and Nutrition, 36*(4), 443–447.

Emborg, C. (1999). Mortality and causes of death in eating disorders in Denmark 1970–1993: A case register study. *International Journal of Eating Disorders, 25*(3), 243–251.

Fairburn, C. G., & Beglin, S. J. (1990). Studies of the epidemiology of bulimia nervosa. *American Journal of Psychiatry, 147*(4), 401–408.

Favaro, A., Caregaro, L., Tenconi, E., Bosello, R., & Santonastaso, P. (2009). Time trends in age at onset of anorexia nervosa and bulimia nervosa. *Journal of Clinical Psychiatry, 70*(12), 1715–1721.

Fichter, M. M., Quadflieg, N., & Gnutzmann, A. (1998). Binge eating disorder: Treatment outcome over a 6-year course. *Journal of Psychosomatic Research, 44*(3–4), 385–405.

Fombonne, E. (1995). Anorexia nervosa. No evidence of an increase. *British Journal of Psychiatry, 166*(4), 462–471.

Garfinkel, P. E. (2002). Eating disorders. *Canadian Journal of Psychiatry—Revue Canadienne de Psychiatrie, 47*(3), 225–226.

Goodwin, R. D., Hoven, C. W., & Spitzer, R. L. (2003). Diabetes and eating disorders in primary care. *International Journal of Eating Disorders, 33*(1), 85–91.

Government of Canada. (2006). *The human face of mental health and mental illness in Canada.* Ottawa, ON, Canada: Author.

Halvorsen, I., Andersen, A., & Heyerdahl, S. (2004). Good outcome of adolescent onset anorexia nervosa after systematic treatment: Intermediate to long-term follow-up of a representative county-sample. *European Child and Adolescent Psychiatry, 13*(5), 295–306.

Harbottle, E. J., Birmingham, C. L., & Sayani, F. (2008). Anorexia nervosa: A survival analysis. *Eating and Weight Disorders, 13*(2), e32–e34.

Harpaz-Rotem, I., Leslie, D. L., Martin, A., & Rosenheck, R. A. (2005). Changes in child and adolescent inpatient psychiatric admission diagnoses between 1995 and 2000. *Social Psychiatry and Psychiatric Epidemiology, 40*(8), 642–647.

Harris, E. C., & Barraclough, B. (1997). Suicide as an outcome for mental disorders: A meta-analysis. *British Journal of Psychiatry, 170*, 205–228.

Hoek, H. W. (2006). Incidence, prevalence and mortality of anorexia nervosa and other eating disorders. *Current Opinion in Psychiatry, 19*(4), 389–394.

Hoek, H. W., & van Hoeken, D. (2003). Review of the prevalence and incidence of eating disorders. *International Journal of Eating Disorders, 34*(4), 383–396.

Hoek, H. W., van Harten, P. N., Hermans, K. M., Katzman, M. A., Matroos, G. E., & Susser, E. S. (2005). The incidence of anorexia nervosa on Curacao. *American Journal of Psychiatry, 162*(4), 748–752.

Hsu, L. K. (1996). Epidemiology of the eating disorders. *Psychiatric Clinics of North America, 19*(4), 681–700.

Hudson, J. I., Hiripi, E., Pope, H. G., Jr., & Kessler, R. C. (2007). The prevalence and correlates of eating disorders in the National Comorbidity Survey Replication. *Biological Psychiatry, 61*(3), 348–358.

Iafusco, D., Vanelli, M., Gugliotta, M., Iovane, B., Chiari, G., & Prisco, F. (2004). Prevalence of eating disorders in young patients with type 1 diabetes from two different Italian cities. *Diabetes Care, 27*(9), 2278.

Isomaa, R., Isomaa, A. L., Marttunen, M., Kaltiala-Heino, R., & Björkqvist, K. (2009). The prevalence, incidence and development of eating disorders in Finnish adolescents: A two-step 3-year follow-up study. *European Eating Disorders Review, 17*(3), 199–207.

Joergensen, J. (1992). The epidemiology of eating disorders in Fyn County, Denmark, 1977–1986. *Acta Psychiatrica Scandinavica, 85*(1), 30–34.

Jones, D. J., Fox, M. M., Babigian, H. M., & Hutton, H. E. (1980). Epidemiology of anorexia nervosa in Monroe County, New York: 1960–1976. *Psychosomatic Medicine, 42*(6), 551–558.

Keel, P., & Mitchell, J. (1997). Outcome in bulimia nervosa. *American Journal of Psychiatry, 154*(3), 313–321.

Kendell, R. E., Hall, D. J., Hailey, A., & Babigian, H. M. (1973). The epidemiology of anorexia nervosa. *Psychological Medicine, 3*(2), 200–203.

Keski-Rahkonen, A., Hoek, H. W., Linna, M. S., Raevuori, A., Sihvola, E., Bulik, C. M., et al. (2009). Incidence and outcomes of bulimia nervosa: A nationwide population-based study. *Psychological Medicine, 39*(5), 823–831.

Keski-Rahkonen, A., Hoek, H. W., Susser, E. S., Linna, M. S., Sihvola, E., Raevuori, A., et al. (2007). Epidemiology and course of anorexia nervosa in the community. *American Journal of Psychiatry, 164*(8), 1259–1265.

Kessler, R. C. (2000). Psychiatric epidemiology: Selected recent advances and future directions. *Bulletin of the World Health Organization, 78*(4), 464–474.

Kessler, R. C., Avenevoli, S., Costello, E. J., Green, J. G., Gruber, M. J., Heeringa, S., et al. (2009). Design and field procedures in the U.S. National Comorbidity Survey Replication Adolescent Supplement (NCS-A). *International Journal of Methods in Psychiatric Research, 18*(2), 69–83.

Kjelsas, E., Bjornstrom, C., & Götestam, K. G. (2004). Prevalence of eating disorders in female and male adolescents (14–15 years). *Eating Behaviors, 5*(1), 13–25.

Knopf, D., Park, M. J., & Paul Mulye, T. (2008). *The mental health of adolescents: A national profile 2008.* San Francisco: National Adolescent Health Information Center, University of California, San Francisco.

Krauth, C., Buser, K., & Vogel, H. (2002). How high are the costs of eating disorders–anorexia nervosa and bulimia nervosa—for German society? *European Journal of Health Economics, 3*(4), 244–250.

Kuboki, T., Nomura, S., Ide, M., Suematsu, H., & Araki, S. (1996). Epidemiological data on anorexia nervosa in Japan. *Psychiatry Research, 62*(1), 11–16.

Lahortiga-Ramos, F., De Irala-Estevez, J., Cano-Prous, A., Gual-Garcia, P., Martinez-Gonzalez, M. A., & Cervera-Enguix, S. (2005). Incidence of eating disorders in Navarra (Spain). *European Psychiatry, 20*(2), 179–185.

Last, J. M., & International Epidemiological Association. (2001). *A dictionary of epidemiology* (4th ed.). New York: Oxford University Press.

Lock, J., Couturier, J., & Agras, W. S. (2008). Costs of remission and recovery using family therapy for adolescent anorexia nervosa: A descriptive report. *Brunner-Mazel Eating Disorders Monograph Series, 16*(4), 322–330.

Lock, J., & Litt, I. (2003). What predicts maintenance of weight for adolescents medically hospitalized for anorexia nervosa? *Eating Disorders, 11*(1), 1–7.

Lucas, A. R., Beard, C. M., O'Fallon, W. M., & Kurland, L. T. (1988). Anorexia nervosa in Rochester, Minnesota: A 45-year study. *Mayo Clinic Proceedings, 63*(5), 433–442.

Lucas, A. R., Beard, C. M., O'Fallon, W. M., & Kurland, L. T. (1991). 50-year trends in the incidence of anorexia nervosa in Rochester, Minn.: A population-based study. *American Journal of Psychiatry, 148*(7), 917–922.

Lucas, A. R., Crowson, C. S., O'Fallon, W. M., & Melton, L. J., III. (1999). The ups and downs of anorexia nervosa. *International Journal of Eating Disorders, 26*(4), 397–405.

Machado, P. P., Machado, B. C., Gonçalves, S., & Hoek, H. W. (2007). The prevalence of eating disorders not otherwise specified. *International Journal of Eating Disorders, 40*(3), 212–217.

Madden, S., Morris, A., Zurynski, Y. A., Kohn, M., & Elliot, E. J. (2009). Burden of eating disorders in 5–13-year-old children in Australia. *Medical Journal of Australia, 190*(8), 410–414.

Marchi, M., & Cohen, P. (1990). Early childhood eating behaviors and adolescent eating disorders. *Journal of the American Academy of Child and Adolescent Psychiatry, 29*(1), 112–117.

Millar, H. R., Wardell, F., Vyvyan, J. P., Naji, S. A., Prescott, G. J., & Eagles, J. M. (2005). Anorexia nervosa mortality in Northeast Scotland, 1965–1999. *American Journal of Psychiatry, 162*(4), 753–757.

Milos, G. F., Spindler, A. M., Buddeberg, C., & Crameri, A. (2003). Axes I and II comorbidity and treatment experiences in eating disorder subjects. *Psychotherapy and Psychosomatics, 72*(5), 276–285.

Mitrany, E., Lubin, F., Chetrit, A., & Modan, B. (1995). Eating disorders among Jewish female adolescents in Israel: A 5-year study. *Journal of Adolescent Health, 16*(6), 454–457.

Moller-Madsen, S., Nystrup, J., & Nielsen, S. (1996). Mortality in anorexia nervosa in Denmark during the period 1970–1987. *Acta Psychiatrica Scandinavica, 94*(6), 454–459.

Muir, A., & Palmer, R. L. (2004). An audit of a British sample of death certificates in which anorexia nervosa is listed as a cause of death. *International Journal of Eating Disorders, 36*(3), 356–360.

Munk-Jorgensen, P., Moller-Madsen, S., Nielsen, S., & Nystrup, J. (1995). Incidence of eating disorders in psychiatric hospitals and wards in Denmark, 1970–1993. *Acta Psychiatrica Scandinavica, 92*(2), 91–96.

Neumark-Sztainer, D., Story, M., Resnick, M. D., Garwick, A., & Blum, R. W. (1995). Body dissatisfaction and unhealthy weight-control practices among adolescents with and without chronic illness: A population-based study. *Archives of Pediatrics and Adolescent Medicine, 149*(12), 1330–1335.

Nicholls, D., & Bryant-Waugh, R. (2009). Eating disorders of infancy and childhood: Definition, symptomatology, epidemiology, and comorbidity. *Child and Adolescent Psychiatric Clinics of North America, 18*(1), 17–30.

Nicholls, D., Chater, R., & Lask, B. (2000). Children into DSM don't go: A comparison of classification systems for eating disorders in childhood and early adolescence. *International Journal of Eating Disorders, 28*(3), 317–324.

Nielsen, S. (1990). The epidemiology of anorexia nervosa in Denmark from 1973 to 1987: A nationwide register study of psychiatric admission. *Acta Psychiatrica Scandinavica, 81*(6), 507–514.

Nielsen, S., Emborg, C., & Molbak, A. G. (2002). Mortality in concurrent type 1 diabetes and anorexia nervosa. *Diabetes Care, 25*(2), 309–312.

Nielsen, S., Moller-Madsen, S., Isager, T., Jorgensen, J., Pagsberg, K., & Theander, S. (1998). Standardized mortality in eating disorders—a quantitative summary of previously published and new evidence. *Journal of Psychosomatic Research, 44*(3–4), 413–434.

Nilsson, K., & Hagglof, B. (2005). Long-term follow-up of adolescent onset anorexia nervosa in Northern Sweden. *European Eating Disorders Review, 13,* 89–100.

Nobakht, M., & Dezhkam, M. (2000). An epidemiological study of eating disorders in Iran. *International Journal of Eating Disorders, 28*(3), 265–271.

Pagsberg, A. K., & Wang, A. R. (1994). Epidemiology of anorexia nervosa and bulimia nervosa in Bornholm County, Denmark, 1970–1989. *Acta Psychiatrica Scandinavica, 90*(4), 259–265.

Papadopoulos, F. C., Ekbom, A., Brandt, L., & Ekselius, L. (2009). Excess mortality, causes of death and prognostic factors in anorexia nervosa. *British Journal of Psychiatry, 194*(1), 10–17.

Pawluck, D. E., & Gorey, K. M. (1998). Secular trends in the incidence of anorexia nervosa: Integrative review of population-based studies. *International Journal of Eating Disorders, 23*(4), 347–352.

Peebles, R., Wilson, J. L., & Lock, J. D. (2006). How do children with eating disorders differ from adolescents with eating disorders at initial evaluation? *Journal of Adolescent Health, 39*(6), 800–805.

Pelaez Fernandez, M. A., Labrador, F. J., & Raich, R. M. (2007). Prevalence of eating disorders among adolescent and young adult scholastic population in the region of Madrid (Spain). *Journal of Psychosomatic Research, 62*(6), 681–690.

Powers, P. S., Malone, J. I., Coovert, D. L., & Schulman, R. G. (1990). Insulin-dependent diabetes mellitus and eating disorders: A prevalence study. *Comprehensive Psychiatry, 31*(3), 205–210.

Preti, A., Girolamo, G., Vilagut, G., Alonso, J., Graaf, R., Bruffaerts, R., et al. (2009). The epidemiology of eating disorders in six European countries: Results of the ESEMeD-WMH project. *Journal of Psychiatric Research, 43*(14), 1125–1132.

Raevuori, A., Hoek, H. W., Susser, E., Kaprio, J., Rissanen, A., & Keski-Rahkonen, A. (2009). Epidemiology of anorexia nervosa in men: A nationwide study of Finnish twins. *PLoS ONE* [Electronic resource], *4*(2), e4402.

Rastam, M., Gillberg, C., & Garton, M. (1989). Anorexia nervosa in a Swedish urban region: A population-based study. *British Journal of Psychiatry, 155,* 642–646.

Raymond, N. C., Chang, P. N., Crow, S. J., Mitchell, J. E., Dieperink, B. S., Beck, M. M., et al. (2000). Eating disorders in patients with cystic fibrosis. *Journal of Adolescence, 23*(3), 359–363.

Robergeau, K., Joseph, J., & Silber, T. J. (2006). Hospitalization of children and adolescents for eating disorders in the State of New York. *Journal of Adolescent Health, 39*(6), 806–810.

Rodriguez-Cano, T., Beato-Fernandez, L., & Belmonte-Llario, A. (2005). New contributions to the prevalence of eating disorders in Spanish adolescents: Detection of false negatives. *European Psychiatry: The Journal of the Association of European Psychiatrists, 20*(2), 173–178.

Rothman, K. J., Greenland, S., & Lash, T. L. (2008). *Modern epidemiology* (3rd ed.). Philadelphia: Wolters Kluwer Health/Lippincott Williams & Wilkins.

Saccomani, L., Savoini, M., Cirrincione, M., Vercellino, F., & Ravera, G. (1998). Long-term outcome of children and adolescents with anorexia nervosa: Study of comorbidity. *Journal of Psychosomatic Research, 44*(5), 565–571.

Salbach-Andrae, H., Schneider, N., Seifert, K., Pfeiffer, E., Lenz, K., Lehmkuhl, U., et al. (2009). Short-term outcome of anorexia nervosa in adolescents after inpatient treatment: A prospective study. *European Child and Adolescent Psychiatry, 18*(11), 701–704.

Sancho, C., Arija, M. V., Asorey, O., & Canals, J. (2007). Epidemiology of eating disorders: A two year follow up in an early adolescent school population. *European Child and Adolescent Psychiatry, 16*(8), 495–504.

Shearer, J. E., & Bryon, M. (2004). The nature and prevalence of eating disorders and eating disturbance in adolescents with cystic fibrosis. *Journal of the Royal Society of Medicine, 97*(Suppl. 44), 36–42.

Signorini, A., De Filippo, E., Panico, S., De Caprio, C., Pasanisi, F., & Contaldo, F. (2007). Long-term mortality in anorexia nervosa: A report after an 8-year follow-up and a review of the most recent literature. *European Journal of Clinical Nutrition, 61*(1), 119–122.

Simon, J., Schmidt, U., & Pilling, S. (2005). The health service use and cost of eating disorders. *Psychological Medicine, 35*(11), 1543–1551.

Smith, F. M., Latchford, G., Hall, R. M., Millner, P. A., & Dickson, R. A. (2002). Indications of disordered eating behaviour in adolescent patients with idiopathic scoliosis. *Journal of Bone and Joint Surgery—British, 84*(3), 392–394.

Smith, F. M., Latchford, G. J., Hall, R. M., & Dickson, R. A. (2008). Do chronic medical conditions increase the risk of eating disorder?: A cross-sectional investigation of eating pathology in adolescent females with scoliosis and diabetes. *Journal of Adolescent Health, 42*(1), 58–63.

Soundy, T. J., Lucas, A. R., Suman, V. J., & Melton, L. J., III. (1995). Bulimia nervosa in Rochester, Minnesota, from 1980 to 1990. *Psychological Medicine, 25*(5), 1065–1071.

Steinhausen, H.-C. (1997). Outcome of anorexia nervosa in the younger patient. *Journal of Child Psychology and Psychiatry and Allied Disciplines, 38*(3), 271–276.

Steinhausen, H.-C. (2002). The outcome of anorexia nervosa in the 20th century. *American Journal of Psychiatry, 159*(8), 1284–1293.

Steinhausen, H.-C. (2009). Outcome of eating disorders. *Child and Adolescent Psychiatric Clinics of North America, 18*(1), 225–242.

Steinhausen, H.-C., Boyadjieva, S., Griogoroiu-Serbanescu, M., & Neumarker, K. J. (2003). The outcome of adolescent eating disorders: Findings from an international collaborative study. *European Child and Adolescent Psychiatry, 12*(Suppl. 1), I91–I98.

Stice, E., Marti, C. N., Shaw, H., & Jaconis, M. (2009). An 8-year longitudinal study of the natural history of threshold, subthreshold, and partial eating disorders from a community sample of adolescents. *Journal of Abnormal Psychology, 118*(3), 587–597.

Striegel-Moore, R. H. (2005). Health services research in anorexia nervosa. *International Journal of Eating Disorders, 37*(Suppl.), S31–S34; discussion, S41–S32.

Striegel-Moore, R. H., DeBar, L., Wilson, G. T., Dickerson, J., Rosselli, F., Perrin, N., et al. (2008). Health services use in eating disorders. *Psychological Medicine, 38*(10), 1465–1474.

Strober, M., Freeman, R., & Morrell, W. (1997). The long-term course of severe anorexia nervosa in adolescents: Survival analysis of recovery, relapse, and outcome predictors over 10–15 years in a prospective study. *International Journal of Eating Disorders, 22*(4), 339–360.

Su, J. C., & Birmingham, C. L. (2003). Anorexia nervosa: The cost of long-term disability. *Eating and Weight Disorders, 8*(1), 76–79.

Sullivan, P. (1995). Mortality in anorexia nervosa. *American Journal of Psychiatry, 152*(7), 1073–1074.

Suris, J. C., Michaud, P. A., Akre, C., & Sawyer, S. M. (2008). Health risk behaviors in adolescents with chronic conditions. *Pediatrics, 122*(5), e1113–e1118.

Szmukler, G. I. (1985). The epidemiology of anorexia nervosa and bulimia. *Journal of Psychiatric Research, 19*(2–3), 143–153.

Szmukler, G. I., & Russell, G. F. M. (1986). Outcome and prognosis of anorexia nervosa. In K. D. Brownell & J. P. Foreyt (Eds.), *Handbook of eating disorders* (pp. 283–300). New York: Basic Books.

Tanaka, H., Kiriike, N., Nagata, T., & Riku, K. (2001). Outcome of severe anorexia nervosa patients receiving inpatient treatment in Japan: An 8-year follow-up study. *Psychiatry and Clinical Neurosciences, 55*(4), 389–396.

Theander, S. (1970). Anorexia nervosa: A psychiatric investigation of 94 female patients. *Acta Psychiatrica Scandinavica, 214*(Suppl.), 1–194.

Theander, S. (1985). Outcome and prognosis in anorexia nervosa and bulimia: Some results of previous investigations, compared with those of a Swedish long-term study. *Journal of Psychiatric Research, 19*(2–3), 493–508.

Tseng, M. M., Fang, D., Lee, M. B., Chie, W. C., Liu, J. P., & Chen, W. J. (2007). Two-phase survey of eating disorders in gifted dance and non-dance high-school students in Taiwan. *Psychological Medicine, 37*(8), 1085–1096.

Turnbull, S., Ward, A., Treasure, J., Jick, H., & Derby, L. (1996). The demand for eating disorder care: An epidemiological study using the general practice research database. *British Journal of Psychiatry, 169*(6), 705–712.

van Son, G. E., van Hoeken, D., Bartelds, A. I., van Furth, E. F., & Hoek, H. W. (2006a). Time trends in the incidence of eating disorders: A primary care study in the Netherlands. *International Journal of Eating Disorders, 39*(7), 565–569.

van Son, G. E., van Hoeken, D., Bartelds, A. I., van Furth, E. F., & Hoek, H. W. (2006b). Urbanisation and the incidence of eating disorders. *British Journal of Psychiatry, 189*, 562–563.

Wakeling, A. (1996). Epidemiology of anorexia nervosa. *Psychiatry Research, 62*(1), 3–9.

Walford, G., & McCune, N. (1991). Long-term outcome in early-onset anorexia nervosa. *British Journal of Psychiatry, 159*, 383–389.

Warnke, I., & Rossler, W. (2008). Length of stay by ICD-based diagnostic groups as basis for the remuneration of psychiatric inpatient care in Switzerland? *Swiss Medical Weekly, 138*(35–36), 520–527.

Watanabe, S., Terazawa, K., Asari, M., Matsubara, K., Shiono, H., & Shimizu, K. (2008). An autopsy case of sudden death due to acute gastric dilatation without rupture. *Forensic Science International, 180*(2–3), e6–e10.

Willi, J., Giacometti, G., & Limacher, B. (1990). Update on the epidemiology of anorexia nervosa in a defined region of Switzerland. *American Journal of Psychiatry, 147*(11), 1514–1517.

Willi, J., & Grossmann, S. (1983). Epidemiology of anorexia nervosa in a defined region of Switzerland. *American Journal of Psychiatry, 140*(5), 564–567.

Williams, P., Tarnopolsky, A., & Hand, D. (1980). Case definition and case identification in psychiatric epidemiology: Review and assessment. *Psychological Medicine, 10*(1), 101–114.

CHAPTER 6

Course and Outcome

Hans-Christoph Steinhausen

In this chapter, separately for anorexia nervosa (AN) and bulimia nervosa (BN), a review is provided first on the limited knowledge of the natural course and the effects of intervention studies. This is followed by a summarizing review of the various studies on the outcome and prognosis of the eating disorders. These studies cover a wide age range and are not restricted to childhood and adolescence. Because of the specific age at manifestation of AN, it is also possible to report specifically on the course of the disorder in patients with adolescent onset. Because BN is less common at this young age, the literature on the outcome of this disorder does not allow such a distinction.

Anorexia Nervosa

Studies of Natural Course

There are only a few studies addressing the natural history of eating behavior, attitudes, and disorders. The majority of these studies are based on questionnaires that deal with eating attitudes and behavior; only a minority have assessed eating disorders that fulfill clinical criteria of diagnoses and assessment. Among the latter, more information is provided on the natural course of BN than on AN. In conjunction with other studies on eating attitudes and behavior, they provide some limited evidence that a substantial percentage of subjects at risk and untreated cases remain stable with regard to their condition across a considerable time span (Rathner, 1992). Findings from the Victorian Adolescent Health Cohort Study in Australia (Patton, Coffey, & Sawyer, 2003) and from Oregon in the United States (Lewinsohn, Striegel-Moore, & Seeley, 2000) show that 11 and 30% of subjects, respectively, had a persistent eating disorder by young adulthood.

Follow-Up Effects of Interventions

Despite the large number of treatment studies in AN, controlled intervention studies with sufficient follow-up periods are rare. Various reviews of pharmacotherapy indicate that no drug has yet been demonstrated to have clinically significant use in AN (Heebink & Halmi, 1995; Kotler & Walsh, 2000; Mitchell, Peterson, Myers, & Wonderlich, 2001).

So far, no study has assessed the long-term effects of any medication. Furthermore, various psychotherapeutic approaches have been commonly advocated for the treatment of AN. However, very few controlled studies have been performed so far and the long-term effects are mostly unknown.

A study by Crisp and colleagues (1997) shows that outcome in a treatment group is better than in a waiting list control group. Furthermore, the authors of the Maudsley treatment studies initially showed that adolescent patients suffering from AN with a relatively short history of their illness responded significantly better to family therapy than to individual supportive therapy (Russell, Szmukler, Dare, & Eisler, 1987). This is also the only study that has documented the stability of treatment effects over at least a 5-year period (Eisler et al., 1997). For the older patients with more chronic AN and BN, the benefits of the treatment were less clear-cut. There was a trend for these patients to respond more favorably to individual supportive therapy. Additional research showed that conjoint family sessions and family counseling as two different forms of family therapy produced similar results in terms of symptomatic relief (Eisler et al., 2000). Another group of researchers (Robin, Siegel, Koepke, Moye, & Tice, 1994; Robin, Siegel, & Moye, 1995) compared behavioral systems therapy versus ego-oriented individual therapy. They found that both treatments produced significant reductions in negative communication and parent–adolescent conflict, eating attitudes, and psychopathology, and that the improvements in eating-related conflict were maintained at 1-year follow-up.

The clinical application of cognitive-behavioral principles has gained extensive support through controlled trials only in BN; the efficacy of similar strategies in AN still has to be established. There is sufficient evidence only from the earlier generation of controlled studies based on behavioral interventions that operant conditioning is an effective short-term method of weight restoration in AN (Bemis, 1987).

Outcomes

So far, the most exhaustive review of the outcome of AN in the 20th century has been the one I have provided (Steinhausen, 2002). In this review, a total of 119 study series covering 5,590 patients that were published in the English and German literature were analyzed in regard to mortality, global outcome, and other psychiatric disorders at follow-up. A precise description of the review methodology is beyond the scope of this chapter but can be found in the published article.

In this review, the four major outcome parameters of mortality, recovery, improvement, and chronicity and the other psychiatric disorders were analyzed. There were rather wide ranges of these parameters in the various studies so that the following findings represent only a central trend. The mean crude mortality rate amounted to 5.0%. In the surviving patients, on average, full recovery was found in only less than half of the patients, whereas a third improved and 20% developed a chronic course of the disorder. Outcome was slightly better for the core symptoms, with normalization of weight occurring in almost 60% of the patients, normalization of menstruation in 57%, and normalization of eating behavior in 47% of the former patients.

Besides the anorexic symptoms, additional psychiatric disorders were seen in a large proportion of the patients at follow-up. Frequent diagnoses were neurotic disorders (25.5%), including anxiety disorders and phobias; affective disorders (24.1%); substance use disorders (14.6%); obsessive–compulsive disorder (12.0%); and unspecified personality disorders including borderline states (17.4%). A few studies reported a high rate of obsessive–compulsive personality disorder (31.4%) and a less pronounced rate of histrionic personality disorder (16.6%), and schizophrenia (4.6%) was only rarely observed at follow-up.

The analyses of the data controlled also for three major effect variables that might have affected outcome. Only the four major outcome parameters and studies that reported these variables were considered for these analyses. The three major effect variables included duration of follow-up (< 4 years, 4–10 years, > 10 years), age at onset of the disorder (adolescence only versus mixed samples with onset in adolescence and adulthood), and time period of study (1950–1979, 1980–1989, 1990–1999).

Findings for duration of follow-up were highly significant, and all four global outcome effect sizes were large. With increasing duration of follow-up, mortality rates increased. In the surviving patients, there was a strong tendency toward recovery with increasing duration of follow-up. The rate of recovery increased, whereas the rates of improvement and chronicity declined. The mortality rate was much lower in the group of younger patients in comparison with the group with a much wider age range at onset of illness. The rates of recovery, improvement, and chronicity were more favorable in the group with the younger patients.

Mortality showed a complex pattern of time trends. It was absent for both very short and very extended study courses in the early studies (with only one study each), from 1950 through 1979, whereas it increased linearly in the studies from 1980 to 1989 and from 1990 to 1999, with the highest rate for the most extended studies reported for 1980–1989. There were few differences between the studies for 1980–1989 and the studies for 1990–1999 on the other outcome measures—recovery, improvement, and chronicity—whereas the studies from 1950–1979 primarily stood out because of high recovery rates and low rates of improvement and chronicity during short-term courses (< 4 years). For all four outcome measures, the effect sizes for duration of follow-up were markedly stronger than for time period.

Prognostic Factors

Besides follow-up data, a considerable number of outcome studies also provided some information on prognosis. However, there was a rather substantial variability as to the type and number of prognostic factors considered for analysis in the various studies. For the majority of the prognostic factors, the findings were considerably heterogeneous. This interpretation applies to the ambiguous findings regarding age at onset of illness as a within-sample factor. In addition, most studies indicated that a short duration of symptoms before treatment resulted in a favorable outcome. The impact of the duration of inpatient treatment is unclear because of ambiguous findings across the outcome studies, and no definite conclusions could be drawn as to whether greater weight loss at presentation had long-term effects on outcome.

In addition, the analyses showed quite clearly that vomiting, BN, and purgative abuse imply an unfavorable prognosis, whereas hyperactivity and dieting as weight-reduction measures did not have any prognostic significance. A small number of studies also showed that premorbid developmental and clinical abnormalities, including eating disorders during childhood, carry the risk for a poor outcome of AN. However, a good parent–child relationship may protect the patient from a poor outcome.

Furthermore, the data clearly showed that chronicity of AN leads to poor outcome, a finding that implies that there are patients in whom treatment is refractory. Some studies provided evidence that the features of histrionic personality disorder indicate a favorable outcome. Furthermore, the features of coexisting obsessive–compulsive personality or compulsivity add to chronicity. In a recent 12-year course and outcome predictors analysis based on a parsimonious empirically based model, four predictors of outcome explaining 45% of the variance were identified—that is, sexual problems, impulsivity, long duration of inpatient treatment, and long duration of an eating disorder (Fichter, Quadflieg, & Hedlund, 2006). Clearly, chronicity is the major background factor in these findings. Finally, no definite conclusions can be drawn from the outcome studies as to the relevance of socioeconomic status.

Adolescent Patients

The outcome findings reported so far in the previous sections have mostly included the full age range at onset of the disorder. When only the adolescent age range at onset was considered in the analyses, it became clear that the course of the disorder in these young patients might be different from the course in patients with later onset of the disorder. The smaller series of young patients in my review of follow-up studies (Steinhausen, 2002) showed a less serious outcome, as compared with a mixed group of studies containing patients with either adolescent- or later-onset of AN. However, adolescent onset was not unequivocally supported as a favorable prognostic factor in all studies.

Some more recent findings based on the (so far) largest outcome study performed with patients who had an adolescent onset of AN provide additional new insights. Within the International Collaborative Outcome Study of Eating Disorders in Adolescence (ICOSEDA), my associates and I studied the clinical features, treatment, and outcome in consecutive cohorts of adolescent patients at five sites in the former West Berlin and East Berlin, Zurich, Sofia, and Bucharest (Steinhausen, Boyadjieva, Grigoroiu-Serbanescu, & Neumärker, 2003). All samples consisted of series of consecutively admitted patients who were initially seen in the 1980s and early 1990s at the five sites. All 338 patients fulfilled the criteria of the International Classification of Diseases (ICD-10) for the various forms of eating disorders. The samples were predominantly composed of patients with AN, with only the Berlin sample and the Zurich sample having 10% each of patients suffering from either BN or atypical eating disorders. Almost all of the patients were female (between 90 and 100%). The mean age at admission for the entire sample was 14.7 ($\pm$ 1.9 SD) years, and the mean age at onset of the disorder was 13.9 ($\pm$ 1.7 SD) years. It was impossible to reassess the whole cohort at follow-up so that extensive attrition analysis had to be performed. As a result of comparisons across 92 individual items, it was concluded that dropout was not due to any serious selection bias. The final follow-up sample constituted a total of 241 patients, which was reassessed with semistructured personal interviews at a mean age of 21.8 ($\pm$ 3.2 SD) years after a mean follow-up period of 6.4 ($\pm$ 3.0 SD) years.

In this collaborative study with quite diverse cultural sites and health systems, the provided treatment varied considerably both in terms of types of intervention and quantity of treatment. There were also some differences in outcome across sites, but these are not reported here. On average, the entire sample had spent 6% of the total follow-up period as inpatients and/or 23% as outpatients. Taken together, the total time spent in any form of treatment amounted to 30% of the entire follow-up period. Half of the sample required a second hospitalization, a quarter a third, 10% a fourth, and 5% a fifth hospitalization. Significant predictors of readmission were a combination of family psychopathology, history, and treatment variables, including paternal alcoholism, history of AN in the family, eating disorder in infancy, periodic overactivity, lower weight increase at first admission, and lower body mass index (BMI) at first discharge. Clearly, readmissions carried the risk for later poor psychosocial and psychiatric outcomes (Steinhausen, Grigoroiu-Serbanescu, Boyadjieva, Neumärker, & Winkler Metzke, 2008).

In this rather young ICOSEDA sample, the average crude mortality rate was only 2.9%, and thus was lower than calculated for the previously reported analysis of the literature, which was 5% (Steinhausen, 2002). The outcome of the eating disorder itself was also more favorable. About 80% of the sample had a normalization of the core symptoms weight, eating behavior, and menstruation at follow-up. On the diagnostic level, a total of 70% were free from any eating disorder, whereas 10% still suffered from AN and another 20% had either BN or an atypical eating disorder.

A good or fair psychosocial outcome was observed in a mean proportion of 71% of the former patients, with only a statistical trend for any differences across sites. Three-quarters of the entire sample did not have another psychiatric disorder at follow-up. These other psychiatric disorders in the sample were affective disorders (N = 25), obsessive–compulsive disorder (N = 8), anxiety disorder (N = 8), somatoform disorders (N = 9), substance abuse (N = 3), schizophrenia (N = 2), and other disorders (N = 21). Among those who had an eating disorder at follow-up, 40% also had an associated other psychiatric disorder. The outcome was worse if one combines the criteria. Only slightly more than half of the patients were free from both an eating disorder and any other psychiatric disorder. In considering the most complex outcome measure, that is, the combination of being free from an eating disorder and any other psychiatric disorder and enjoying a good or fair psychosocial outcome, then only half of the sample fulfilled this optimal criterion of mental health.

In addition to outcome, prognostic factors were also analyzed in the ICOSEDA. In contrast with previous studies, an exhaustive list of potential predictors of outcome was tested and various outcome criteria were considered. In addition, multiple regression analyses were performed in order to control for an overlap of prognostic factors and to identify the essential associations. In these extended analyses, only a few out of 17 predictors were significant. The BMI at follow-up was predicted by the BMI at initial assessment and treatment adherence (in terms of a negative association with rejection of premature termination of treatment). A more complex criterion, namely, an eating disorder score composed of five core symptoms (i.e., dieting, vomiting, bulimic episodes, laxative abuse, and menstruation) was more abnormal with longer duration of outpatient treatment and rejections of premature termination of treatments. The same two variables and a psychiatric disorder other than the eating disorder at follow-up jointly also predicted the total outcome score, which was composed of the eating disorder symptoms and five additional psychosocial items reflecting sexuality and the quality of social relationships (Steinhausen et al., 2003).

These findings clearly show that the consideration of a large list of prognostic factors in rather parsimonious analytical models resulted in only very few significant predictors of the outcome in this rather young sample of patients. Irrespective of the outcome criteria, the most consistent finding was the unfavorable role played by rejection or premature termination of treatment for the long-term course of the eating disorders. Second, the findings point to a treatment-refractory subgroup because the outcome deteriorated with increasing duration of outpatient treatment. Both findings are indicative of the pivotal function of treatment variables in the outcome of adolescent eating disorders.

There are a few more recent European outcome studies on adolescent patients supporting the general finding that the course of AN is more favorable in this young age group in comparison with older patients. In a controlled study in Germany with a prospective 10-year follow-up, 69% were fully recovered and none of the patients had died. However, half of the patients had an axis I disorder, whereas almost a quarter met the full criteria for a personality disorder, and depressive, anxious, and obsessive–compulsive features were more common in the long-term recovered patients than in the controls (Herpertz-Dahlmann et al., 2001; Holtkamp, Müller, Heussen, Remschmidt, & Herpertz-Dahlmann, 2005). Similarly, a 9-year follow-up study in Norway found a high recovery rate of 82% and no mortality but frequent axis I diagnoses at follow-up and substantially more internalizing problems in former patients than in their siblings (Halvorsen, Andersen, & Heyerdahl, 2004, 2005). A favorable outcome of adolescent-onset AN in terms of recovery was also reported in two studies from Sweden. However, these findings were associated with poor psychosocial outcomes, frequent depression, and other psychiatric problems in a sizeable proportion of the subjects (Ivarsson, Rastom, Wentz, Gillberg, & Gillberg, 2000; Nilsson & Hagglof, 2005; Wentz, Gillberg, Gillberg, & Rastam, 2001).

Conclusions

The analysis of a large body of follow-up studies leads to various conclusions as to the long-term course of AN. A first, rather general, conclusion has to emphasize that AN is a mental illness with a serious course and outcome in many of the afflicted individuals. This conclusion is based on the high crude mortality rate that increases with length of follow-up and is corroborated by an analysis of an almost 18-fold increase in mortality in patients with AN, including a high suicide rate (Nielsen et al., 1998) and other register-based findings of an increased rate of premature death due to AN (Birmingham, Su, Hlynsky, Goldner, & Gao, 2005; Millar et al., 2005). This conclusion is also supported by the high rate of chronic courses, which may be expected in approximately 20% of cases across all ages at onset of the disorder. The seriousness of the course of AN is further documented by the fact that at follow-up more than half of the patients showed either a complete or a partial eating disorder in combination with another psychiatric disorder or another psychiatric disorder without an eating disorder. A 40% probability of a comorbid mental disorder can be expected in the younger patients with an eating disorder at follow-up.

The second conclusion has to address the mitigating factors of the outcome of AN. Age at onset of the disorder and duration of follow-up are definitely important. Analyses based on the entire set of studies indicate that onset of the disorder during adolescence is associated with lower crude mortality rates and a better outcome of the eating disorder per se. However, there is a relatively high rate of other psychiatric disorders in former adolescent patients at follow-up. It is less certain whether other psychiatric disorders including comorbid disorder at follow-up occur at a lower rate than in patients who are older at onset of the disorder. The data based on comparable methods are simply lacking for this type of comparison. Furthermore, it must also be kept in mind that onset of AN before puberty has a very poor outcome, as shown in clinical reports (Russell, 1992).

The other mitigating factor, namely, duration of follow-up, shows a clear trend of an improved global outcome of AN with increasing course so that there is also substantial hope, even for persons with some rather complicated cases.

Third, there is only very limited knowledge of how intervention actually affects the course of AN. It may be that an early intervention, short duration of inpatient treatment, and adherence to the treatment program contribute to a more favorable prognosis. However, all these variables may only reflect more latent clinical factors in terms of severity of the disorder and patient characteristics. Clearly, the scarcity of controlled intervention studies with a sufficient duration of follow-up represents a major obstacle in the field of outcome research in AN. A notable exception is the Maudsley family therapy study with its documentation that treatment effects were kept at a 5-year follow-up (Eisler et al., 1997).

Finally, our understanding of the prognosis of AN has serious limitations. Quite obviously, vomiting, bulimia and purgative abuse, chronicity, and obsessive–compulsive features are unfavorable prognostic factors, whereas hysterical personality features are the only favorable prognostic factor that has been documented with very little conflicting evidence in the literature. However, the lack of replication of the factors in the data of the ICOSEDA data set for patients with adolescent onset and a rigorous control of overlapping effects of various prognostic factors asks for a more conservative interpretation. In the same way, the variability in findings on various other prognostic factors preclude any delineation of clear and simple rules as to the individual prognosis in a patient suffering from AN.

Despite the fact that more recent prospective outcome studies (Herzog et al., 1999; Steinhausen, Seidel, & Winkler Metzke, 2000; Strober, Freeman, & Morrell, 1997) have analyzed time trends of certain features of AN and thus focused more on the process rather than on the outcome, much has still to be learned about the continuity and discontinuity of AN and the factors influencing this process.

Bulimia Nervosa

The characteristic peak of onset of BN occurs in early adulthood. Thus, there is only a rather small body of literature on BN in adolescence. So far, separate follow-up studies on this group of young patients are completely missing. Furthermore, the available outcome studies do not allow the separation of findings that are relevant for adolescent patients only. Therefore, the following description reports findings on the course and prognosis of BN without consideration of separate age groups.

Natural Course

There are only a small series of longitudinal studies that have used either screening measures or a two-stage approach with a sequence of screening and interview that provide information on the natural history of BN. Several screening studies indicate that, in general, there is remarkable stability of symptoms and diagnoses over time (Drewnowski, Yee, & Krahn, 1988; Johnson, Tobin, & Lipkin, 1989; Patton, Coffey, & Sawyer, 2003; Steinhausen, Gavez, & Winkler Metzke, 2005; Striegel-Moore, Silberstein, Frensch, & Rodin 1989; Yager, Landsverk, & Edelstein, 1987).

Studies using the two-stage approach consolidate the impression of stability in the natural course of BN. In a consecutive series of adult patients who were attending a general practice, King (1989) found a high stability of diagnostic status at follow-up 12–18 months later. At the second follow-up 2–3 years after the first assessment (King, 1991), three out of five of the original patients were still diagnosed as suffering from BN, and there was little change in patients with the full syndrome of BN or in those with partial syndromes between the first and second follow-up. Lewinsohn and colleagues (2000) observed an increase of lifetime prevalence rates for BN of 0.8% in adolescence to 2.8% in young adulthood.

In a large sample of female adolescents Patton and colleagues (2003) diagnosed BN or partial syndromes and calculated a mean point prevalence rate for these two categories of 2.1% across the teens and 1.9% in young adulthood. Finally, Keller, Herzog, Lavori, Bradburn, and Mahoney (1992) also reported very high rates of chronicity, relapse recurrence, and psychosocial morbidity in 30 women with BN. Their findings show that almost one-third of the subjects remained in the index episode after entry into the study.

Intervention Effects on Course

There are various intervention studies in BN. In most of these studies there is a strong emphasis on treatment evaluation with rather short follow-up periods. The majority of studies, performed in the 1990s, compared different types of intervention. Both interpersonal therapy and cognitive-behavioral therapy were found superior to cognitive-behavioral therapy without cognitive components (Fairburn, Jones, Peveler, Hope, & O'Connor, 1993; Fairburn et al., 1995). Further studies proved that cognitive-behavioral therapy was superior to interpersonal therapy (Fairburn, Kirk, O'Connor, & Cooper, 1986; Wilson, Agras, Fairburn, Walsh, & Kraemer, 2002) or found no significant differences in the effects of either cognitive-behavioral therapy or the combination of cognitive-behavioral therapy and hypnotherapy (Griffiths, Channon-Little, & Hadzi-Pavlovic, 1995). In another study by Bailer and colleagues (2004), more patients became symptom-free with the use of a self-help manual rather than with cognitive-behavioral therapy. Even physical activity, but not diet counseling, has been shown superior to cognitive-behavioral therapy (Sundgot-Borgen, Rosenvinge, Bahr, & Sundgot-Schneider, 2002).

In a study on the optimization of cognitive-behavioral therapy (Treasure et al., 1996), one group used a self-help manual and additional cognitive-behavioral therapy if that was felt necessary. Another group of patients received cognitive-behavioral therapy only. There were no significant differences between the two approaches. In a study on the effectiveness of either the antidepressant fluoxetine or interpersonal therapy after a first inefficient phase of cognitive-behavioral therapy (Mitchell et al., 2002), no significant differences between the two approaches were found.

When comparing the effects of the antidepressant desipramine and cognitive-behavioral therapy, or a combination of both measures (Agras et al., 1994), cognitive-behavioral therapy or the combined intervention resulted in a stronger reduction of symptoms than pure antidepressant treatment after 24 weeks. Adding exposure with response prevention to cognitive-behavioral therapy did not result in improved results (Carter, McIntosh, Joyce, Sullivan, & Bulik, 2003). Another study (Laessle et al., 1991) revealed that in comparison with a coping with stress program, diet counseling led to a more rapid improvement of eating behavior and to reduction and abstinence of binge attacks.

Two studies on the effects of family therapy revealed controversial findings. In a study by Russell and colleagues (1987) it was found that family intervention was inferior to individual psychotherapy, whereas family therapy was shown to be superior in another study (Le Grange, Crosby, Rathouz, & Leventhal, 2007). No significant differences were found in the effectiveness of group versus individual psychotherapy (Nevonen & Broberg, 2006). Finally, a positive effect of control visits after treatment on the course of BN has been documented (Lacey, 1992).

In their meta-analysis of 26 studies on cognitive-behavioral therapy of BN, Lewandowski, Gebing, Anthony, and O'Brian (1997) revealed large effect sizes for both cognitive-behavioral and cognition-attitudinal outcome measures. However, follow-up effect sizes were less favorable and the diversity of time spans and outcome measures used to calculate follow-up effect sizes limited their utility.

Outcomes

So far, the most exhaustive review on the outcome of BN has been provided recently by Steinhausen and Weber (2009). In this review, a total of 79 patient samples entered into the analyses. Findings had been published between 1981 and 2007 in the English literature. The published reports were composed of 5,653 patients (group mean size = 71.6, SD = 113.4, range = 4–884) and there were considerable differences in design, group size, methods, duration of follow-up, and missing data. Diagnostic classification changed considerably over the period of the studies. Based on 46 studies containing 2,508 patients, mean age at onset was 17.2 (SD = 1.7, range = 14.3–23.2) years and mean age at follow-up was 28.4 (SD = 4.3, range = 16.6–38.0) years in 39 studies containing 2,478 patients. Mean duration of follow-up varied between 6 months and 12.5 years (mean = 3.2, SD = 3.3) in 77 studies containing 5,239 patients. In 66 studies containing 3,830 patients a total of 75 (1.9 %) males were included. Besides data on outcome, a total of 35 studies included information on prognostic factors and 14 studies dealt exclusively with prognostic factors.

The three-level classification of global outcome in terms of recovery, improvement, and chronicity was used in a total of 27 studies and was supplemented by the crossover rate in six studies. Based on this procedure, close to 45% of the patients on average showed full recovery from BN whereas 27% improved considerably and 23% had a chronic protracted course. In another 27 studies, only two outcome parameters were used. There were 19 studies that used recovery and chronicity supplemented by crossover to another eating disorder as an indicator of course of the disorder. In these studies, recovery increased to almost 60% on average, some 30% of the patients had a chronic course, and the remaining 10% were marked by a crossover to another eating disorder.

A further eight studies used a two-level classification and found a mean of 42% of the patients to be recovered and 41% to be improved. There was no information on crossover to another eating disorder and quite a substantial amount of missing outcome information in these studies. A single outcome criterion only was used in a further 25 studies. According to these studies, the mean recovery rate amounted to 42% in 15 studies, whereas the mean improvement rate was two-thirds in just two studies, and chronicity was 51% on average in eight studies. Eight among these studies provided additional information on crossover to another eating disorder, which was almost 32% on average.

Detailed information on crossover diagnoses was available in 23 studies. Among more than a fifth of the patients with crossover, a majority of 16% changed to eating disorders not otherwise specified (EDNOS), which in most cases was a subclinical manifestation of BN, and only some 6% of the patients developed the full clinical picture of AN. Only a few patients developed binge-eating disorders (BEDs). Mortality was reported in 76 studies, and there were 14 deaths among 4,309 patients, leading to a crude mortality rate of 0.32%.

Various comorbidities were present at follow-up. The former patients most frequently suffered from affective disorders (22.5%), followed by so-called neurotic disorders, including mostly anxiety disorders (16.2%). Unspecific personality disorders and/or borderline personality disorders (15.3%) were also quite frequent. Substance use disorders (7.3%) were less frequently seen, and obsessive–compulsive disorders (1%), schizophrenias, or psychoses (1%) were described only in a single study.

In accordance with previous analyses in AN (Steinhausen, 2002), the following effect variables were analyzed: dropout rate, duration of follow-up, and type of intervention. The dropout rate had a strong impact on rates of recovery and crossover of diagnoses. The rate of recovered patients at follow-up was lower with high dropout rates and the reverse was true for crossover. There was a medium effect size on improvement rate and no significant effect on chronicity.

Duration of follow-up was categorized as follows: (1) less than 4 years, (2) 4–9 years, and (3) 10 and more years. Studies with variable length of course were not considered for analyses of effects. In case there was more than one report based on the same cohort, only the last report with the longest duration of follow-up was considered for the analyses. The effect of duration of follow-up was most potent among the three effect variables. The effect size on recovery, chronicity, and crossover was strong, and it was medium on improvement. Post hoc comparisons indicated that the recovery rate was strongest after 4 years but less strong before, and later at 10 and more years, of the course of the disorder. The figures on improvement showed the highest rates before 4 years of follow-up, whereas the rate of chronic patients was also highest before 4 years of follow-up. A considerable number of crossover diagnoses were seen only in patients with a long-term follow-up beyond 10 years.

The third independent variable was type of intervention. Because of limited data, the classification had to be restricted to the following three types: (1) (nonbehavioral) psychotherapy, (2) (unspecified) medical therapy, and (3) (cognitive) behavioral therapy. The effects of intervention on outcome in a small sample of 10 patient series were strong. There was a clear gradient of effects on recovery, with psychotherapy ranking highest, followed by medical therapy and behavioral therapy. The gradient of recovery was just the reverse, and there was no real eminent difference in the proportion of chronic patients across intervention types, except that it was higher with behavioral therapy than with nonbehavioral psychotherapy. The effect of treatment type on chronicity was only weak. Crossover was observed most frequently with behavioral therapy, less frequently with medical therapy, and not with psychotherapy.

In addition to outcome, a large list of prognostic factors has been studied in BN. A detailed description is beyond the scope of this chapter. The review by Steinhausen and Weber (2009) describes the findings grouped into the following categories: specific characteristics of the disorder or the patients, history of the patients, family history and environment, social factors, and treatment factors. From these analyses it had to be concluded that the majority of these factors did not prove to have any significant effect on the disorder. Only few of the significant factors were replicated, and many studies even came up with controversial findings.

Conclusions

The understanding of the outcome of BN is severely hampered by a lack of commonly accepted outcome criteria. Different three-level or two-level classifications or single criteria have been used in the literature on the outcome of BN. Given the wide acceptance of the distinction between recovery, improvement, and chronicity as a classification of diseases in general and in the review on the course of AN in particular by Steinhausen (2002), findings based on this classification should be considered those with highest face validity. Thus, this classification was also used in the review by Steinhausen and Weber (2009) on the outcome of BN. Findings on mean recovery rates in BN (45%) and AN (46%) (Steinhausen, 2002) were remarkably similar. In addition, the mean improvement rates (27 vs. 33%) and the mean chronicity rates (23 vs. 20%) are not widely apart from each other in the two largest reviews. However, these figures represent only central trends and there is a large variation across studies in both reviews. Furthermore, the different criteria for outcome in the studies on the course of BN add to the uncertainty. Thus, studies relying on other schemes of classification resulted in higher or similar mean rates of recovery or higher mean rates of improvement and chronicity.

According to the recent review by Steinhausen and Weber (2009), crossover diagnoses in the course of BN are very common. However, again because of differences in the designs of the outcome studies, it is difficult to indicate precisely the mean rate of crossover diagnoses, which lies between a low of 10% and a high of 32%, depending on different criteria for outcome. Obviously, the most common crossover at follow-up has been to EDNOS, followed by AN, and the least to BED. However, the low rate of BED may be partially due to underreporting because the term was not yet introduced when many of the older outcome studies were performed.

Quite obviously, mortality rates differ markedly in the two eating disorders as calculated in the two major reviews by the author. With a mean crude mortality rate of 0.3%, including a number of deaths without any cause due to the basic disorder, BN is definitely a less fatal disorder than AN, with a mean crude mortality rate of 5%. However, the frequencies of comorbid psychiatric disorders are high in both disorders. Affective and neurotic/anxiety disorders ranked highest, and there was a sizeable proportion of patients with personality disorders at follow-up. Although the crude figures of comorbid disorders are even higher in AN, these differences should not be overestimated because many studies do not clearly indicate the criteria for assessment or diagnosis.

Based on the findings presented earlier, several conclusions may be drawn from the analyses of three central variables with an effect on outcome of BN. First, there is some evidence that, perhaps counter to expectation, patients who drop out from follow-up studies may have a more favorable course of BN. Staying in the follow-up cohort may reflect the patients' continuous need for further treatment. Thus, one might argue that the outcome of representative samples of patients without sample loss may even be more favorable than derived from the data thus far.

Second, duration of follow-up is the variable with the strongest impact on outcome. The distribution of data did not allow for a more fine-grained analysis, particularly before 4 years of follow-up. However, it seems that there is a curvilinear course of BN, particularly if one considers the curve of crossover diagnoses to be part of the chronic courses. Then it becomes obvious that the mean recovery rate peaks in the 4- to 9-year interval and declines thereafter, whereas the chronic plus crossover rates follow the reverse pattern and the rates of improvement remain relatively stable across time. According to these data, the developmental trajectory of BN is rather different from the course of AN, which shows a linear relationship indicating better outcome with increasing duration of follow-up (Steinhausen, 2002). However, it must be taken into consideration that all these data were derived from a composition of cross-sectional samples only. The few larger longitudinal BN outcome studies with repeated assessments over extended follow-up tend to provide a more favorable picture with increasing duration of follow-up (Fichter & Quadflieg, 2004; Herzog et al., 1999). These findings, however, may not be representative because they are based on patients who had been treated in clinical expert centers.

Third, the analyses of both effect variables and intervention studies allow conclusions on the role of treatment in BN. This is in contrast to the studies on AN including only a paucity of facts on the impact of interventions on outcome (Steinhausen, 2002). In the entire data set of studies on the outcome of BN there were strong effects indicating a clear superiority of psychotherapy over medical therapy and behavioral therapy. However, this finding is overshadowed by the lack of clear descriptions of the type and modalities of treatment that were employed in the various studies. Furthermore, because of methodological shortcomings and/or controversial findings, intervention studies provide only limited evidence of which treatments may actually contribute to a positive outcome. Standards of intervention studies, such as controlled randomization or a waiting control group, are almost entirely missing in the literature because of problems with clinical practicality. At least for cognitive-behavioral therapy, there is some limited evidence that it may contribute to more favorable outcomes for BN. Clearly, this field of research is in need of further, more sophisticated research.

Finally, there are a large number of studies dealing with prognostic factors in various domains. Despite the considerable effort that has been invested in this area of research, the majority of these factors did not prove to have any significant effect on the disorders. Information on prediction models, excluded variables, or nonsignificant factors was mostly missing in the reports. Most frequently, prognostic factors were seen in isolation. In the outcome literature on AN, it has been shown that favorable, unfavorable, or nonsignificant prognostic factors may be extracted from the various study reports (Steinhausen, 2002). However, multivariate analyses with consideration of a large group of factors in a large sample of patients with AN have clearly shown that very few variables really have an effect on outcome if their covariation is considered (Steinhausen et al., 2003). Thus, most of the findings on prognostic factors in BN must be considered as insufficiently controlled. Certainly, this field is also in need of further refinement of research. On the basis of the existing literature, a concentration on treatment factors seems most promising. However, one has to consider the likely nature of study data that preclude any delineation of rules as to an individual prognosis in a given patient.

Acknowledgments

This chapter is based in part on two updated reviews by the author (Steinhausen, 2002; Steinhausen & Weber 2009).

References

Agras, W. S., Rossiter, E. M., Arnow, B., Telch, C. F., Raeburn, S. D., Bruce, B., et al. 1994). One-year follow-up of psychosocial and pharmacologic treatments for bulimia nervosa. *Journal of Clinical Psychiatry, 55,* 179–183.

Bailer, U., de Zwaan, M., Leisch, F., Strnad, A., Lennkh-Wolfsberg, C., El-Giamal, N., et al.

(2004). Guided self-help versus cognitive-behavioural group therapy in the treatment of bulimia nervosa. *International Journal of Eating Disorders, 35*, 522–537.

Bemis, K. M. (1987). The present status of operant conditioning for the treatment of anorexia nervosa. *Behavior Modification, 11*, 432–463.

Birmingham, C. L., Su, J., Hlynsky, J. A., Goldner, E. M., & Gao, M. (2005). The mortality rate from anorexia nervosa. *International Journal of Eating Disorders, 38*(2), 143–146.

Carter, F. A., McIntosh, V. V., Joyce, P. R., Sullivan, P. F., & Bulik, C. M. (2003). Role exposure with response prevention in cognitive-behavioral therapy for bulimia nervosa: Three-year follow-up results. *International Journal of Eating Disorders, 33*, 127–135.

Crisp, A. H., Norton, K., Gowers, S., Halek, C., Bowyer, C., Yeldhau, D., et al. (1997). A controlled study of the effects of therapies aimed at adolescent and family psychopathology in anorexia nervosa. *British Journal of Psychiatry, 159*, 325–333.

Drewnowski, A., Yee, D. K., & Krahn, D. D. (1988). Bulimia in college women—Incidence and recovery rates. *American Journal of Psychiatry, 145*, 733–735.

Eisler, I., Dare, C., Hodes, M., Russell, G., Dodge, E., & Le Grange, D. (2000). Family therapy for adolescent anorexia nervosa: The results of a controlled comparison of two family interventions. *Journal of Child Psychology and Psychiatry, 41*(6), 727–736.

Eisler, I., Dare, C., Russell, G. F., Szmukler, G., Le Grange, D., & Dodge, E. (1997). Family and individual therapy in anorexia nervosa: A 5-year follow- up. *Archives of General Psychiatry, 54*(11), 1025–1030.

Fairburn, C. G., Jones, R., Peveler, R. C., Hope, R. A., & O'Connor, M. E. (1993). Psychotherapy and bulimia nervosa: Longer-term effects of interpersonal psychotherapy, behavior therapy and cognitive behavior therapy. *Archives of General Psychiatry, 50*, 419–428.

Fairburn, C. G., Kirk, J., O'Connor, M. E., & Cooper, P. J. (1986). A comparison of two psychological treatments for bulimia nervosa. *Behavior Research and Therapy, 24*, 629–643.

Fairburn, C. G., Norman, P. A., Welch, S. L., O'Connor, M. E., Doll, H. A., & Peveler, R. C. (1995). A prospective study of outcome in bulimia nervosa and the long-term effects of three psychological treatments. *Archives of General Psychiatry, 52*, 304–312.

Fichter, M. M., & Quadflieg, N. (2004). Twelve-year course and outcome of bulimia nervosa. *Psychological Medicine, 34*, 1395–1406.

Fichter, M. M., Quadflieg, N., & Hedlund, S. (2006). Twelve-year course and outcome predictors of anorexia nervosa. *International Journal of Eating Disorders, 39*(2), 87–100.

Griffiths, R., Channon-Little, L., & Hadzi-Pavlovic, D. (1995). Hypnotizablility and outcome in the treatment of bulimia nervosa. *Contemporary Hypnosis, 2*, 165–172.

Halvorsen, I., Andersen, A., & Heyerdahl, S. (2004). Good outcome of adolescent onset anorexia nervosa after systematic treatment: Intermediate to long-term follow-up of a representative county-sample. *European Child and Adolescent Psychiatry, 13*(5), 295–306.

Halvorsen, I., Andersen, A., & Heyerdahl, S.(2005). Girls with anorexia nervosa as young adults: Self-reported and parent-reported emotional and behavioural problems compared with siblings. *European Child and Adolescent Psychiatry, 14*(7), 397–406.

Heebink, D. M., & Halmi, K. A. (1995). Psychopharmacology in adolescents with eating disorders. In H.-C. Steinhausen (Ed.), *Eating disorders in adolescence* (pp. 271–286). Berlin, New York: Walter de Gruyter.

Herpertz-Dahlmann, B., Müller, B., Herpertz, S., Heussen, N., Hebebrand, J., & Remschmidt, H. (2001). Prospective 10-year follow-up in adolescent anorexia nervosa: Course, outcome, psychiatric comorbidity, and psychosocial adaptation. *Journal of Child Psychology and Psychiatry, 42*(5), 603–612.

Herzog, D. B., Dorrer, D., Keel, P. K., Selwyn, S. E., Ekeblad, E., Flores, A. T., et al. (1999). Recovery and relapse in anorexia and bulimia nervosa: A 7.5-year follow-up study. *Journal of the American Academy of Child and Adolescent Psychiatry, 38*, 829–837.

Holtkamp, K., Müller, B., Heussen, N., Remschmidt, H., & Herpertz-Dahlmann, B. (2005). Depression, anxiety, and obsessionality in long-term recovered patients with adolescent-onset anorexia nervosa. *European Child and Adolescent Psychiatry, 14*(2), 106–110.

Ivarsson, T., Rastom, M., Wentz, E., Gillberg, I. C., & Gillberg, C. (2000). Depressive disorders in teenage-onset anorexia nervosa: A controlled longitudinal, partly community-based study. *Comprehensive Psychiatry, 41*(5), 398–403.

Johnson, C., Tobin, D. L., & Lipkin, J. (1989). Epidemiologic changes in bulimic behaviour among female adolescents over a five-year period. *International Journal of Eating Disorders, 8*, 647–655.

Keller, M. B., Herzog, D. B., Lavori, P. W., Bradburn, I. S., & Mahoney, E. S. (1992). The naturalistic history of bulimia nervosa: Extraordinarily high rates of chronicity, elapse, recurrence, and psychosocial morbidity. *International Journal of Eating Disorders, 12*(1), 1–9.

King, M. B. (1989). Eating disorders in a general practice population: Prevalence, characteristics and follow-up at 18 months. *Psychological Medicine, 14*(Monograph Suppl.), 1–34.

King, M. B. (1991). The natural history of eating pathology in attenders to primary medical care. *International Journal of Eating Disorders, 10*, 379–388.

Kotler, L. A., & Walsh, B. T. (2000). Eating disorders in children and adolescents: Pharmacological therapies. *European Child and Adolescent Psychiatry, 9*(Suppl.1), I108–I116.

Lacey, J. H. (1992). Long-term follow-up of bulimic patients treated in integrated behavioural and psychodynamic treatment programmes. In W. Herzog, H. C. Deter, & W. Vandereycken (Eds.), *The course of eating disorders: Long-term follow-up studies of anorexia and bulimia nervosa* (pp. 150–173). Berlin: Springer.

Laessle, R. G., Beumont, P. J. V., Butow, P., Lennerts, W., O'Connor, M. E, Pirke, K. M., et al. (1991). A comparison of nutritional management with stress management in the treatment of bulimia nervosa. *British Journal of Psychiatry, 159*, 250–261.

Le Grange, D., Crosby, R. D., Rathouz, P. J.,

& Leventhal, B. L. (2007). A randomized controlled comparison of family-based treatment and supportive psychotherapy for adolescent bulimia nervosa. *Archives of General Psychiatry, 64*, 1049–1056.

Lewandowski, L. M., Gebing, T. A., Anthony, J. L., & O'Brian, W. H. (1997). Meta-analysis of cognitive-behavioral treatment studies for bulimia. *Clinical Psychology Review, 17*(7), 703–718.

Lewinsohn, P. M., Striegel-Moore, R. H., & Seeley, J. R. (2000). Epidemiology and natural course of eating disorders in young women from adolescence to young adulthood. *Journal of the Academy of Child and Adolescent Psychiatry, 39*, 1284–1292.

Millar, H. R., Wardell, F., Vyvyan, J. P., Naji, S. A., Prescott, G. J., & Eagles, J. M. (2005). Anorexia nervosa mortality in Northeast Scotland, 1965–1999. *American Journal of Psychiatry, 162*(4), 753–757.

Mitchell, J. E., Halmi, K., Wilson, G. T., Agras, W. S., Kraemer, H., & Crow, S. J. (2002). A randomized secondary treatment study of women with bulimia nervosa who fail to respond to CBT. *International Journal of Eating Disorders, 32*, 271–281.

Mitchell, J. E., Peterson, G. B., Myers, T., & Wonderlich, S. (2001). Combining pharmacotherapy and psychotherapy in the treatment of patients with eating disorders. *Psychiatric Clinics of North America, 24*, 315–323.

Nevonen, L., & Broberg, A. G. (2006). A comparison of sequenced individual and group psychotherapy for patients with bulimia nervosa. *International Journal of Eating Disorders, 39*, 117–127.

Nielsen, S., Møller-Madsen, S., Isager, T., Jørgensen, J., Pagsberg, K., & Theander, S. (1998). Standardized mortality in eating disorders: A quantitative summary of previously published and new evidence. *Journal of Psychosomatic Research, 44*(3–4), 413–434.

Nilsson, K., & Hagglof, B. (2005). Long-term follow-up of adolescent onset anorexia nervosa in Northern Sweden. *European Eating Disorders Review, 13*, 89–100.

Patton, G. C., Coffey, C., & Sawyer, S. M. (2003). The outcome of adolescent eating disorders: Findings from the Victorian adolescent health cohort study. *European*

Child and Adolescent Psychiatry, 12(Suppl. 1), 25–29.

Rathner, G. (1992). Aspects of the natural history of normal and disordered eating and some methodological considerations. In W. Herzog, H.-C. Deter, & W. Vandereycken (Eds.), *The course of eating disorders: Long-term follow-up studies of anorexia and bulimia nervosa* (pp. 273–303). Berlin: Springer.

Robin, A. L., Siegel, P. T., Koepke, T., Moye, A. W., & Tice, S. (1994). Family therapy versus individual therapy for adolescent females with anorexia nervosa. *Journal of Developmental and Behavioral Pediatrics, 15*(2), 111–116.

Robin, A. L., Siegel, P. T., & Moye, A. (1995). Family versus individual therapy for anorexia: Impact on family conflict. *International Journal of Eating Disorders, 17*(4), 313–322.

Russell, G. (1992). Anorexia nervosa of early onset and its impact on puberty. In P. J. Cooper & A. Stein (Eds.), *Feeding problems and eating disorders in children and adolescents* (pp. 85–112). Philadelphia: Harwood Academic.

Russell, G. F. M., Szmukler, G. I., Dare, C., & Eisler, I. (1987). An evaluation of family therapy in anorexia nervosa and bulimia nervosa. *Archives of General Psychiatry, 44*, 1047–1056.

Steinhausen, H.-C. (2002). The outcome of anorexia nervosa in the twentieth century. *Amercan Journal of Psychiatry, 159*, 1284–1293.

Steinhausen, H.-C., Boyadjieva, S., Griogoroiu-Serbanescu, M., & Neumärker, K.-J. (2003). The outcome of adolescent eating disorders: Findings from an international collaborative study. In K.-J. Neumärker & H.-C. Steinhausen (Eds.), *Eating disorders in young people. European Child and Adolescent Psychiatry, 12*(Suppl. 1), 91–98.

Steinhausen, H.-C., Gavez, S., & Winkler Metzke, C. (2005). Psychosocial correlates, outcome, and stability of abnormal adolescent eating behavior in community samples of young people. *International Journal of Eating Disorders, 37*, 1–8.

Steinhausen, H.-C., Grigoroiu-Serbanescu, M., Boyadjieva, S., Neumärker, K.-J., & Winkler Metzke, C. (2008). Course and predictors of rehospitalization in adolescent anorexia nervosa in a multisite study. *International Journal of Eating Disorders, 41*(1), 29–36.

Steinhausen, H.-C., Seidel, R., & Winkler Metzke, C. (2000). Evaluation of treatment and intermediate and long-term outcome of adolescent eating disorder. *Psychosomatic Medicine, 30*, 1089–1098.

Steinhausen, H.-C., & Weber, S. (2009). The outcome of bulimia nervosa: Findings from a quarter of a century of research. *American Journal of Psychiatry, 166*, 1331–1341.

Striegel-Moore, R. H., Silberstein, L. R., Frensch, P., & Rodin, J. (1989). A prospective study of disordered eating among college students. *International Journal of Eating Disorders, 8*(5), 523–532.

Strober, M., Freeman, R., & Morrell, W. (1997). The long-term course of severe anorexia nervosa in adolescents: Survival analysis of recovery, relapse, and outcome predictors over 10–15 years in a prospective study. *International Journal of Eating Disorders, 22*, 339–360.

Sundgot-Borgen, J., Rosenvinge, J. H., Bahr, R., & Sundgot-Schneider, L. (2002). The effect of exercise, cognitive therapy and nutritional counseling in treating bulimia nervosa. *Medicine and Science in Sports and Exercise, 34*, 190–194.

Treasure, J., Schmidt, U., Troop, N., Tiller, J., Todd, G., & Turnbull, S. (1996). Sequential treatment for bulimia nervosa incorporating a self-care manual. *British Journal of Psychiatry, 168*, 94–98.

Wentz, E., Gillberg, C., Gillberg, I. C., & Rastam, M. (2001). Ten-year follow-up of adolescent-onset anorexia nervosa: Psychiatric disorders and overall functioning scales. *Journal of Child Psychology and Psychiatry, 42*(5), 613–622.

Wilson, G. T., Agras, W. S., Fairburn, C. G., Walsh, B. T., & Kraemer, H. (2002). Cognitive-behavioral therapy for bulimia nervosa: Time course and mechanisms of change. *Journal of Consulting and Clinical Psychology, 70*, 267–274.

Yager, J., Landsverk, J., & Edelstein, C. K. (1987). A 20-month follow-up study of 628 women with eating disorders: I. Course and severity. *American Journal of Psychiatry, 144*, 86–94.

PART III

DIAGNOSIS AND CLASSIFICATION

CHAPTER 7

Diagnosis and Classification of Disordered Eating in Childhood

Rachel Bryant-Waugh
Dasha Nicholls

In this chapter we focus on issues related to the diagnosis and classification of disordered feeding and eating in children below the age of 13. Consistent with the wider focus of this book, our attention is primarily directed to presentations of disordered feeding or eating, conceptualized as behavioral or mental disorders, rather than eating difficulties that result directly from a medical condition. We start by making some general comments about feeding and eating in childhood, moving on to a discussion of the current state of play with regard to diagnosis and classification of childhood feeding and eating disorders. We refer to the main feeding and eating disturbances described in the literature and discuss current difficulties in matching presentations seen in clinical practice with existing diagnostic categories. At the time of writing, revisions are in progress to the two main diagnostic systems used by mental health professionals (DSM-IV-TR [American Psychiatric Association, 2000]; ICD-10 [World Health Organization, 1992]), with scheduled publication dates of 2013 and 2015 for DSM-5 and ICD-11, respectively. In line with these efforts, there has been a recent increase in discussion and debate about a number of issues relating to classification and diagnosis, including those relevant to childhood presentations. We include in this chapter mention of what we regard as the main pertinent issues to emerge in this respect, and by doing so aim to inform the reader of possible future directions and developments.

Background

Before addressing the diagnosis and classification of disordered eating in childhood it is important to consider the question, What is normal feeding and eating? Although there has been a considerable amount of research into factors that influence and shape children's eating behaviors in general (e.g., Kral & Rauh, 2010; Pearson, Biddle, & Gorely, 2009; Wardle, Carnell, & Cooke, 2005), as well as studies of factors affecting weight gain and growth (e.g., Birch & Davison, 2001; Scaglioni, Salvioni, & Galimberti, 2008), there is a surprisingly limited amount of data available on the eating patterns of ordinary children, that is, children not seen in clinical settings (Nicklas et al., 2004; Popkin & Duffey, 2010). Typically, people hold idiosyncratic and often strong views about what constitutes "normal" eating, usually influenced by their own experiences and upbringing. Parents of children with problem eating often describe having had to endure the opinions of well-meaning friends and relatives about how their child "should" be eating. Equally, in our experience, some clinicians promote passionately held views about children's eating behavior, or objectives to be reached, without much in the way of research evidence to back up their opinions. Being clear about "normal" childhood eating as a basis for establishing what might be abnormal or disordered is not straightforward.

Normal, that is, unproblematic, feeding and eating depends on the successful integration of a number of physiological systems and areas of function. A biopsychosocial model to understand the complex interplay of factors is relevant, as problem-free childhood eating relies on the successful integration of aspects of both physical and psychological functions (to include behavioral, emotional, and cognitive factors) as well as on aspects of interpersonal relationships. It is perhaps unsurprising that early in life mild to moderate feeding problems are relatively common, given the complexity of the task and the need for feeding behavior to become established, to develop, and to adapt in an interpersonal context.

An additional consideration is that many eating behaviors in childhood experienced as problematic by parents or caregivers are relatively common, developmentally normal, and usually transient. Most are mild, but some become chronic and clinically significant. Some eating behaviors are normal at certain developmental stages, but less so at others—for example, a wariness and avoidance of new foods is developmentally normal in toddlers (Birch 1998), but food neophobia in a child of age 10 or 11 is likely to be more problematic. At present there is little to alert the clinician to combinations of presenting features that may suggest a poorer prognosis, so important opportunities for preventative intervention may be missed.

It is therefore difficult to settle on a definition of "normal eating" in childhood, but for the purposes of this chapter we propose that it might be understood as feeding or eating consistent with the child's growing, developing, and functioning at an appropriate developmental level. By implication, problem or disordered feeding or eating could then be defined as feeding or eating patterns or behaviors that result in disruption to expected growth, development, and/or functioning. In practice, and consistent with this broad definition, issues that cause concern and lead to clinical presentation vary, including feeding or eating patterns and behaviors associated with impairment to physical function or that cause physical harm (examples include disordered eating resulting in growth delay where overall energy intake is consistently low, or resulting in a specific nutritional deficiency such as iron deficiency anemia where there is a very restricted range of accepted foods); concerns and difficulties about eating that cause the child distress (examples include presentations where the child is fearful of certain foods and avoids them at all costs, or where significant and distressing shame and embarrassment is experienced because of being restricted to age-inappropriate foods); and situations in which the child's eating significantly interferes with family life (examples include families being unable to eat out together, or where there is significant parental disagreement about how to manage the child's difficulty, associated with conflict and family discord).

Ruling out direct medical causes (such as inadequate swallow function, gastroesophageal reflux, or other medical conditions that may directly account for an eating problem at the time of presentation), we generally find it helpful to assess four clear areas of risk in determining whether a child has a clinically significant eating problem:

- Nutritional adequacy of diet—Is the child at short- and/or longer-term physical risk if current nutritional intake continues?
- Impact of feeding/eating disturbance on weight, growth, and physical development/function—Is overall intake insufficient to sustain healthy growth and weight gain? Is the texture or type of diet holding the child back in terms of developing appropriate biting and chewing skills?
- Impact of feeding/eating disturbance on social and emotional development/function—Is the child refusing to mix with peers at mealtimes or missing out on social occasions? Is the child experiencing increasing anxiety or distress in relation to his or her eating problems?
- Impact of feeding/eating disturbance on interaction with caregiver and family function—Is there a breakdown in relationships in the family concerning food and eating? Are caregivers unable to agree about management, thus contributing to family tension and conflict?

In our experience if one of these factors is present, there is sufficient justification to intervene and to regard the eating disturbance as clinically significant. Again, however, there is surprisingly little literature on the long-term impact of highly restricted diets and few long-term follow-up studies of feeding problems from which to gauge the risk of significant harm (Mikkilä et al., 2007; Moore et al., 2005).

Returning to the issue of what constitutes disordered eating, another important factor for consideration is whether parental perception of an eating problem is consistent with clinical opinion. This is not always the case, and there has been some debate about the importance (or otherwise) of the discrepancy between parental perception and report of an eating problem and clinical opinion or objective measurement of the eating difficulty. There has to date been limited research in this area, which in turn has been limited to exploring specific types of problem feeding behavior only. For example, a well-designed prospective study of 135 children aiming to validate parental reports of picky eating by using objective measures found that picky eating reported by parents was indeed associated with a consistent pattern of limited eating starting in infancy (Jacobi, Agras, Bryson, & Hammer, 2003). Important considerations in the debate about the significance of a discrepancy in perception between parents and clinicians include the fact that a wide range of variables unrelated to the child have been shown to be linked to the likelihood of parents viewing their child as having a feeding or eating problem. For example, in a longitudinal study of 99 women by Farrow and Blissett (2006), maternal reports of feeding difficulties were predicted by certain maternal core beliefs during pregnancy, and self-esteem and social isolation beliefs postnatally were also found to contribute significantly to maternal reports of problem feeding. These authors furthermore demonstrated that although a correlation was found between maternal reports of feeding problems and the observations of the research team, correlation coefficients were relatively weak, and that maternal core beliefs and level of self-esteem failed to significantly predict independent observations of feeding problems.

Another important consideration includes the common observation that parental behaviors such as mealtime management are affected by a perception of the child's having an eating problem (which in turn can affect the child's eating behavior) and difficulties in objective measurement of childhood eating problems generally. The few available standardized assessment measures relating to eating attitudes and behaviors of children ages 0–12 years tend to rely on parent report, with only a few studies reporting direct observational measures (e.g., Ammaniti, Ambruzzi, Lucarelli, Cimino, & D'Olimpio, 2004). In clinical practice, we may consider it appropriate to intervene in a situation where we do not think that the child at the time of presentation has a severe feeding or eating difficulty but where parental anxiety is extremely high and associated parental management strategies appear likely to exacerbate the difficulty. Thus we would regard it sensible to both take account of parental perception of the nature and severity of the eating problem and form our own clinical opinion in this regard, recognizing that the former might well influence the interaction around food between parents and child and in this way is relevant to clinical consideration of a child's eating. Coming back to implications for diagnosis and the determination of when a child has a "disorder," this highlights why there have been calls to reconsider the diagnosis of feeding problems in children in an interpersonal context (Davies et al., 2006).

We have mentioned that childhood eating can usefully be understood within a biopsychosocial model comprising physical, psychological, and interactional domains. Given that these domains are interrelated and that difficulties can arise in one or more concurrently, it is perhaps not difficult to see why children with eating problems tend to be seen for treatment by a relatively wide range of clinical services and professionals. Clinics for children with feeding and eating problems are commonly led by pediatric gastroenterologists, speech/language pathologists, dietitians, or mental health professionals, and most are multidisciplinary in terms of team composition. The focus of assessment and intervention tends to vary between clinics with three main areas of interest: those with an emphasis on the management of underlying or associated medical conditions; those focusing on oral/motor skills and/or swallow function; and those working with emotional, behavioral, and interactional aspects of eating difficulties.

Irrespective of the main focus of assessment and management within different clinics, multidisciplinary team composition is very helpful because of the complex integration of systems and functions required to sustain normal, developing eating patterns and behaviors. However, in relation to diagnosis and classification of childhood feeding and eating disturbances, the fact that children may have been seen by a number of different professionals has inevitably contributed to a lack of consistency in terminology and classification, which in turn has, in our view, had a negative effect on treatment and outcome research.

To summarize, in this section we have raised a number of issues, each of which is relevant to a consideration of the diagnosis and classification of disordered eating in childhood:

- It is difficult to be clear as to what constitutes "normal" childhood eating, and there are limited data to help define the edges of a disorder, or "caseness."
- We have suggested that a biopsychosocial model is needed to understand the complex interplay of factors related to the establishment and maintenance of normal feeding and eating in childhood. This can make it difficult to locate some forms of eating disturbance solely in the child as a behavioral or mental disorder, even

when there is an absence of a medical condition that might directly account for the eating difficulty at the time of presentation.

- We have considered the fact that childhood eating patterns or behaviors experienced by parents as problematic might be developmentally normal and short-lived, and reflected that it can be difficult to tell at the time of presentation which might become chronic or severe.
- We have suggested a working definition for "problem" or "disordered eating" in childhood (i.e., feeding or eating patterns or behaviors that result in disruption to expected growth, development, and/or functioning) and have suggested that four main domains might usefully be considered by clinicians in determining the clinical significance of and need to intervene in a presentation of problem eating: nutritional adequacy of intake; impact of feeding/eating disturbance on weight, growth, and physical development/function; impact of feeding/eating disturbance on social and emotional development/function; impact of feeding/eating disturbance on interaction with caregiver and family functioning.
- We have considered the importance of a discrepancy between parental and clinician views about the nature and severity of the eating problem and have suggested that both need to be taken into account, as parental perception might directly influence the child's eating.
- Finally, we have referred to the fact that children with eating difficulties are seen in a range of different settings by different professionals and suggested that this has contributed to a wide array of descriptive and diagnostic terms being used, often for very similar presentations.

Current Diagnostic Categories for Childhood Feeding and Eating Disturbances

In this section we consider the main published diagnostic systems with available categories for classifying disordered eating in childhood. As well as making reference to the current DSM-IV-TR and ICD-10 systems, we have included others that we believe to be of relevance to mental health professionals working in pediatric settings (e.g., DC:0–3R [Zero to Three, 2005]); Rome III criteria (Drossman et al., 2006)). These other systems are perhaps not usually discussed in relation to diagnosis and classification of eating disorders in older populations. However, there are a number of reasons why we consider it appropriate to discuss them here: boundaries between somatic and psychological aspects of presentation are often blurred in younger patients; there are well-recognized arguments for the need for developmentally based approaches to the classification of behavioral, developmental, and mental health difficulties in the early years; and we still have a long way to go in elucidating and understanding the links and pathways between early feeding problems, childhood eating disturbances, and eating disorders in adolescence and adulthood. Mental health practitioners seeing the full range of disordered eating presentations in childhood and researchers interested in this age group, arguably, need to have an awareness of a range of relevant classification strategies.

Turning first to the two main diagnostic systems used by mental health practitioners, current categories for eating disturbances as mental or behavioral disorders are limited to:

- In DSM-IV-TR (American Psychiatric Association, 2000):
  - o *Eating disorders*: anorexia nervosa 307.1; bulimia nervosa 307.51; eating disorder not otherwise specified 307.50.
  - o *Feeding and eating disorders of infancy or early childhood*: pica 307.52; rumination disorder 307.53; feeding disorder of infancy or early childhood 307.59.
- In ICD-10 (World Health Organization, 1992):
  - o *Eating disorders* (F50)—in the section "Behavioural syndromes associated with physiological disturbances and physical factors": anorexia nervosa F50.0; atypical anorexia nervosa F50.1; bulimia nervosa F50.2; atypical bulimia nervosa F50.3; overeating associated with other psychological disturbance F50.4; vomiting associated with other psychological disturbance F50.5; other eating disorder F50.8; eating disorder, unspecified F50.9.
  - o *Other behavioural and emotional disorders with onset usually occurring in childhood and adolescence* (F98)—in the section "Behavioural and emotional disorders with onset usually occurring in childhood and adolescence": feeding disorder of infancy and childhood F98.2; pica of infancy and childhood F98.3.

Thus the two main diagnostic systems allow for diagnosis of childhood presentations of anorexia nervosa (AN), bulimia nervosa (BN) and variants of these; of broadly defined feeding disorders characterized by poor weight gain; and of pica and rumination disorder. (*Note:* ICD-10 also has categories for childhood feeding and eating problems *not* classified as behavioral or mental disorders; these are mentioned later in this section.) However, there are many other presentations that are familiar to clinicians working in pediatric mental health settings that currently do not fit well within these options. In addition, there has been a strongly held view that the two main systems are problematic in relation to psychiatric presentations in very young children, thus leading to the development of alternative diagnostic classification systems for psychiatric disorders in preschool children (Postert, Averbeck-Holocher, Beyer, Müller, & Furniss, 2009). For the sake of completeness in this discussion of feeding and eating disorders in childhood it is therefore important to include two further classification systems: "Zero to Three," commonly identified as DC:0–3R, which is a diagnostic classification system of mental health and developmental disorders of infancy and early childhood (Zero to Three, 2005); and Research Diagnostic Criteria—Preschool Age (RDC-PA), which attempts to set out clear, developmentally appropriate criteria to guide diagnosis of psychiatric disorders in children from 0 to 5 years of age (Task Force on Research Diagnostic Criteria: Infancy and Preschool, 2003). The original Zero to Three criteria were published in 1994, but were thought to lack the operationalized criteria required for reliable research investigations. This led to the publication of RDC-PA in 2003, which in turn contributed to the revised version of Zero to Three published in 2005. Both RDC-PA and DC:0–3R are intended to complement rather than replace DSM and ICD systems, and both provide separate criteria for six subcategories of feeding disorder as follows:

- In DC:0–3R (Zero to Three, 2005):
  - o *Feeding behavior disorder*: feeding disorder of state regulation; feeding disorder of caregiver–infant reciprocity; infantile anorexia; sensory food aversions; feeding disorder associated with concurrent medical condition; feeding disorder associated with insults to the gastrointestinal tract.

- In RDC-PA (Task Force on Research Diagnostic Criteria: Infancy and Preschool, 2003):
  - *Feeding and eating disorders of infancy or early childhood*: feeding disorder of state regulation; feeding disorder of caregiver–infant reciprocity; infantile anorexia; sensory food aversions; feeding disorder associated with concurrent medical condition; posttraumatic feeding disorder.

These subclassifications of psychiatric feeding disorders in infants and younger children are of relevance to a consideration of disordered eating in middle childhood, as some of the presentations described in this older age range, such as selective eating (Nicholls, Christie, Randall, & Lask, 2001), food avoidance emotional disorder (Higgs, Goodyer, & Birch, 1989), and functional dysphagia (Nicholls & Bryant-Waugh, 2009) appear to be similar to the subcategories outlined in DC:0–3R and RDC-PA and may differ only in developmental expression (in the three examples given there are similarities to sensory food aversions, infantile anorexia, and posttraumatic feeding disorder, respectively). In turn, this is of relevance to this book on eating disorders, as such presentations are currently diagnosed by some clinicians as eating disorder not otherwise specified (EDNOS).

One other published classification system deserves mention here, namely, the Rome III Diagnostic Criteria for Functional Gastrointestinal Disorders (Drossman et al., 2006). These criteria have been drawn up by the Rome Foundation and represent an international collaborative effort to classify "functional" gastrointestinal disorders (FGIDs). Unlike DSM-IV-TR, DC:0–3R, and RDC-PA, Rome III is not a classification scheme for psychiatric disorders, but a classification scheme for gastrointestinal (GI) disorders, that is, disorders expressed physically and presenting to physicians, where no obvious organic cause can be determined. As we have argued earlier, and as is increasingly accepted in wider clinical practice, there is a general shift away from biomedical reductionism and Cartesian mind–body dualism toward biopsychosocial models of illness and disease, and the Rome criteria have been conceptualized and developed in line with this trend. The first Rome criteria were published in 1989, with pediatric criteria added in the second and third versions. Although these criteria are not specifically for eating disturbances, there is an overlap between some of the presentations they cover and presentations seen in pediatric mental health settings for children's eating disturbances. Rome III currently includes the following categories relevant to children:

- *G. Childhood functional GI disorders: infant/toddler*: G1 infant regurgitation; G2 infant rumination syndrome; G3 cyclic vomiting syndrome; G4 infant colic; G5 functional diarrhea; G6 infant dyschezia; G7 functional constipation.
- *H. Childhood functional GI disorders: child/adolescent*: H1 vomiting and aerophagia (H1a adolescent rumination syndrome; H1b cyclic vomiting syndrome; H1c aerophagia); H2 abdominal pain related functional GI disorders (H2a functional dyspepsia; H2b irritable bowel syndrome; H2c abdominal migraine; H2d childhood functional abdominal pain; H2d1 childhood functional abdominal pain syndrome); H3 constipation and incontinence (H3a functional constipation; H3b nonretentive fecal incontinence).

Diagnostic categories of particular interest in the discussion in this chapter are functional dyspepsia and the childhood functional abdominal pain categories. A diagnosis of functional dyspepsia requires persistent or recurrent pain or discomfort in the upper abdomen, and childhood functional abdominal pain requires episodic or continuous abdominal pain. In childhood functional abdominal pain syndrome, this is associated with some loss of daily function and additional somatic symptoms such as sleep problems or headaches. Children presenting with eating disturbances in pediatric mental health settings might well give abdominal pain, for which there is no obvious organic cause, as a reason why they do not want to eat. It is not difficult to see how the boundaries between some of the childhood presentations described in the eating disorders literature, such as food avoidance emotional disorder (see below) or some EDNOS presentations (e.g., children who have what appears to be an AN-type of illness but who do not endorse weight/shape concerns, instead insisting that they can't eat because their stomachs hurt or they feel uncomfortable all the time) and some of these FGIDs become blurred.

Curiously, in Rome III there does not appear to be a place for rumination behaviors in childhood, with criteria provided for rumination syndrome in adolescence and infancy only. In relation to younger children, three of the Rome categories overlap with psychiatric categories already discussed, namely infant regurgitation and infant rumination syndrome with rumination disorder (DSM-IV-TR) and infant colic with feeding disorder of state regulation (DC:0–3R and RDC-PA).

Finally, in this discussion of potential diagnostic categories for disordered eating in childhood we return briefly to the ICD-10 system. This contains two further sections worth mention:

- *Feeding problems of newborn* (P92)—in the section "Other disorders originating in the perinatal period (P90–P96)," which is a subset of "Certain conditions originating in the perinatal period": vomiting in newborn (P92.0); regurgitation and rumination in newborn (P92.1); slow feeding of newborn (P92.2); underfeeding of newborn (P92.3); overfeeding of newborn (P92.4); neonatal difficulty in feeding at breast (P92.5); other feeding problems of newborn (P92.8); feeding problem of newborn, unspecified (P92.9).
- *Symptoms and signs concerning food and fluid intake* (R63)—in the section "General symptoms and signs (R50–R69)," which is a subset of "Symptoms, signs and abnormal clinical and laboratory findings, not elsewhere classified": anorexia (R63.0); polydipsia (R63.1); polyphagia (R63.2); feeding difficulties and mismanagement (R63.3); abnormal weight loss (R63.4); abnormal weight gain (R63.5); other symptoms and signs concerning food and fluid intake (R63.8).

These categories are intended to exclude instances of feeding and eating difficulties of "nonorganic" origin; however, in practice this can be difficult to determine. Overlaps are evident between some presentations under "feeding problems of newborn" and the psychiatric diagnoses "rumination disorder" (DSM-IV-TR); "feeding disorder of state regulation" (DC:0–3R and RDC-PA); "feeding disorder of caregiver–infant reciprocity" (DC:0–3R and RDC-PA); and "infantile anorexia" (DC:0–3R and RDC-PA). The listing of a range of symptoms and signs associated with food and fluid intake may also result in inconsistencies and confusion about how best to diagnose some childhood presentations of eating disturbances.

To summarize this section, we have reviewed the main published diagnostic systems, which have categories for classifying disordered eating in childhood as mental, behavioral, and developmental disorders (DSM-IV-TR, ICD-10, DC:0–3R, and RDC-PA). We have also referred to the pediatric sections of the Rome III system for diagnosing and classifying functional GI disorders as well as some of the other categories in ICD-10, not conceptualized as behavioral or mental disorders but covering disturbances in feeding and eating seen in childhood. Our aim in doing so has been to highlight the overlap between the various systems, which use different terminology to describe potentially very similar presentations, as well as to highlight the complexities in teasing out somatic and psychological aspects of presentations in childhood. Given this situation, it is perhaps unsurprising that the whole area of classification and diagnosis of disordered eating in childhood is something of a muddle.

Clinical Presentations and Current Diagnostic Criteria

A review of the literature on disordered eating in childhood quickly reveals discrepancies between descriptions of common presentations to clinics seeing children with feeding or eating disturbances deemed to be "nonorganic" and available diagnostic categories in mental/behavioral disorder classification schemes. Commonly described feeding problems in younger children include refusal of solid foods, difficulties in making transitions in the weaning process, poor appetite and disinterest in food, food faddiness, lack of opportunity to develop age-appropriate oral/motor skills, failure to progress to age-appropriate self-feeding, and in some cases complete refusal of oral intake (Bryant-Waugh & Piepenstock, 2008). Such presentations may or may not meet formal DSM-IV-TR or ICD-10 criteria for feeding disorder (discussed in a later section).

In older children a range of fussy, faddy, restrictive, and avoidant eating disturbances have been described, as well as AN and related disorders. BN appears relatively rare in children under the age of 13 seen in clinical settings, although, interestingly, many adult patients with BN describe a childhood onset. Studies of time trends in age at onset of both AN and BN have concluded that it is decreasing (e.g., Favaro, Caregaro, Tenconi, Bosello, & Santonastaso, 2009).

Approaching feeding and eating disturbances in children through the lens of "mental disorder," it is then possible to diagnose feeding disorder (FD), rumination disorder (RD), pica, AN and its variants (EDNOS/atypical AN) and also to identify three predominant variants of eating difficulty that have been described in the literature, but are less easily placed within existing diagnostic categories, as follows: those with little interest in food and eating, or whose desire to eat is impaired, where intake is inadequate in terms of overall energy intake; those displaying an aversive response to food or engagement in fear-based avoidance; and those with a more sensory-based avoidance. These are discussed in turn at the end of this section. First, we discuss childhood presentations falling into the main formal feeding and eating diagnostic categories.

Anorexia Nervosa

In order to receive a formal diagnosis of AN, children must of course fulfill all diagnostic criteria and so, by definition, have a clinical presentation very similar to that of adolescent and adult patients. In our clinic we have seen children with full AN from the age of 7–8 years and older. In these early presentations all criteria can be met; there is no expectation that the amenorrhea criterion should apply to prepubertal girls, and the physical and cognitive criteria can be endorsed in even these young patients when carefully assessed clinically or when age-appropriate diagnostic assessment tools are used (Bryant-Waugh, Cooper, Taylor, & Lask, 1996). However, children vary in their capacity to report, describe, understand, and appreciate the meaning of their disturbed eating behaviors and thoughts (Bravender et al., 2007). In addition, the weight criterion is very difficult to apply consistently, and the health consequences of weight loss are not easily or uniformly associated with reaching specific weight thresholds. (For a more detailed discussion, see Bravender et al., 2007, 2010.) Furthermore, a diagnosis of AN currently relies heavily on self-report, unlike many childhood psychiatric disorders that require a multi-informant perspective to validate the diagnosis. Most childhood presentations of AN are characterized by restriction and exercise, rather than associated with bingeing and purging, with other typical aspects of presentation including food preoccupations, guilt related to eating, concern about eating with others, and often low self-esteem. In boys, concern related to fitness and health is often part of the clinical picture, with stated reasons for dietary restriction often more explicitly related to health concerns. Many boys engage in overexercising, and there is often an association with obsessive–compulsive traits.

Bulimia Nervosa

In our clinical experience, full presentations of BN in children below the age of 13 are relatively rare, although we have seen a few 11- and 12-year-olds, who are usually postmenarchal. As with AN, in order to receive a formal diagnosis, children must fulfill all diagnostic criteria, and therefore their presentation is essentially similar to that of adults. However, there are similar issues to those discussed earlier in relation to cognitive aspects; it can be difficult to endorse the requirement that self-evaluation is unduly influenced by shape and weight in some children based on patient report, and a sense of loss of control, which is required for an overeating episode to qualify as a binge, is a complex construct to assess in a child. In addition, calls have been made to lower the frequency thresholds for bingeing and purging to enable younger patients to meet the criteria at a reduced level of symptom severity. One recent study has, for example, demonstrated that child and adolescent patients not meeting the full criteria for BN nevertheless present with relatively high levels of medical complications, arguing for the criteria to be broadened to better capture clinical significance (Peebles, Hardy, Wilson, & Lock, 2010). For a fuller discussion of developmental considerations relating to the criteria for BN, see the two papers published by the Workgroup for Classification of Eating Disorders in Children and Adolescents (Bravender et al., 2007, 2010). In relation to presenting features in very young patients with BN, our experience suggests that vomiting is more common than laxative misuse as a compensatory behavior.

EDNOS/Atypical AN and BN

Due to the wording of current criteria taking insufficient account of developmental differences between children, adolescents, and adults, many childhood presentations do not fully meet the formal criteria for AN or BN, and so receive an atypical or EDNOS diagnosis. It is in our view extremely important to be able to distinguish between childhood presentations characterized by low weight and restricted intake that are associated with weight and/or shape concerns and those that are not. In some children unable to endorse cognitive criteria, behavioral indicators point strongly to a determination to avoid weight gain, whereas in others there appears to be no avoidance of intake for reasons of weight or shape or an intact sense of being underweight. We would diagnose the former as EDNOS, but not the latter, as there is no evidence of core eating disorder psychopathology. We have mentioned that full BN presentations are relatively unusual in those of age 12 and under; in particular, frequency criteria are often not met, resulting in an EDNOS diagnosis. Again, we argue for the need to establish that some core psychopathology is present to warrant an EDNOS diagnosis—for example, a child who overeats and vomits would not be included. A number of authors have emphasized that although eating disorders symptoms are reduced in either frequency or severity, EDNOS may be no less severe in terms of clinical severity, inasmuch as patients not meeting full the criteria are more likely to have comorbid disorders (Schmidt et al., 2008).

In DSM-IV-TR research criteria are provided for binge-eating disorder (BED), proposed as a specific subtype of EDNOS. BED therefore has a different status from the formal clinical categories of AN, BN, and EDNOS, and we mention it only briefly here. There has been some discussion about the assessment of binge eating in children with proposals for provisional BED research criteria for children; the consensus view on the basis of existing research is that loss of control over eating may be more important than the amount eaten, at least in relation to reported distress and other associated difficulties (Marcus & Kalarchian, 2003; Tanofsky-Kraff, Marcus, Yanovski, & Yanovski, 2008). Nevertheless, the reliable and consistent assessment of a sense loss of control in children remains a challenge.

EDNOS has become a catchall diagnosis, which is, unhelpfully, inconsistently applied. Our practice has always been to reserve the eating disorder diagnoses of AN, BN, and EDNOS for children in whom some level of eating disorder psychopathology is apparent, placing others in what we have termed "other childhood eating disturbances," discussed further below.

Feeding Disorder of Infancy or Early Childhood

There are well-recognized difficulties in matching presentations of feeding and eating disturbances in young children to feeding disorder (FD) criteria (Bryant-Waugh, Markham, Kreipe, & Walsh, 2010). In practice, many children seen at feeding clinics or programs do not qualify (Williams, Riegel, & Kerwin, 2009), partly because of the requirement that there should be a significant failure to gain weight or there should be a significant loss of weight, and partly due to the requirement that the disorder should be "nonorganic." As we have mentioned, this can be difficult to determine, and there appears to have been confusion among clinicians as to how the DSM-IV-TR stipulation, that the disturbance "should not be due to an associated gastrointestinal or other general medical condition" (APA, 2000), should be interpreted. The ICD-10 wording specifying that there should be "no evidence of organic disease sufficient to account for the disturbance alone" (WHO, 1992) is slightly more specific, as it does not rule out the possibility that there may have been precipitating or underlying medical problems. Feeding problems generally have multifactorial causes, and even where there is a concurrent contributory medical condition, there is often a significant behavioral or relationship component. For this reason, the inclusion of "feeding disorder associated with concurrent medical condition" in DC: 0–3R and RDC-PA can be justified.

Rumination Disorder

Rumination disorder (RD) is included as a diagnostic category in the DSM but not in the ICD system. It is placed in the section "Feeding disorders of infancy or early childhood," yet one of the criteria stipulates that the diagnosis should not be given if the behavior occurs exclusively during the course of AN or BN, suggesting that it is a diagnosis that can be given to adolescent or adult patients. Many clinicians may have encountered older patients who show regurgitation, rechewing, and/or reswallowing characteristic of rumination, and as indicated by the Rome III system, including criteria for rumination syndrome in infants, adolescents, and adults, it can and does occur across the age range, with slightly different features. DSM criteria for RD also specify that the disturbance should have been preceded by a period of "normal functioning," whereas Rome III does not. From a clinical point of view, the diagnosis is not particularly helpful in guiding appropriate treatment interventions, as the behavior can have a number of different functions depending on the age of the patient at presentation and the context in which it occurs. Common functions include self-stimulation (for example, in the context of mental retardation), anxiety management, and emotion regulation.

Pica

Pica is included in both DSM-IV-TR and ICD-10, but not in Rome III. This disorder is characterized by the eating of "nonnutritive" substances. Again, it is included in both the main diagnostic systems as a disorder of infancy or early childhood, yet it is well documented as occurring across the age range to include older children, adolescents, and adults. Matching presentations to the diagnosis is not particularly problematic, although there is some potential for confusion about the meaning of the term "nonnutritive": some diet foods are of no nutritional value and therefore nonnutritive; however, ingestion of diet foods is not included as pica. There is also potential for confusion about the inclusion of food items in a form not usually consumed by humans—for example, raw potatoes. In general, however, pica is a discrete, relatively easily identified behavior.

"Other" Feeding and Eating Disturbances

As discussed, many childhood presentations of disordered eating do not fit the aforementioned diagnostic categories. Leaving aside overfeeding or overeating associated with obesity, and disordered eating that can directly be accounted for by an ongoing medical condition or syndrome, there are a number of presentations that are typically (but not exclusively) seen in childhood. These presentations are characterized by avoidance or restriction of intake, but there is no evidence that weight or shape concerns play any role in the development or maintenance of such disturbances. Avoidant or restrictive behaviors related to intake do not appear to be associated with avoidance of weight gain, and, as mentioned, three predominant variants emerge, as discussed in the following sections. It does not seem appropriate to include these presentations as developmental variants of an AN or BN, nor to include them in EDNOS, as core eating disorder psychopathology is absent.

Presentations Characterized by Little Interest in Food/Eating

A number of subtypes of feeding disorder associated with behavioral symptoms seen in early childhood have been incorporated into the DC:0–3R and RDC-PA systems. One of these, infantile anorexia, is characterized by a lack of interest in food, refusal to eat adequate amounts of food, and a failure to communicate hunger. Such children show growth deficiency or a downward trend in weight percentiles. Its onset is described as occurring before the age of 3 years (Chatoor, 2009). Children with this presentation may well meet the formal criteria for FD, but interesting parallels have also been described in children seen at an older age. For example, our group has described a difficulty seen in children referred to in middle childhood as "restrictive eating" (Bryant-Waugh & Lask, 2007). Such children typically eat much less than their peers, often seem to lack interest in food or not be hungry, do not restrict their diet in terms of variety or texture, and their weight and height are usually on the lower percentiles. They often need prompting to eat and would forget to eat if not supervised. These children do not have abnormal cognitions or preoccupations regarding weight or shape and generally seem well in terms of mood and general functioning. Often this pattern is long-standing, but the child first presents in middle or later childhood. Such children sometimes have delayed puberty due to suboptimal energy intake and a failure to increase intake in line with growth spurts. Other common precipitants to clinic presentation include increased concern about growth, parental anxiety about the small amount eaten, or family conflict in relation to how best to manage the child's eating. The relationship between this presentation and that of infantile anorexia is unclear.

Food avoidance emotional disorder (FAED) is similarly a presentation characterized by little interest in food or eating, in which the child's desire to eat is impaired and in which intake is inadequate in terms of overall energy intake. This presentation is distinguished from restrictive eating in that it is a change from previous eating behavior, usually associated with significant weight loss and faltering growth. FAED is a term first used by Higgs and colleagues in the late 1980s to describe a group of children who appeared similar to children with AN in that they had an emotional disorder with marked food avoidance and significant weight loss as prominent features, but did not display the weight/shape concerns or cognitive distortions characteristic of a formal eating disorder (Higgs et al., 1989). It is interesting to note that in the original article the disorder was described as being characterized by "a history of food avoidance or difficulty such as food fads or restrictions," suggesting a long-standing problem with origins in early childhood. Our group and others have added to the description of this presentation (Bryant-Waugh & Lask, 2007; Casper, 2000), noting an association with other anxiety-based behaviors such as school refusal and a tendency for a wide range of reasons to be given to account for the food refusal (Nicholls & Bryant-Waugh, 2009). The lack of endorsement of weight or shape concerns brings FAED into overlap with a presentation in older individuals that has been termed non-fat-phobic anorexia nervosa (NFP-AN) (Becker, Thomas, & Pike 2009); in these patients fear of fatness appears to be absent and is not recognized as a contributory factor to restriction of intake. The relationship of FAED to AN, to NFP-AN, or to the conditions described earlier in younger children, remains uncertain; 20–30% of those under age 13 have this type of presentation (Madden, Morris, Zurynski, Kohn, & Elliot, 2009; Nicholls, Lynn, & Viner, in press).

Presentations Characterized by Aversion or Fear-Based Avoidance

Again, starting with subtypes of feeding disorder included in early childhood diagnostic systems, a presentation characterized by a child's refusing to eat solid food after experiencing significant choking, gagging, reflux, or vomiting has been identified. In RDC-PA, termed "posttraumatic feeding disorder" and in DC:0–3R "feeding disorder associated with insults to the gastrointestinal tract." The presentation has been described in latency-aged children, but also in infants and toddlers; hence its inclusion in diagnostic systems covering the early years. It typically involves a marked resistance to oral intake in young children and a more explicit fearful avoidance in older children, which can result in extreme weight loss. A number of terms, including "functional dysphagia," "globus hystericus," and "food phobia" have been used to describe similar presentations (Bryant-Waugh et al., 2010; Chatoor, 2009). We have previously described functional dysphagia in children below the age of 13, as avoidance of normal intake or texture of diet related to fear of choking or swallowing, which often follows a traumatic experience of choking, but where there is no evidence of abnormal cognitions about weight/shape.

There are a number of other childhood presentations that are essentially specific phobias associated with extremely limited intake. There may be a specific fear related to one or more foods or food types that can rapidly escalate and generalize (e.g., a child with an extreme and irrational fear of being poisoned by unrefined sugar who restricts intake to a few foods regarded as safe, despite the fact that a much wider range of foods do not contain sugar). Some children show a specific fear related to the consequences of eating (for example, a phobia of vomiting or diarrhea), which leads to an avoidance of food as the child attempts to manage perceived risk. The consequences of food avoidance can vary in severity; we have seen a number of extremely physically compromised children at our eating disorders service with such presentations. Sometimes these children are mistakenly believed to have AN as they strenuously avoid eating a normal amount or variety of food, which is accompanied in most cases by significant weight loss. However, abnormal cognitions about weight and shape are not present. It can be argued that these presentations are not helpfully classified as feeding or eating disorders, as they are essentially anxiety disorders, yet the main presenting feature is a clinically significant eating disturbance.

Presentations Characterized by Sensory-Based Avoidance

"Sensory food aversion" is a subtype of feeding disorder included in DC:0–3R and RDC-PA. This presentation is characterized by avoidance of eating or restriction of intake based on the sensory aspects of food. These may include taste, texture, smell, appearance, and/or temperature. This form of eating disturbance has also been well described in older children; we have called it "selective eating" (Bryant-Waugh & Lask, 2007), others have used different terms, such as perseverant eating, food neophobia, and food aversion (Chatoor, 2009). There are clear parallels between the presentation in infants and toddlers and in older children, although these have not been systematically studied. When it first presents in older children, they have been eating only a narrow range of food for a number of years in the majority of cases. It is extremely difficult to get these children to try new foods, but there is no evidence of abnormal cognitions about weight or shape. Developmental or anxiety factors can contribute to the presentation, which may fluctuate in severity in relation to environmental stressors. It is seen in children who have an autism spectrum disorder, but also in children who do not. It can be associated with clinically significant nutritional deficiencies, although in general weight is in the normal range, as these children will eat without difficulty as long as they are offered their preferred foods. It can also hold back social development, contribute to emotional distress and embarrassment in older children, and have a significant negative impact on family relationships and functioning. At present, such presentations have no place in the DSM-IV-TR or ICD-10 system. They do not meet the criteria for FD, as weight is not usually an issue, and they seem inappropriate to include as EDNOS or an atypical eating disorder.

To summarize this section on clinical presentations and highlight the problems in relation to current diagnostic criteria, we have seen that some children meet the criteria for existing formal diagnostic categories of AN, BN, EDNOS/atypical eating disorder, FD, RD, and pica. We have also seen that many children do not, but despite this have clinically significant presentations of disordered eating associated with risks that warrant intervention. We have briefly presented some of the arguments in relation to the need to make the criteria for AN, BN, and EDNOS more developmentally sensitive, and discussed how the "other" presentations can be broadly classified into three different groups, which appear to occur across childhood. We have argued that such presentations do not belong in EDNOS. We have suggested that the field generally lacks coordinated momentum and believe that inconsistent use of terms and classificatory systems has hampered research and contributed to a poorly developed evidence base for the treatment of disordered eating in childhood, little by way of clinical guidelines for management, and limited knowledge about outcomes. There are also limited longitudinal data on well-defined subgroups and prognosis is unclear, thus it is not always clear how best to focus clinical attention, making it likely that important preventative opportunities are lost. The field is short on robust assessment tools (in relation to both measures and protocols), making it difficult to obtain reliable incidence and prevalence rates. Inconsistencies in terminology and classification and inadequacies related to the wording of current diagnostic criteria have been major contributors to this unsatisfactory situation.

Future Directions

Inevitably, and helpfully, given the problems outlined earlier and the process of revision of the DSM and ICD systems, a number of suggestions have been put forward to improve the current situation. The Workgroup for Classification of Eating Disorders in Children and Adolescents (WCEDCA), a self-appointed international group of clinicians and researchers working with patients in this age range, has argued that behavioral indicators should be allowed to substitute for internally referenced cognitive criteria and that clinicians need to be alerted to developmental limitations that may preclude endorsement of cognitive criteria; that previous growth and maturational trajectory is important in determining healthy weight status in children and that this should be reflected in the wording of criteria; that for younger patients lower thresholds of weight loss for AN and of binge eating and compensatory behavior frequency for BN should be included in revisions; that multiple physical systems need to be evaluated for clinical management of eating disorders in children, but no single system should be required for diagnosis; and that the experience of loss of control should be the hallmark of binge-eating behavior in children (Bravender et al., 2007, 2010). These recommendations have been broadly supported by research investigating empirically derived categories in child and adolescent patients (Eddy et al., 2010). With regard to younger children, other groups have similarly made suggestions and recommendations intended to move the field forward. For example, Dovey, Farrow, Martin, Isherwood, and Halford (2009) have proposed a system for classifying childhood food refusal behaviors, which they put forward as an extension of previously published classification systems. This includes five main subtypes as follows: selective food refusal, fear-based food refusal, appetite-awareness-autonomy-based food refusal, learning-dependent food refusal, and medical complications food refusal.

Initial suggestions for revisions to DSM-IV-TR criteria are now in the public domain, and at the time of writing a period of consultation and field testing is in progress in advance of settling on final criteria and categories to be published in DSM-5. A main aim of the Eating Disorders Work Group has been to reduce the number of patients receiving a diagnosis of EDNOS, as these have consistently been reported as outnumbering those in the AN and BN categories together. The main proposals include the following: widening the criteria for AN and BN with the possibility of including criteria for "behaviorally similar" variants of AN, BN, and BED; moving BED into a formal diagnostic category; moving pica and RD out of disorders of infancy and childhood; and replacing FD with avoidant/restrictive food intake disorder (ARFID), a diagnosis not restricted to childhood, with descriptions of three main subtypes intended to promote further evaluation, research, and clarification of whether these are indeed distinct subtypes. The wording of ARFID criteria is also intended to overcome some of the current difficulties relating to FD criteria. In relation to placement in the classification scheme, the current proposal is to have feeding and eating disorders placed together, to include AN, BN, BED, pica, RD, ARFID, and what is hoped to be a smaller category of feeding and eating disorders or conditions not elsewhere classified.

In relation to proposals for ICD-11, as with DSM-5, a case has been made to reorganize existing categories rather than make radical changes to existing categories or criteria. This approach has been further developed and simplified to include specifiers such as intellectual ability, life cycle, and personality to help with more detailed categorization (Kingdon et al., 2010). Thus, division into child and adolescent versus adult disorders would be eliminated. Other suggestions include combining feeding and eating disorders, locating this section within the "emotional disorders," rather than on the "behavioral disorders" grouping, making developmental modifications to wording, and attempting to better capture some of the "other" presentations such as FAED (Nicholls & Arcelus, 2010).

Our hope for the future is that it will be possible to improve on the establishment of a shared means of communicating about different presentations of disordered eating in childhood and that we will be able to classify some well-recognized presentations that are not currently captured by diagnostic criteria. We advocate moving away from the distinction between feeding and eating, since all eating involves relationships and interaction, and we think it likely that many of the presentations that have been described in this chapter also present in adulthood, their expression but not their nature being determined by developmental stage. We look forward to a situation that will promote research essential for the development of treatment interventions and for improvement of our knowledge about course, prognosis, and outcome.

References

American Psychiatric Association. (2000). *Diagnostic and statistical manual of mental disorders* (4th ed., text rev.). Washington, DC: Author.

Ammaniti, M., Ambruzzi, A. M., Lucarelli, L., Cimino, S., & D'Olimpio, F. (2004). Malnutrition and dysfunctional mother–child feeding interactions: Clinical assessment and research implications. *Journal of the American College of Nutrition, 23,* 259–271.

Becker, A. E., Thomas, J. J., & Pike, K. M. (2009). Should non-fat-phobic anorexia nervosa be included in DSM-V? *International Journal of Eating Disorders, 42.* 620–635.

Birch, L.L. (1998). Development of food acceptance patterns in the first years o f life. *Proceedings of the Nutrition Society, 57,* 617–624.

Birch, L. L., & Davison, K. K. (2001). Family environmental factors influencing the developing behavioral controls of food intake and childhood overweight. *Pediatric Clinics of North America, 48,* 893–907.

Bravender, T., Bryant-Waugh, R., Herzog, D., Katzman, D., Kreipe, R. D., Lask, B., et al. (2007). Classification of child and adolescent eating disturbances. *International Journal of Eating Disorders, 40,* S117–S122.

Bravender, T., Bryant-Waugh, R., Herzog, D., Katzman, D., Kreipe, R. D., Lask, B., et al. (2010). Classification of eating disturbance in children and adolescents: Proposed changes for the DSM-V. *European Eating Disorders Review, 18,* 79–89.

Bryant-Waugh, R., Cooper P., Taylor, C., & Lask, B. (1996). The use of the Eating Disorder Examination in children: A pilot study. *International Journal of Eating Disorders, 19,* 391–401.

Bryant-Waugh, R., & Lask, B. (2007). Overview of the eating disorders. In B. Lask & R. Bryant-Waugh (Eds.), *Eating disorders in childhood and adolescence* (3rd ed., pp. 35–50). London: Routledge.

Bryant-Waugh, R., Markham, L., Kreipe, R. E., & Walsh, B. T. (2010). Feeding and eating disorders in childhood. *International Journal of Eating Disorders, 43:* 98–111.

Bryant-Waugh, R., & Piepenstock, E. (2008). Childhood disorders: Feeding and related disorders of infancy or early childhood. In A. Tasman, J. Kay, J. A. Lieberman, M. B. First, & M. Maj (Eds.), *Psychiatry* (3rd ed., pp. 830–846). New York: Wiley.

Casper, R. C. (2000). Eating disturbances and eating disorders in childhood. In F. E. Bloom & D. Kupfer (Eds.), *Psychopharmcology: The fourth generation of progress.* New York: Raven Press.

Chatoor, I. (2009). *Diagnosis and treatment of feeding disorders in infants, toddlers and young children.* Washington, DC: Zero to Three.

Davies, W. H., Berlin, K. S., Sato, A. F., Fischer, E. A., Arvedson, J. C., Satter, E., et al. (2006). Reconceptualizing feeding and feeding disorders in interpersonal context: The case for a relational disorder. *Journal of Family Psychology, 20,* 409–417.

Dovey, T. M., Farrow, C. V., Martin, C. I., Isherwood, E., & Halford, J. C. G. (2009). When does food refusal require professional intervention? *Current Nutrition and Food Science, 5,* 160–171.

Drossman, D. A., Corazziari, E., Delvaux, M., Spiller, R. C., Talley, N. J., Thompson, W. G., et al. (2006). *Rome III: The functional gastrointestinal disorders* (3rd ed.). McLean, VA: Degnon.

Eddy, K. T., Le Grange, D., Crosby, R., Hoste, R. R., Celio Doyle, A., Smyth, A., et al. (2010). Diagnostic classification of eating disorders in children and adolescents: How does DSM-IV-TR compare to empirically derived categories? *Journal of the American Academy of Child and Adolescent Psychiatry, 49,* 277–287.

Farrow, C., & Blissett, J. (2006). Maternal cognitions, psychopathologic symptoms and infant temperament as predictors of early infant feeding problems: A longitudinal study. *International Journal of Eating Disorders, 39,* 128–134.

Favaro, A., Caregaro, L., Tenconi, E., Bosello, R., & Santonastaso, P. (2009). Time trends in age at onset of anorexia nervosa and bulimia nervosa. *Journal of Clinical Psychiatry, 70,* 1715–1721.

Higgs, J. F., Goodyer, I. M., & Birch, J. (1989). Anorexia nervosa and food avoidance emotional disorder. *Archives of Disease in Childhood, 64,* 346–351.

Jacobi, C., Agras, W. S., Bryson, S., & Hammer, L. D. (2003). Behavioral validation, precursors, and concomitants of picky eating in childhood. *Journal of the American Academy for Child and Adolescent Psychiatry, 42,* 76–84.

Kingdon, D., Afghan, S., Arnold, R., Faruqui, R., Friedman, T., Jones, I., et al. (2010). A diagnostic system using broad categories with clinically relevant specifiers: Lessons for ICD-11. *International Journal of Social Psychiatry, 56,* 326–335.

Kral, T. V., & Rauh, E. M. (2010). Eating behaviors of children in the context of their family environment. *Physiology and Behavior, 100,* 567–573.

Madden, S., Morris, A., Zurynski, Y. A., Kohn, M., & Elliot, E. J. (2009). Burden of eating disorders in 5–15-year-old children in Australia. *Medical Journal of Australia, 190*(8), 410–414.

Marcus, M. D., & Kalarchian, M. A. (2003). Binge eating in children and adolescents. *International Journal of Eating Disorders, 34,* S47–S57.

Mikkilä, V., Räsänen, L., Raitakari, O. T., Marniemi, J., Pietinen, P., Rönnemaa, T., et al. (2007). Major dietary patterns and cardiovascular risk factors from childhood to adulthood: The Cardiovascular Risk in Young Finns Study. *British Journal of Nutrition, 98,* 218–225.

Moore, L. L., Singer, M. R., Bradlee, M. L., Djoussé, L., Proctor, M. H., Cupples, L. A., et al. (2005). Intake of fruits, vegetables, and dairy products in early childhood and subsequent blood pressure change. *Epidemiology, 16,* 4–11.

Nicholls, D., & Arcelus, J. (2010). Making eating disorders classification work in ICD-11. *European Eating Disorders Review, 18,* 247–250.

Nicholls, D., & Bryant-Waugh, R. (2009). Eating disorders of infancy and childhood: Definition, symptomatology, epidemiology and comorbidity. *Child and Adolescent Psychiatric Clinics of North America, 18,* 17–30.

Nicholls, D., Christie, D., Randall, L., & Lask, B. (2001). Selective eating: Symptom, disorder or normal variant. *Clinical Child Psychology and Psychiatry, 6,* 257–270.

Nicholls, D. E., Lynn, R., & Viner, R. M. (in press). Childhood eating disorders: British national surveillance study. *British Journal of Psychiatry.*

Nicklas, T. A., Morales, M., Linares, A., Yang, S. J., Baranowski, T., DeMoor, C., et al. (2004). Children's meal patterns have changed over a 21-year period: The Bogalusa Heart Study. *Journal of the American Dietetic Association, 104,* 753–761.

Pearson, N., Biddle, S. J., & Gorely, T. (2009). Family correlates of fruit and vegetable consumption in children and adolescents: A systematic review. *Public Health Nutrition, 12,* 267–283.

Peebles, R., Hardy, K. K., Wilson, J. L., & Lock, J. D. (2010). Are diagnostic criteria for eating disorders markers of medical severity? *Pediatrics, 125,* e1193–e1201.

Popkin, B. M., & Duffey, K. J. (2010). Does hunger and satiety drive eating anymore? Increasing eating occasions and decreasing time between eating occasions in the United States. *American Journal of Clinical Nutrition, 91,* 1342–1347.

Postert, C., Averbeck-Holocher, M., Beyer, T., Müller, J., & Furniss, T. (2009). Five systems of psychiatric classification for preschool children: Do differences in validity, usefulness and reliability make for competitive or complimentary constellations? *Child Psychiatry and Human Development, 40,* 25–41.

Scaglioni, S., Salvioni, M., & Galimberti, C. (2008). Influence of parental attitudes in the development of children's eating behavior. *British Journal of Nutrition, 99,* S22–S25.

Schmidt, U., Lee, S., Perkins, S., Eisler, I., Treasure, J., Beecham, J., et al. (2008). Do adolescents with eating disorder not otherwise specified or full-syndrome bulimia nervosa differ in clinical severity, comorbidity, risk factors, treatment outcome or cost? *International Journal of Eating Disorders, 41,* 498–504.

Tanofsky-Kraff, M., Marcus, M. D., Yanovski, S. Z., & Yanovski, J. A. (2008). Loss of control eating disorder in children age 12 years and younger: Proposed research criteria. *Eating Behaviors, 9,* 360–365.

Task Force on Research Diagnostic Criteria: Infancy and Preschool. (2003). Research diagnostic criteria for infants and preschool children: The process and empirical support. *Journal of the American Academy of Child and Adolescent Psychiatry, 42,* 1504–1512.

Wardle, J., Carnell, S., & Cooke, L. (2005). Parental control over feeding and children's fruit and vegetable intake: How are they related? *Journal of the American Dietetic Association, 105,* 227–232.

Williams, K., Riegel, K., & Kerwin, M. (2009). Feeding disorder of infancy or early childhood: How often is it seen in feeding programs? *Journal of Child Health Care, 38,* 123–136.

World Health Organization. (1992). *The ICD-10 classification of mental and behavioural disorders: Clinical descriptions and diagnostic guidelines.* Geneva: Author.

Zero to Three. (2005). *Diagnostic classification of mental health and developmental disorders of infancy and early childhood* (rev. ed.; DC:0–3R). Washington, DC: Zero to Three Press.

CHAPTER 8

Diagnosis and Classification of Eating Disorders in Adolescence

Kamryn T. Eddy
David B. Herzog
Nancy L. Zucker

Eating disorders are psychiatric illnesses defined by severe disturbances in eating behavior and disruptions in the experience of the body that intrude upon cognition and impact functioning. The current *Diagnostic and Statistical Manual of Mental Disorders*, fourth edition, text revision (DSM-IV-TR; American Psychiatric Association, 2000) includes three eating disorder diagnoses: anorexia nervosa (AN) and bulimia nervosa (BN), each with specific criteria sets, and eating disorder not otherwise specified (EDNOS), a broader diagnosis without specific criteria that is intended to capture clinically significant eating disorder presentations that do not meet the criteria for AN or BN. The stated purpose of the DSM-IV-TR classification system is to "provide clear descriptions of diagnostic categories in order to enable clinicians and investigators to diagnose, communicate about, study, and treat people with mental disorders" (American Psychiatric Association, 2000, p. xxxvii). This classification system is in evolution, and it is expected that a revised version of DSM (DSM-5) will be published in 2013. The goal of this chapter is to examine the state of the evidence regarding the current system in regard to the diagnosis of eating disorders in adolescents to provide a gauge to examine how the current diagnostic system is fulfilling its purpose.

In the current system, although there are shared features across the eating disorders, including preoccupation with food and/or weight and shape, there are notable differences in clinical presentation by eating disorder type. For example, both AN and BN are characterized by a relentless desire for thinness; however, AN is marked by extreme weight loss, disturbance in the experience of the body, and a debilitating fear of weight gain, whereas the hallmarks of BN are binge eating and compensatory behaviors, with body weight typically within the normal weight range. EDNOS is a heterogeneous diagnosis that includes clinical presentations that narrowly miss meeting the full criteria for AN or BN, as well as a range of other symptom clusters, some of which have been recommended for consideration as a formal diagnostic category (e.g., binge-eating disorder [BED]). Although AN and BN have received the most research attention, EDNOS is the most common eating disorder diagnosis in clinical settings.

The onset of eating disorders typically occurs during adolescence and they are most often observed in adolescent and young adult females (American Psychiatric Association, 2000). They may be chronic and relapsing conditions and are often associated with psychiatric comorbidity and medical sequelae. The current diagnostic criteria for eating disorders are intended to apply to individuals across the age span, although developmentally sensitive accommodations are recommended.

In this chapter we present the DSM-IV-TR criteria for diagnosing eating disorders in adolescents, discuss the application of these criteria to eating disturbances in adolescents, review the literature that addresses the nosology of eating disorders in adolescents, and conclude with suggestions for future research in this area.

DSM-IV-TR Diagnostic Criteria for Eating Disorders

Anorexia Nervosa

DSM-IV-TR AN is characterized by a person's refusal to maintain a minimally healthy body weight, intense fear of weight gain, body image disturbance, and amenorrhea (American Psychiatric Association, 2000). Individuals with AN lose weight (or fail to gain weight during a period of growth), reaching an unhealthy low body weight; as a guideline, DSM-IV-TR operationalizes this low weight criterion as less than 85% of that expected for age, height, and gender. Accompanying the hallmark low weight is an extreme fear of weight gain and a disturbance in the experience of the body. Body image disturbance may include misperception of one's body shape or size (e.g., as being larger than it is), overvaluation of weight and shape in regard to self-worth, and failure to appreciate the seriousness of the current low body weight. In postmenarcheal females, these symptoms are accompanied by the loss of three consecutive menstrual periods, and in premenarcheal females, these symptoms may delay the onset of menses.

DSM-IV-TR distinguishes between two subtypes of AN—restricting and binge-eating/purging—based on the presence or absence of bulimic symptoms. Longitudinal studies suggest that individuals with AN may alternate between periods of restricting eating and subsequent periods of binge eating and purging during the course of their illness (Eddy et al., 2002; Eddy, Dorer, et al., 2008). Relative to the restricting type, the binge-eating/purging type may be more associated with comorbid impulsivity, including substance use disorders, cluster B personality disorders, mood lability, and suicidality (American Psychiatric Association, 2000). Individuals with binge-eating/purging type may develop more severe medical complications relative to the restricting subtype, as binge/purge behaviors compound their low weight. Thus, although both subtypes are associated with increased mortality risk, the binge-eating/purging type may be particularly associated with poorer prognoses, including chronic illness and premature death (Peat, Mitchell, Hoek, & Wonderlich, 2009).

Bulimia Nervosa

DSM-IV-TR BN is characterized by recurrent episodes of binge eating, inappropriate compensatory behaviors (e.g., self-induced vomiting, misuse of laxatives/diuretics/enemas, excessive exercising, or strict dieting/fasting) to prevent weight gain, and overconcern with weight and shape. "Binge eating" is defined as the consumption of an objectively large amount of food in a discrete period of time, accompanied by the subjective sense that one has lost control over the ability to stop eating or to refrain from initiating a binge-eating episode. The amount of food that defines a binge currently lacks an objective criterion and is judged relative to the inappropriateness of the amount of food, given the context in which the food is eaten. DSM-IV-TR indicates a frequency threshold of an average of twice weekly over a 3-month period. In addition to the binge–purge behaviors, BN is associated with beliefs that overemphasize the importance of weight and shape to self-esteem or self-worth.

DSM-IV-TR recognizes two subtypes of BN—purging and nonpurging—based on the type of associated compensatory behaviors. Most individuals with BN are diagnosed with the purging type (i.e., compensatory behaviors including vomiting, use of laxatives or diuretics). Although individuals with BN often use more than one type of compensatory behavior, the majority engage in self-induced vomiting (American Psychiatric Association, 2000). Purging-type BN may be associated with more medical morbidity and psychiatric comorbidity, as compared with the nonpurging type. Furthermore, there is some evidence to suggest that the use of multiple *types* of purging behaviors is associated with increased body image disturbance, dietary restraint, and eating concerns (Edler, Haedt, & Keel, 2007).

Eating Disorder Not Otherwise Specified

EDNOS is the diagnostic category used to describe individuals with clinically significant eating disturbances that do not fit into the narrowly defined AN or BN criteria sets. This is a comparatively large and heterogeneous diagnostic group; approximately half of the individuals presenting for eating disorders treatment in the community meet the criteria for EDNOS (e.g., Eddy, Celio Doyle, et al., 2008; Fairburn & Bohn, 2005). Because there are no specific criteria for EDNOS, the boundaries of the disorder are not clear. DSM-IV-TR provides examples of EDNOS, but this list is not exhaustive. A subset of those with EDNOS have symptom presentations that closely align with AN or BN but fall outside these diagnoses because of missing one criterion (e.g., amenorrhea, binge/purge frequency). Other examples of EDNOS symptom clusters include patients who binge eat but do not engage in compensatory behaviors, individuals who purge but do not have objective binge-eating episodes, those who engage in chewing and spitting, and those who regularly engage in nighttime eating.

Although EDNOS is the most prevalent eating disorder, research on the epidemiology, course, and outcome of this heterogeneous diagnostic group is limited. Within the category of EDNOS, the one symptom cluster presentation that has received comparatively more attention is BED.

Binge-Eating Disorder

BED was formally recognized in 1994 with the publication of DSM-IV when it was introduced as a specific example within the heterogeneous category of EDNOS. DSM-IV-TR provides research criteria for BED. As a new diagnosis in need of further study, BED has received significant research and clinical attention during the last 15 years and has been recommended for inclusion as a separate diagnosis in DSM-5.

BED is characterized by recurrent binge eating (objective overeating accompanied by the subjective experience of loss of control over eating) and associated distress in the absence of the regular compensatory behaviors that characterize BN. The binge episodes may involve a cluster of symptoms, including eating more rapidly than normal, eating until feeling uncomfortably full, eating large amounts in the absence of physical hunger, eating in secret due to embarrassment about overeating, and feeling disgusted, depressed, or guilty after eating. The phenomenon of binge eating in patients with BED is similar to that of individuals with BN. However, in BN, binge eating may be thought to represent lapses in overcontrol in the context of overall dietary restraint; in BED, binge eating may be more likely to occur in the context of generally chaotic food patterns and overeating (Wilfley, Schwartz, Spurrell, & Fairburn, 2000). Furthermore, whereas BN typically occurs in individuals of normal weight, BED is more often associated with overweight and obesity and is found at increased rates in populations seeking weight-loss treatment (Marcus & Kalarchian, 2003; Striegel-Moore & Franko, 2003).

Applying Diagnostic Criteria for Eating Disorders to Youth

The eating disorders most typically first develop during adolescence and often persist into adulthood. Yet physical and cognitive maturation that occur over the course of adolescence challenge the application of these diagnostic criteria to eating disturbances in youth. For example, the diagnosis of AN requires low body weight and amenorrhea. The delineation of low body weight in growing adolescents can be challenging. Various guidelines have been proposed, including percentage of ideal body weight, a body mass index (BMI) centile cutoff, or consideration of prior weight gain trajectory using deviations from a prior growth curve as an index of aberrant development (Bravender et al., 2007). Recent position statements emphasize the importance of this latter strategy, given the limited value of weight cutoffs relative to an adolescent's unique developmental history of weight loss and gain. Furthermore, as the onset of eating disorders may occur prior to full pubertal maturation, having a criterion such as amenorrhea is developmentally inappropriate. Notwithstanding, it is increasingly recognized that there is much individual variation in the effects of malnourishment on the body, leading some researchers to recommend that the essence of this criterion be changed to a more general medical criterion reflecting the ill effects of weight loss on the body (Bravender et al., 2007, 2010). At the same time, given this variability, many individuals experience significant weight loss, yet because of individual differences do not evidence laboratory abnormalities. In addition, review of the literature suggests that the presence of amenorrhea reflects nutritional status for some but does not generally differentiate low-weight individuals with eating disorders with regard to relevant psychological characteristics and thus may be nonspecific as a diagnostic criterion (Attia & Roberto, 2009). However, this research focuses on adults and adolescents who have reached menarche, which limits generalizability to younger patients. Finally, the regularity of the menstrual cycle is influenced by numerous factors (e.g., stress, affective disorders), suggesting that amenorrhea is not pathognomonic of AN. Combined, these factors question the utility of amenhorrea, certainly for adolescents but potentially for adults as well.

In addition, both AN and BN include cognitive symptoms in their criteria sets, which may be developmentally incongruous for younger adolescents. Brain structure and function continue to evolve into early adulthood, with associated complex cognitive capacities such as risk appraisal and abstract reasoning evidencing signs of continual maturation throughout this period. Diverse trajectories of maturation, in general, combined with differences between adolescents and adults may challenge the validity of the cognitive criteria constructs in youth (Becker, Eddy, & Perloe, 2009; Bravender et al., 2007). As currently worded, existing cognitive criteria demand future risk appraisal (as in criteria that describe denial of illness) and the ability to compare and contrast multiple abstract concepts (as in the criterion that requires that individuals rank order the facets of their self-worth). Without reference to more concrete or behavioral indicators for these parameters, cognitive criteria may not be validly assessed in many young individuals.

In regard to the behavioral criteria for BN and BED, several questions emerge. In adults and youth alike, the twice weekly frequency criterion for binge eating and compensatory behaviors required for the diagnoses is not empirically based and may be too strict a threshold (see Wilson & Sysko, 2009, for a recent review). Furthermore, how to quantify an objectively large amount of food can be difficult, particularly in growing youth. At issue is not just the variability and large amounts of food needed to support optimal growth, but also that adolescents often cannot control access to foodstuffs and thus may be constrained from eating all that they would if food were freely available. Some investigators have argued that the subjective experience of loss of control over eating, rather than the amount of food consumed, be used to define binge eating in youth (e.g., Shomaker et al., 2010; Tanofsky-Kraff, Marcus, Yanovski, & Yanovski, 2008). However, this may also present a challenge in diagnosing younger patients where the assessment of the loss of control, a complex and abstract construct, may also be difficult to reliably and validly assess in adolescents and children. The Workgroup for the Classification of Eating Disorders in Children and Adolescents (WCEDCA) has suggested that across the diagnostic criteria for eating disorders a more lenient threshold for diagnosis be applied in youth, which would allow some whose eating disorder presentations narrowly miss the full criteria for AN or BN (or BED) to be classified with those full-syndrome disorders rather than within the heterogeneous category of EDNOS (Bravender et al., 2007, 2010). This suggestion also has the advantage of promoting early detection, diagnosis, and treatment of clinically significant eating disorder pathology in youth.

Nosological Research on Eating Disorders in Youth

In addition to providing clinicians and researchers a common language for describing psychopathology, diagnostic classification systems convey information in regard to prognosis, course, and treatment approaches. Yet the value of a classification system is determined by its validity and the degree to which it captures the full range of clinical presentations. This issue is particularly salient for children and adolescents seeking treatment for eating disorders, as recent evidence suggests that poor sensitivity in detecting threshold eating disorder cases may have harmful health implications for children and adolescents (Peebles, Hardy, Wilson, & Lock, 2010). Furthermore, research examining the "fit" of the nosological system to observed clinical presentations is critical, given the influence of diagnostic classification systems in guiding research and clinical practice.

At present, the DSM-IV-TR does not make specific provisions for the diagnosis of eating disorders in children and adolescents and demonstrates little recognition that eating disorders in these younger patients may differ from those observed in adults (Bravender et al., 2007). A limited amount of empirical work has been conducted to examine the appropriateness and applicability of the DSM-IV-TR categories to youth.

Available evidence indicates the challenges inherent in applying existing criteria to these developmental periods. A number of descriptive reports on adolescent clinical samples indicate the predominance of EDNOS in these samples (Eddy, Celio Doyle, et al., 2008; O'Toole, De Socio, Munoz, Crosby, & Wonderlich, 2009; Peebles, Wilson, & Lock, 2006). Although the predominance of EDNOS is not unique to children, what may distinguish these findings is that children and adolescents may fail to meet the current diagnostic criteria because of the developmental limitations of existing criteria sets. For example, EDNOS presentations in children and adolescents commonly resemble AN or BN, falling short by narrowly missed criteria (e.g., Binford & Le Grange, 2005; Eddy, Celio Doyle, et al., 2008). As youth may be more likely to minimize or deny the cognitive eating disorder criteria than their adult counterparts (e.g., Fisher, Schneider, Burns, Symons, & Mandel, 2001), some of these children diagnosed with EDNOS may actually be diagnosed with AN or BN if the criteria were to be framed with consideration of developmental capacities.

Building on the descriptive studies, empirical approaches to examining the "fit" of DSM-IV-TR categories to eating disorder presentations in youth have begun to utilize advanced statistical techniques such as latent class or latent profile analysis (LCA/LPA; Lazarsfeld & Henry, 1968). LCA/LPA posits that a heterogeneous group can be reduced to a finite number of homogeneous (underlying or latent) subgroups through minimizing associations among responses across multiple indicators (e.g., eating disorder features) (Wonderlich et al., 2007). In doing so, LCA/LPA identifies the number and composition of unobserved mutually exclusive latent groups. (LPA has the advantage of allowing for continuous indicators, whereas LCA is limited to categorical indicators.) Several recent reports have applied LCA/LPA to clinical samples that include adolescents with eating disorders (Eddy et al., 2010; O'Toole et al., 2009; Pinhas et al., 2008). In a U.S. clinical eating disorders sample (N = 401; ages 7–19, mean = 15.14 ± 2.35 years), Eddy and colleagues (2010) identified three groups of individuals with eating disorders—a group characterized by binge eating and purging (and mostly of normal weight), a group characterized by excessive exercise and extreme eating disorder cognitions, and a group characterized by minimal eating disorder behaviors or cognitions; notably, low-weight patients in this sample were included in the latter two latent groups. These findings were similar to those of O'Toole and colleagues (2009), who identified four latent groups in their clinical sample (N = 323; ages 6.1–18.7 years, mean = 13.3 years): two groups resembled BN but were differentiated from each other by degree of cognitive eating disorder symptoms, and two groups resembled AN, but were differentiated from each other by degree of cognitive eating disorder symptoms. Indeed, in this sample, the low-weight group with minimal eating disorder symptoms represented the largest subgroup (n = 123, 38.1% of sample). Although these statistical approaches may offer novel and more empirically based methods of characterizing eating disorder syndromes, using these approaches within a developmental framework would require that groups identified in late adolescence be verified in early adolescent and child samples.

Work by a large international survey conducted by child psychiatrists in Australia, Canada, and England complements the studies of older adolescents and begins to address this goal. Pinhas and colleagues (2008) identified two groups of children and young adolescents (ages 5–13; mean age approximately 11.5 years) with eating disorders using LCA. One of these identified groups resembled typical AN, and the other the authors termed "food avoidant emotional eating disorder" characterized by weight loss and minimal eating disorder behaviors or cognitions along with an increase in somatic complaints. Taken together, the findings from these preliminary studies begin to suggest ways that eating disorder presentations may be expressed differently across the developmental spectrum. Most notably, this work suggests that it may be important to recognize subgroups with eating disorder symptoms who have minimal eating disorder cognitions that are considered hallmarks of typical eating disorders. Such groups may have alternative expressions of disordered eating that more closely match their level of cognitive development.

Conclusion and Future Directions

The current classification system for eating disorders assumes that AN, BN, and EDNOS can be diagnosed in adolescents using the same criteria set that is applied to adults. Many adolescents do have eating disorders that are symptomatically similar to those observed in adults. However, clinical wisdom and ongoing adolescent-focused research suggests that for some adolescents, there are important differences in presentation. Because of developmental differences, lower thresholds for diagnosing eating disorders in adolescents are warranted to promote early detection and intervention. If the DSM-5 Eating Disorder Workgroup's proposal to broaden (or lower) the thresholds for AN, BN, and BED across the age spectrum is borne out in DSM-5, this represents significant progress toward early identification. In addition, there needs to be recognition that the cognitive symptoms are difficult to assess in younger patients and a lack of endorsement may have multiple meanings. Whether the expression of minimal cognitive symptoms reflects a developmental variant of the full-syndrome eating disorders observed in adulthood or, rather, a different eating disorder (or illness) is a question in need of further study. Sensitive measurement tools that consider self-report and informant-report (e.g., parent, clinician) of both behaviors and cognitions are needed to comprehensively assess eating disorder pathology in youth.

A notable limitation of this review is the exclusive focus on DSM-IV-TR diagnostic categories without consideration of alternative classification systems such as the International Classification of Diseases (ICD-10; World Health Organization, 1992). Furthermore, this chapter focuses on adolescent eating disorders; a discussion of childhood eating and feeding disorders is presented elsewhere (see Bryant-Waugh & Nicholls, Chapter 7, this volume).

Nevertheless, in preparation for DSM-5, continued research aimed at describing adolescent presentations is needed. Longitudinal studies that follow youth with eating disorders during adolescence have the potential to inform clinicians and researchers about the course of these illnesses and to address the importance of these nosological distinctions (e.g., on the basis of cognitive symptom endorsement) with regard to treatment outcome. Research is needed to clarify the continuity between adolescent and adult eating disorders. Furthermore, at present it is not clear where to draw the outer boundaries of the eating disorders. On what basis are disturbances in eating behaviors or related cognitions impairing or clinically distressing, particularly to adolescents who may have more difficulty articulating this than their adult counterparts? Other types of empirical approaches to the study of classification, such as taxometric analyses, may be useful in addressing whether the relationship between different eating disorder diagnostic groups (or empirically derived classes) is truly discontinuous and qualitative (taxonic) versus continuous and quantitative (dimensional). Only then we come closer to "carving nature at its joints" (Pickles & Angold, 2003).

References

American Psychiatric Association. (2000). *Diagnostic and statistical manual of mental disorders* (4th ed., text rev.). Washington, DC: Author.

Attia, E., & Roberto, C. A. (2009). Should amenorrhea be a diagnostic criterion for anorexia nervosa? *International Journal of Eating Disorders, 42,* 581–589.

Becker, A. E., Eddy, K. T., & Perloe, A. (2009). Clarifying criteria for cognitive signs and symptoms for eating disorders in DSM-5. *International Journal of Eating Disorders, 42,* 611–619.

Binford, R. B., & Le Grange, D. (2005). Adolescents with bulimia nervosa and eating disorder not otherwise specified–purging only. *International Journal of Eating Disorders, 38,* 157–161.

Bravender, T., Bryant-Waugh, R., Herzog, D., Katzman, D., Kreipe, R. D., Lask, B., et al. (2007). Classification of child and adolescent eating disturbances. Workgroup for Classification of Eating Disorders in Children and Adolescents (WCEDCA). *International Journal of Eating Disorders, 40,* S117–S122.

Bravender, T., Bryant-Waugh, R., Herzog, D., Katzman, D., Kreipe, R. D., Lask, B., et al. (2010). Classification of eating disturbance in children and adolescents: Proposed changes for the DSM-V. *European Eating Disorders Review, 18*(2), 79–89.

Eddy, K. T., Celio Doyle, A., Hoste, R. R., Herzog, D. B., & Le Grange, D. (2008). Eating disorder not otherwise specified (EDNOS): An examination of EDNOS presentations in adolescents. *Journal of the American Academy of Child and Adolescent Psychiatry, 47,* 156–164.

Eddy, K. T., Dorer, D. J., Franko, D. L., Tahilani, K., Thompson-Brenner, H., & Herzog, D. B. (2008). Longitudinal diagnostic crossover of anorexia and bulimia nervosa: Implications for DSM-5. *American Journal of Psychiatry, 165,* 245–250.

Eddy, K. T., Keel, P. K., Dorer, D. J., Delinsky, S. S., Franko, D. L., & Herzog, D. B. (2002). Longitudinal comparison of anorexia nervosa subtypes. *International Journal of Eating Disorders, 31*(2), 191–201.

Eddy, K. T., Le Grange, D., Crosby, R. D., Hoste, R. R., Celio Doyle, A., Smyth, A., et al. (2010). Diagnostic classification of eating disorders in children and adolescents: How does DSM-IV compare to empirically-derived categories? *Journal of the American Academy of Child and Adolescent Psychiatry, 49,* 277–287.

Edler, C., Haedt, A. A., & Keel, P. K. (2007). The use of multiple purging methods as an indicator of eating disorder severity. *International Journal of Eating Disorders, 40,* 515–520.

Fairburn, C. G., & Bohn, K. (2005). Eating disorder NOS (EDNOS): An example of the troublesome "not otherwise specified (NOS)" category in DSM-IV. *Behaviour Research and Therapy, 43,* 691–701.

Fisher, M., Schneider, M., Burns, J., Symons, H., & Mandel, F. S. (2001). Differences between adolescents and young adults at presentation to an eating disorders program. *Journal of Adolescent Health, 28,* 222–227.

Lazarsfeld, P. F., & Henry, N. W. (1968). *Latent structure analysis.* Boston: Houghton Mifflin.

Marcus, M. D., & Kalarchian, M. A. (2003). Binge eating in children and adolescents. *International Journal of Eating Disorders, 34,* S47–S57.

O'Toole, J. K., De Socio, J. E., Munoz, D. J., Crosby, R. D., & Wonderlich, S. A. (2009,

March). *Eating disorders in children and adolescents: Diagnostic differences and challenges.* Oral presentation at the Conference on the Classification and Diagnosis of Eating Disorders, Washington, DC.

Peat, C., Mitchell, J. E., Hoek, H. W., & Wonderlich, S. A. (2009). Validity and utility of subtyping anorexia nervosa. *International Journal of Eating Disorders, 42*, 590–594.

Peebles, R., Hardy, K. K., Wilson, J. L., & Lock, J. D. (2010). Are diagnostic criteria for eating disorders markers of medical severity? *Pediatrics, 125*, 1193–1201.

Peebles, R., Wilson, J. L., & Lock, J. D. (2006). How do children with eating disorders differ from adolescents with eating disorders at initial evaluation? *Journal of Adolescent Health, 39*, 800–805.

Pickles, A., & Angold, A. (2003). Natural categories or fundamental dimensions: On carving nature at the joints and the rearticulation of psychopathology. *Development and Psychopathology, 15*, 529–551.

Pinhas, L., Madden, S., Katzman, D. K., Lynne, R., Morris, A., & Nicholls, D. (2008, May). *Restrictive eating disorders in children: Global findings from the International Network of Pediatric Surveillance Units.* Paper presented at the International Conference on Eating Disorders. Seattle, WA.

Shomaker, L. B., Tanofsky-Kraff, M., Elliot, C., Wolkoff, L. E., Columbo, K. M., Ranzenhofer, L. M., et al. (2010). Salience of loss of control for pediatric binge episodes: Does size really matter? *International Journal of Eating Disorders, 43*(8), 707–716.

Striegel-Moore, R. H., & Franko, D. L. (2003). Epidemiology of binge eating disorder. *International Journal of Eating Disorders, 34*, S19–S29.

Tanofsky-Kraff, M., Marcus, M. D., Yanovski, S. Z., & Yanovski, J. A. (2008). Loss of control eating disorder in children age 12 years and younger: Proposed research criteria. *Eating Behaviors, 9*, 360–365.

Wilfley, D. E., Schwartz, M. B., Spurrell, E. B., & Fairburn, C. G. (2000). Using the Eating Disorder Examination to identify the specific psychopathology of binge eating disorder. *International Journal of Eating Disorders, 27*, 259–269.

Wilson, G. T., & Sysko, R. (2009). Frequency of binge eating episodes in bulimia nervosa and binge eating disorder: Diagnostic considerations. *International Journal of Eating Disorders, 42*, 603–610.

Wonderlich, S. A., Joiner, T. E., Keel, P. K., Williamson, D. A., & Crosby, R. D. (2007). Eating disorder diagnoses: Empirical approaches to classification. *American Psychologist, 62*, 167–180.

World Health Organization. (1992). *International classification of diseases, 10th revision* (ICD-10). Geneva: Author.

■ PART IV ■

MEDICAL ISSUES AND ASSESSMENT

CHAPTER 9

Medical Issues Unique to Children and Adolescents

Debra K. Katzman
Sheri M. Findlay

It is essential for clinicians caring for children and adolescents with eating disorders to be knowledgeable about the medical complications associated with these serious and potentially life-threatening conditions. Knowledge of the physical effects of eating disorder behaviors allows the clinician to better educate the patient and family and understand the critical role nutritional rehabilitation plays in treatment of these disorders. Improved medical knowledge also offers the potential to improve patient outcomes through early identification and the prompt recognition of medical complications and intervention.

Restrictive eating and binge–purge behaviors associated with eating disorders have the potential to affect all organ systems in the growing body. Clinicians should be aware of the acute and long-term medical complications caused by these disorders. Several of the changes discussed in this chapter are adaptations to malnutrition and reflect the body's attempts to maintain homeostasis. These adaptations however, can pose serious immediate threats such as cardiac arrhythmias and metabolic derangements or long-term problems such as growth impairment and low bone mineral density. Although the complications discussed here are categorized by organ system, it is important to recognize that the medical complications are unlikely to exist in isolation and can occur in multiple organ systems simultaneously. In addition, dysfunction in one organ system is likely to have consequences in other organ systems.

Fluid and Electrolyte Abnormalities

Acute changes in hydration status and serum electrolytes can pose serious threats to a young person with an eating disorder. Hypokalemia is one of the most common and harmful metabolic complications of an eating disorder. The reported frequency of hypokalemia varies, depending on the age of the patients and the study setting. In adolescents treated as inpatients, the frequency of hypokalemia has been reported to be as high as 50% (Alvin, Zogheib, Rey, & Losay, 1993), whereas most studies of outpatients have shown a frequency between 4 and 20% in adolescents and young adults with bulimia nervosa (BN) or anorexia nervosa (AN)—binge–purge subtype (Greenfeld, Mickley, Quinlan, & Roloff, 1995; Miller, Grinspoon, et al., 2005; Palla & Litt, 1988; Wolfe, Metzger, Levine, & Jimerson, 2001). In patients with AN who do not vomit or use laxatives, the frequency of hypokalemia is very low (Greenfeld et al., 1995; Palla & Litt, 1988). Most of the pathological consequences of hypokalemia are due to total body potassium depletion that results from gastrointestinal losses (vomiting, laxative-induced diarrhea), transcellular shifts, and decreased intake or malnutrition. Acute consequences of hypokalemia can result in cardiac arrhythmias, including life-threatening ventricular dysrhythmias. Chronic hypokalemia can cause intestinal dysmotility and constipation, muscle myopathy, and nephropathy that results in chronic renal failure.

Hyponatremia has been reported in adolescents with AN and can be due to excessive consumption of water or "water loading," dehydration with total body sodium depletion, or, rarely, inappropriate secretion of antidiuretic hormone (Caregaro, Di Pascoli, Favaro, Nardi, & Santonastaso, 1993; Challier & Carbrol, 1995). Hyponatremia, when severe and occurring quickly, can result in seizures. Case reports in the adult literature describe central pontine myelinolysis resulting from the rapid correction of hyponatremia (Amann, Schafer, Sterr, Arnold, & Grunze, 2001; Santonastaso, Sala, & Favaro, 1998). Other electrolyte abnormalities include hypochloremia and alkalosis, most commonly encountered in patients who engage in purging behaviors (Alvin et al., 1993; Miller, Grieco, & Klibanski, 2005; Palla & Litt, 1988). Although there are no specific reports on the clinical implications of hypochloremic metabolic alkalosis in patients with eating disorders, lethargy, dehydration, impaired cognitive function, muscle wasting, and renal dysfunction and failure have been reported in children and adolescents with other medical disorders and hypochloremic metabolic alkalosis. The refeeding syndrome is a constellation of medical sequelae resulting from fluid and electrolyte imbalances as a result of reintroducing nutrition to a patient following a period of adaption to prolonged starvation and malnutrition (Solomon & Kirby, 1990). The symptoms range from mild to severe, depending on the degree of starvation. Multiple organ systems can be involved, including cardiac, respiratory, neurological, and hematological. Multisystem organ failure and death can occur.

The hallmark of the refeeding syndrome is fluid and electrolyte dysregulation, severe hypophosphatemia, hypokalemia, hypomagnesemia, abnormal glucose metabolism, and deficiencies in vitamins and trace elements. Hypophosphatemia can result in serious cardiac, neurological, and hematological dysfunction. Several articles have documented the occurrence of this syndrome in children and adolescents with AN (Kohn, Golden, & Shenker, 1998; O'Connor & Goldin, in press; Ornstein, Golden, Jacobson, & Shenker, 2003). The risk of hypophosphatemia is highest in the most severely malnourished patients and appears to be present during the first week of refeeding. Ornstein and colleagues (2003) reported that 27.5% of inpatient adolescents undergoing refeeding developed hypophosphatemia, with the nadir occurring on day 4 of hospitalization. Reviews on the subject routinely recommend that refeeding severely malnourished patients needs to be done with close medical supervision, including monitoring of the cardiovascular system and regular examination of metabolic and neurological status (Katzman, 2005; Kohn et al., 1998; Ornstein et al., 2003).

Metabolic Alterations

Alterations in energy metabolism are observed in patients with AN. The basal metabolic rate (BMR) is reduced in low-weight patients with AN (Obarzanek, Lesem, & Jimerson, 1994; Platte et al., 1994). The decrease in BMR may be due to a number of factors, including a change in body composition and a down-regulation of cellular metabolism. Several physiological mechanisms have been proposed, including reduction of activity of the sympathetic nervous system, alterations in peripheral thyroid metabolism, lowered insulin secretion, and a decrease in leptin levels (Muller, Focker, Holtkamp, Herpertz-Dahlmann, & Hebebrand, 2009).

Mild hypoglycemia is common and usually asymptomatic in patients with AN. There are many hypotheses on the development of hypoglycemia in patients with AN. The major risk factors identified are low body weight, excessive exercise, and infection. The precise pathogenesis has not been elucidated, but several mechanisms, including depletion of liver glycogen, defective gluconeogenesis, and failure of glucagon secretion have been proposed. Other findings suggest that a rapid increase of energy intake can cause reactive hypoglycemia with an associated elevated level of insulin secretion.

Hyperaminoacidemia has been reported in children with AN, reflecting a marasmic pattern of protein–energy undernutrition (Moyano, Vilaseca, Artuch, & Lambruschini, 1998). Cystine and arginine have been shown to be lower in patients with AN as compared with reference values, suggesting that this deficiency may have an impact on oxidative functions, which is one of the ways that the cells in the body create energy for essential bodily functions (Moyano et al., 1998). Although counterintuitive in considering the caloric restriction state found in AN, normal plasma total protein and albumin levels have been reported in adolescents with eating disorders (Palla & Litt, 1988). Currently, there are no biological mechanisms that explain this.

Hypercholesterolemia is common in adolescents with AN, despite emaciation (Palla & Litt, 1988). Elevated cholesterol concentrations in AN are generally the result of accelerated cholesterol synthesis in this population (Weinbrenner et al., 2004). Increased lipolysis, decreased endogenous cholesterol synthesis, and decreased bile–acid synthesis and turnover that results in decreased cholesterol catabolism are the suggested mechanisms of hypercholesterolemia in AN. The long-term implications of the hypercholesterolemia in AN are unknown. As with other metabolic changes, return to normal levels is expected after weight restoration.

Vitamins and minerals are necessary for normal functioning and growth. Although vitamin and mineral deficiencies are rare in patients with eating disorders, subclinical iron, calcium, and zinc deficiencies have been reported (Fisher et al., 1995). Clinicians should consider monitoring these nutrients as potential causes of metabolic abnormalities in adolescents with eating disorders.

Renal Complications

Renal abnormalities reported in adolescents with eating disorders include elevated blood urea nitrogen (BUN) and creatinine, thought to be partially due to dehydration or volume depletion and may also be due to a reduced glomerular filtration rate and problems with concentrating urine. In addition, pyuria, hematuria, and proteinuria have also been reported in adolescents with AN (Palla & Litt, 1988). More recently, there was a study that showed that 17% of adolescents with AN had nocturnal enuresis. In addition, this study demonstrated a high frequency of day- and nighttime urinary incontinence symptoms in this population. It was hypothesized that both decreased functional bladder capacity and detrusor muscle instability may be responsible for contributing to nocturnal enuresis (Kanbur et al., in press).

In the adult literature there are case reports of kidney stones and chronic renal failure, thought to be secondary to chronic hypokalemia due to long-standing purging (Abdel-Rahman & Moorthy, 1997; Yasuhara et al., 2005). In the pediatric population there are case reports of acute renal failure thought to be secondary to acute rhabdomy-olysis, which is the rapid breakdown of skeletal muscle and the release of myoglobin, which can be harmful to the kidneys and lead to renal failure (Wada, Nagase, Koike, Kugai, & Nagata, 1992).

Cardiovascular and Respiratory Complications

Complications of the cardiovascular system are serious and potentially life-threatening consequences of AN and BN in children and adolescents. The effect of starvation on the heart is likely responsible for the majority of acute medical admissions to the hospital for children and adolescents with eating disorders.

Studies have documented bradycardia in children and adolescents with low weight secondary to an eating disorder. Prevalence rates in this patient population range from 30 to 60%, depending on the study population and definition used (Alvin et al., 1993; Lupoglazoff et al., 2001; Miller, Grieco, et al., 2005; Misra et al., 2004; Mont et al., 2003; Palla & Litt, 1988). Bradycardia can cause fatigue, weakness, dizziness, palpita-tions, shortness of breath, and, in some cases, cardiac arrest. Other markers of cardio-vascular compromise, such as hypotension and orthostatic heart rate and blood pressure changes, are also well documented. Electrocardiographic and Holter monitor changes are frequently seen and include sinus bradycardia, low voltages and prolongation of the QTc interval and QTc dispersion (Alvin et al., 1993; Galetta et al., 2002; Lupoglazoff et al., 2001; Mont et al., 2003; Palla & Litt, 1988; Swenne & Larsson, 1999; Ulger et al., 2006; Vanderdokt, Lambert, Montero, Boland, & Brohet, 2001). The aforementioned studies that have evaluated the response to refeeding have reassuringly demonstrated that all deteriorations in cardiac functioning have returned to normal following weight restoration.

Structural and functional heart changes in patients with AN have been documented on both chest x-ray and echocardiogram. On chest x-ray the heart silhouette appears small (Moodie & Salcedo, 1983; Silverman, 1983), and echocardiograms have confirmed that weight loss results in loss of cardiac mass, specifically a reduced left ventricular volume and diminished thickness of cardiac walls (de Simone et al., 1994; Galetta et al., 2005; Lupoglazoff et al., 2001; Mont et al., 2003; Ramacciotti, Coli, Biadi, & Dell'Osso, 2003; Romano et al., 2003; Ulger et al., 2006). Despite the loss of cardiac muscle, func-tion is generally normal, patients are asymptomatic, and the findings are reversible with weight restoration. Other frequent findings on an echocardiogram are mitral valve pro-lapse and pericardial effusion. There is one case report of medical compromise with pericardial effusion in an adolescent with AN (Polli et al., 2006); however, no other functional abnormalities have been reported (Alvin et al., 1993; de Simone et al., 1994; Lupoglazoff et al., 2001; Ramacciotti et al., 2003).

Less evidence exists on the effect of starvation associated with eating disorders on pulmonary functioning. There is one report involving adolescents suggesting that there is some measurable decline in pulmonary functioning present in patients with chronic malnutrition (Ziora et al., 2008) (a recently published abstract described respiratory acidosis in medically compromised adolescents with AN; Kerem, Riskin, Everin, Srugo, & Kugelman, 2010). There are a few articles in the adult literature suggesting an increased risk of emphysema-like changes in the lungs of patients with chronic AN (Cook, Coxson, Mason, & Bai, 2001; Coxson et al., 2004; Gardenghi et al., 2009). One case report described asymptomatic pneumomediastinum in an adolescent with AN and self-induced vomiting (Overby & Litt, 1988). A possible explanation is that starvation and malnutrition may predispose a person to changes within the lung interstitium, leading to the formation of bullae and emphysema, which adds to the risk of spontaneous pneumomediastinum after vomiting (Hochlehnert et al., 2010).

Oral and Gastrointestinal Complications

The digestive tract is invariably affected by the presence of an eating disorder. Dysfunction can occur along the entire gastrointestinal tract and can be a result of starvation, purging, binge eating, or the use of laxatives or enemas. In addition, functional gastrointestinal symptoms with negative work-up—such as pain, lack of appetite, bloating, and early satiety—are extremely common in this clinical population (Boyd, Abraham, & Kellow, 2005; Chami, Andersen, Crowell, Schuster, & Whitehead, 1995). It is important to recognize the full extent of possible gastrointestinal pathology in order to safely evaluate, but to avoid overinvestigation of, digestive complaints in the young person with an eating disorder. In the assessment of gastrointestinal complaints in the young person with an eating disorder, the history and physical examination usually does not reveal any markers of more serious gastrointestinal pathology such as upper or lower gastrointestinal bleeding, diarrhea, spontaneous emesis, or jaundice. Laboratory investigations should not reveal markers of inflammation or infection such as an elevated erythrocyte sedimentation rate, an elevated white blood cell count, or the presence of anemia. If these are present, it is critical to investigate thoroughly for more serious consequences of the eating disorder or other causes of the symptoms.

The oral cavity is adversely affected by binge eating and purging, but can also be affected by starving, dehydration, the use of antidepressant medication, and dental hygiene practices (Ohrn, Enzell, & Angmar-Mansson, 1999; Roberts & Tylenda, 1989). Studies on dental complications generally involve adult patients; however, pediatric clinicians can educate patients and families about the complications. The most common dental complication is dental enamel erosion or perimylolysis on the lingual, palatal, and posterior occlusal surfaces of the teeth, which worsens with frequency and duration of vomiting (Touyz et al., 1993). This is a result of low-pH gastric contents coming in contact with dental enamel. Gingival disease and xerostomatia (reduced saliva production) is common in patients with either AN or BN, in association with dehydration and the use of antidepressant medication (Ohrn et al., 1999). Salivary gland enlargement, particularly of the parotid or submandibular glands, and hyperamylasemia are associated with purging behaviors and are proportional to the frequency of purging behaviors (Gwirtsman et al., 1989; Touyz et al., 1993).

Symptoms of upper gastrointestinal tract dysfunction are very common in children and adolescents with AN or BN. Few studies have investigated esophageal dysfunction or injury, and those that have, have not shown any increased rates of poor esophageal motility or mucosal injury, even in patients with frequent bulimic symptoms (Nickl, Brazer, Rockwell, & Smith, 1996; Stacher et al., 1986). Adolescents with BN who present with hematemesis may have the Mallory-Weiss syndrome, which consists of tears at the junction of the esophagus and the stomach (Silber, 2005). In patients who vomit, the increase in intragastric pressure predisposes them to the development of these tears, possibly resulting in hematemesis. There are a few isolated case reports of dramatic complications such as esophageal perforation (Overby & Litt, 1988; Palla & Litt, 1988). Delayed gastric emptying is common in children and adolescents with AN or BN. The presenting symptoms include fullness, bloating, and lack of appetite (Benini et al., 2004; Hutson & Wald, 1990; McCallum et al., 1985; Robinson, Clarke, & Barrett, 1988; Stacher et al., 1986). Randomized controlled trials in adults with eating disorders comparing prokinetic agents to placebos are inconclusive. To date, evidence suggests that nutritional rehabilitation accelerates gastric motility.

Despite the frequency of dyspepsia symptoms (Chami et al., 1995; Palla & Litt, 1988), there have not been any studies suggesting that gastroesophageal reflux disease is more common in adolescents with eating disorders. Similarly, there is no evidence that patients with eating disorders experience a higher rate of peptic ulcer disease or gastritis, and there are no increased rates of helicobacter pylori infection (Hill, Hill, Humphries, Maloney, & McClain, 1999; Sherman et al., 1993).

Gastric dilation, with or without rupture, is a rare but potentially lethal complication of severe binge eating that has been described in a few case reports of teenagers with eating disorders (Holtkamp, Mogharrebi, Hanishch, Schumpelick, & Herpertz-Dahlmann, 2002; Nakao et al., 2000; Sinicina, Pantkratz, Buttner, & Mall, 2005). Patients with superior mesenteric artery syndrome, in which the duodenum is compressed by the superior mesenteric artery, present with gastric dilatation, vomiting, and abdominal pain. Although this is a rare complication, if left untreated, it can be fatal (Adson, Mitchell, & Trenkner, 1997).

Symptoms of lower digestive tract dysfunction are also very common. The majority of adolescents with eating disorders report symptoms of constipation (Chami et al., 1995; Kamal et al., 1991; Palla & Litt, 1988; Waldholtz & Andersen, 1990). Various mechanisms contribute to the constipation, including reduced food and fluid intake, electrolyte abnormalities, and slowed colonic transit time (Chiarioni et al., 2000; Zipfel et al., 2006). The treatment of lower gastrointestinal dysfunction can be challenging, as traditional constipation treatments have not been shown to be effective and can cause iatrogenic complications, including possible laxative dependence, in this patient population. As with most other gastrointestinal symptoms, constipation resolves with nutritional rehabilitation, fluid and electrolyte balance, and weight gain.

Rectal prolapse has been reported in the adult eating disorder literature but not in the child and adolescent eating disorder literature to date (Dreznik, Vishne, Kristt, Alper, & Ramadan, 2001; Malik, Stratton, & Sweeney, 1997). The misuse of laxatives has been found to be present in about one-third of adolescents with AN (Stock, Goldberg, Corbett, & Katzman, 2002; Turner, Batik, Palmer, Forbes, & McDermott, 2000). The possible complications depend on the amount and type of laxatives misused. Reports of complications include dehydration, electrolyte abnormalities, chronic diarrhea, kidney stones, and possible pancreatic damage (Baker & Sandle, 1996; Brown, Treasure, & Campbell, 2001; Meyers et al., 1990). Withdrawal from laxatives has not been reported in pediatric eating disorders, but in the adult literature rebound constipation, fluid retention, edema, and congestive heart failure have been described (Meyers et al., 1990; Riley, Brown, & Walker, 1996).

In the adult literature, dysfunction of the pancreas and pancreatitis (both acute and chronic) have been reported in patients with AN or BN; however, there are no case reports for the pediatric population (Backett, 1985; Cox, Cannon, Ament, Phillips, & Schaffer, 1983; Morris, Stephenson, Herring, & Marti, 2004; Nordgren & von Scheele, 1977; Wesson, Sparaco, & Smith, 2008). Increases in liver function tests, specifically serum aspartate aminotransferase (AST), alanine aminotransferase (ALT), lactate dehydrogenase (LDH) and gamma-glutamyl transpeptidase (GGT) can occur as a result of refeeding, as a manifestation of excessive calories and fat deposition in the liver, or may be due to severe malnutrition before refeeding has occurred (Fong et al., 2008; Montagnese et al., 2007; Narayanan, Gaudiani, Harris, & Mehler, 2010; Sherman, Leslie, Goldberg, Rybczynski, & St. Louis, 1994; Tsukamoto et al., 2008). The elevations are usually mild and improve with nutritional rehabilitation and weight gain. Two studies showed that the degree of elevation of transaminases was inversely proportional to the severity of emaciation (Fong et al., 2008; Ozawa, Shimizu, & Shishiba, 1998). There are case reports of severe liver dysfunction and liver failure in adolescents and adults (de Caprio et al., 2006; Furuta et al., 1999; Narayanan et al., 2010; Rautou et al., 2008).

Hematological and Infectious Complications

A recent detailed review (Hutter, Ganepola, & Hofmann, 2009), reported that the hematological complications of AN included possible deficits in all cell lines. Normocytic anemia is the most frequent finding and present in 21–39% of patients. Micronutrients such as folic acid, vitamin B_{12} and iron are generally found to be normal in patients with AN, thus microcytosis and macrocytosis are infrequently encountered. Leukocytopenia is found in about one-third of patients with AN. Lymphocytopenia and neutropenia can occur alone or simultaneously, although severe deficits are rare. Mild reductions in platelet counts are found in 5–11% of patients, but coagulation remains normal.

The deficits in all three cell lines are related to bone marrow atrophy and in severe cases a condition called "gelatinous transformation," which describes the histological appearance of the bone marrow associated with atrophy of fat cells and depletion of the normal cell line precursors. The bone marrow abnormalities are thought to be related to chronic malnutrition and reduced body fat stores and can exist in as many as 50% of patients with AN with normal peripheral blood cell counts. Deficits in red and white blood cells, platelets, and bone marrow are all reversible with nutritional rehabilitation (Hutter et al., 2009). Although few studies have included patients with BN in evaluating hematological changes in patients with eating disorders, one study showed no increased risk of anemia in adult women with BN (Wolfe et al., 2001).

In addition to alterations of white blood cells and cell-mediated immunity, defective bactericidal activity of granulocytes, low complement levels, and changes in cytokines have been reported in patients with AN (Pomeroy et al., 1997). Despite this, there is no evidence to suggest that patients with AN are at increased risk for infection. Of clinical importance, however, is that many of the normal clinical responses to infection (e.g., fever and increased heart rate) may not be present in adolescents with AN. Clinicians should be extremely vigilant if they suspect an infection in an adolescent with an eating disorder.

Endocrine Complications

The impact of chronic malnutrition on the hormonal systems can have a profound and possibly irreversible effect on the growth and development of children and adolescents. Several literature reviews have been conducted documenting the wide extent of possible changes (Gianotti et al., 2002; Krassas, 2003; Misra & Klibanski, 2010; Munoz & Argente, 2002; Stoving, Hangaard, Hansen-Nord, & Hagen, 1999).

Thyroid dysfunction in both AN and BN is common. In patients with AN the expected finding is the "low T_3 syndrome" with a low triiodothyronine (T_3), a normal or low-normal thyroxine (T_4), and a normal thyroid-stimulating hormone (TSH) (Onur et al., 2005; Palla & Litt, 1988; Tamai et al., 1986). The underlying mechanisms accounting for the low T_3 are not fully understood, but likely include a reduced peripheral conversion of T_4 to T_3 and a concurrent increase in production of the inactive rT_3 from T_4 (Kiyohara, Tamai, Takaichi, Nakagawa, & Kumagai, 1989). Although random TSH levels are usually normal, there is evidence of hypothalamic dysfunction with a blunted and/or delayed TSH response to thyrotropin-releasing hormone administration. The thyroid gland itself shows diffuse atrophy in adults with AN (Stoving, Bennedbaek, Hegedus, & Hagen, 2001). The abnormalities of thyroid functioning appear to be fully reversible with refeeding (Misra & Klibanski, 2010; Stoving et al., 1999). In patients with BN, the thyroid abnormalities are less consistent and depend on the patient's nutritional status (Altemus, Hetherington, Kennedy, Licinio, & Gold, 1996; Fichter, Pirke, Pollinger, Wolfram, & Brunner, 1990). However, even in patients of normal weight with BN there can be similar abnormalities as those found in patients with AN. None of these studies of BN have focused on children and adolescents.

Abnormalities of reproductive hormones are also expected with suppression of the hypothalamic-pituitary-gonadal axis in both girls and boys with AN. Hypogonadotropic-hypogonadism is the norm for patients with AN (Estour et al., 2010; Misra & Klibanski, 2010; Nogal, Pniewska-Siark, & Lewinski, 2008). In girls, this presents clinically as primary or secondary amenorrhea, pubertal delay, and growth failure, and in boys, pubertal delay and growth failure. Laboratory assessment can reveal prepubertal levels of luteinizing hormone (LH), follicle stimulating hormone (FSH), estradiol, and testosterone (Misra et al., 2008; Munoz & Argente, 2002; Palla & Litt, 1988; Tomova, Makker, Kirilov, Agarwal, & Kumanov, 2007). A variety of factors may contribute to amenorrhea in adolescents with AN: weight loss, decreased body fat, hypoleptinemia, excessive exercising, emotional disturbances, and abnormal eating attitudes and behaviors. These factors interfere with the onset of menarche and normal sexual development in the premenarcheal girl and cause secondary amenorrhea and delayed sexual development in the postmenarcheal girl. For patients with BN, the reproductive axis can be normal, or abnormalities can be similar to those found in patients with AN (Fichter et al., 1990;

Palla & Litt, 1988). Clinically, adolescents with BN can have normal menstrual function, irregular menstrual function, or amenorrhea (Austin et al., 2008). Recovery of the reproductive hormones' abnormalities in menstrual function is expected with weight restoration, improved emotional states, decrease in excessive exercise behavior, and improved eating attitudes and behaviors.

Abnormalities of the growth hormone (GH) and insulinlike growth factor-1 (IGF-1) have been studied in patients with AN, yet much remains unknown. Basal secretion of GH is usually elevated whereas IGF-1 levels are reduced, and it is thought that a state of GH resistance exists in this malnourished population (Munoz & Argente, 2002; Prabhakaran et al., 2008; Stoving et al., 1999). Despite an abundance of abnormalities in the hormone systems that control growth and development, the clinical relevance of these abnormalities for patient care is uncertain. It is not clear whether there can be permanent growth failure in children and adolescents with eating disorders. For instance, studies have shown that the onset of AN before the pubertal growth spurt, coupled with marked weight loss and prolonged duration of illness, can adversely affect the adolescent's ultimate adult height, whereas the onset of AN after peak height velocity may not substantially affect the adolescent's stature (Prabhakaran et al., 2008; Roze et al., 2007). Thus, it appears that early treatment is critical to avoid delayed or irreversible effects on the adolescent's pubertal growth and development.

Hypercortisolemia has also been found to be present in adolescents with AN and is believed to be associated with both hypothalamic dysregulation and peripheral cortisol resistance (Munoz & Argente, 2002; Stoving et al., 1999). The clinical significance of these abnormalities is unknown.

Decreased Bone-Mineral Density

The increased risk of low bone-mineral density in females and males with AN and in adolescents with BN and a history of low weight or amenorrhea is well documented in the literature (Bredella et al., 2008; Castro, Toro, Lazaro, Pons, & Halperin, 2002; Hofman, Landewe-Cleuren, Wojciechowski, & Kruseman, 2009; Katzman, 2005; Katzman & Golden, 2008; Mehler, Sabel, Watson, & Andersen, 2008; Misra et al., 2008). Low bone-mineral density, one of the most profound, earliest medical complications of AN, is prevalent in adolescents with AN. Reduced bone-mineral density is associated with reduced bone turnover and decreased bone formation and bone-resorption markers. Adolescents with BN with a history of low weight or amenorrhea are also at risk of impaired bone-mineral density.

Low bone-mineral density is one of the earliest medical complications found in girls with AN, often evident in the first year of the illness (Bachrach, Guido, Katzman, Litt, & Marcus, 1990; Jagielska et al., 2002). The etiology of the bone loss is related to both increased bone breakdown and decreased bone formation. The pathophysiology for low bone-mineral density in adolescents is multifactorial (Willer et al., 2009) and complex and includes decreased bone accretion, high cortisol levels, hypoestrogenemia, low testosterone levels, low levels of IGF-1, low calcium and vitamin D intake, abnormal levels of gastrointestinal peptides (Misra et al., 2008), and low body weight (Hofman et al., 2009; Katzman, 2005; Lawson et al., 2010; Mehler et al., 2008; Misra et al., 2008; Winston, Alwazeer, & Bankart, 2008).

The low bone-mineral density associated with AN has been shown to be at least partially reversible. Essential factors in improvement of low bone density are weight restoration and resumption of menstruation (Bass et al., 2005; Castro et al., 2002; De Alvaro et al., 2007; Dominguez et al., 2007; Gleich et al., 2001; Katzman, 2005; Legroux-Gerot, Vignau, Collier, & Cortet, 2008; Misra et al., 2008). The prevention and treatment of low bone-mineral density in AN have been studied, and to date there is no convincing evidence for the use of pharmacotherapy (Mehler & MacKenzie, 2009). Estrogen replacement therapy has not been shown to be effective in the prevention of progressive bone loss or enhancement of bone mineralization (Katzman, 2005; Sim et al., 2010). Supplementation with calcium and vitamin D are recommended, although the evidence for these interventions is less definitive. Currently, there are no evidence- or consensus-based guidelines for the dose of vitamin D required in adolescents with AN. The literature suggests that exercise protects against osteopenia in adults with AN; however, this has not been confirmed for adolescents.

Other medications that have been investigated for treatment of low bone density in adolescents with AN are dehydroepiandrosterone, alendronate, biphosphonates, and IGF-1. No studies have shown clear benefits for these medications and none are yet recommended for routine use (Golden et al., 2002, 2005; Katzman, 2005; Mehler & MacKenzie, 2009).

Neurological Complications

Literature on the effect of eating disorders on the central nervous system in children and adolescents has been mounting, but much remains unknown. The malnutrition associated with AN has been clearly shown to cause structural brain changes, including an increase in the cerebrospinal fluid volumes and a loss of gray matter and white matter volumes (Kerem & Katzman, 2003; Nogal et al., 2008). Persistent deficits in gray matter and elevated cerebrospinal fluid volumes, but normal white matter volumes, have been reported among weight-restored participants with adolescent-onset AN. These findings suggest that structural brain abnormalities are not completely reversible for this group. Low weight and high cortisol levels are associated with greater structural brain abnormalities. Young women with adolescent-onset AN have also been shown to have abnormal cognitive function. Abnormal menstrual function is associated with cognitive deficits, which improve with the resumption of menstruation. The severity of these changes appears to be related to duration of illness and degree of weight loss. The degree of reversibility of these changes is not fully known, as studies have revealed conflicting results. The clinical relevance of these changes also remains unknown, as changes in cognitive functioning, mood, or personality have not been directly linked to these abnormalities.

Other neuroimaging techniques, including positron emission tomography and single photon emission computed tomography scans, have been used to measure cerebral glucose metabolism and cerebral blood flow, respectively, to compare the brains of young people with AN with healthy controls (Lask et al., 2005). Various changes have been noted, such as a reduction of cerebral blood flow to the temporal lobe in about 75% of young people with AN, which does not appear to be fully reversible with weight restoration. It is hypothesized that some of the abnormalities found with functional neuroimaging may represent a primary deficit, which may predispose a person to eating disorders, and other changes may be secondary to starvation (see Kaye, Chapter 2, this volume). Currently, the clinical implications of the aforementioned neurological findings are unknown; however, it is important to educate patients and families about possible changes to brain structure and function associated with untreated eating disorders.

There have been several articles reporting neurological symptoms in patients with eating disorders. One study surveyed more than 100 adult patients and found that about half of them reported neurological symptoms, most commonly generalized muscle weakness and peripheral neuropathy (Patchell, Fellows, & Humphries, 1994). There are also case reports of foot drop associated with nerve compression due to weight loss (Kershenbaum, Jaffa, Zeman, & Boniface, 1997) and a reversible metabolic myopathy (McLoughlin et al., 2000). All of these reported complications are thought to be reversible with nutritional rehabilitation.

Dermatological and Hair Complications

The impact of eating disorders on the skin and hair does not pose the serious acute and chronic health risks as does the impact on other organ systems; however, patients can frequently be distressed by such changes more than by other medical complications. A review of the literature published in 2002 concluded that there are as many as 40 different cutaneous manifestations of eating disorders (Tyler, Wiseman, Crawford, & Birmingham, 2002); however, most are uncommon as individual entities. Only one study focused on children and adolescents, which found that the most commonly encountered complications are xerosis and dermatographism, hypertrichosis, lanugo hair, acrocyanosis, telogen effluvium, and brittle nails (Mehler et al., 2001). Several studies in adults with eating disorders revealed very similar findings (Glorio et al., 2000; Strumia, 2005; Strumia, Varotti, Manzato, & Gualandi, 2001), but also document the presence of Russell's sign (callous formation on the dorsum of the hand secondary to trauma to the hand as a result of using the fingers to stimulate the gag reflux to vomit), cheilitis, carotenoderma, and generalized pruritus.

Conclusion

AN and BN are associated with numerous medical complications in children and adolescents. Their consequences can range from mild to life threatening. Some of the complications are markers of malnutrition and pose minimal threat, but are nonetheless relevant for clinicians to be aware of, as they can be used therapeutically to educate patients and families about the effects of malnutrition on the growing body. Furthermore, resolution of these symptoms can serve as markers of physical recovery. Other complications are far more serious and can result in acute medical compromise or long-term disability or death. Nutritional rehabilitation and elimination of restrictive and binge and purge behaviors have the ability to ameliorate the medical complications associated with eating disorders. Treatment of the cognitive and behavioral symptoms of restricting, bingeing, and purging is challenging. In untreated or partially treated patients, permanent sequelae involving poor growth, low bone-mineral density and long-term impact to the structure and function of the brain are possible consequences.

References

Abdel-Rahman, E. M., & Moorthy, A. V. (1997). End-stage renal disease (ESRD) in patients with eating disorders. *Clinical Nephrology, 47*(2), 106–111.

Adson, D. E., Mitchell, J., & Trenkner, S. (1997). The superior mesenteric artery syndrome and acute gastric dilatation in eating disorders: A report of two cases and a review of the literature. *International Journal of Eating Disorders, 21*(2), 103–114.

Altemus, M., Hetherington, M., Kennedy, B., Licinio, J., & Gold, P. W. (1996). Thyroid function in bulimia nervosa. *Psychoneuroendocrinology, 21*(3), 249–261.

Alvin, P., Zogheib, J., Rey, C., & Losay, J. (1993). Severe complications and mortality in mental eating disorders in adolescence: On 99 hospitalized patients. *Archives Francaises de Pediatric, 50*(9), 755–762.

Amann, B., Schafer, M., Sterr, A., Arnold, S., & Grunze, H. (2001). Central pontine myelinolysis in a patient with anorexia nervosa. *International Journal of Eating Disorders, 30*(4), 462–466.

Austin, S. B., Ziyadeh, N. J., Vohra, S., Forman, S., Gordon, C. M., Prokop, L. A., et al. (2008). Irregular menses linked to vomiting in a nonclinical sample: Findings from the National Eating Disorders Screening Program in high schools. *Journal of Adolescent Health, 42*(5), 450–457.

Bachrach, L. K., Guido, D., Katzman, D., Litt, I. F., & Marcus, R. (1990). Decreased bone density in adolescent girls with anorexia nervosa. *Pediatrics, 86*(3), 440–447.

Backett, S. A. (1985). Acute pancreatitis and gastric dilatation in a patient with anorexia nervosa. *Postgraduate Medical Journal, 61*(711), 39–40.

Baker, E., & Sandle, G. (1996). Complications of laxative abuse. *Annual Review of Medicine, 47*, 127–134.

Bass, S. L., Saxon, L., Corral, A. M., Rodda, C. P., Stauss, B. J., Reidpath, D., et al. (2005). Near normalisation of lumbar spine bone density in young women with osteopenia recovered from adolescent onset anorexia nervosa: A longitudinal study. *Journal of Pediatric Endocrinology and Metabolism, 18*(9), 897–907.

Benini, L., Todesco, T., Dalle Grave, R., Deiorio, F., Salandini, L., & Vantini, I. (2004). Gastric emptying in patients with restricting and binge/purging subtypes of anorexia nervosa. *American Journal of Gastroenterology, 99*(8), 1448–1454.

Boyd, C., Abraham, S., & Kellow, J. (2005). Psychological features are important predictors of functional gastrointestinal disorders in patients with eating disorders. *Scandanavian Journal of Gastroenterology, 40*(8), 929–935.

Bredella, M. A., Misra, M., Miller, K. K., Madisch, I., Sarwar, A., Cheung, A., et al. (2008). Distal radius in adolescent girls with anorexia nervosa: Trabecular structure analysis with high-resolution flat-panel volume CT. *Radiology, 249*(3), 938–946.

Brown, N. W., Treasure, J. L., & Campbell, I. C. (2001). Evidence for long-term pancreatic damage caused by laxative abuse in subjects recovered from anorexia nervosa. *International Journal of Eating Disorders, 29*(2), 236–238.

Caregaro, L., Di Pascoli, L., Favaro, A., Nardi, M., & Santonastaso, P. (1993). Sodium depletion and hemoconcentration: Overlooked complications in patients with anorexia nervosa. *Nutrition, 21*(4), 438–445.

Castro, J., Toro, J., Lazaro, L., Pons, R., & Halperin, I. (2002). Bone mineral density in male adolescents with anorexia nervosa. *Journal of the American Academy of Child and Adolescent Psychiatry, 41*(5), 613–618.

Challier, P., & Carbrol, S. (1995). Severe hyponatremia associated with anorexia nervosa: Role of inappropriate antidiuretic hormone secretion. *Archives of Pediatric and Adolescent Medicine, 2*(10), 977–979.

Chami, T. N., Andersen, A. E., Crowell, M. D., Schuster, M. M., & Whitehead, W. E. (1995). Gastrointestinal symptoms in bulimia nervosa: Effects of treatment. *American Journal of Gastroenterology, 90*(1), 88–92.

Chiarioni, G., Bassotti, G., Monsignori, A., Menegotti, M., Salandini, L., Di Matteo, G., et al. (2000). Anorectal dysfunction in constipated women with anorexia nervosa. *Mayo Clinic Proceedings, 75*(10), 1015–1019.

Cook, V. J., Coxson, H. O., Mason, A. G., & Bai, T. R. (2001). Bullae, bronchiectasis and nutritional emphysema in severe anorexia nervosa. *Canadian Respiratory Journal, 8*(5), 361–365.

Cox, K. L., Cannon, R. A., Ament, M. E., Phillips, H. E., & Schaffer, C. B. (1983). Biochemical and ultrasonic abnormalities of the pancreas in anorexia nervosa. *Digestive Diseases and Sciences, 28*(3), 225–229.

Coxson, H., Chan, I. H., Mago, J. R., Hlynsky, J. A., Nakano, Y., & Birmingham, C. L. (2004). Early emphysema in patients with anorexia nervosa. *American Journal of Respiratory and Critical Care Medicine, 170*(7), 748–752.

De Alvaro, M. T., Muñoz-Calvo, M. T., Barrios, V., Martinez, G., Martos-Moreno, A., Hawkins, F., et al. (2007). Regional fat distribution in adolescents with anorexia nervosa: Effect of duration of malnutrition and weight recovery. *European Journal of Endocrinology, 157*(4), 473–479.

de Caprio, C., Alfano, A., Senatore, I., Zarella, L., Pasanisi, F., & Contaldo, F. (2006). Severe acute liver damage in anorexia nervosa: Two case reports. *Nutrition, 22*(5), 572–575.

de Simone, G., Scalfi, L., Galderisi, M., Celentano, A., Di Biase, G., Tammaro, P., et al. (1994). Cardiac abnormalities in young women with anorexia nervosa. *British Heart Journal, 71*(3), 287–292.

Dominguez, J., Goodman, L., Sen Gupta, S., Mayer, L., Etu, S. F., Walsh, B. T., et al. (2007). Treatment of anorexia nervosa is associated with increases in bone mineral density, and recovery is a biphasic process involving both nutrition and return of menses. *American Journal of Clinical Nutrition, 86*(1), 92–99.

Dreznik, Z., Vishne, T., Kristt, D., Alper, D., & Ramadan, E. (2001). Rectal prolapse: A possibly underrecognized complication of anorexia nervosa amenable to surgical correction. *International Journal of Psychiatry in Medicine 31*(3), 347–352.

Estour, B., Germain, N., Diconne, E., Frere, D., Cottet-Emard, J. M., Carrot, G., et al. (2010). Hormonal profile heterogeneity and short-term physical risk in restrictive anorexia nervosa. *Journal of Clinical Endocrinology and Metabolism, 95*(5), 2203–2210.

Fichter, M. M., Pirke, K. M., Pollinger, J., Wolfram, G., & Brunner, E. (1990). Disturbances in the hypothalamo-pituitary-adrenal and other neuroendocrine axes in bulimia. *Biological Psychiatry, 27*(9), 1021–1037.

Fisher, M., Golden, N. H., Katzman, D. K., Kreipe, R. E., Rees, J., Schebendach, J., et al. (1995). Eating disorders in adolescents: A background paper. *Journal of Adolescent Health, 16*(6), 420–437.

Fong, H. F., Divasta, A. D., Difabio, D., Ringelheim, J., Jonas, M. M., & Gordon, C. M. (2008). Prevalence and predictors of abnormal liver enzymes in young women with anorexia nervosa. *Journal of Pediatrics, 153*(2), 247–253.

Furuta, S., Ozawa, Y., Maejima, K., Tashiro, H., Kitahora, T., Hasegawa, K., et al. (1999). Anorexia nervosa with severe liver dysfunction and subsequent critical complications. *Internal Medicine, 38*(7), 575–579.

Galetta, F., Franzoni, F., Cupisti, A., Belliti, D., Prattichizzo, F., & Rolla, M. (2002). QT interval dispersion in young women with anorexia nervosa. *Journal of Pediatrics, 140*(4), 456–460.

Galetta, F., Franzoni, F., Cupisti, A., Morelli, E., Santoro, G., & Pentimone, F. (2005). Early detection of cardiac dysfunction in patients with anorexia nervosa by tissue Doppler imaging. *International Journal of Cardiology, 101*(1), 33–37.

Gardenghi, G., Boni, E., Todisco, P., Manara, F., Borghesi, A., & Tantucci, C. (2009). Respiratory function in patients with stable anorexia nervosa. *Chest, 136*(5), 1356–1363.

Gianotti, L., Lanfranco, F., Ramunni, J., Destefanis, S., Ghigo, E., & Arvat, E. (2002).

GH/IGF-I axis in anorexia nervosa. *Eating and Weight Disorders, 7*(2), 94–105.

Gleich, L. L., Gluckman, J. L., Nemunaitis, J., Suen, J. Y., Hanna, E., Wolf, G. T., et al. (2001). Clinical experience with HLA-B7 plasmid DNA/lipid complex in advanced squamous cell carcinoma of the head and neck. *Archives of Otolaryngology—Head and Neck Surgery, 127*(7), 775–779.

Glorio, R., Allevato, M., De Pablo, A., Abbruzzese, M., Carmona, L., Savarin, M., et al. (2000). Prevalence of cutaneous manifestations in 200 patients with eating disorders. *International Journal of Dermatology, 39*(5), 348–353.

Golden, N. H., Iglesias, E. A., Jacobson, M. S., Carey, D., Meyer, W., Schebendach, J., et al. (2005). Alendronate for the treatment of osteopenia in anorexia nervosa: A randomized, double-blind, placebo-controlled trial. *Journal of Clinical Endocrinology and Metabolism, 90*(6), 3179–3185.

Golden, N. H., Lanzkowsky, L., Schebendach, J., Palestro, C. J., Jacobson, M. S., & Shenker, I. R. (2002). The effect of estrogen-progestin treatment on bone mineral density in anorexia nervosa. *Journal of Pediatric and Adolescent Gynecology, 15*(3), 135–143.

Gordon, C. M., Grace, E., Emans, S. J., Feldman, H. A., Goodman, E., Becker, K. A., et al. (2002). Effects of oral dehydroepiandrosterone on bone density in young women with anorexia nervosa: A randomized trial. *Journal of Clinical Endocrinology and Metabolism, 87*(11), 4935–4941.

Greenfeld, D., Mickley, D., Quinlan, D. M., & Roloff, P. (1995). Hypokalemia in outpatients with eating disorders. *American Journal of Psychiatry, 152*(1), 60–63.

Gwirtsman, H. E., Kaye, W. H., George, D. T., Jimerson, D. C., Ebert, M. H., & Gold, P. W. (1989). Central and peripheral ACTH and cortisol levels in anorexia nervosa and bulimia. *Archives of General Psychiatry, 46*(1), 61–69.

Hill, K., Hill, D., Humphries, L. L., Maloney, M., & McClain, C. (1999). A role for helicobacter pylori in the gastrointestinal complaints of eating disorder in patients.

International Journal of Eating Disorders, 25(1), 109–112.

Hochlehnert, A., Lowe, B., Bludau, H. B., Borst, M., Zipfel, S., & Herzog, W. (2010). Spontaneous pneumomediastinum in anorexia nervosa: A case report and review of the literature on pneumomediastinum and pneumothorax. *European Eating Disorders Review, 2*, 107–115.

Hofman, M., Landewe-Cleuren, S., Wojciechowski, F., & Kruseman, A. N. (2009). Prevalence and clinical determinants of low bone mineral density in anorexia nervosa. *European Journal of Internal Medicine, 20*(1), 80–84.

Holtkamp, K., Mogharrebi, R., Hanishch, C., Schumpelick, V., & Herpertz-Dahlmann, B. (2002). Gastric dilatation in a girl with former obesity and atypical anorexia nervosa. *International Journal of Eating Disorders, 32*(3), 372–376.

Hutson, W., & Wald, A. (1990). Gastric emptying in patients with bulimia nervosa and anorexia nervosa. *American Journal of Gastroenterology, 85*(1), 41–46.

Hutter, G., Ganepola, S., & Hofmann, W. K. (2009). The hemotology of anorexia nervosa. *International Journal of Eating Disorders, 42*(4), 293–300.

Jagielska, G., Wolanczyk, T., Komender, J., Tomaszewicz-Libudzic, C., Przedlacki, J., & Ostrowski, K. (2002). Bone mineral density in adolescent girls with anorexia nervosa: A cross-sectional study. *European Child and Adolescent Psychiatry, 11*(2), 57–62.

Kamal, N., Chami, T., Andersen, A., Rosell, F. A., Schuster, M. M., & Whitehead, W. E. (1991). Delayed gastrointestinal transit times in anorexia nervosa and bulimia nervosa. *Gastroenterology, 101*(5), 1320–1324.

Kanbur, N., Pinhas, L., Lorenzo, A., Farhat, W., Licht, C., & Katzman, D. K. (in press). Nocturnal enuresis in adolescents with anorexia nervosa: Prevalence, potential causes, and pathophysiology. *International Journal of Eating Disorders.*

Katzman, D. K. (2005). Medical complications in adolescents with anorexia nervosa: A review of the literature. *International Jour-*

nal of Eating Disorders, 37(Suppl.), S52–S59; discussion, S59–S87.

Katzman, D. K., & Golden, N. H. (2008). Anorexia nervosa and bulimia nervosa. In L. Neinstein, C. Gordon, D. K. Katzman, D. S. Rosen, & E. R. Woods (Eds.), *Adolescent health care: A practical guide* (5th ed., pp. 477–494). Philadelphia: Lippincott, Williams & Wilkins.

Kerem, N., Riskin, A., Everin, E., Srugo, I., & Kugelman, A. (2010). *The effect of malnutrition on venous blood gases in adolescents with anorexia nervosa hospitalized for medical stabilization: A retrospective review.* Paper presented at the International Conference on Eating Disorders, Salzburg, Austria.

Kerem, N. C., & Katzman, D. K. (2003). Brain structure and function in adolescents with anorexia nervosa. *Adolescent Medicine, 14*(1), 109–118.

Kershenbaum, A., Jaffa, T., Zeman, A., & Boniface, S. (1997). Bilateral foot-drop in a patient with anorexia nervosa. *International Journal of Eating Disorders, 22*(3), 335–337.

Kiyohara, K., Tamai, H., Takaichi, Y., Nakagawa, T., & Kumagai, L. F. (1989). Decreased thyroidal triiodothyronine secretion in patients with anorexia nervosa: Influence of weight recovery. *American Journal of Clinical Nutrition, 50*(4), 767–772.

Kohn, M. R., Golden, N. H., & Shenker, I. R. (1998). Cardiac arrest and delirium: Presentations of the refeeding syndrome in severely malnourished adolescents with anorexia nervosa. *Journal of Adolescent Health, 22*(3), 239–243.

Krassas, G. (2003). Endocrine abnormalities in anorexia nervosa. *Pediatric Endocrinology Reviews, 1*(1), 46–54.

Lask, B., Gordon, I., Christie, D., Frampton, I., Chowdhury, U., & Watkins, B. (2005). Functional neuroimaging in early-onset anorexia nervosa. *International Journal of Eating Disorders, 37*(Suppl.), S49–S51; discussion, S49–S87.

Lawson, E. A., Miller, K. K., Bredella, M. A., Phan, C., Misra, M., Meenaghan, E., et al. (2010). Hormone predictors of abnormal bone microarchitecture in women with anorexia nervosa. *Bone, 46*(2), 458–463.

Legroux-Gerot, I., Vignau, J., Collier, F., & Cortet, B. (2008). Factors influencing changes in bone mineral density in patients with anorexia nervosa-related osteoporosis: The effect of hormone replacement therapy. *Calcified Tissue International, 83*(5), 315–323.

Lupoglazoff, J. M., Berkane, N., Denjoy, I., Maillard, G., Leheuzey, M. F., Mouren-Simeoni, M. C., et al. (2001). Cardiac consequences of adolescent anorexia nervosa. *Archives des Maladies du Coeur et der Vaisseaux, 94*(5), 494–498.

Malik, M., Stratton, J., & Sweeney, W. (1997). Rectal prolapse associated with bulimia nervosa: Report of seven cases. *Diseases of the Colon and Rectum, 40*(11), 1382–1385.

McCallum, R., Grill, B., Lange, R., Planky, M., Glass, E., & Greenfeld, D. (1985). Definition of a gastric emptying abnormality in patients with anorexia nervosa. *Digestive Diseases and Sciences, 8*, 713–722.

McLoughlin, D. M., Wassif, W. S., Morton, J., Spargo, E., Peters, T. J., & Russell, G. F. (2000). Metabolic abnormalities associated with skeletal myopathy in severe anorexia nervosa. *Nutrition, 16*(3), 192–196.

Mehler, C., Wewetzer, C., Schulze, U., Warnke, A., Theisen, F., & Dittmann, R. W. (2001). Olanzapine in children and adolescents with chronic anorexia nervosa: A study of five cases. *European Child and Adolescent Psychiatry, 10*(2), 151–157.

Mehler, P. S., & MacKenzie, T. D. (2009). Treatment of osteopenia and osteoporosis in anorexia nervosa: A systematic review of the literature. *International Journal of Eating Disorders, 42*(3), 195–201.

Mehler, P. S., Sabel, A. L., Watson, T., & Andersen, A. (2008). High risk of osteoporosis in male patients with eating disorders. *International Journal of Eating Disorders, 41*(7), 666–672.

Meyers, A. M., Feldman, C., Sonnekus, M. I., Ninin, D. T., Margolius, L. P., & Whalley, N. A. (1990). Chronic laxative abusers with pseudo-idiopathic oedema and autonomous pseudo-Bartter's syndrome: A spectrum of metabolic madness, or new lights on an old disease. *South African Medical Journal, 78*(11), 631–636.

Miller, K. K., Grieco, K. A., & Klibanski, A. (2005). Testosterone administration in women with anorexia nervosa. *Journal of Clinical Endocrinology and Metabolism, 90*(3), 1428–1433.

Miller, K. K., Grinspoon, S. K., Ciampa, J., Hier, J., Herzog, D., & Klibanski, A. (2005). Medical findings in outpatients with anorexia nervosa. *Archives of Internal Medicine, 165*(5), 561–566.

Misra, M., Aggarwal, A., Miller, K. K., Almazan, C., Worley, M., Soyka, L. A., et al. (2004). Effects of anorexia nervosa on clinical, hematologic, biochemical, and bone density parameters in community-dwelling adolescent girls. *Pediatrics, 114*(6), 1574–1583.

Misra, M., Katzman, D. K., Cord, J., Manning, S. J., Mendes, N., Herzog, D. B., et al. (2008). Bone metabolism in adolescent boys with anorexia nervosa. *Journal of Clinical Endocrinology and Metabolism, 93*(8), 3029–3036.

Misra, M., & Klibanski, A. (2010). Neuroendocrine consequences of anorexia nervosa in adolescents. *Endocrine Reviews, 17,* 197–214.

Mont, L., Castro, J., Herreros, B., Pare, C., Azqueta, M., Magrina, J., et al. (2003). Reversibility of cardiac abnormalities in adolescents with anorexia nervosa after weight recovery. *Journal of the American Academy of Child and Adolescent Psychiatry, 42*(7), 808–813.

Montagnese, C., Scalfi, L., Signorini, A., De Filippo, E., Pasanisi, F., & Contaldo, F. (2007). Cholinesterase and other serum liver enzymes in underweight outpatients with eating disorders. *International Journal of Eating Disorders, 40*(8), 746–750.

Moodie, D., & Salcedo, E. (1983). Cardiac function in adolescents and young adults with anorexia nervosa. *Journal of Adolescent Health, 4*(1), 9–14.

Morris, L. G., Stephenson, K. E., Herring, S., & Marti, J. L. (2004). Recurrent acute pancreatitis in anorexia and bulimia. *Journal of the Pancreas, 5*(4), 231–234.

Moyano, D., Vilaseca, M. A., Artuch, R., & Lambruschini, N. (1998). Plasma amino acids in anorexia nervosa. *European Journal of Clinical Nutrition, 52*(9), 684–689.

Muller, T. D., Focker, M., Holtkamp, K., Herpertz-Dahlmann, B., & Hebebrand, J. (2009). Leptin-mediated neuroendocrine alterations in anorexia nervosa: Somatic and behavioral implications. *Child and Adolescent Psychiatric Clinics of North America, 18*(1), 117–129.

Munoz, M. T., & Argente, J. (2002). Anorexia nervosa in female adolescents: Endocrine and bone mineral density disturbances. *European Journal of Endocrinology, 147*(3), 275–286.

Nakao, A., Isozaki, H., Iwagaki, H., Kanagawa, T., Takakura, N., & Tanaka, N. (2000). Gastric perforation caused by a bulimic attack in an anorexia nervosa patient: Report of a case. *Surgery Today, 30*(5), 435–437.

Narayanan, V., Gaudiani, J. L., Harris, R. H., & Mehler, P. S. (2010). Liver function test abnormalities in anorexia nervosa: Cause of effect. *International Journal of Eating Disorders, 43*(4), 378–381.

Nickl, N. J., Brazer, S. R., Rockwell, K., & Smith, J. W. (1996). Patterns of esophageal motility in patients with stable bulimia. *American Journal of Gastroenterology, 91*(12), 2544–2547.

Nogal, P., Pniewska-Siark, B., & Lewinski, A. (2008). Evaluation of selected clinical and diagnostic parameters in girls with anorexia nervosa. *Neuro Endocrinology Letters, 29*(6), 879–883.

Nordgren, L., & von Scheele, C. (1977). Hepatic and pancreatic dysfunction in anorexia nervosa: A report of two cases. *Biological Psychiatry, 12*(5), 681–686.

Obarzanek, E., Lesem, M. D., & Jimerson, D. C. (1994). Resting metabolic rate of anorexia nervosa patients during weight gain. *American Journal of Clinical Nutrition, 60*(5), 666–675.

O'Connor, G., & Goldin, J. (in press). The refeeding syndrome and glucose load. *International Journal of Eating Disorders.*

Ohrn, R., Enzell, K., & Angmar-Mansson, B.

(1999). Oral status of 81 subjects with eating disorders. *European Journal of Oral Sciences, 107*(3), 157–163.

Onur, S., Haas, V., Bosy-Westphal, A., Hauer, M., Paul, T., Nutzinger, D., et al. (2005). L-tri-iodothyronine is a major determinant of resting energy expenditure in underweight patients with anorexia nervosa and during weight gain. *European Journal of Endocrinology, 152*(2), 179–184.

Ornstein, R. M., Golden, N. H., Jacobson, M. S., & Shenker, I. R. (2003). Hypophosphatemia during nutritional rehabilitation in anorexia nervosa: Implications for refeeding and monitoring. *Journal of Adolescent Health, 32*(1), 83–88.

Overby, K. J., & Litt, I. F. (1988). Mediastinal emphysema in an adolescent with anorexia nervosa and self-induced emesis. *Pediatrics, 81*(1), 134–136.

Ozawa, Y., Shimizu, T., & Shishiba, Y. (1998). Elevation of serum aminotransferase as a sign of multiorgan-disorders in severely emaciated anorexia nervosa. *Internal Medicine, 37*, 32–39.

Palla, B., & Litt, I. F. (1988). Medical complications of eating disorders in adolescents. *Pediatrics, 81*(5), 613–623.

Patchell, R. A., Fellows, H. A., & Humphries, L. L. (1994). Neurologic complications of anorexia nervosa. *Acta Neurologica Scandandavica, 89*(2), 116–116.

Platte, P., Pirke, K. M., Trimborn, P., Pietsch, K., Krieg, J. C., & Fichter, M. M. (1994). Resting metabolic rate and total energy expenditure in acute and weight recovered patients with anorexia nervosa and in healthy young women. *International Journal of Eating Disorders, 16*(1), 45–52.

Polli, N., Blengino, S., Moro, M., Zappulli, D., Scacchi, M., & Cavagnini, F. (2006). Pericardial effusion requiring pericardiocentesis in a girl with anorexia nervosa. *International Journal of Eating Disorders, 39*(7), 609–611.

Pomeroy, C., Mitchell, J., Eckert, E., Raymond, N., Crosby, R., & Dalmasso, A. P. (1997). Effect of body weight and caloric restriction on serum complement proteins, including factor D/adipsin: Studies in anorexia nervosa and obesity. *Clinical and Experimental Immunology, 108*(3), 507–515.

Prabhakaran, R., Misra, M., Miller, K. K., Kruczek, K., Sundaralingam, S., Herzog, D. B., et al. (2008). Determinants of height in adolescent girls with anorexia nervosa. *Pediatrics, 121*(6), e1517–e1523.

Ramacciotti, C., Coli, E., Biadi, O., & Dell'Osso, L. (2003). Silent pericardial effusion in a sample of anorexic patients. *Eating and Weight Disorders, 8*(1), 68–71.

Rautou, P. E., Cazals-Hatem, D., Moreau, R., Francoz, C., Feldmann, G., Lebrec, D., et al. (2008). Acute liver cell damage in patients with anorexia nervosa: A possible role of starvation-induced hepatocyte autophagy. *Gastroenterology, 135*(3), 840–848, 848 e841–e843.

Riley, J. A., Brown, R. A., & Walker, B. E. (1996). Congestive cardiac failure following laxative withdrawal. *Postgraduate Medical Journal, 72*, 491–492.

Roberts, M. W., & Tylenda, C. A. (1989). Dental aspects of anorexia and bulimia nervosa. *Pediatrician, 16*, 178–184.

Robinson, P. H., Clarke, M., & Barrett, J. (1988). Determinants of delayed gastric emptying in anorexia nervosa and bulimia nervosa. *Gut, 29*(4), 458–464.

Romano, C., Chinali, M., Pasanisi, F., Greco, R., Celentano, A., Rocco, A., et al. (2003). Reduced hemodynamic load and cardiac hypotrophy in patients with anorexia nervosa. *American Journal of Clinical Nutrition, 77*(2), 308–312.

Roze, C., Doyen, C., Le Heuzey, M. F., Armoogum, P., Mouren, M. C., & Leger, J. (2007). Predictors of late menarche and adult height in children with anorexia nervosa. *Clinical Endocrinology, 67*(3), 462–467.

Santonastaso, P., Sala, A., & Favaro, A. (1998). Water intoxication in anorexia nervosa: A case report. *International Journal of Eating Disorders, 24*(4), 439–442.

Sherman, P., Leslie, K., Golderg, E., MacMillan, J., Hunt, R., & Ernst, P. (1993). Helicobacter pylori infection in adolescents with eating disorders and dyspeptic symptoms. *Journal of Pediatrics, 122*(5, Pt. 1), 824–826.

Sherman, P., Leslie, K., Goldberg, E., Rybczynski, J., & St. Louis, P. (1994). Hypercarotenemia and transaminitis in female adolescents with eating disorders: A prospective, controlled study. *Journal of Adolescent Health, 15*(3), 205–209.

Silber, T. J. (2005). Anorexia nervosa among children and adolescents. *Advances in Pediatrics, 52,* 49–76.

Silverman, J. A. (1983). *Medical consequences of starvation: The malnutrition of anorexia nervosa: Caveat medicus, in anorexia nervosa: Recent developments in research.* New York: Liss.

Sim, L. A., McGovern, L., Elamin, M. B., Swiglo, B. A., Erwin, P. J., & Montori, V. M. (2010). Effect on bone health of estrogen preparations in premenopausal women with anorexia nervosa: A systematic review and meta-analyses. *International Journal of Eating Disorders, 43*(3), 218–225.

Sinicina, I., Pantkratz, H., Buttner, A., & Mall, G. (2005). Death due to neurogenic shock following gastric rupture in an anorexia nervosa patient. *Forensic/Science International, 155*(1), 7–12.

Solomon, S. M., & Kirby, D. F. (1990). The refeeding syndrome: A review. *Journal of Parenteral and Enteral Nutrition, 14*(1), 90–97.

Stacher, G., Kiss, A., Wiesnagrotzki, S., Bergmann, H., Hobart, J., & Schneider, C. (1986). Oesophageal and gastric motility disorders in patients categorised as having primary anorexia nervosa. *Gut, 27*(10), 1120–1126.

Stock, S. L., Goldberg, E., Corbett, S., & Katzman, D. K. (2002). Substance use in female adolescents with eating disorders. *Journal of Adolescent Health, 31*(2), 176–182.

Stoving, R. K., Bennedbaek, F. N., Hegedus, L., & Hagen, C. (2001). Evidence of diffuse atrophy of the thyroid gland in patients with anorexia nervosa. *International Journal of Eating Disorders, 29*(2), 230–235.

Stoving, R. K., Hangaard, J., Hansen-Nord, M., & Hagen, C. (1999). A review of endocrine changes in anorexia nervosa. *Journal of Psychiatric Research, 33*(2), 139–152.

Strumia, R. (2005). Dermatologic signs in patients with eating disorders. *American Journal of Clinical Dermatology, 6*(3), 165–173.

Strumia, R., Varotti, E., Manzato, E., & Gualandi, M. (2001). Skin signs in anorexia nervosa. *Dermatology, 203*(4), 314–317.

Swenne, I., & Larsson, P. T. (1999). Heart risk associated with weight loss in anorexia nervosa and eating disorders: Risk factors for QTc interval prolongation and dispersion. *Acta Paediatrica, 88*(3), 304–309.

Tamai, H., Mori, K., Matsubayashi, S., Kiyohara, K., Nakagawa, T., Okimura, M. C., et al. (1986). Hypothalamic-pituitary-thyroidal dysfunctions in anorexia nervosa. *Psychotherapy and Psychosomatics, 46*(3), 127–131.

Tomova, A., Makker, K., Kirilov, G., Agarwal, A., & Kumanov, P. (2007). Disturbances in gonadal axis in women with anorexia nervosa. *Eating and Weight Disorders, 12*(4), e92–e97.

Touyz, S. W., Liew, V., Tseng, P., Frisken, K., Williams, H., & Beumont, P. (1993). Oral and dental complications in dieting disorders. *International Journal of Eating Disorders, 14*(3), 341–347.

Tsukamoto, M., Tanaka, D., Arai, M., Ishii, N., Ohta, D., Horiki, N., et al. (2008). Hepatocellular injuries observed in patients with an eating disorder prior to nutritional treatment. *Internal Medicine, 47*(16), 1447–1450.

Turner, J., Batik, M., Palmer, L. J., Forbes, D., & McDermott, B. M. (2000). Detection and importance of laxative use in adolescents with anorexia nervosa. *Journal of the American Academy of Child and Adolescent Psychiatry, 39*(3), 378–385.

Tyler, I., Wiseman, M. C., Crawford, R. I., & Birmingham, C. L. (2002). Cutaneous manifestations of eating disorders. *Journal of Cutaneous Medicine and Surgery, 6*(4), 345–353.

Ulger, Z., Gurses, D., Ozyurek, A. R., Arikan, C., Levent, E., & Aydogdu, S. (2006). Follow-up of cardiac abnormalities in female adolescents with anorexia nervosa after refeeding. *Acta Cardiologica, 61*(1), 43–49.

Vanderdokt, O., Lambert, M., Montero, M.

C., Boland, B., & Brohet, C. (2001). The 12-electrocardiogram in anorexia nervosa: A report of two cases followed by a retrospective study. *Journal of Electrocardiology, 34*, 233–242.

Wada, S., Nagase, T., Koike, Y., Kugai, N., & Nagata, N. (1992). A case of anorexia nervosa with acute renal failure induced by rhabdomyolysis: Possible involvement of hypophosphatemia or phosphate depletion. *Internal Medecine, 31*(4), 478–482.

Waldholtz, B. D., & Andersen, A. E. (1990). Gastrointestinal symptoms in anorexia nervosa: A prospective study. *Gastroenterology, 98*(6), 1415–1419.

Weinbrenner, T., Zuger, M., Jacoby, G. E., Herpertz, S., Liedtke, R., Sudhop, T., et al. (2004). Lipoprotein metabolism in patients with anorexia nervosa: A case-control study investigating the mechanisms leading to hypercholesterolaemia. *British Journal of Nutrition, 91*(6), 959–969.

Wesson, R., Sparaco, A., & Smith, M. (2008). Chronic pancreatitis in a patient with malnutrition due to anorexia nervosa. *Journal of the Pancreas, 9*(3), 327–331.

Willer, C. J., Speliotes, E. K., Loos, R. J., Li, S., Lindgren, C. M., Heid, I. M., et al. (2009). Six new loci associated with body mass index highlight a neuronal influence on body weight regulation. *Nature Genetics, 41*(1), 25–34.

Winston, A. P., Alwazeer, A. E., & Bankart, M. J. (2008). Screening for osteoporosis in anorexia nervosa: Prevalence and predictors of reduced bone mineral density. *International Journal of Eating Disorders, 41*(3), 284–287.

Wolfe, B. E., Metzger, E. D., Levine, J. M., & Jimerson, D. C. (2001). Laboratory screening for electrolyte abnormalities and anemia in bulimia nervosa: A controlled study. *International Journal of Eating Disorders, 30*(3), 288–293.

Yasuhara, D., Naruo, T., Taguchi, S., Umekita, Y., Yoshida, H., & Nozoe, S. (2005). "Endstage kidney" in longstanding bulimia nervosa. *International Journal of Eating Disorders, 38*(4), 383–385.

Ziora, K., Ziora, D., Oswiecimska, J., Roczniak, W., Machura, E., Dworniczak, S., et al. (2008). Spirometric parameters in malnourished girls with anorexia nervosa. *Journal of Physiology and Pharmacology, 59*(Suppl. 6), 801–807.

Zipfel, S., Sammet, I., Rapps, N., Herzog, W., Herpertz, S., & Martens, U. (2006). Gastrointestinal disturbances in eating disorders: Clinical and neurobiological aspects. *Autonomic Neuroscience, 129*(1–2), 99–106.

CHAPTER 10

Assessment of Eating Disorders in Children and Adolescents

Katharine L. Loeb
Melanie Brown
Michal Munk Goldstein

Accurate assessment of the cardinal features of eating disorders is essential for case identification, which, in turn, has implications for early intervention, long considered to confer significant prognostic advantage (Deter & Herzog, 1994; Ratnasuriya, Eisler, Szmukler, & Russell, 1991; Schoemaker, 1997). This is especially important for adolescents, who represent the highest-risk group for anorexia nervosa (AN) and bulimia nervosa (BN) in light of the positively skewed distributions for prevalence and onset across age (Ackard, Fulkerson, & Neumark-Sztainer, 2007; Hoek, 2006; Hoek & van Hoeken, 2003; Lewinsohn, Striegel-Moore, & Seeley, 2001; Lucas, Beard, O'Fallon, & Kurland, 1991). Identifying subsyndromal or atypical variants of AN and BN is equally important from a public health perspective, as such presentations may portend ultimate conversion to full-blown disorders for a subset of individuals (Ben-Tovim et al., 2001; Herzog, Hopkins, & Burns, 1993; King, 1989; Le Grange, Loeb, Van Orman, & Jellar, 2004; Patton, Johnson-Sabine, Wood, Mann, & Wakeling, 1990; Yager, Landsverk, & Edelstein, 1987); moreover, they are clinically significant in their own right, carrying liabilities in the medical, psychiatric, and psychosocial domains similar to their higher-threshold diagnostic counterparts (Andersen, Bowers, & Watson, 2001; Bunnell, Shenker, Nussbaum, Jacobson, & Cooper, 1990; Cachelin & Maher, 1998; Crow, Agras, Halmi, Mitchell, & Kraemer, 2002; Garfinkel et al., 1996; McIntosh et al., 2004; Peebles, Hardy, Wilson, & Lock, 2010; Ricca et al., 2001; Watson & Andersen, 2003). Such cases of eating disorders not otherwise specified (EDNOS) dominate treatment-seeking samples, particularly among children and adolescents. Beyond early case identification and targeted intervention for high-risk and already diagnosed youth with eating disorders, an arsenal of sound assessment tools and methods is also necessary for tracking the effectiveness of treatment and making corresponding decisions about appropriate levels of care, and for tertiary prevention by monitoring signs of potential relapse. To address the range of purposes, the ideal assessment tools would yield diagnostic decisions with algorithms corresponding to widely used criteria, such as the *Diagnostic and Statistical Manual of Mental Disorders*

(DSM-IV-TR; American Psychiatric Association, 2000), as well as severity indices that encompass both diagnostic symptoms (e.g., pathological shape and weight concerns) and associated features of illness such as dietary restraint.

The assessment of eating disorders in children and adolescents poses particular challenges relative to adult assessment. Some of these difficulties, such as reliance on self-report with an ego-syntonic disorder, are present with adults as well, but are potentiated in youth because of factors including cognitive limitations inherent to normal developmental stage—with implications for endorsement of abstract psychological symptoms (e.g., undue influence of shape and weight on self-evaluation), dynamic definitions of health (e.g., expected weight) during the physical maturation process, variability in timing of pubertal markers (e.g., menarche) that relate to diagnostic criteria, and increased motivation for deliberate denial and minimization of symptoms to avoid externally (i.e., parent-) imposed intervention efforts. (For a comprehensive review of these issues and corresponding recommendations for changes to DSM-5, see Bravender et al., 2007, 2010.) The task of effective assessment tools for eating disorders in youth is threefold: to accurately measure the associated physiological, behavioral, and cognitive symptoms, to interpret the raw findings against the backdrop of normal child and adolescent development, and, when necessary, to capitalize on input from multiple informants (Kraemer et al., 2003), such as parents, to mitigate the potential for obfuscated symptom profiles. Although child and adolescent patients often deny, minimize, and lack insight into their symptoms (Arnow, Sanders, & Steiner, 1999; Couturier & Lock, 2006a; Fisher, Schneider, Burns, Symons, & Mandel, 2001; Fosson, Knibbs, Bryant-Waugh, & Lask, 1987; Viglione, Muratori, Maestro, Brunori, & Picchi, 2006), as well as fear the implications of their symptoms endorsement, parents can report observable, behavioral indicators of the psychological features of the illness, consider information reported by reliable third parties, such as teachers, and report "clues" to behavioral symptoms, even secretive ones like binge eating (see Table 10.1). Measures of eating disorder symptoms in youth should also be sensitive enough to ascertain intent, separate from manifest behavior (e.g., Bryant-Waugh, Cooper, Taylor, & Lask, 1996). For example, minors can be forced into treatment by their parents and generally have less autonomy over food choices; as such, they may be temporarily weight restored while fully intending to reengage in self-starvation when supervision is reduced.

Specific Assessment Challenges and Considerations in the Diagnosis of Eating Disorder Symptoms in Youth

Assessment of the Physiological Criteria

Low Weight

Even the relatively objective criteria for AN, namely, low weight and amenorrhea, are subject to interpretation and misrepresentation in childhood and adolescence. The AN criterion "refusal to maintain body weight at or above a minimally normal weight for age and height" does not specify how to establish "normal weight," for which there are various definitions for children and adolescents. For example, it is unclear whether universal (e.g., body mass index [BMI]-for-age percentile ranges) or individualized (e.g., deviations from personally established growth curve trajectories) reference points have

TABLE 10.1. Patients versus Parents as Informants: Clinical Case Examples

Patients	Parents
"I don't need treatment. My parents are the problem."	"She won't listen to her pediatrician, who says since she's been underweight and missing her period for so long, she can develop osteoporosis." "She says she'll be fat at the target weight set by her doctor."
"I'm not scared of gaining weight."	"She won't eat more than 500 calories a day." "She screams and throws food at us when we try to get her to eat." "She ran out of the house when we tried to have her eat a decent dinner, and we couldn't find her for hours. We had to call the police."
"I'm fine with my body."	"She wears only baggy clothes." "She tells me every day that she is fat." "I removed the full-length mirror from her room because she would spend so much time in front of it, looking upset."
"I'm fine with my weight."	"She weighs herself several times a day." "She tells me she wants to lose more weight."
"I eat lunch at school."	"Her teacher called me, concerned because she never eats lunch."
"Shape and weight are as important to me as they are to any of my friends."	"She says that she hates herself because she is so fat."
"I'm an athlete. I'm not exercising to lose weight."	"Her coach says she trains beyond what her teammates do."
"I just exercise to stay healthy."	"Her doctor told her she can't exercise, but I see her doing everything she can to burn calories—she even stands instead of sitting whenever possible." "One night, I woke up and found her using the treadmill at 2:00 A.M.." "She used to go out with friends if she finished her homework early, but now she goes running instead."
"I'm not bingeing."	"I find junk food and empty wrappers hidden in her room." "I find large amounts of food missing from the kitchen in the mornings, especially after nights when she skips dinner."
"I'm not vomiting."	"She runs to the bathroom right after meals, and our housekeeper finds vomit residue on the toilet." "She says she stopped, but the pediatrician says her potassium is still low."
"I'm getting my period regularly."	"I haven't bought sanitary products for her in 6 months."

superior clinical utility, and there have been recommendations to adopt the latter strategy for children and adolescents (Bravender et al., 2010). There are also inconsistencies across universal standards. A study of a sample of 224 children and adolescents with a range of eating disorder diagnoses compared rates of AN versus EDNOS on the basis of four different methods for calculating a reference point or range for expected weight from which to determine low-weight status (Loeb et al., in press). Investigators using the 50th percentile of weight for age, height, and gender according to the 1966–1970 National Center for Health Statistics (NCHS; 1973) data found that 53% of the subsample was below the 85% cutoff for normal body weight recommended by DSM-IV (American Psychiatric Association, 2000). Applying the weight corresponding to the 50th percentile of BMI-for-age according to the more recent NCHS data as a proxy for normal weight (National Center for Health Statistics, 2000), it was found that 43% met the strict AN criterion by falling below 85% of that reference point. With a cutoff of BMI < 17.5 from the ICD-10 criteria (World Health Organization, 2007), the percentage defined as AN rose to 66%. Using the medical guideline of underweight for children defined as being below the 5th percentile of BMI-for-age (NCHS), the percentage diagnosed with AN fell to a low of 27%. The striking variability is purely a function of the range of definitions of "normal weight" in children and adolescents. This study also found that the first method (percentage of ideal body weight calculated using the weight corresponding to the 50th percentile of BMI-for-age according to newer NCHS norms as a proxy for ideal)—with a cutoff similar to the DSM-IV (American Psychiatric Association, 2000) recommendation of 85%—had the greatest predictive validity for treatment outcome, and in turn, the best clinical utility among the assessment strategies. However, it is important to note that life-threatening medical complications of malnutrition can occur in individuals who do not fall below this threshold (Madden, Morris, Zurynksi, Kohn, & Elliot, 2009).

Another challenge is that normal weight is a moving target, as children and adolescents age chronologically and grow in stature; an adolescent may gain 10 pounds in treatment but not change her weight status if she also ages 1 year and grows 2 inches during the course of the intervention. In addition to the difficulty in establishing and accounting for the dynamic nature of normal reference points, the very measurement of weight is vulnerable to significant error. Variability across scales, time of day, and levels of undress is compounded by methods patients employ to artificially inflate weight, including water-loading and the hiding of weighted objects in clothing and body cavities. This carries greater implications for assessing weight throughout treatment than when obtaining weight and weight history at an initial evaluation, for which self-report among adolescents with eating disorders has been found to be accurate (Swenne, Belfrage, Thurfjell, & Engström, 2005).

Amenorrhea

Menstrual status, the other "objective" criterion, is also difficult to assess. First, menstrual irregularities are common in adolescence, particularly following menarche (Watson & Andersen, 2003). Second, it may be difficult at young ages to distinguish between primary amenorrhea and the naturalistic timing of menarche, especially in the context of an eating disorder (Vyver, Steinegger, & Katzman, 2008). This is problematic for both case identification and measurement of treatment outcome. Although the recommended age to diagnose primary amenorrhea in the general population is 16 (van Hooff et al., 1998), earlier detection is important if an eating disorder is the suspected culprit (Bravender et al., 2007). Third, assessment of menstrual status often relies on patient report and is therefore subject to misrepresentation as a function of denial or deliberate deception. As with weight, however, patients are more likely to exhibit motivated deception for within-treatment assessments that have bearing on critical decisions regarding the intensity or continued duration of intervention; at the initial evaluation self-reported menstrual status has been shown to be fairly consistent with—although an insufficient proxy for—information obtained in a medical interview and examination (Swenne et al., 2005). Given the amenorrhea criterion's long history of controversy (Cachelin & Maher, 1998; Dalle Grave, Calugi, & Marchesini, 2008; Garfinkel et al., 1996; Mitchell, Cook-Myers & Wonderlich, 2005; Pinheiro et al., 2007; Roberto, Steinglass, Mayer, Attia, & Walsh, 2008; Thomas, Vartanian, & Brownell, 2009), and its limited ability to mark the severity of the illness or associated psychopathology (Andersen et al., 2001; Cachelin & Maher, 1998; Garfinkel et al., 1996; Watson & Andersen, 2003), researchers have suggested eliminating it as a criterion from DSM-5 for children and adolescents (Bravender et al., 2007) and even across the age spectrum (Mitchell et al., 2005). Another recommendation is to consider amenorrhea as one of multiple indicators of the ill effects of malnutrition in determining the diagnosis of AN in youth (Bravender et al., 2010; Hebebrand, Casper, Treasure, & Schweiger, 2004). Regardless, it will remain a common associated feature of AN, and even of BN in younger patients (Binford & Le Grange, 2005), and therefore accurate assessment of menstrual status represents a current challenge in the field.

Assessment of the Behavioral Criteria

Binge Eating

Binge eating as defined in DSM-IV-TR (American Psychiatric Association, 2000) encompasses two main features: the act (consuming an excessively large amount of food in a discrete period of time) and the subjective experience (a sense of loss of control during the episode). The act is often private or furtive, and the experience internal, rendering some form of self-report—whether elicited by questionnaire or interview—imperative in the assessment of binge eating. By extension, parent–child agreement on reports of the child's binge eating is poor (Johnson, Grieve, Adams, & Sandy, 1999; Pendley & Bates, 1996; Steinberg et al., 2004; Tanofsky-Kraff, Yanovski, & Yanovski, 2005), which bears relevance for identifying BN and AN, binge-eating/purging type. However, the identification of indirect behavioral indicators and correlates of binge eating, such as hiding food or secretive eating—which can often be described by parents—is considered important in case identification of disorders such as binge eating disorder (BED) in children and adolescents (Marcus & Kalarchian, 2003). As for adults, measures of binge eating for children and adolescents should adequately capture both relevant constructs (size and loss of control) and either allow an interviewer to determine whether the raw responses qualify as binge eating and at what frequency, or provide some guidelines and definitions in a questionnaire for the patient so as to avoid subjective categorizations and counts based on what he or she experiences as most salient. For example, loss of control during the consumption of a small amount of a forbidden food may be self-reported as a binge-eating episode but would not correspond to the DSM-IV (American Psychiatric Association, 2000) definition. This likely accounts for the higher rates of binge eating found via questionnaires as compared with semistructured interviews (e.g., Fairburn & Beglin, 1994).

Research shows that loss of control is a concept that younger patients can understand and endorse, especially if developmentally sensitive metaphors, such as "like a ball rolling down a hill, going faster and faster" (Bryant-Waugh et al., 1996; Tanofsky-Kraff et al., 2004), are used as prompts. In fact, loss of control may be the more clinically significant and valid marker of disordered eating among youth, relative to quantity consumed (Marcus & Kalarchian, 2003). When well-assessed, a pattern of maladaptive eating and associated behaviors can emerge in a subset of children and adolescents that mirrors eating disorders in adults (Tanofsky-Kraff et al., 2007).

Inappropriate Compensatory Mechanisms

Inappropriate compensatory mechanisms referenced in DSM-IV-TR (American Psychiatric Association, 2000) include purging (self-induced vomiting, laxative misuse, diuretic misuse, enema misuse) and nonpurging (fasting, excessive exercise) behaviors. Like binge eating, purging tends to occur in private, and nonpurging mechanisms are often intentionally obscured by the patient ("I ate lunch today" or "I'm just going to swim practice"). Parent–child agreement therefore tends to be poor in reporting these behaviors (Steinberg et al., 2004; Tanofsky-Kraff et al., 2005). Another significant challenge is the assessment of the intent behind these symptoms in younger patients, who might not be able to reason about, or articulate their reasons for engaging in, such behaviors (Bryant-Waugh et al., 1996). Purging can be associated with medical complications such as hypokalemia; although rare, hypokalemia holds significant medical risk and potassium should be routinely evaluated at baseline. However, although potentially indicating the presence of purging, hypokalemia is not strongly or reliably correlated with frequency (Imbierowicz et al., 2004).

Assessment of the Cognitive Criteria

The cognitive criteria for eating disorders include an intense fear of weight gain (AN), disturbance in the experience of shape and weight (AN), undue influence of shape and weight on self-evaluation (AN and BN), and denial of the seriousness of low weight (AN). Children and adolescents, especially those with AN-spectrum disorder, exhibit denial and minimization of these psychological features (Arnow et al., 1999; Fosson et al., 1987); in addition, they display a discrepancy between their diagnostic profile and the symptom endorsement that would be expected by their diagnosis on measures of dietary restraint, shape and weight concerns, and pathological eating attitudes (Couturier & Lock, 2006a; Viglione et al., 2006). In contrast to this picture, parents often report having observed behavioral indicators of these phenomena in their offspring (Arnow et al., 1999), which have been recommended as allowable substitutes for direct symptom endorsement in the upcoming DSM-5 (Bravender et al., 2007, 2010). One study (Couturier, Lock, Forsberg, Vanderheyden, & Yen, 2007) showed mixed results of parent–child agreement in a clinical sample, with adolescents with AN-spectrum disorder scoring lower than parents rated them on dietary restraint and weight concern, but not on shape concern or eating concern. Patients with BN-spectrum disorder showed a different pattern, scoring higher in direct report than in parent report on dietary restraint and shape concern, but not on weight concern or eating concern. In the same study clinician ratings were significantly and consistently lower than patient ratings for AN, but for BN they were equivalent. In a nonclinical sample (Pendley & Bates, 1996) adolescents scored higher than maternal report on measures of the psychological features of eating disorders. Collectively, these data highlight the importance of developing algorithms to incorporate data from multiple informants for accurate case identification and assessment (Kraemer et al., 2003). Table 10.2 summarizes issues and recommendations for the assessment of diagnostic criteria in children and adolescents.

Eating Disorders Measures Designed for or Used with Children and Adolescents

The following instruments have been used to assess disordered eating behaviors and cognitions in children and adolescents. The measures detailed in this chapter assess either a full range of diagnostic symptoms across eating disorders or the specific symptoms of a single eating disorder. We review interview, self-report, parent report, and other instruments. This chapter focuses exclusively on diagnostic assessment of eating disorder symptoms in children and adolescents.

Interview Measures

Eating Disorder Examination

The Eating Disorder Examination (EDE; Cooper & Fairburn, 1987; Fairburn & Cooper, 1993; Fairburn, Cooper, & O'Connor, 2008) is highly regarded as the "gold standard" for assessing eating disorder psychopathology (Wilson, 1993). The EDE is a standardized, semistructured, investigator-based interview that assesses the frequency and severity of behavioral and attitudinal symptoms of disordered eating, including eating concern, shape concern, weight concern, and dietary restraint—corresponding to the four subscales of the measure—as well as binge eating and compensatory behaviors. It was designed to identify clinical levels of eating disorder symptoms in adults but is commonly used for assessment of disordered eating in adolescents. The EDE has also been adapted for younger populations in the Child Version of the EDE (ChEDE; Bryant-Waugh et al., 1996; see the following section).

The EDE was created by Cooper and Fairburn (1987) and is currently in its 16th version (Fairburn, Cooper, & O'Connor, 2008). Revisions were introduced to address changes in diagnostic criteria as well as improve psychometric properties. The 12th version of the EDE (Fairburn & Cooper, 1993) was revised in order to specifically diagnose AN and BN based on DSM-IV diagnostic criteria (American Psychiatric Association, 2000) and has been widely used in clinical research, particularly as an outcome measure in treatment studies. The most recent (16th) version of the EDE (Fairburn et al., 2008) includes a module for assessing BED based on DSM-IV diagnostic criteria (American Psychiatric Association, 2000).

TABLE 10.2. Summary of Issues and Recommendations for the Assessment of Diagnostic Criteria in Children and Adolescents

Symptom	Featured in which disorder(s)	Assessment-related implications for differential diagnosis	Recommended method(s) of assessment for children and adolescents
Physiological domain			
Low weight (weight below 85% expected)	AN	AN-B/P type vs. BN (BN requires normal weight); AN vs. EDNOS (expected weight may vary as a function of individual growth curves)	1. Calculate BMI[a] from height (on stadiometer) and weight (on physician's scale), ideally obtained as a gown weight. 2. Reference BMI-for-age percentiles on the CDC website.[b] 3. Compare weight at current BMI to weight corresponding to the 50th percentile BMI-for-age and sex (as a proxy for expected weight).[c] 4. Calculate current weight as a percentage of expected weight.[d]
Amenorrhea (absence of 3 expected menstrual cycles)	AN	AN vs. EDNOS (not applicable for boys and premenarcheal females; oligomenorrhea common in adolescent females)	Medical interview/examination. Assess for primary amenorrhea prior to the standard recommended age of 16. In cases of secondary amenorrhea when premorbid cycles were irregular, consider pattern of historical cycle lengths to assess whether three expected periods were missed.
Behavioral domain			
Binge eating (discrete episodes of excessive eating accompanied by loss of control)	AN-B/P type, BN, BED	BN or BED vs. EDNOS (based on quantity consumed, presence of loss of control, and frequency of behavior)	Self-report (using developmentally sensitive metaphors as prompts, particularly for sense of loss of control); parental report that incorporates direct observation, evidence of secretive binge eating, and behavioral indicators of loss of control, while keeping in mind that parent report likely underestimates presence and frequency of binge eating overall
Purging (self-induced vomiting, laxative/ diuretic misuse)	AN-B/P type, BN-purging type	BN vs. EDNOS (based on frequency)	Self-report; parental report that includes evidence of purging such as finding vomit residue in the bathroom; chem-screen panel/potassium level (as a rare but medically important indicator of presence of purging, but not necessarily frequency); a developmentally sensitive assessment of intent
Fasting	AN-restricting type, BN-nonpurging type	AN or BN vs. EDNOS (based on frequency)	Self-report; parental report regarding skipped or refused meals and snacks; a developmentally sensitive assessment of intent
Excessive exercise	AN-restricting type, BN-nonpurging type	AN or BN vs. EDNOS (based on frequency)	Self-report; parental report that incorporates direct observation and input from coaches/dance instructors as applicable; a developmentally sensitive assessment of intent

(cont.)

TABLE 10.2. *(cont.)*

Symptom	Featured in which disorder(s)	Assessment-related implications for differential diagnosis	Recommended method(s) of assessment for children and adolescents
Cognitive domain			
Fear of weight gain	AN	AN vs. EDNOS (denial and minimization among children and adolescents may obscure direct symptom endorsement)	Self-report; parental report of behavioral indicators such as fear responses and refusal to eat high-caloric foods and severe self-directed dietary restriction
Disturbance in experience of shape and weight	AN	AN vs. EDNOS (denial and minimization among children and adolescents may obscure direct symptom endorsement)	Self-report; parental report of behavioral indicators such as body checking rituals and frequent weighing
Self-evaluation unduly influenced by shape and/or weight	AN, BN	AN vs. EDNOS (normal limitations in abstract cognitive skills among children and adolescents may limit ability to endorse symptom)	Self-report; parental report of changes and narrowing in self-definition of their child
Denial of the seriousness of low body weight	AN	AN vs. EDNOS (poor risk appraisal is normative among adolescents, yielding potential false positives)	Self-report; parent report of behavioral indicators including active rejection of medical prescriptions for weight gain

[a]Weight in kilograms/(height in meters)^2.
[b]*apps.nccd.cdc.gov/dnpabmi.*
[c]*www.cdc.gov/growthcharts/clinical_charts.htm#Set1.*
[d]If an individual child's historical (i.e., prior to the onset of eating disorders symptoms) BMI-for-age percentile was stable, within normal limits (5th–84th percentile), and associated with good health, the weight corresponding to that percentile for the current age should be used as the "expected" weight (instead of the weight corresponding to the population-based 50th percentile for current age).

The EDE's semistructured interview is administered by an extensively trained interviewer. Its time frame for most items is the past 28 days, although diagnostic symptoms are assessed for the time frames required by eating disorder criteria (e.g., 3 months for AN and BN). Questions are scored on a 7-point scale, with higher scores indicating greater eating pathology. The EDE produces individual scores on each of the items, four subscale scores, and a summary (global) score.

The psychometric properties of the EDE have been well established for adult populations. The reliability of the EDE with adults has been evidenced by good internal consistency (Beumont, Kopec-Schrader, Talbot, & Touyz, 1993; Cooper, Cooper, & Fairburn, 1989) and interrater reliability (Cooper & Fairburn, 1987; Rosen, Vara, Wendt, & Leitenberg, 1990; Wilson & Smith, 1989). The discriminant validity (Cooper et al., 1989; Rosen et al., 1990; Wilson & Smith, 1989) and concurrent validity (Rosen et al., 1990) have also been demonstrated for the EDE for adults. In a study of the reliability of the EDE in adult women, Rizvi, Peterson, Crow, and Agras (2000) found acceptable test–retest reliability over 2–7 days for all of the EDE subscales and high interrater reliability. Only subjective bulimic episodes and days showed low test–retest reliability (Rizvi et al., 2000). Good interrater reliability and test–retest reliability (over 6–14 days) for the EDE has also been shown in adult patients with BED (Grilo, Masheb, Lorano-Blanco, & Barry, 2004).

Several studies have investigated ways to improve the EDE for use in children and adolescents. Adolescents with AN tend to report much lower scores than expected as compared with adolescents with BN, and this difference is hypothesized to be due to high levels of denial, minimization, and shame in the early stages of eating disorders in young people (Couturier et al., 2007). Couturier and colleagues (2007) investigated the use of multiple informants in assessing eating disorders in children and adolescents using the EDE. In addition to a clinician obtaining a child interview using the EDE, parents completed a slightly modified version of the EDE in which the wording was altered slightly to inquire about the parents' perspective on their child's symptoms. The clinician who conducted the interview also provided a clinical summary score based on information from both the child and the parents, factoring in the clinician's judgment as well. The three scores from the child, the parents, and the clinician were compared to determine if the additional information obtained from multiple informants would assist in making a more accurate clinical judgment. For patients with AN or eating disorder not otherwise specified with a restrictive pattern (EDNOS-R), the child scores were significantly lower than clinician scores on all subscales and significantly lower than parent scores on the Restraint and Weight Concern subscales, suggesting minimization or denial on the part of the child. On the basis of this finding, parent and clinician ratings appear to be particularly important in diagnosis for child AN and EDNOS-R patient groups. Parents may also underestimate symptoms for young patients with AN or EDNOS-R, inasmuch as parent scores were significantly lower than clinician scores on all subscales except the Weight Concern subscale. Some differences were found between child and parent scores for patients with BN, but no differences were found between child and clinician scores. The use of multiple informants seems to be less crucial for the diagnosis of patients with BN. In another study of the EDE for use in young people, Couturier and Lock (2006b) investigated whether the addition of eight supplementary items that had been developed by the authors of the EDE for Version 14.3 (Fairburn & Cooper, 2000) would improve the assessment of symptoms of AN in adolescents. Although some of the items increased baseline subscale scores and internal consistency, the scores were still well below the expected scores that would adequately capture the level of eating pathology. Couturier and Lock concluded that the addition of the items still did not modify the EDE sufficiently to address problems of denial and minimization in adolescents with AN.

Child Version of the EDE

The Child Version of the EDE (ChEDE; Bryant-Waugh et al., 1996) was adapted from the EDE with the goal of making the EDE more comprehensible to younger individuals, and hence more accurate, in the assessment of disordered eating symptoms in children and adolescents. Four modifications were made to the EDE for this purpose (Christie, Watkins, & Lask, 2000). First, the language of the interview is modified, rendering it more understandable to children. Second, a diary of events is created by parents and provided to the child to be used as a memory aide during the interview. Third, *intention* is assessed, in addition to actual behavior, inasmuch as a child may not be in control of what he or she would like to do if unsupervised. For example, a child may wish to skip a meal due to weight or shape concerns, but adult caregivers do not allow this behavior. Fourth, the importance of shape and weight is evaluated using a sort task rather than through direct questioning. This modification addresses the issue that children may not be developmentally able to think in the abstract and self-evaluative ways that are necessary to answer the corresponding items from the original interview.

Watkins, Frampton, Lask, and Bryant-Waugh (2005) have shown preliminary support for the reliability and validity of the ChEDE. These authors found the ChEDE to have high internal consistency and interrater reliability for a sample of children and adolescents ages 8–14 years. In this study, the ChEDE also differentiated individuals with AN from controls and individuals with other eating problems, lending support to the validity of the measure. Wade, Byrne, and Bryant-Waugh (2008) investigated the norms and validity of the EDE modified for children based on recommendations for use with children (Bryant-Waugh et al., 1996) using a sample of young and mid-adolescent girls ages 12–15 years. Wade and colleagues found that the total score across all 22 items of the EDE and the Shape Concern subscale score of the EDE had good internal reliability for the sample. However, the other subscales of the EDE were found to have an unstable factor structure and poor internal reliabilities. Factor analysis revealed an alternative eight-item weight and shape concern subscale with good internal reliability. Significant differences in eating-related problems and cognitions were found between 12- and 13-year-old girls and 14- and 16-year-old girls, indicating that increased levels of disordered eating symptoms are associated with developmental change. Strong associations were found between threshold diagnostic measures of behaviors and the importance of weight and shape. The subscales of the EDE were also found to be strongly associated with the Body Dissatisfaction and Ineffectiveness scales of the Eating Disorder Inventory (EDI; Garner, Olmsted, & Polivy, 1983).

Overall, the diagnostic items discriminated between age groups and the presence of eating disorder behaviors. Wade and colleagues (2008) concluded that the modified version of the EDE should perform well as a diagnostic and predictive measure of eating disorders in young adolescents, given the importance of weight and shape in the diagnosis and prediction of disordered eating, but that the individual subscales of the EDE should be used and interpreted with caution for this population.

Structured Interview for Anorexic and Bulimic Syndromes for Expert Rating

The Structured Interview for Anorexic and Bulimic Syndromes for Expert Rating (SIAB-EX; Fichter, Herpertz, Quadflieg, & Herpertz-Dahlmann, 1998) is a semistructured, standardized, expert-rated interview that covers a wider range of specific and general psychopathology related to eating disorders than the EDE, including body image disturbance, bulimic symptoms, substance abuse, social integration, sexuality, depression, anxiety, and compulsion. The stability of the factor structure as well as good interrater reliability, internal consistency, convergent validity, and discriminant validity have all been demonstrated for adults (Fichter et al., 1998; Fichter & Quadflieg, 2000, 2001).

Interview for the Diagnosis of Eating Disorders

The Interview for the Diagnosis of Eating Disorders (IDED; Kutlesic, Williamson, Gleaves, Barbin, & Murphy-Eberenz, 1998) was originally developed by Williamson (1990) and has been modified to create its current version, the IDED-IV (Kutlesic et al., 1998). Unlike the SIAB-EX, which assesses more general psychopathology related to disordered eating, the IDED is specifically designed for the differential diagnosis of AN, BN, and BED, as set out in DSM-IV. The IDED has been shown to be both reliable and valid in the diagnosis of eating disorders (Kutlesic et al., 1998). Kutlesic and colleagues (1998) established good internal consistency and interrater reliability for the measure and found support for its content, concurrent, and discriminant validity.

Children's Binge Eating Disorder Scale

The Children's Binge Eating Disorder Scale (C-BEDS; Shapiro et al., 2007) is a brief, simple structured interview that was designed to measure binge eating in children. An interview format provides more accurate information about binge episodes than self-report questionnaires because the interviewer can explain the concept of loss of control, a diagnostic criterion for defining a binge episode (Shapiro et al., 2007). Although adults often have difficulty in understanding what is meant by loss of control in eating, understanding loss of control is even more challenging for children. The C-BEDS offers an easy, developmentally appropriate screening instrument for identifying binge eating in children. Studies of the psychometric properties of the C-BEDS are needed to establish its reliability and validity.

Clinical Eating Disorders Rating Instrument

The Clinical Eating Disorders Rating Instrument (CEDRI; Palmer, Christie, Cordle, Davies, & Kenrick, 1987) is a semistructured interview that was developed as a clinical rating scale to assess the behaviors and beliefs in AN and BN using a sample of adult and adolescent patients with eating disorders and controls. It was designed to be administered by a clinician and rates eating attitudes and behaviors as well as features of general psychopathology. Palmer and colleagues (1987) provided evidence of adequate interrater reliability of the CEDRI. The validity of the measure has also been demonstrated by its ability to discriminate between individuals with clinical eating disorders (AN and BN) and dieters not suffering from eating disorders (Palmer, Robertson, Cain, & Black, 1996).

Rating of Anorexia and Bulimia Interview

The Rating of Anorexia and Bulimia Interview (RAB; Clinton & Norring, 1999) is a Swedish semistructured interview designed to address clinical utility in terms of diagnosis, treatment planning, and outcome evaluation, as well as research utility (Clinton & Norring, 1999). Nevonen, Broberg, Clinton, and Norring (2003) modified the RAB to create the Rating of Anorexia and Bulimia Interview—Revised version (RAB-R) to address some of the original RAB's psychometric shortcomings, including a subscale that had poor internal consistency scores and problematic diagnostic discrimination. The

RAB-R consists of 36 items comprising six subscales: (1) Anorexic Eating Behavior, (2) Body Shape and Weight Preoccupation, (3) Bulimic Symptoms, (4) Partner Relationships, (5) Parental Relationships, and (6) Peer Relationships. In addition, the RAB-R includes 34 items that cover other relevant clinical problem areas. The RAB-R demonstrated satisfactory internal consistency, interrater reliability, and test–retest reliability, as well as good concurrent and criterion validity (Nevonen et al., 2003). A teenage version of the RAB (RAB-T) and the RAB-R have been used in a 3-year follow-up study of adolescents in Finland (Isomaa, Isomaa, Marttunen, Kaltiala-Heino, & Björkqvist, 2009).

Self-Report Measures Originally Developed for an Adult Population but Used with Children and Adolescents

Eating Attitudes Test

The Eating Attitudes Test (EAT; Garner & Garfinkel, 1979; Garner, Olmsted, Bohr, & Garfinkel, 1982) is a self-report questionnaire that has been widely used to assesses eating attitudes and behaviors for the purpose of identifying eating disorder symptoms. The original version, the EAT-40 (Garner & Garfinkel, 1979), is a 40-item self-report questionnaire that was developed to detect symptoms of AN. The EAT uses a 6-point, forced choice Likert scale and yields a total score based on the sum of the scores on the 40 items. Higher scores indicate higher levels of eating pathology, and a cutoff of 30 is used to identify disordered eating. Factor analysis of the EAT-40 revealed seven factors (Garner & Garfinkel, 1979): (1) food preoccupation, (2) body image for thinness, (3) vomiting and laxative abuse, (4) dieting, (5) slow eating, (6) clandestine eating, and (7) perceived social pressure to gain weight. A shorter, 26-item version of the EAT (EAT-26; Garner et al., 1982) was created on the basis of factor analysis that allowed for elimination of 14 items that did not substantially affect the correlation of the EAT-26 with the original EAT-40 ($r = .98$). The EAT-26 has three subscales identified by factor analysis—(1) Dieting, (2) Bulimia and Food Preoccupation, and (3) Oral Control, which are related to bulimia, weight, body image variables and psychological symptoms. Although both versions of the EAT are very useful in assessing symptoms, they are not diagnostic instruments. The EAT is easily administered and scored and provides an efficient screening measure for eating disorder symptoms. The EAT has been adapted for children by Maloney, Mcguire, and Daniels (1988) as the Children's Eating Attitudes Test (ChEAT).

In developing the original EAT-40, Garner and Garfinkel (1979) showed that the measure had good internal consistency using a sample of adult patients with AN (alpha = 0.79) as well as using a pool of adult patients with AN and psychiatric controls (alpha = 0.94). Garner and Garfinkel also demonstrated discriminant validity and predictive validity of the EAT-40 when distinguishing controls from anorexic patients. Garner and colleagues (1982) found that the shorter EAT-26 also had good internal consistency (alpha = 0.90) for a sample of adult patients with AN and indicated that both the EAT-26 and the EAT-40 show acceptable criterion-related validity in predicting group membership. Garner and colleagues found that bulimic and restricter subtypes of AN were differentiated, as on the factor-derived subscale scores of the EAT-26 but not on the total score. However, another study suggests that the EAT does not discriminate between AN and BN (Williamson, Prather, McKenzie, & Blouin, 1990). Carter and Moss (1984) found that the EAT did not effectively identify or discriminate AN and BN in a sample of college females, although good test–retest reliability was shown for the EAT (r = .84). Given these findings, the EAT is most effective in measuring disordered eating symptoms in general as opposed to differential diagnosis of eating disorders.

Evidence of the reliability and validity of EAT in samples of children and adolescents is more limited. The concurrent validity of the EAT was supported in a sample of adolescent boys and girls (Rosen, Silberg, & Gross, 1988). Rosen and colleagues also found that normative results of eating and weight attitudes as measured by the EAT for boys and girls differed dramatically by gender but not by age. A Bulgarian version of the EAT demonstrated validity in differentiating adolescent patients with AN from normal controls (Boyadjieva & Steinhausen, 1996).

Eating Disorder Examination–Questionnaire

The Eating Disorder Examination–Questionnaire (EDE-Q; Fairburn & Beglin, 1994) is a self-report measure that was adapted from the interview-based EDE. The current version of the EDE-Q is the EDE-Q 6.0 (Fairburn & Beglin, 2008). In contrast to the EDE, the EDE-Q requires no specialized training to administer and is less time-consuming, thus rendering the EDE-Q more efficient in both clinical and research settings. The EDE-Q consists of 36 items that are scored on a 7-point scale. Like the EDE, the EDE-Q measures disordered eating over a 28-day period, with some symptoms being assessed for 2- and 3-month periods as well. The EDE-Q uses the four subscales from the EDE, (1) Eating Concern, (2) Shape Concern, (3) Weight Concern, and (4) Dietary Restraint, and also assesses for binge eating and compensatory behaviors.

The psychometric properties of the EDE-Q have been well examined in adult populations. The EDE-Q has been found to have good internal consistency and test–retest reliability in use with adults (Luce & Crowther, 1999). Both its concurrent validity (Black & Wilson, 1996; Fairburn & Beglin, 1994; Wilfley, Schwartz, Spurrell, & Fairburn, 1997) and its discriminant validity (Wilson, Nonas, & Rosenblum, 1993) have been demonstrated with adults. In an adult community sample, the EDE-Q was shown to have good concurrent validity and acceptable criterion validity (Mond, Hay, Rodgers, Owen, & Beumont, 2004).

Although evidence suggests that the EDE-Q is both a reliable and valid measure, some significant differences have been found, for both adults and adolescents, between scores from the EDE and the EDE-Q that are related to differences in administration of the two measures (Binford, Le Grange, & Jellar, 2005). Studies comparing the EDE and the EDE-Q have found that the EDE-Q does not measure binge eating and shape concerns as precisely as the EDE, although self-induced vomiting and laxative misuse appear to be measured similarly using the EDE and the EQE-Q (Binford et al., 2005). The differences are likely to be due to the ability of the interviewer to clarify and make rating judgments about more complex, subjective concepts, such as binge size and self-evaluation related to weight and shape, using the EDE.

Two studies have examined the correspondence of the EDE with the EDE-Q in adolescents (Binford et al., 2005; Passi, Bryson, & Lock, 2003). In a study of adolescents with AN, Passi and colleagues (2003) found high correlation between scores from the EDE and the EDE-Q, but also found significant differences in scores from all of the subscales except Dietary Restraint, with the EDE-Q consistently overestimating pathology relative to the EDE. The differences between the interviewer-based EDE and the self-reported EDE-Q in the adolescent sample reflect similar findings in studies of adults and suggest that the EDE is a more accurate measure, given that some of the complex concepts in the subscales are more precisely assessed with the assistance of a trained interviewer (Binford et al., 2005; Passi et al., 2003). Binford and colleagues (2005) also compared the EDE and the EDE-Q in a sample of adolescent patients with AN, BN, and partial-threshold BN. The EDE-Q was found to perform similarly to the EDE on three of the four subscales, Dietary Restraint, Shape Concerns, and Weight Concerns, and only the Eating Concern subscale scores were significantly different between the two measures for individuals with full-syndrome BN. Both instruments were in agreement on purging frequency and self-induced vomiting. Overall, preliminary findings support use of the EDE-Q in adolescent populations, although strong evidence suggests that the interview format of the EDE is superior to the questionnaire version in providing the most accurate information about disordered eating in youth.

Eating Disorder Diagnostic Scale

The Eating Disorder Diagnostic Scale (EDDS; Stice, Telch, & Rizvi, 2000) is a brief self-report scale developed for the purpose of diagnosing AN, BN, and BED. The EDDS consists of 22 items that assess DSM-IV symptoms across 3-month and 6-month periods using a combination of Likert, yes–no, frequency, and write-in response formats. Responses can be used to diagnose AN, BN, or BED based on DSM-IV criteria. The reliability and validity of the EDDS has been demonstrated in samples of both adolescents and adults. Using a sample of female participants ages 13–65 years, Stice and colleagues (2000) showed that diagnoses derived from the scale exhibited temporal stability (test–retest mean kappa = 0.80) and criterion validity when compared with interview diagnoses (mean kappa = 0.83). The EDDS also exhibited good test–retest reliability (r = .87) and internal consistency (mean alpha = 0.89) and demonstrated convergent validity for the overall symptom composite (Stice et al., 2000). Additional studies using adolescent and young adult women by Stice, Fisher, and Martinez (2004) supported the robust psychometric properties of the EDDS. The EDDS was found to have good internal consistency and to possess criterion, convergent, and predictive validity (Stice et al., 2004). Preliminary support for the validity of EDDS with adolescents was found in a large sample of girls (N = 387) and boys (N = 359) in Hong Kong (Lee et al., 2007). Lee and colleagues (2007) found good internal consistency of items related to each of the four factors of the scale, namely, body dissatisfaction, bingeing behaviors, bingeing frequency, and compensatory behaviors. Good internal reliability for both girls and boys was shown, although test–retest reliability was poor over a 1-month period. The unexpectedly high prevalence of identified eating disorders in the study led the investigators to suspect the possibility of a high false-positive rate for detection of eating disorders in adolescents using the measure, and Lee and colleagues recommended exercising caution in determining clinically significant cases.

Eating Disorder Inventory

The original version of the Eating Disorder Inventory (EDI; Garner et al., 1983) is a self-report questionnaire that assesses disordered eating using eight subscales. The subscales allow for the evaluation of behaviors and psychological features associated with AN and BN. The 64 items in the EDI are scored using a 6-point, forced choice Likert scale ranging from *always* to *never*. Higher scores indicate more pathological attitudes and behaviors. The original subscales of the EDI are (1) Drive for Thinness, (2) Bulimia, (3) Body Dissatisfaction, (4) Ineffectiveness, (5) Perfectionism, (6) Interpersonal Distrust, (7) Interoceptive Awareness, and (8) Maturity Fears. The first three subscales assess attitudes and behavior related to eating and body shape, and the remaining five subscales measure traits that are associated with AN. The EDI-2 (Garner, 1991) added 27 items to the original 64 items, for a total of 91 items, and created three additional subscales: (9) Asceticism, (10) Impulse Regulation, and (11) Social Insecurity. A third version of the EDI, the EDI-3 (Garner, 2004), utilized rational and empirical methodology to update the measure to reflect the current understanding of eating disorders (Cumella, 2006). The EDI-3 retains the 91 items of the EDI-2 but divides the measure into 12 individual subscales that yield six composite scores. The 12 subscales are divided into eating disorder risk scales and psychological scales. The six composite scores of the EDI-3 are (1) Eating Disorder Risk, (2) Ineffectiveness, (3) Interpersonal Problems, (4) Affective Problems, (5) Overcontrol, and (6) General Psychological Maladjustment. The EDI-3 includes three response-style indicators to assist in determining the validity of responding, a Symptom Checklist (EDI-3SC) that assesses symptom frequency and history, and a Referral Form (EDI-3-RF). The EDI-3-RF is a shortened form of the EDI-3 that assesses only Drive for Thinness, Bulimia, and Body Dissatisfaction and provides an Eating Disorder Risk composite score.

The reliability and validity of the EDI used with adults have been supported, particularly for the eight original subscales of the EDI. Garner and colleagues (1983) established that the original version of the EDI has good internal consistency. The EDI also demonstrated convergent and discriminant validity of the subscales and was shown to discriminate between adult AN and comparison groups, providing evidence of construct validity of the EDI (Garner et al., 1983). Another study supported good test–retest reliability of the EDI across five of the eight subscales (Drive for Thinness, Body Dissatisfaction, Ineffectiveness, Perfectionism, and Interpersonal Distrust) and for the total score, but less stability was found for the Bulimia, Interoceptive Awareness, and Maturity Fears subscales (Crowther, Lilly, Crawford, & Shepard, 1992). Eberenz and Gleaves (1994) found support for the reliability and factor structure of the original eight subscales, but not for the three additional subscales of the EDI-2, in a sample of adult patients with eating disorders.

Some studies have also examined the psychometric properties of the EDI in children and adolescents. Shore and Porter (1990) investigated norms and reliability of the EDI in a sample of 11- to 18-year-old girls and boys. Echoing results from Crowther and colleagues' (1992) study with adults, six of the eight subscales of the EDI were found to demonstrate adequate reliability, with internal consistency measured by an alpha greater than 0.70, but the Bulimia and Maturity Fears subscales showed inadequate reliability. Significant gender differences on the Body Dissatisfaction, Drive for Thinness, and Interoceptive Awareness subscales were noted, supporting the notion that girls are more at risk for the development of eating disorders than boys. McCarthy, Simmons, Smith, Tomlinson, and Hill (2002) also conducted a 3-year study of female adolescents and found evidence for the reliability and validity of the EDI-2. The EDI-2 showed adequate internal consistency for the five subscales of the EDI-2 that were studied, Drive for Thinness, Body Dissatisfaction, Ineffectiveness, Perfectionism, and Interpersonal Distrust (alpha coefficients ranging from 0.60 to 0.92), with the Perfectionism and Interpersonal Distrust subscales displaying the lowest internal consistency. The subscales showed stability over time, with the exception of the Body Dissatisfaction subscale, which increased across the 3-year period for a young adolescent sample. The five-factor model reflected by the five subscales tested also fit the data well.

A large-scale investigation of a nonclinical sample involving a total of 1,323 French adolescents tested the construct validity of the EDI in five separate studies (Maïano, Morin, Monthuy-Blanc, Garbarino, & Stephan, 2009). The first study revealed that the clarity of three-fourths of the items in the original French version of the EDI was unsatisfactory when used with adolescents. An evaluation and modification of the instrument produced the EDI for adolescents (EDI-A). The EDI-A is a shortened 24-item scale that presents content and wording in a manner that is easily understandable to adolescents. The remaining four studies in the investigation analyzed the EDI-A and found support for its factorial validity, measurement invariance, reliability, convergent and discriminant validity, thus providing evidence of the construct validity of the EDI-A.

Bulimic Investigatory Test, Edinburgh

The Bulimic Investigatory Test, Edinburgh (BITE; Henderson & Freeman, 1987) is a brief self-report questionnaire that assesses bulimic behaviors and is used to identify individuals with symptoms of bulimia or binge eating. The 33 items of the BITE consist of (1) a Symptom subscale that assesses the degree of symptoms present and (2) a Severity subscale that indicates the severity of binge eating and purging behaviors based on frequency. Items are answered in a binary yes–no format.

Henderson and Freeman (1987) found that the BITE demonstrates satisfactory reliability and validity with its use in adult women. The internal consistency of the Symptom subscale and the Severity subscale was evidenced by alpha coefficients of 0.96 and 0.62, respectively, and test–retest reliability was also demonstrated. The BITE showed sensitivity to changes in both symptoms and behaviors and was able to clearly distinguish binge eaters from normal subjects. The internal consistency of the BITE has been demonstrated with 18- to 24-year-old Turkish university students (alpha = 0.86) (Kiziltan, Karabudak, Unver, Sezgin, & Unal, 2006). A study of bulimic symptoms in adolescent girls and boys found differences in the factor structure of the BITE based on gender (Ricciardelli, Williams, & Kiernan, 1999). For girls one factor related to overall bulimic symptoms was found that is consistent with the original scale, but for boys two factors, (1) emotional and rigid/disruptive eating style and (2) food preoccupation and bingeing, emerged. Ricciardelli and colleagues suggest that the presence of the second factor of food preoccupation and bingeing that is not associated with high levels of emotional distress for boys indicates that boys experience a form of binge eating that may be less problematic Ricciardelli and colleagues (1999) hypothesized that binge eating may be more socially acceptable for boys, and therefore some binge eating in boys is not associated with negative emotional outcomes.

Bulimia Test—Revised

The Bulimia Test—Revised (BULIT-R; Thelen, Farmer, Wonderlich, & Smith, 1991) is a self-report measure that was developed to assess BN on the basis of criteria set out in the DSM-III-R (American Psychiatric Association, 1987). The original version of the measure, the Bulimia Test (BULIT; Smith & Thelen, 1984), was revised to reflect changes in diagnostic criteria in DSM-III-R from DSM-III (American Psychiatric Association, 1980). The BULIT-R has been shown to be a valid measure based on DSM-IV criteria for BN as well (Thelen, Mintz, & Vander Wal, 1996). The BULIT-R is a 36-item questionnaire that is scored using a five-point Likert scale. Scoring is based on 28 items that reflect DSM criteria, and the remaining eight items are related to specific weight-control behaviors.

The reliability and validity of the BULIT-R have been demonstrated in both adults and adolescents. Thelen and colleagues (1991) provided evidence of the validity of the BULIT-R in predicting group membership, using female bulimic and control subjects, and showed test–retest reliability ($r = .95$) and validity in predicting the diagnosis in an adult female nonclinical sample. The BULIT-R has also been found to have high internal consistency (alpha = 0.98) and has demonstrated validity in identifying individuals who meet the diagnosis for BN based on DSM-IV criteria in a sample of adolescent and adult females (Thelen et al., 1996). Thelen and colleagues identified five factors—(1) bingeing and control, (2) radical weight loss and body image, (3) laxative and diuretic use, (3) self-induced vomiting, and (5) exercise for the BULIT-R—using a sample of adult females. However, evidence suggests that a four-factor model of (1) bingeing, (2) control, (3) normative weight loss (dieting and exercise), and (4) extreme weight loss behaviors is a better fit for adolescent boys and girls (Vincent, McCabe, & Ricciardelli, 1999). Bingeing and control were found to be separate factors for adolescent boys and girls, in contrast to a combined bingeing and control factor found in adults (Vincent et al., 1999). Vincent et al. also showed good internal consistency for girls (alpha = 0.90), for boys (alpha = 0.88), and for the total sample (alpha = 0.88) and adequate concurrent validity for the BULIT-R with adolescents. A study of female adolescents over a 3-year period found strong evidence of high internal consistency (alpha coefficients ranging from 0.93 to 0.95), stability, and factor invariance for the BULIT-R across both younger and older adolescent samples and over time (McCarthy et al., 2002).

Minnesota Eating Behavior Survey

The Minnesota Eating Behavior Survey (MEBS; Klump, McGue, & Iacono, 2000; von Ranson, Klump, Iacono, & McGue, 2005) is a brief, 30-item self-report inventory that assesses behaviors and attitudes associated with AN, BN, and BED. It was developed specifically for the Minnesota Twin Family Study (MTFS) to measure disordered eating longitudinally and across cohorts with an age range of 11 years to adulthood. The MTFS is a longitudinal study of more than 700 families with 11-year-old or 17-year-old twin girls. Because the sample of individuals ranged from prepubescent children to adults, an assessment tool was needed that was brief, simple, and easily understood across developmental levels for children, adolescents, and adults. The MEBS was developed by identifying 23 items from three EDI subscales (Body Dissatisfaction, Bulimia, and Drive for Thinness) that measure disordered eating cognitions and behaviors rather than personality traits. Two items were also added from the Interoceptive Awareness subscale of the EDI, and five items were developed separately to assess compensatory behaviors, including self-induced vomiting, abuse of laxatives, diuretics, and diet pills, and exercise. The language of items that were drawn from the EDI was simplified to make them more comprehensible to children. The measure was further simplified by limiting responses on a number of items to true or false. The MEBS provides a total score that indexes eating pathology overall as well as four subscale scores. The subscales of the MEBS are (1) Body Dissatisfaction, (2) Weight Preoccupation, (3) Binge Eating, and (4) Compensatory Behavior.

Klump and colleagues (2000) found good stability of the subscales across a 3-year interval and showed that the MEBS discriminated between eating-disordered and non-eating-disordered individuals. The Compensatory Behavior subscale was not found to be reliable in the 11-year-old twin cohort, however. The low frequency of endorsement for the Compensatory Behavior subscale, along with its poor reliability, suggests that compensatory behaviors are difficult to assess in children. Von Ranson and colleagues (2005) investigated the psychometric properties of the MEBS using a large community sample of girls, women, and men participating in the MTFS. Internal consistency was good for the total score and the Body Dissatisfaction and Weight Preoccupation subscales (alpha ranging from 0.71 to 0.85). The Binge Eating subscale showed adequate internal consistency, with alphas at about 0.70, but the Compensatory Behavior subscale showed much lower reliability (alphas ranging from 0.40 to 0.71). Test–retest reliability was good for the MEBS total scores and the subscales measuring attitudes (i.e., Body Dissatisfaction and Weight Preoccupation), but subscales measuring behaviors (i.e., Compensatory Behavior and Binge Eating) were less stable over a 3-year period. Among girls with an eating disorder diagnosis, all scales but the Body Dissatisfaction subscale showed a lack of stability over time. Von Ranson and colleagues found that the MEBS had good factor convergence and demonstrated evidence for concurrent and criterion validity of the MEBS. Mixed support for the reliability and validity of the MEBS was found in a study including Canadian university women (von Ranson, Cassin, Bramfield, & Fung, 2007). Although some evidence for adequate internal consistency and convergent and discriminant validity was found, the Compensatory Behavior subscale demonstrated low reliability and validity coefficients. In addition, the original factor structure was found to be questionable because the Compensatory Behavior and Weight Preoccupation subscales were two factors that did not fit the data well.

Questionnaire for Eating Disorder Diagnoses

The Questionnaire for Eating Disorder Diagnoses (Q-EDD; Mintz, O'Halloran, Mulholland, & Schneider, 1997) was designed specifically to operationalize DSM-IV criteria for the diagnoses of eating disorders in a self-report questionnaire format. The Q-EDD is a revision of the Weight Management Questionnaire (WMQ; Mintz & Betz, 1988, revision of Ousley, 1986, DSM-III questionnaire). Mintz and colleagues (1997) updated the WMQ, which is based on DSM-III-R criteria, to reflect changes in eating disorder diagnoses in the DSM-IV. The Q-EDD contains 50 questions that take approximately 5–10 minutes to complete. Questions relate to specific DSM-IV criteria, which allows for categorical identification of eating disorders based on a flowchart of decision rules used in scoring. The Q-EDD assesses frequency of behaviors as well as categorical information. Individuals are classified according to diagnostic categories that reflect DSM-IV. Two broad categories of non-eating-disordered and eating-disordered each encompass multiple subcategories. The non-eating-disordered category consists of asymptomatic and symptomatic subtypes. The eating-disorder category is broken down into diagnostic categories of AN, BN, and four EDNOS categories of subthreshold BN, menstruating AN, nonbingeing BN, and BED.

Mintz and colleagues (1988) found support for the psychometric properties of the Q-EDD in a sample of adult women. Test–retest reliability was found to be adequate over a 2-week period but less stable over a 1- to 3-month period. Interscorer reliability was very good, with 100% agreement demonstrated. Convergent validity was shown by comparing Q-EDD diagnoses with scores on the BULIT-R and the EAT. Excellent support was demonstrated for the criterion validity of the Q-EDD when diagnoses using the Q-EDD were compared with clinical interviews and clinical judgment.

SCOFF Questionnaire

The SCOFF questionnaire (Morgan, Reid, & Lacy, 1999) is a five-question screening questionnaire that addresses the core features of AN and BN. The acronym SCOFF comes from the following five questions:

1. Do you make yourself **S**ick because you feel uncomfortably full?
2. Do you worry that you have lost **C**ontrol over how much you eat?
3. Have you recently lost more than **O**ne stone (14 pounds) in a 3-month period?
4. Do you believe yourself to be **F**at when others say you are too thin?
5. Would you say that **F**ood dominates your life?

The questions can be administered orally or in written form. Hill, Reid, Morgan, and Lacey (2010) summarized the initial development, testing and validation, and the new developments and limitations of the SCOFF. The initial development of the SCOFF demonstrated the instrument's sensitivity and specificity to identify true and false cases in an adult female sample of cases and controls (Morgan et al., 1999). Perry and colleagues (2002) compared written delivery of the SCOFF with oral delivery using female and male adult students to investigate the reliability of the measure in the two formats. The written form of the SCOFF was found to exhibit good reliability as compared with oral administration of the measure. Although good agreement was demonstrated between the two formats (written vs. oral), the written format tended to produce higher scores, possibly due to increased willingness to disclose in writing as compared with direct interaction with the administrator. Some differences were also found on the basis of the order of administration of the formats, with greater consistency between the two formats being found when written administration preceded verbal administration. In terms of clinical utility and validity in a primary care population, the SCOFF has shown high sensitivity and specificity in identifying cases of AN and BN and acceptable sensitivity and specificity in identifying EDNOS in adult females (Luck et al., 2002). The SCOFF has been validated in primary care settings in both the United Kingdom and the United States by comparing it with results from other established eating disorder measures such as the Q-EDD and the EDE-Q (Hill et al., 2010). A study of children and adolescents in Barcelona, Spain, investigated the psychometric properties of a Catalan version of the SCOFF (Muro-Sans, Amador-Campos, & Morgan, 2008). The SCOFF demonstrated moderate reliability, low-to-moderate concurrent validity, and gender differences in both total SCOFF scores and factor structure for the measure in the sample of Spanish females and male youths.

Stirling Eating Disorder Scales

The Stirling Eating Disorder Scales (SEDS; Williams et al., 1994; Williams & Power, 1996) is an 80-item self-report instrument that was developed to measure the cognitive and behavioral symptoms of AN and BN. Each of the items is answered as either true or false. The measure consists of eight subscales that assess (1) Anorexic Dietary Cognitions, (2) Anorexic Dietary Behaviors, (3) Bulimic Dietary Cognitions, (4) Bulimic Dietary Behaviors, (5) Perceived External Control, (6) Low Assertiveness, (7) Low Self-esteem, and (8) Self-directed Hostility.

Williams and colleagues (1994) found evidence of the reliability and validity of the SEDS for adults when developing the measure. Internal consistency for each of the eight subscales was shown to be high (alpha greater than 0.80). Test–retest reliability was found to be very good with correlation coefficients for the eight subscales, as well as the overall score of the SEDS ranging from 0.85 to 0.98. Williams and colleagues also demonstrated group validity and concurrent validity for the SEDS. Gamble and colleagues (2006) investigated the psychometric properties of the SEDS in adult patients with eating disorders and found good internal consistency for the overall SEDS score, indicating that it is a reliable measure of eating disorder psychopathology in general, but found variation in the internal consistency of the individual subscales. Only five of the eight subscales demonstrated acceptable levels of internal consistency with alpha greater than 0.70. The Assertiveness, Anorexic Cognitions, and Anorexic Behaviors subscales did not show good internal consistency. The SEDS demonstrated good concurrent validity when compared with the EDE, but the factor structure of the eight subscales could not be replicated in the study (Gamble et al., 2006). Openshaw and Waller (2005) also found that the internal consistency of the overall SEDS total score was good (alpha = 0.84) for a clinical sample of women, but the internal consistency of the subscales was inadequate, with alpha coefficients ranging from 0.45 to 0.67 for all of the subscales except the Perceived External Control subscale (alpha = 0.74). In an investigation of the psychometric properties of the SEDS with adolescents, the SEDS was found to have both high internal consistency for the eight scales (all alpha coefficients greater than 0.70) as well as good criterion and discriminant validity for a sample of adolescent patients with eating disorders and age-matched controls (Campbell, Lawrence, Serpell, Lask, & Neiderman, 2002).

Survey of Eating Disorders

The Survey of Eating Disorders (SEDs; Götestam & Agras, 1995) was initially developed to assess prevalence rates of various eating disorders in an adult Norwegian population. The measure consists of 36 items, six of which are demographic questions. The SEDs was further modified by Ghaderi and Scott (2002), in which a definition of binge eating was provided to responders, based on DSM-IV criteria, and the questions relating to purging were combined in four questions.

Ghaderi and Scott (2002) found that there were no significant differences between the diagnoses concluded from the SEDs and EDE, indicating high predictive value of the measure. At times the SEDs did underdiagnose participants—for instance, diagnosing individuals with BED, in contrast to the EDE, with which they were diagnosed as having BN—and at other times overdiagnosed people—for example, diagnosing them as having BN, as opposed to the findings of the EDE, with which they were diagnosed with EDNOS. Test–retest reliability was very high, in that all students were reclassified into the same categories they were in the first time they took the SEDs, with approximately a 2-week interval between tests. Concurrent validity was also good, in that students who met a diagnosis on the SEDs also had significantly elevated scores on the EDI (Ghaderi &

Scott, 2002). The SEDs has also been used with adolescents. For example, Kjelsås, Bjørnstrøm, and Götestam (2004) used the questionnaire in a study assessing the prevalence of eating disorders in adolescents.

Self-Report Measures Developed for Children and Adolescents

Children's EAT

The Children's EAT (ChEAT; Maloney et al., 1988) is a modified version of the Eating Attitudes Test–26 (EAT-26; Garner & Garfinkel, 1979) that was developed for adults. The language of the EAT-26 was simplified for the ChEAT, which was initially developed and used with children ages 8–13 years. Test–retest reliability ranged between 0.75 and 0.88 for students in grades 3 to 6, with an overall reliability score of 0.81. Internal reliability scores ranged from 0.68 to 0.80, and when a question yielding negative correlations (item 19) with the rest of the items was removed, the overall internal consistency score was 0.76. No pattern of younger children yielding more unreliable scores was evident, suggesting that this measure may be reliably used for children as young as 8 years old (Maloney et al., 1988).

Smolak and Levine (1994) further studied the psychometric properties of the ChEAT. Cronbach's alpha was 0.88 (range for the children in grades 6–8 was 0.78–0.91), when item 19 was deleted, and 0.89 (ranging between 0.81 and 0.92), when three items with low correlations were deleted from the scale. Unlike Maloney and colleagues (1988), Smolak and Levine found that Cronbach's alpha reliability scores did increase with grade level, and therefore suggested that this measure should be further modified if used with younger children. They also found moderate significant correlations between the ChEAT and weight measurement behavior as well as body dissatisfaction, indicating concurrent validity. A factor analysis conducted by Smolak and Levine showed that there are primarily four underlying factors to the measure. They labeled the four factors "dieting," "restricting and purging" (which is not on the EAT), "food preoccupation," and "oral control." Lattimore and Halford (2003) have assessed the utility of the suggested cutoff score of 20 on the ChEAT and found that this score was not an accurate indication of disordered eating. Erickson and Gerstle (2007) found that for certain ages a cutoff score of 25 seemed more accurate.

A modified version of the ChEAT was used with a Spanish sample, from which six questions were removed as they were seen as being non–age appropriate (Sancho, Asorey, Arija, & Canals, 2005). This version also yielded good reliability (Cronbach's alpha was 0.71, and 0.73 when the equivalent to item 19 was removed) and fair test–retest reliability ($r = .56$). Concurrent reliability was measured through correlations with the Body Area Satisfaction Scale (Cash, 1997); correlations on these measures were nonsignificant for males (–.19) and low for females (–.106) (Sancho et al., 2005).

Child EDE-Q

The Child EDE-Q (ChEDE-Q; Decaluwé, 1999; Decaluwé & Braet, 1999, as cited in Decaluwé & Braet, 2004) was adapted from a measure developed for adults, the EDE-Q (Fairburn & Beglin, 1994). Although not many studies have assessed the psychometric properties of the ChEDE-Q, a study by Decaluwé and Braet (2004), which incorporated use of the ChEDE-Q, reported Cronbach's alpha scores ranging from 0.62 to 0.88 on the different subscales. Each of the subscales significantly correlated with the ChEDE subscales; however, significant differences between the ChEDE interview and ChEDE-Q were evident in identification of adolescents with binge eating (Decaluwé & Braet, 2004). This may be a limitation of the questionnaire, although more data on the psychometric properties of the measure seem necessary.

EDI for Children

The EDI for Children (EDI-C; Garner, 1991, 2004) is a modified version of the Eating Disorder Inventory–2 and was specifically formulated for children and adolescents. The measure consists of 91 statements with forced choice responses, which factors into 11 subscales. Examples of the subscales include "Drive for Thinness," "Maturity Fears," and "Interpersonal Distrust" (Thurfjell et al., 2004). The subscales fall into three categories that are (1) attitudes and behaviors relating to eating, weight, and shape; (2) psychological traits accompanying eating disorders; and (3) tendencies observed among patients with eating disorders (Eklund, Paavonen, & Almqvist, 2005). A study conducted on Swedish nonclinical adolescent and preadolescent males and females yielded Cronbach's alpha total scores ranging between 0.79 and 0.93. Individual subscale Cronbach's alpha scores ranged from 0.33 to 0.93 (Thurfjell et al., 2004). In a study conducted by Eklund and colleagues (2005), the EDI-C was administered to children in grades 4–10. Twenty-seven items were dropped from the 11-factor model and reanalysis established five factors accounting for 49% of the variance. The factors the authors derived were "Drive for Thinness," "Emotional Distractibility," "Self-Esteem," "Overeating," and "Maturity Fears." Interestingly, these differ from the factors on the EDI and the EDI-2. The five factors yielded good internal consistency scores ranging between 0.63 and 0.91. Thus, it has been suggested that the five underlying factors may increase reliability, in contrast to the 11 factors that underlie the EDI-2 (Eklund et al., 2005).

Kids' Eating Disorders Survey

The Kids' Eating Disorders Survey (KEDS; Childress, Jarrell, & Brewerton, 1993) is a 14-item self-report measure, adapted from the Eating Symptoms Inventory (Whitaker et al., 1989), which was based on DSM-III criteria. The KEDS was developed specifically for children, especially to assess binge eating, fasting, use of diuretics, diet pills, or laxatives. Answers include yes, no, and ? choices. In addition, there is a question assessing weight and body image dissatisfaction through analysis of responses to eight figure choices, which differ by gender. Factor analysis indicated two underlying factors accounting for 33.8% of the total variance of the measure. The first factor relates to eating and weight dissatisfaction, whereas the second factor relates to behaviors used to control weight. Frequent binge eating (defined as eating large amounts of food more than 12 times) and body dissatisfaction did not load highly onto any factor (<0.40) (Childress et al., 1993).

Fifth- through eighth-graders were assessed in order to analyze psychometric properties of the KEDS (Childress et al., 1993). Internal consistency scores, as measured by Cronbach's alpha, ranged from 0.68 to 0.77 for the different grades. Test–retest reliability over 4 months yielded a Spearman correlation coefficient of 0.83 for the total group and was slightly higher for boys (0.85, $p < .05$) than for girls (0.77, $p < .05$) (Childress et al., 1993). Recently, the measure has been translated and used in a Spanish population (Zúñiga & Padrón, 2009). Factor analysis indicated two underlying factors to the measure which accounted for 74.4% of variance. Cronbach's alpha for the Spanish version of the measure was 0.92, where the body dissatisfaction factor yielded a score of 0.91 and the purging/restricting scale 0.87. The KEDS demonstrated 0.83 correlation coefficient with the EAT-40, indicating good convergent validity (Zúñiga & Padrón, 2009).

McKnight Risk Factor Survey III

The McKnight Risk Factor Survey III (MRFS-III; Shisslak et al., 1999) followed after two pilot studies of the MRFS. It was developed to assess risk and protective factors for developing eating disorders specifically in female adolescents. Thus, the measure covers a range of behaviors and symptoms (i.e., parents involvement with school, smoking), and here we focus primarily on the psychometric properties relating to eating disordered behaviors. The elementary school version of the MRFS-III consists of 75 items, and the middle school version consists of 79 items. Test–retest reliability, internal consistency, and convergent validity properties were assessed in elementary school, middle school, and high school students. In terms of the eating disordered items, the Psychological Weight Control Behavior Scale and the Overconcern with Weight and Shape Scale yielded good test–retest reliability scores as well as good Cronbach's alpha scores, with coefficients for the former scale ranging between 0.76 and 0.93 for the three groups of students and Cronbach's alpha scores ranging between 0.86 and 0.90. For the latter scale, coefficients ranged from 0.79 to 0.90 for the three groups, respectively, and Cronbach's alpha scores ranged between 0.82 and 0.87. However, the Eating Disorder (Binge Scale) rendered a relatively low test–retest reliability range of 0.43 to 0.67 and Cronbach's alpha scores ranging between 0.43 and 0.62, as did the Purge Scale, on which test–retest reliability coefficients ranged between 0.45 and 0.81 and Cronbach's alpha ranged from 0.62 to 0.68. Convergent validity was partially measured by comparing correlations between the Weight Concerns Scale (WCS; Killen et al., 1994) and the MRFS-III. Correlations with the Overconcern with Shape and Weight Scale ranged between 0.74 and 0.88 in elementary, middle, and high school students, respectively. Reliability of the measure was not significantly different when a subset of the population was administered an oral version of the test instead of the written version, indicating that this measure may be used with children with reading difficulties (Shisslak et al., 1999).

Questionnaire for Eating and Weight Patterns—Adolescent Version

The Questionnaire for Eating and Weight Patterns—Adolescent Version (QEWP-A; Johnson, Grieve, Adams, & Sandy, 1999) was developed as based on the Questionnaire for Eating and Weight Patterns (QEWP; Spitzer et al., 1992), which was developed specifically to assess BED according to DSM-IV research criteria. The measure consists of 13 items relating to the behavioral components of BED. The QEWP-A was adapted from this version, specifically to assess binge eating in adolescents. Essentially, the modifications included simplification of the language and the combination of two questions, thus reducing the number of questions from 13 to 12. Some response choices for questions are on a 2-point scale (yes–no), whereas others are on a 5-point scale. The psychometric properties were initially assessed with children and adolescents ranging in age from 10 to

18 years. The measure classifies adolescents as no diagnosis (ND), nonclinical binge eating (NBE), and binge eating disorder (BED). Concordance between the QEWP-A and the QEWP-P (Johnson et al., 1999) (a parent version of the QEWP-A, see a later section) was assessed (Johnson et al., 1999). Of adolescent and parental reports 81.6% were concordant in the first category, 15.5% of reports in the second category, and 25% concordance was evident in the last category. Overall kappa scores were 0.19. The low rates of agreement, Johnson and colleagues (1999) suggest, may indicate that parents are unaware of the eating-disordered behaviors that are occurring, leading to the conclusion that direct assessment of the adolescent is essential. Similar results were found by Steinberg and colleagues (2004) in concordance rates between 6- to 12-year-old children and their parents, filling out the QEWP-A and the QEWP-P.

Test–retest reliability of the QEWP-A was also assessed (Johnson, Kirk, & Reed, 2001). Results of a study including 12- to 18-year-old males and females indicated that test–retest reliability was more stable for males than for females over a 3-week period. In fact, 33% of females changed from a baseline categorization of nonclinical binge eating (NCBE) to a no diagnosis (ND) categorization (Johnson et al., 2001). Concurrent validity of the measure was assessed by using it as a predictor of depression, using the Children's Depression Inventory (CDI; Kovacs, 1982, as cited in Johnson et al., 1999), and eating attitudes, using the children's version of the Eating Attitudes Test (ChEAT; Maloney et al., 1988). Results indicated that those classified as having BED, per the QEWP-A, had significantly higher scores on both the CDI and the ChEAT (Johnson et al., 1999).

When the QEWP-A was compared with the ChEDE, little agreement was evident between the two measures for the number or type of eating episodes that had occurred in the past month between the QEWP-A and the ChEDE ($p < .05$). When the ChEDE was set as the criterion, the QEWP-A evidenced a range of 0–41% sensitivity for Objective Overeating, Loss of Control, Subjective Bulimic Episodes, and Objective Bulimic Episodes, and specificity ranged from 83 to 91% (Tanofsky-Kraff et al., 2003). (For more information on how the QEWP-A compares with the YEDE-Q, see the following section detailing the YEDE-Q.)

Youth EDE-Q

The Youth EDE-Q (YEDE-Q; Goldschmidt, Doyle, & Wilfley, 2007) was developed based on the EDE-Q (Fairburn & Beglin, 1994), with a goal to clarify the concepts of "loss of control" and "large amounts of food" for the adolescent population. Instructions that have been used to assist adults in defining a binge (Goldfein, Devlin, & Kamenetz, 2005) were modified by providing visuals, vignettes, and examples of large food amounts. The measure is set at a third-grade reading level. The psychometric properties were assessed in a population of 12- to 17-year-olds, and the authors have suggested that the measure be used for these ages until further studies are conducted. As in the original EDE (Cooper & Fairburn, 1987), the four subscales include Restraint, Weight Concerns, Eating Concern, and Shape Concern. Cronbach's alpha scores ranged from 0.63 to 0.89, with the Restraint scale yielding the lowest alpha level. Convergent validity was assessed by comparing the YEDE-Q with the ChEDE and the QEWP-A (Johnson et al., 1999). Analysis of the YEDE-Q and ChEDE subscales and global scales indicated significant correlations between the measures (scale range: 0.58–0.84). Moreover, significant correlations were evident on the measures between Objective Bulimic Episodes (OBE) days, with females exhibiting significantly more agreement on the two measures as compared with males, and OBE days. No significant correlations were evident between measures for Subjective Bulimic Episodes (SBE), Objective Overeating (OO), and driven exercise; the YEDE-Q generated significantly higher ratings on these scales than did the ChEDE. Between 62.9 and 80% of participants scored within a one-point difference on the ChEDE and the YEDE-Q on each of the subscales, and there was a significant difference in classification of high- and low-risk groups per the two measures. In reference to the ChEDE, the YEDE-Q identified only 8.6% false positives and no false negatives (Goldschmidt et al., 2007).

When compared with the QEWP-A, the YEDE-Q did show significant correlations in terms of weight and shape concern but not in terms of OBE days or episodes of driven exercise (Goldschmidt et al., 2007). Goldschmidt and colleagues (2007) indicate that the YEDE-Q may be a promising measure in terms of flagging adolescents with eating-disordered behaviors, but more extensive interviews should be conducted to render the most accurate diagnoses.

Parent Measures (Interview and Self-Report)

Anorectic Behavior Observation Scale

The Anorectic Behavior Observation Scale (ABOS; Vandereycken & Meerman, 1984) is a 30-item self-report measure whereby parents (though can be other family members, such as spouses) complete questions regarding an individual with response choices of yes, no, or not sure. Higher scores indicate greater pathology. Vandereycken's (1992) study, assessing the reliability and validity of the measure, was conducted with parents of females between the ages of 12 and 37. A cutoff score of 19 yielded 90% sensitivity and 89.6% specificity rates. Factor analysis indicated three underlying factors, (1) Eating Behavior, Weight and Food Concern, Denial of Problems, (2) Bulimic-like Behavior, and (3) Hyperactivity. Cronbach's alpha for these subscales ranged between 0.69 and 0.80. Use of the ABOS with a German sample showed high total internal consistency (alpha = 0.95), although lower reliability for the total scores of each subsample (.52 for a clinical eating disorder subsample and .76 for a nonclinical school-based sample). In this German version of the ABOS, a cutoff score of 23 demonstrated the best sensitivity and specificity. In the German sample as well, factor analysis of the measure revealed three underlying factors (Salbach-Andrae et al., 2009). In a Japanese population in which 102 relatives of clinical patients were sampled, three underlying factors were indicated as well, although they differed from the factors described by Vandereycken (1992), which Uehara and colleagues (2002) attribute to cultural differences.

Questionnaire for Eating and Weight Patterns—Parent Version

The Questionnaire for Eating and Weight Patterns—Parent Version (QEWP-P; Johnson et al., 1999) utilizes the same questions as the QEWP-A. The questions were modified so that they are directed to parents, referencing their children (i.e., During the past 6 months, did your child ever eat what most people, like his or her friends, would think was a really big amount of food?) The QEWP-P evidenced low concordance rates with the QEWP-A (see QEWP-A in an earlier section). The authors suggest that this is consistent with binge eating and bulimia being very private, and parents being unaware of these disordered eating behaviors (Johnson et al., 1999).

When compared with Ch-EDE, the QEWP-P identified more participants as having BED, BN, or subclinical ED (Tanofsky-Kraff et al., 2005) ($p = .02$). Differences between identification of eating episodes were also notable between the two measures. The QEWP-P evidenced 30% sensitivity and 79% specificity for the diagnosis of Objective Overeating without loss of control, and 50% sensitivity and 83% specificity for the diagnosis of Binge Eating, when the ChEDE was used as the criterion method. Significant correlations were evident between the two measures on several items. These include the comparison of ChEDE Eating Concern subscale and the QEWP-P question asking parents how bad their child felt about loss of control over eating, the ChEDE Shape Concern and Weight Concern, and the QEWP-P question regarding importance of shape and weight (Tanofsky-Kraff et al., 2005). Tanofsky-Kraff and colleagues (2005) suggest this may indicate that parents have a limited sense of what occurs in terms of their children's private eating habits, characteristic of binge eating, and thus parental measures of binge eating or bulimia may have limited utility. However, parents may have a sense of how bad their children are feeling.

Parent Version of the EDE

The Parent Version of the EDE (P-EDE; Loeb, 2008) was developed to improve eating disorders case identification in children and adolescents by employing multiple informants (parents) in the assessment of eating habits, behaviors, and attitudes and inquiring about behavioral or observable indicators of the psychological features of eating disorders (such as shape and weight concerns), which may not be readily endorsed by direct report in youth (Bravender et al., 2010). The P-EDE is based on the EDE, 16th edition (Fairburn, Cooper, & O'Conner, 2008), and was adapted in consultation with its first author. Psychometric studies are currently under way. The P-EDE interviewer is asked to secure symptom ratings for a third party (the child or adolescent), with the parent(s) or guardian(s) serving as informant. In general, an item is to be rated as present if the parent or guardian has (1) observed the phenomenon directly, (2) heard the child report the phenomenon, or (3) heard reports of the phenomenon by a reliable third-party observer such as a housekeeper or the child's sibling, friend, or teacher. Although general rating practice dictates erring on the side of less pathology if in doubt, for this interview, if a child has either denied or failed to report a symptom, but the parent has other evidence that the symptom is present, this additional evidence should trump the child's report. In addition, the P-EDE asks parents to exercise their best judgment—factoring in all sources of information, including their own extrapolation—in determining the data (e.g., number of days, manifestations of severity) that will ultimately inform the interviewer's rating. If there are days in the month for which the parent has no information, the rating is prorated to obtain a 28-day frequency. Either one or both parents may be interviewed. Applied collectively, these decision rules can ideally maximize the sensitivity and specificity of each item. The reason for these decision rules, which permit more extrapolation and subjective judgment than the original EDE, is the dual challenge of rating eating disorder symptoms (as these disorders are typically associated with high levels of denial, minimization, and deceit), and doing so within a child and adolescent population (in which insight into symptoms is further reduced and there may be increased motivation to deny symptoms).

The format for most items on the P-EDE is a stem question on the phenomenon of interest, a query on the data the parent has (e.g., What exactly have you observed or has been reported to you?), and an assessment of the child's intent if the symptom is rated positively. Whereas the original EDE assesses intent pertaining to, for instance, shape and weight concerns for many items (e.g., Dietary Restraint should be related to shape and weight, not exclusively to another variable like overall health, to be rated positively on the EDE), the P-EDE inquires about whether the child has indicated a reason for engaging in the symptom. In the absence of a stated reason for the symptom endorsement (i.e., if the child has neither volunteered nor been asked for a reason, or has refused to answer when asked), the interviewer still rates the number of days on which the symptom occurred, but marks a separate code indicating that intent could not be established. If intent is ascertained even for one day, it may be inferred for the other days on which the symptom occurred.

The P-EDE begins with an orientation to the child's environment, including caregivers who may have conveyed valuable information to the parent, followed by a detailed growth history against which the interviewer can determine if the current height and weight represent a deviation from a previously healthy trend and a possible indicator of a current AN-spectrum diagnosis. An item on Refusal to Maintain a Normal Body Weight, corresponding to DSM-IV (American Psychiatric Association, 2000) criterion A for AN, is added to assess the phenomenon by asking about verbal rejections of maintaining or achieving a healthy weight as well as passive (e.g., refusing to eat) and active (e.g., throwing a tantrum, threatening to self-harm if made to eat) resistance to attempts by the parents or professional to increase the child's weight or prevent him or her from losing additional weight; some of these indicators are also relevant to Fear of Weight Gain, the item corresponding to DSM-IV (American Psychiatric Association, 2000) criterion B for AN. An item is also added to assess Denial of the Seriousness of Low Body Weight, corresponding to DSM-IV (American Psychiatric Association, 2000) criterion C for AN. Menstrual Status inquires about information obtained from physicians, as well as whether the parent has any evidence (e.g., not needing to purchase sanitary products; see the case example in Table 10.1) that amenorrhea may be present.

The Overeating section is expanded to include the assessment of evidence of secretive binge eating, such as parents finding large amounts of food missing from the kitchen, which they have reason to believe their child has consumed, or finding food or empty wrappers in the child's room. In addition, Loss of Control is assessed by parents' observations of the child expressing this subjective experience, as well as by behavioral indicators of and features associated with loss of control over eating, some drawn or adapted from the working DSM-IV (American Psychiatric Association, 2000) criteria for BED. Ratings are made using both traditional and expanded definitions of Loss of Control. Finally, two types of subjective bulimic episodes (overeating subjectively regarded, but actually normal–small amounts of food, accompanied by Loss of Control) are evaluated—the internally driven type that is captured in the original EDE, and an externally imposed type to account for meals and snacks that parents or treatment providers demand that the child eat.

Inappropriate compensatory behaviors such as self-induced vomiting are assessed by querying parents about their general knowledge of these behaviors as well as clues to their presence. For example, evidence of vomiting can include finding vomit residue in the child's bathroom or containers of vomit in the child's room; in addition, if there is an established history of self-induced vomiting, hypokalemia or furtive trips to the bathroom during a meal or immediately after eating are also considered valid indicators according to the P-EDE. Excessive Exercise is determined by the presence of at least two of three constructs: excessive duration, excessive intensity, and compulsive quality. Each of these is determined by detailed questions about behavior and attitudes of the offspring. If a child participates in sports or dance, information is elicited about his or her duration and intensity of exercise and training relative to the activity of his or her peers. Items pertinent to the Shape Concern, Weight Concern, and Eating Concern subscales have been revised to include—in addition to rating parents' report of child utterances consistent with each symptom—behavioral indicators of the psychological features of eating disorders, including body checking and talking excessively about food, eating, calories, shape, and weight.

Early research has been conducted comparing the P-EDE to the EDE on a sample of 50 children and adolescents between the ages of 9 and 18 (mean age = 14.03, SD = 2.13) who were seen at the Eating and Weight Disorders Program at Mount Sinai School of Medicine with symptoms of AN for participation in a study comparing family-based treatment with individual supportive psychotherapy in the prevention of full AN (Loeb et al., 2009). The sample was predominantly female (90%) and white (75%). The body mass indices (BMI) of participants ranged from 13.2 to 22.1 (M = 17.12, SD = 1.90), with 38% of participants at less than 85% of their ideal body weight. The EDE and P-EDE were administered to all participants and their parents, respectively. Cohen's kappas were used to make pairwise comparisons between DSM-IV criteria A–D for AN as generated by the two interviews. In addition, paired-sample t-tests were used to compare child and parent scores on the subscales and continuous diagnostic items.

Cohen's kappas indicated that agreement between parent and child reports for Criteria A (Refusal to Maintain a Normal Body Weight; kappa = 0.307), B (Fear of Weight Gain; kappa = 0.210), and C (Disturbance in the Experience of Shape/Weight; kappa = 0.368) were poor. In contrast, agreement between parent and child reports for criterion D (Amenorrhea) was good (kappa = 0.795). On the Restraint subscale, parent scores were significantly higher than child scores (p = .009). With regard to psychological diagnostic items, parent scores were also significantly higher than child scores on the Importance of Weight diagnostic item at months 1 to 3 (p = .000) and the Importance of Shape diagnostic item at months 1 to 3 (p = .007 for month 1; p = .000 for months 2–3). No other significant differences for subscales or diagnostic items were found.

Overall, parents reported greater levels of pathology than their children, suggesting denial and minimization on the part of patients, although the possibility that parents were overestimating the extent of their offspring's eating pathology must also be considered. This study highlights the importance of using complementary data from multiple informants in the assessment and diagnosis of youth with eating disorders. Although this may be less crucial in assessing the severity of AN symptoms, the kappa findings of poor agreement on AN criteria A–C indicate that it is crucial to understand and resolve discrepancies that carry implications for early and accurate diagnosis of this pernicious disorder.

Parent Version of the EDEQ

A Parent Version of the EDE-Q (P-EDEQ), a questionnaire version of the P-EDE, has also been developed (Loeb, 2007), which is based on the EDE-Q (Fairburn & Beglin, 1994). Like the P-EDE, the P-EDEQ asks parents to rate their child's symptoms, although the scope of modifications to capture behavioral indicators and other child/adolescent symptom manifestations is more limited. Psychometric research on the P-EDEQ is under way. An early study was conducted comparing the P-EDE with the P-EDEQ in a sample of with 24 children and adolescents (ages 11–17 years) with symptoms of AN included in the same study described earlier. For each of the four subscale scores (Restraint, Eating Concern, Shape Concern, and Weight Concern), parents' reports indicated significantly greater psychopathology than children's self-reports. In regard to diagnostic items, there were also significant discrepancies. Parent scores were significantly higher than child scores on Fear of Weight Gain, Feelings of Fatness, Importance of Weight, and Importance of Shape. Agreement between parent and child reports for criteria C and D was poor (kappa = 0.319 and 0.333, respectively).

Other

Branched Eating Disorders Test

The Branched Eating Disorders Test (BET; Selzer, Hamill, Bowes, & Patton, 1996), was developed in order to address the shortcomings of self-report measures and interviews. The BET is a branched questionnaire administered by computer. It is written at a 12-year-old level. It consists of 47 questions, which are followed up by more specific questions regarding frequency, duration, and severity of the endorsed response. In a study conducted by Selzer and colleagues (1996), the BET was used with 653 students in grades 5–8. Based on a comparison with the EDE (Fairburn & Cooper, 1993), the BET indicated sensitivity of 0.70 and specificity of 0.99 in categorizing a nonclinical sample as being at high or low risk for developing an eating disorder. Kappa scores ranged from 0.52 to 1.0 in comparing the BET and EDE, with self-worth contingent on weight rendering the lowest kappa scores and fear of fatness and body image distortion yielding the highest.

Conclusions

The accurate assessment of eating disorders in youth faces several challenges, including those unique to eating disorders more broadly and those specific to developmental differences in children and adolescents as compared with adults. Using parents as informants may theoretically minimize some error in direct assessment, but potentially prove inadequate for secretive behaviors like binge eating. Overall, there is a wealth of interview- and questionnaire-based instruments with demonstrated psychometric properties available for use within both community and clinical youth samples, and appropriate for epidemiological, clinical, and treatment research. These measures may be used to generate diagnoses, assess associated features and related psychopathology, and track response to treatment in younger patients, who represent the age group at highest risk for onset of eating disorders, and, in turn, are where our most aggressive case identification efforts should be focused.

References

Ackard, D. M., Fulkerson, J. A., & Neumark-Sztainer, D. (2007). Prevalence and utility of DSM-IV eating disorder diagnostic criteria among youth. *International Journal of Eating Disorders, 40*, 409–417.

American Psychiatric Association. (1980). *Diagnostic and statistical manual of mental disorders* (3rd ed.). Washington, DC: Author.

American Psychiatric Association. (1987). *Diagnostic and statistical manual of mental disorders* (3rd ed., text rev.). Washington, DC: Author.

American Psychiatric Association. (2000). *Diagnostic and statistical manual of mental disorders* (4th ed., text rev.). Washington, DC: Author.

Andersen, A. E., Bowers, W. A., & Watson, T. (2001). A slimming program for eating disorders not otherwise specified: Reconceptualizing a confusing, residual diagnostic category. *Psychiatry Clinics of North America, 24*, 271–280.

Arnow, B., Sanders, M. J., & Steiner, H. (1999). Premenarcheal versus postmenarcheal anorexia nervosa: A comparative study. *Clinical Child Psychology and Psychiatry, 4*, 403–414.

Ben-Tovim, D. I., Walker, K., Gilchrist, P., Freeman, R., Kalucy, R., & Esterman, A. (2001). Outcome in patients with eating disorders: A 5-year study. *Lancet, 357*, 1254–1257.

Beumont, P., Kopec-Schrader, E., Talbot, P., & Touyz, S. (1993). Measuring the specific psychopathology of eating disorder patients. *Australian and New Zealand Journal of Psychiatry, 27*, 506–511.

Binford, R. B., & Le Grange, D. (2005). Adolescents with bulimia nervosa and eating disorder not otherwise specified—purging only. *International Journal of Eating Disorders, 38*, 157–161.

Binford, R. B., Le Grange, D., & Jellar, C. C. (2005). Eating Disorders Examination versus Eating Disorders Examination—Questionnaire in adolescents with full and partial-syndrome bulimia nervosa and anorexia nervosa. *International Journal of Eating Disorders, 37*, 44–49.

Black, C. M., & Wilson, G. T. (1996). Assessment of eating disorders: Interview versus questionnaire. *International Journal of Eating Disorders, 20*, 43–50.

Boyadjieva, S., & Steinhausen, H.-C. (1996). The Eating Attitudes Test and the Eating Disorders Inventory in four Bulgarian clinical and nonclinical samples. *International Journal of Eating Disorders, 19*, 93–98.

Bravender, T., Bryant-Waugh, R., Herzog, D., Katzman, D., Kreipe, R. D., Lask, B., et al. (2007). Classification of child and adolescent eating disturbances. Workgroup for Classifications of Eating Disorders in Children and Adolescents (WCEDCA). *International Journal of Eating Disorders, 40*(Suppl.), S117–S122.

Bravender, T., Bryant-Waugh, R., Herzog, D., Katzman, D., Kreipe, R. D., Lask B., et al. (2010). Classification of eating disturbance in children and adolescents: Proposed changes for the DSM-V. *European Eating Disorders Review, 18*(2), 79–89.

Bryant-Waugh, R., Cooper, P., Taylor, C., & Lask, B. (1996). The use of the Eating Disorder Examination with children: A pilot study. *International Journal of Eating Disorders, 6*, 1–8.

Bunnell, D. W., Shenker, I. R., Nussbaum, M. P., Jacobson, M. S., & Cooper, P. (1990). Subclinical versus formal eating disorders: Differentiating psychological features. *International Journal of Eating Disorders, 9*, 357–362.

Cachelin, F. M., & Maher, B. A. (1998). Is amenorrhea a critical criterion for anorexia nervosa? *Journal of Psychosomatic Research, 44*, 435–440.

Campbell, M., Lawrence, B., Serpell, L., Lask, B., & Neiderman, M. (2002). Validating the Striving Eating Disorders Scales (SEDS) in an adolescent population. *Eating Behaviors, 3*, 285–293.

Carter, P., & Moss, R. (1984). Screening for anorexia and bulimia nervosa in a college population: Problems and limitations. *Addictive Behaviors, 9*, 417–419.

Cash, T. F. (1997). *The body image workbook: An 8-step program for learning to like your looks.* Oakland, CA: New Harbinger.

Childress, A. C., Jarrell, M. P., & Brewerton, T. (1993). The Kids' Eating Disorders Survey (KEDS): Internal consistency, component analysis, and reliability. *Eating Disorders, 1*, 123–133.

Christie, D., Watkins, B., & Lask, B. (2000). Assessment. In B. Lask & R. Bryant-Waugh (Eds.), *Anorexia nervosa and related eating disorders in childhood and adolescence* (pp. 105–125). East Sussex, UK: Psychology Press.

Clinton, D., & Norring, C. (1999). The Rating of Anorexia and Bulimia (RAB) Interview: Development and preliminary validation. *European Eating Disorders Review, 7*, 362–371.

Cooper, Z., Cooper, P. J., & Fairburn, C. G. (1989). The validity of the Eating Disorder Examination and its subscales. *British Journal of Psychiatry, 154*, 807–812.

Cooper, Z., & Fairburn, C. G. (1987). The Eating Disorder Examination: A semistructured interview for the assessment of the specific psychopathology of eating disorders. *International Journal of Eating Disorders, 6*, 1–8.

Couturier, J., & Lock, J. (2006a). Denial and minimization in adolescents with anorexia nervosa. *International Journal of Eating Disorders, 39*, 212–216.

Couturier, J., & Lock, J. (2006b). Do supplementary items on the Eating Disorder Examination improve the assessment of adolescents with anorexia nervosa? *International Journal of Eating Disorders, 39*, 426–433.

Couturier, J., Lock, J., Forsberg, S., Vanderheyden, D., & Yen, H. (2007). The addition of a parent and clinician component to the Eating Disorder Examination for children and adolescents. *International Journal of Eating Disorders, 40*, 472–475.

Crow, S. J., Agras, W. S., Halmi, K., Mitchell, J. E., & Kraemer, H. C. (2002). Full syndromal versus subthreshold anorexia nervosa, bulimia nervosa, and binge eating disorder: A multicenter study. *International Journal of Eating Disorders, 32*, 309–318.

Crowther, J. H., Lilly, R. S., Crawford, P. A., & Shepard, K. L. (1992). The stability of the Eating Disorder Inventory. *International Journal of Eating Disorders, 12*, 97–101.

Cumella, E. J. (2006). Review of the Eating Disorder Inventory-3. *Journal of Personality Assessment, 87*, 116–117.

Dalle Grave, R., Calugi, S., & Marchesini, G. (2008). Is amenorrhea a clinically useful criterion for the diagnosis of anorexia nervosa? *Behaviour Research and Therapy, 46*, 1290–1294.

Decaluwé, V. (1999). *Child Eating Disorder Examination—Questionnaire.* Dutch translation and adaptation of the Eating Disorder Examination—Questionnaire, authored by C. G. Fairburn & S. J. Beglin. Unpublished manuscript.

Decaluwé, V., & Braet, C. (2004). Assessment of eating disorder psychopathology in obese children and adolescents: Interview versus self-report questionnaire. *Behaviour Research and Therapy, 42*, 799–811.

Deter, H. C., & Herzog, W. (1994). Anorexia nervosa in a long-term perspective: Results of the Heidelberg-Mannheim study. *Psychosomatic Medicine, 56*, 20–27.

Eberenz, K. P., & Gleaves, D. H. (1994). An examination of the internal consistency and factor structure of the Eating Disorder Inventory-2 in a clinical sample. *International Journal of Eating Disorders, 16*, 371–379.

Eklund, K., Paavonen, E. J., & Almqvist, F. (2005). Factor structure of the Eating Disorder Inventory–C. *International Journal of Eating Disorders, 37*, 330–341.

Erickson, S. J., & Gerstle, M. (2007). Developmental considerations in measuring children's disordered eating attitudes and behaviors. *Eating Behaviors, 8*, 224–235.

Fairburn, C. G., & Beglin, S. (2008). Appendix B. Eating Disorder Examination Questionnaire (EDE-Q 6.0) In C. G. Fairburn (Ed.), *Cognitive behavior therapy and eating disorders* (pp. 309–313). New York: Guilford Press.

Fairburn, C. G., & Beglin, S. J. (1994). Assessment of eating disorders: Interview or self-report questionnaire? *International Journal of Eating Disorders, 16*, 363–370.

Fairburn, C. G., & Cooper, Z. (1993). Eating Disorder Examination (12th ed.). In C. G. Fairburn & G. T. Wilson (Eds.), *Binge eating: Nature, assessment, and treatment* (pp. 317–360). New York: Guilford Press.

Fairburn, C. G., & Cooper, Z. (2000). *Eating Disorder Examination* (14th ed., version 14.3). Oxford, UK: University of Oxford.

Fairburn, C. G., Cooper, Z., & O'Connor, M. E. (2008). Appendix A. Eating Disorder Examination (16.0D). In C. G. Fairburn (Ed.), *Cognitive behavior therapy and eating disorders* (pp. 265–308). New York: Guilford Press.

Fichter, M. M., Herpertz, S., Quadflieg, N., & Herpertz-Dahlmann, B. (1998). Structured interview for anorexic and bulimic disorders for DSM-IV and ICD-10 (3rd rev. ed.). *International Journal of Eating Disorders, 24,* 227–249.

Fichter, M. M., & Quadflieg, N. (2000). Comparing self- and expert rating: A self-report screening version (SIAB-S) of the Structured Interview for Anorexic and Bulimic Syndromes for DSM-IV and ICD-10 (SIAB-EX). *European Archives of Psychiatry and Clinical Neuroscience, 250,* 175–185.

Fichter, M., & Quadflieg, N. (2001). The Structured Interview for Anorexic and Bulimic Disorders for DSM-IV and ICD-10 (SIAB-EX): Reliability and validity. *European Psychiatry, 16,* 38–48.

Fisher, M., Schneider, M., Burns, J., Symons, H., & Mandel, F. S. (2001). Differences between adolescents and young adults at presentation to an eating disorders program. *Journal of Adolescent Health, 28,* 222–227.

Fosson, A., Knibbs, J., Bryant-Waugh, R., & Lask, B. (1987). Early onset anorexia nervosa. *Archives of Disease in Childhood, 62,* 114–118.

Gamble, C., Bryant-Waugh, R., Turner, H., Jones, C., Mehta, R., & Graves, A. (2006). An investigation into the psychometric properties of the Stirling Eating Disorder Scales (2006). *Eating Behaviors, 7,* 395–403.

Garfinkel, P. E., Lin, E., Goering, P., Spegg, C., Goldbloom, D., Kennedy, S., et al. (1996). Should amenorrhoea be necessary for the diagnosis of anorexia nervosa?: Evidence from a Canadian community sample. *British Journal of Psychiatry, 68,* 500–506.

Garner, D. M. (1991). *Eating Disorder Inventory–2 manual.* Odessa, FL: Psychological Assessment Resources.

Garner, D. M. (2004). *Eating Disorder Inventory–3 manual.* Lutz, FL: Psychological Assessment Resources.

Garner, D. M., & Garfinkel, P. E. (1979). The Eating Attitudes Test: An index of the symptoms of anorexia nervosa. *Psychological Medicine, 9,* 273–279.

Garner, D. M., Olmsted, M. P., Bohr, Y., & Garfinkel, P. E. (1982). The Eating Attitudes Test: Psychometric features and clinical correlates. *Psychological Medicine, 12,* 871–878.

Garner, D. M., Olmsted, M. P., & Polivy, J. (1983). Development and validation of a multidimensional eating disorder inventory for anorexia nervosa and bulimia. *International Journal of Eating Disorders, 2,* 15–34.

Ghaderi, A., & Scott, B. (2002). The preliminary reliability and validity of the Survey for Eating Disorders (SEDs): A self-report questionnaire for diagnosing eating disorders. *European Eating Disorders Review, 10,* 61–76.

Goldfein, J. A., Devlin, M. J., & Kamenetz, C. (2005). Eating Disorder Examination—Questionnaire with and without instruction to assess binge eating in patients with binge eating disorder. *International Journal of Eating Disorders, 37,* 107–111.

Goldschmidt, A. B., Doyle, A. C. & Wilfley, D. E. (2007). Assessment of binge eating in overweight youth using a questionnaire version of the Child Eating Disorder Examination with instructions. *International Journal of Eating Disorders, 40,* 460–467.

Götestam, K. G., & Agras, W. S. (1995). General population-based epidemiological study of eating disorders in Norway. *International Journal of Eating Disorders, 18,* 119–126.

Grilo, C. M., Masheb, R. M., Lorano-Blanco, C., & Barry, D. T. (2004). Reliability of the Eating Disorder Examination in patients with binge eating disorder. *International Journal of Eating Disorders, 35,* 80–85.

Hebebrand, J., Casper, R., Treasure, J., & Schweiger, U. (2004). The need to revise the diagnostic criteria for anorexia nervosa. *Journal of Neural Transmission, 111*(7), 827–840.

Henderson, M., & Freeman, C. P. L. (1987). A

self-rating scale for bulimia. The "BITE." *British Journal of Psychiatry, 150,* 18–24.

Herzog, D. B., Hopkins, J. D., & Burns, C. D. (1993). A follow-up study of 33 subdiagnostic eating disordered women. *International Journal of Eating Disorders, 14,* 261–267.

Hill, L. S., Reid, F., Morgan, J. F., & Lacey, J. H. (2010). SCOFF, the development of an eating disorder screening questionnaire. *International Journal of Eating Disorders, 43,* 344–351.

Hoek, H. W. (2006). Incidence, prevalence and mortality of anorexia nervosa and other eating disorders. *Current Opinion in Psychiatry, 19,* 389–394.

Hoek, H. W., & van Hoeken, D. (2003). Review of the prevalence and incidence of eating disorders. *International Journal of Eating Disorders, 34,* 383–396.

Imbierowicz, K., Curkovic, I., Braks, K., Geiser, F., Liedtke, R., & Jacoby, G. E. (2004). Effect of weight-regulating practices on potassium level in patients with anorexia or bulimia nervosa. *European Eating Disorders Review, 12*(5), 300–306.

Isomaa, R., Isomaa, A., Marttunen, M., Kaltiala-Heino, R., & Björkqvist, K. (2009). The prevalence, incidence and development of eating disorders in Finnish adolescents—a two-step 3-year follow-up study. *European Eating Disorders Review, 17,* 199–207.

Johnson, W. G., Grieve, F. G., Adams, C. D., & Sandy, J. (1999). Measuring binge eating in adolescents: Adolescent and parent versions of the questionnaire of eating and weight patterns. *International Journal of Eating Disorders, 26,* 301–314.

Johnson, W. G., Kirk, A. A., & Reed, A. E. (2001). Adolescent version of the questionnaire of eating and weight patterns: Reliability and gender differences. *International Journal of Eating Disorders, 29,* 94–96.

Killen, J. D., Taylor, C. B., Hayward, C., Wilson, D. M., Haydel, K. F., Hammer, L. D., et al. (1994). Pursuit of thinness and onset of eating disorder symptoms in a community sample of adolescent girls: A three-year prospective analysis. *International Journal of Eating Disorders, 16,* 227–238.

King, M. B. (1989). Eating disorders in a general practice population: Prevalence, char-

acteristics and follow-up at 12–18 months. *Psychological Medicine 14*(Suppl.), 1–34.

Kiziltan, G., Karabudak, E., Unver, S., Sezgin, E., & Unal, A. (2006). Prevalence of bulimic behaviors and trends in eating attitudes among Turkish late adolescents. *Adolescence, 41,* 677–689.

Kjelsås, E., Bjørnstrøm, C., & Götestam, K. G. (2004). Prevalence of eating disorders in female and male adolescents (14–15 years). *Eating Behaviors, 5,* 13–25.

Klump, K. L., McGue, M., & Iacono, W. G. (2000). Age differences in genetic and environmental influences on eating attitudes and behaviors in preadolescent and adolescent female twins. *Journal of Abnormal Psychology, 109,* 239–251.

Kovacs, M. (1982). *The Children's Depression Inventory.* Unpublished manuscript.

Kraemer, H. C., Measelle, J. R., Ablow, J. C., Essex, M. J., Boyce, W. T., & Kupfer, D. J. (2003). A new approach to integrating data from multiple informants in psychiatric assessment and research: Mixing and matching contexts and perspectives. *American Journal of Psychiatry, 160,* 1566–1577.

Kutlesic, V., Williamson, D. A., Gleaves, D. H., Barbin, J. M., & Murphy-Eberenz, K. P. (1998). The Interview for the Diagnosis of Eating Disorders-IV: Application to DSM-IV diagnostic criteria. *Psychological Assessment, 10,* 41–48.

Lattimore, P. J., & Halford, C. G. (2003). Adolescence and the diet–dieting disparity: Healthy food choice or risky health behaviour? *British Journal of Health Psychology, 8,* 451–463.

Lee, S. W., Stewart, S. M., Striegel-Moore, R. H., Lee, S., Ho, S., Lee, P. W. H., et al. (2007). Validation of the Eating Disorder Diagnostic Scale for use with Hong Kong adolescents. *International Journal of Eating Disorders, 40,* 569–574.

Le Grange, D., Loeb, K. L., Van Orman, S., & Jellar, C. (2004). Bulimia nervosa: A disorder in evolution? *Archives of Pediatric Adolescent Medicine, 158,* 478–482.

Lewinsohn, P. M., Striegel-Moore, R. H., & Seeley, J. R. (2001). Epidemiology and natural course of eating disorders in young women from adolescence to young adulthood. *Journal of the American Academy of Child and Adolescent Psychiatry, 39,* 1284–1292.

Loeb, K. L. (2007). *Eating Disorder Examination Questionnaire—Parent Version (P-EDEQ), Version 1.4.* Unpublished measure.

Loeb, K. L. (2008). *Eating Disorder Examination—Parent Version (P-EDE), Version 1.4.* Unpublished measure.

Loeb, K. L., Le Grange, D., Hildebrandt, T., Greif, R., Lock, J., & Alfano, L. (in press). Eating disorders in youth: Diagnostic variability and predictive validity. *International Journal of Eating Disorders.*

Lucas, A. R., Beard, C. M., O'Fallon, W. M., & Kurland, L. T. (1991). 50-year trends in the incidence of anorexia nervosa in Rochester, Minn.: A population-based study. *American Journal of Psychiatry, 148,* 917–922.

Luce, K. H., & Crowther, J. H. (1999). The reliability of the Eating Disorder Examination: Self-report questionnaire version (EDE-Q). *International Journal of Eating Disorders, 25,* 349–351.

Luck, A. J., Morgan, J. F., Reid, F., O'Brien, A., Brunton, J., Price, C., et al. (2002). The SCOFF questionnaire and clinical interview for eating disorders in general practice: Comparative study. *British Medical Journal, 325,* 755–756.

Madden, S., Morris, A., Zurynski, Y. A., Kohn, M., & Elliot, E. J. (2009). Burden of eating disorders in 5–13-year-old children in Australia. *Medical Journal of Australia, 190,* 410–414.

Maïano, C., Morin, A. J. S., Monthuy-Blanc, J., Garbarino, J., & Stephan, Y. (2009). Eating Disorder Inventory: Assessment of its construct validity in a nonclinical French sample of adolescents. *Journal of Psychopathology and Behavioral Assessment, 31,* 387–404.

Maloney, M. J., Mcguire, J. B., & Daniels, S. R. (1988). Reliability testing of a children's version of the Eating Attitudes Test. *Journal of the American Academy of Child and Adolescent Psychiatry, 27,* 541–543.

Marcus, M. D., & Kalarchian, M. A. (2003). Binge eating in children and adolescents. *International Journal of Eating Disorders, 34*(Suppl.), S47–S57.

McCarthy, D. M., Simmons, J. R., Smith, G. T., Tomlinson, K. L., & Hill, K. K. (2002). Reliability, stability, and factor structure of the Bulimia Test—Revised and Eating Disorder Inventory–2 scales in adolescence. *Assessment, 9,* 382–389.

McIntosh, V. V. W., Jordan, J., Carter, F. A., McKenzie, J. M., Luty, S. E., Bulik, C. M., et al. (2004). Strict versus lenient weight criterion in anorexia nervosa. *European Eating Disorders Review, 12,* 51–60.

Mintz, L. B., & Betz, N. E. (1988). Prevalence and correlates of eating disordered behavior among undergraduate women. *Journal of Consulting Psychology, 35,* 463–471.

Mintz, L. B., O'Halloran, S. M., Mulholland, A. M., & Schneider, P. A. (1997). Questionnaire for Eating Disorder Diagnoses: Reliability and validity of operationalizing DSM-IV criteria into a self-report format. *Journal of Consulting Psychology, 44,* 63–79.

Mitchell, J. E., Cook-Myers, T., & Wonderlich, S. A. (2005). Diagnostic criteria for anorexia nervosa: Looking ahead to DSM-5. *International Journal of Eating Disorders, 37,* S95–S97.

Mond, J. M., Hay, P. J., Rodgers, B., Owen, C., & Beumont, P. J. V. (2004). Validity of the Eating Disorder Examination Questionnaire (EDE-Q) in screening for eating disorders in community samples. *Behavior Research and Therapy, 42,* 551–567.

Morgan, J. F., Reid, F., & Lacy, J. H. (1999). The SCOFF questionnaire: Assessment of a new screening tool for eating disorders. *British Medical Journal, 319,* 1467–1468.

Muro-Sans, P., Amador-Campos, J. A., & Morgan, J. F. (2008). The SCOFF-c: Psychometric properties of the Catalan version in a Spanish adolescent sample. *Journal of Psychosomatic Research, 64,* 81–86.

National Center for Health Statistics. (1973). Height and weight of youths 12–17 years: United States. Retrieved April 1, 2009, from *www.cdc.gov/nchs/data/series/sr_11/ sr11_124.pdf.*

National Center for Health Statistics with the National Center for Chronic Disease Prevention and Health Promotion. (2000). 2000 CDC Growth Charts: United States.

Retrieved April 1, 2009, from *www.cdc. gov/growthcharts*.

Nevonen, L., Broberg, A. G., Clinton, D., & Norring, C. (2003). A measure for the assessment of eating disorders: Reliability and validity studies of the Rating of Anorexia and Bulimia Interview—Revised Version (RAB-R). *Scandinavian Journal of Psychology, 44,* 303–310.

Openshaw, C., & Waller, G. (2005). Psychometric properties of the Stirling Eating Disorder Scales with bulimia nervosa patients. *Eating Behaviors, 6,* 165–168.

Palmer, R., Christie, M., Cordle, C., Davies, D., & Kenrick, J. (1987). The Clinical Eating Disorder Rating Instrument (CEDRI): A preliminary description. *International Journal of Eating Disorders, 6,* 9–16.

Palmer, R., Robertson, D., Cain, M., & Black, S. (1996). The Clinical Eating Disorders Rating Instrument (CEDRI): A validation study. *European Eating Disorders Review, 4,* 149–156.

Passi, V. A., Bryson, S. W., & Lock, J. (2003). Assessment of eating disorders in adolescents with anorexia nervosa: Self-report questionnaire versus interview. *International Journal of Eating Disorders, 33,* 45–54.

Patton, G. C., Johnson-Sabine, E., Wood, K., Mann, A. H., & Wakeling, A. (1990). Abnormal eating attitudes in London schoolgirls—a prospective epidemiological study: Outcome at twelve month follow-up. *Psychological Medicine, 20,* 383–394.

Peebles, R., Hardy, K. K., Wilson, J. L., & Lock, J. D. (2010). Are diagnostic criteria for eating disorders markers of medical severity? *Pediatrics, 125*(5), e1193–e1201.

Pendley, J. S., & Bates, J. E. (1996). Mother/daughter agreement on the Eating Attitudes Test and the Eating Disorder Inventory. *Journal of Early Adolescence, 16,* 179–191.

Perry, L., Morgan, J., Reid, F., Brunton, J., O'Brien, A., Luck, A., et al. (2002). Screening for symptoms of eating disorders: Reliability of the SCOFF screening tool with written compared to oral delivery. *International Journal of Eating Disorders, 32,* 466–472.

Pinheiro, A., Thornton, L., Plotnicov, K. H., Tozzi, T., Klump, K. L., Berrettini, W. H., et al. (2007). Patterns of menstrual disturbance in eating disorders. *International Journal of Eating Disorders, 40,* 424–434.

Ratnasuriya, R., Eisler, I., Szmukler, G. I., & Russell, G. F. (1991). Anorexia nervosa: Outcome and prognostic factors after 20 years. *British Journal of Psychiatry, 158,* 495–496.

Ricca, V., Mannucci, E., Mezzani, B., Di Bernardo, M., Zucchi, T., Paionni, A., et al. (2001). Psychopathological and clinical features of outpatients with an eating disorder not otherwise specified. *Eating and Weight Disorders, 6,* 157–165.

Ricciardelli, L. A., Williams, R. J., & Kiernan, M. J. (1999). Bulimic symptoms in adolescent girls and boys. *International Journal of Eating Disorders, 26,* 217–221.

Rizvi, S. L., Peterson, C. B., Crow, S. J., & Agras, W. S. (2000). Test–retest reliability of the Eating Disorders Examination. *International Journal of Eating Disorders, 28,* 311–316.

Roberto, C. A., Steinglass, J., Mayer, L. E., Attia, E., & Walsh, B. T. (2008). The clinical significant of amenorrhea as a diagnostic criterion for anorexia nervosa. *International Journal of Eating Disorders, 41,* 559–563.

Rosen, J. C., Silberg, N. T., & Gross, J. (1988). Eating Attitudes Test and Eating Disorders Inventory: Norms for adolescent girls and boys. *Journal of Consulting and Clinical Psychology, 56,* 305–308.

Rosen, J. C., Vara, L., Wendt, S., & Leitenberg, H. (1990). Validity studies of the Eating Disorder Examination. *International Journal of Eating Disorders, 9,* 519–528.

Salbach-Andrae, H., Klinkowski, N., Holzhausen, K. F., Frieler, K., Bohnekamp, I., Thiels, C., et al. (2009). The German version of the Anorectic Behavior Observation Scale (ABOS). *European Child and Adolescent Psychiatry, 18,* 321–325.

Sancho, C., Asorey, O., Arija, V., & Canals, J. (2005). Psychometric characteristics of the Children's Eating Attitudes Test in a Spanish sample. *European Eating Disorders Review, 13,* 338–343.

Schoemaker, C. (1997). Does early intervention improve the prognosis in anorexia nervosa?: A systematic review of the treatment–outcome literature. *International Journal of Eating Disorders, 21,* 1–15.

Selzer, R., Hamill, C., Bowes, G., & Patton, G. (1996). The Branched Eating Disorders Test: Validity in a nonclinical population. *International Journal of Eating Disorders, 20,* 57–64.

Shapiro, J. R., Woolson, S. L., Hamer, R. M., Kalarchian, M. A., Marcus, M. D., & Bulik, C. M. (2007). Evaluating binge eating disorder in children: Development of the Children's Binge Eating Disorder Scale (C-BEDS). *International Journal of Eating Disorders, 40,* 82–89.

Shisslak, C. M., Renger, R., Sharpe, T., Crago, M., McKnight, K. M., Gray, N., et al. (1999). Development and evaluation of the McKnight Risk Factor Survey for assessing potential risk and protective factors for disordered eating in preadolescent and adolescent girls. *International Journal of Eating Disorders, 25,* 195–214.

Shore, R. A., & Porter, J. E. (1990). Normative and reliability data for 11 and 18 year olds on the Eating Disorder Inventory. *International Journal of Eating Disorders, 9,* 201–207.

Smith, M. C., & Thelen, M. H. (1984). Development and validation of a test for bulimia. *Journal of Consulting and Clinical Psychology, 52,* 863–872.

Smolak, L., & Levine, M. P. (1994). Psychometric properties of the Children's Eating Attitudes Test. *International Journal of Eating Disorders, 16,* 275–282.

Spitzer, R. L., Devlin, M. J., Walsh, B. T., Hasin, D., Wing, R. R., Marcus, M. D., et al. (1992). Binge eating disorder: A multisite field trial for the diagnostic criteria. *International Journal of Eating Disorders, 11,* 191–203.

Steinberg, E., Tanofsky-Kraff, M., Cohen, M. L., Elberg, J., Freedman, R. J., Semega-Janneh, M., et al. (2004). Comparison of the child and parent forms of the Questionnaire on Eating and Weight Patterns in the assessment of children's eating-disordered behaviors. *International Journal of Eating Disorders, 36,* 183–194.

Stice, E., Fisher, M., & Martinez, E. (2004). Eating Disorder Diagnostic Scale: Additional evidence of reliability and validity. *Psychological Assessment, 16,* 60–71.

Stice, E., Telch, C. F., & Rizvi, S. L. (2000). Development and validation of the Eating Disorder Diagnostic Scale: A brief self-report measure of anorexia, bulimia, and binge-eating disorder. *Psychological Assessment, 12,* 123–131.

Swenne, I., Belfrage, E., Thurfjell, B., & Engström, I. (2005). Accuracy of reported weight and menstrual status in teenage girls with eating disorders *International Journal of Eating Disorders, 38,* 375–379.

Tanofsky-Kraff, M., Goossens, L., Eddy, K. T., Ringham, R., Goldschmidt, A. S., Yanovski, S. Z., et al. (2007). A multisite investigation of binge eating behaviors in children and adolescents. *Journal of Consulting and Clinical Psychology, 75,* 901–913.

Tanofsky-Kraff, M., Morgan, C., Yanovski, S. Z., Marmarosh, C., Wilfley, D. E., & Yanovski, J. A. (2003). Comparison of assessments of children's eating-disordered behaviors by interview and questionnaire. *International Journal of Eating Disorders, 33,* 213–224.

Tanofsky-Kraff, M., Yanovski, S. Z., Wilfley, D. E., Marmarosh, C., Morgan, C. M., & Yanovski, J. A. (2004). Eating disordered behaviors, body fat, and psychopathology in overweight and normal-weight children. *Journal of Consulting and Clinical Psychology, 72,* 53–61.

Tanofsky-Kraff, M., Yanovski, S. Z., & Yanovski, J. A. (2005). Comparison of child interview and parent reports of children's eating disordered behaviors. *Eating Behaviors, 6,* 95–99.

Thelen, M. H., Farmer, J., Wonderlich, S., & Smith, M. (1991). A revision of the Bulimia Test: The BULIT-R. *Psychological Assessment: A Journal of Consulting and Clinical Psychology, 3,* 119–124.

Thelen, M. H., Mintz, L. B., & Vander Wal, J. S. (1996). The Bulimia Test—Revised: Validation with DSM-IV criteria for bulimia nervosa. *Psychological Assessment, 8,* 219–221.

Thomas, J. J., Vartanian, L. R., & Brownell, K. D. (2009). The relationship between eating disorder not otherwise specified (EDNOS) and officially recognized eating disorders: Meta-analysis and implications for DSM. *Psychological Bulletin, 153,* 407–433.

Thurfjell, B., Edlund, B., Arinell, H., Hägglöf, B., Garner, D. M., & Engström, I. (2004). Eating Disorder Inventory for Children (EDI-C): Effects of age and gender in a Swedish sample. *European Eating Disorders Review, 12,* 256–264.

Uehara, T., Takeuchi, K., Ohmori, I., Kawashima, Y., Goto, M., Mikuni, M., et al. (2002). Factor-analytic study of the Anorectic Behavior Observation Scale in Japan: comparisons with the original Belgian study. *Psychiatry Research, 111,* 241–246.

Vandereycken, W. (1992). Validity and reliability of the Anorectic Behavior Observation Scale for parents. *Acta Psychiatrica Scandinavica, 85,* 163–166.

Vandereycken, W., & Meerman, R. (1984). *Anorexia nervosa: A clinician's guide to treatment.* Berlin: Walter de Gruyter.

van Hooff, M. H. A., Voorhorst, F. J., Kaptein, M. B. M., Hirasing, R. A., Koppenaal, C., & Schoemaker, J. (1998). Relationship of the menstrual cycle pattern in 14–17 year old adolescents with gynaecological age, body mass index and historical parameters. *Human Reproduction, 13*(8), 2252–2260.

Viglione, V., Muratori, F., Maestro, S., Brunori, E., & Picchi, L. (2006). Denial of symptoms and psychopathology in adolescent anorexia nervosa. *Psychopathology, 39,* 255–260.

Vincent, M. A., McCabe, M. P., & Ricciardelli, L. A. (1999). Factorial validity of the Bulimia Test—Revised in adolescent boys and girls. *Behavior Research and Therapy, 37,* 1129–1140.

Vitousek, K., & Manke, F. (1994). Personality variables and disorders in anorexia nervosa and bulimia nervosa. *Journal of Abnormal Psychology, 103,* 137–147.

von Ranson, K. M., Cassin, S. E., Bramfield, T. D., & Fung, T. S. (2007). Psychometric properties of the Minnesota Eating Behavior Survey in Canadian university women. *Canadian Journal of Behavioural Science, 39,* 151–159.

von Ranson, K. M., Klump, K. L., Iacono, W. G., & McGue, M. (2005). The Minnesota Eating Behavior Survey: A brief measure of disordered eating attitudes and behaviors. *Eating Behaviors, 6,* 373–392.

Vyver, E., Steinegger, C., & Katzman, D. K. (2008). Eating disorders and menstrual dysfunction in adolescents. *Annals of the New York Academy of Sciences, 1135,* 253–264.

Wade, T. D., Byrne, S., & Bryant-Waugh, R. (2008). The Eating Disorder Examination: Norms and construct validity with young and middle adolescent girls. *International Journal of Eating Disorders, 41,* 551–558.

Watkins, B., Frampton, I., Lask, B., & Bryant-Waugh, R. (2005). Reliability and validity of the child version of the Eating Disorder Examination: A preliminary investigation. *International Journal of Eating Disorders, 38,* 183–187.

Watson, T. L., & Andersen, A. E. (2003). A critical examination of the amenorrhea and weight criteria for diagnosing anorexia nervosa. *Acta Psychiatrica Scandinavica, 108*(Suppl.), 175–82.

Whitaker, A., Davies, M., Shaffer, D., Johnson, J., Abrams, S., Walsh, B. T., et al. (1989). The struggle to be thin: A survey of anorexic and bulimic symptoms in a nonreferred adolescent population. *Psychological Medicine, 19,* 143–163.

Wilfley, D. E., Schwartz, M. B., Spurrell, E. B., & Fairburn, C. G. (1997). Assessing the specific psychopathology of binge eating disorder patients: Interview or self-report? *Behavior Research and Therapy, 35,* 1151–1159.

Williams, G., & Power, K. G. (1996). *Manual of the Stirling Eating Disorder Scales.* London: Psychological Corporation.

Williams, G., Power, K. G., Miller, H. R., Freeman, C. P., Yellowlees, A., Dowds, T., et al. (1994). Development and validation of the Stirling Eating Disorder Scales. *International Journal of Eating Disorders, 16,* 35–43.

Williamson, D. A. (1990). *Assessment of eating disorders: Obesity, anorexia, and bulimia nervosa.* Elmsford, NY: Pergamon Press.

Williamson, D. A., Anderson, D. A., Jackman, L. P., & Jackson, S. R. (1995). Assessment of eating disordered thoughts, feelings and behaviors. In D. B. Allison (Ed.), *Handbook of assessment methods for eating behaviors and weight related problems: Measures, theory and research* (pp. 347–386). Thousand Oaks, CA: Sage.

Williamson, D. A., Prather, R. C., McKenzie, S. J., & Blouin, D. C. (1990). Behavioral assessment procedures can differentiate bulimia nervosa, compulsive overeater, obese, and normal subjects. *Behavioral Assessment, 12,* 239–252.

Wilson, G., & Smith, D. (1989).Assessment of bulimia nervosa: An evaluation of the Eating Disorders Examination. *International Journal of Eating Disorders, 8,* 173–179.

Wilson, G. T. (1993). Assessment of binge eating. In C. G. Fairburn & G. T. Wilson (Eds.), *Binge eating: Nature, assessment, and treatment* (pp. 227–249). New York: Guilford Press.

Wilson, G. T., Nonas, C. A., & Rosenblum, G. D. (1993). Assessment of binge eating in obese patients. *International Journal of Eating Disorders, 13,* 25–33.

World Health Organization. (2007). *International Statistical Classification of Diseases and Related Health Problems,* 10th Revision, Version for 2007. Retrieved April 1, 2009, from *apps.who.int/classifications/apps/icd/icd10online.*

Yager, J., Landsverk, J., & Edelstein, C. K. (1987). A 20-month follow-up study of 628 women with eating disorders: Course and severity. *American Journal of Psychiatry, 144,* 1172–1177.

Zúñiga, O., & Padrón, E. (2009). Translation and psychometric properties of the Kid's Eating Disorders Survey (KEDS)—Spanish version. *Actas Espanolas de Psiquiatria, 37,* 326–329.

PART V

TREATMENT

INTENSIVE TREATMENT PROGRAMS

CHAPTER 11

Improving Connections for Adolescents across High-Intensity Settings for the Treatment of Eating Disorders

Mary Tantillo
Richard Kreipe

I think that the source of hope lies in believing that one has or can move toward a sense of connection.

— JEAN BAKER MILLER (oral presentation, 2004)

G arfinkel and Garner (1982) described a set of predisposing and precipitating factors at the individual, familial, and cultural levels triggering anorexia nervosa (AN), as well as perpetuating factors that sustain it. Though widely varied, the key features of precipitating factors were noted to be a "threat of loss of self-control and/or a threat or actual loss of self-worth" (p. 204). Although these factors remain true 30 years later, details have emerged regarding the importance of biological factors, including genetics, mood, anxiety, neurotransmitter and brain function of both AN and bulimia nervosa (BN), resulting in the view that "eating disorders are presumably brain disorders," even though "little is known about their pathophysiology" (Chavez & Insel, 2007, p. 164). Despite much remaining unknown about the determinants of eating disorders, it is known that eating disorders are not randomly distributed in populations; more than 90% of identified patients are adolescents or young adults at onset, and 90% of those are female.

Thus, although the Worldwide Charter for Action on Eating Disorders classifies eating disorders as "*mental* disorders," they could also be framed as "*developmental* disorders" because their origins are so often—though not always—tied to adolescent growth and development during the transition from childhood to adulthood (Kreipe & Dukarm, 1999). This does not minimize the role played by mental health problems that often underlie eating disorders, but it extends the scope of understanding and intervention to the developmental processes that prepare an adolescent for healthy and rewarding adulthood. Rather than focusing on psychopathology, the developmental challenges that appear to precipitate the onset of an eating disorder and that provide a context for treatment include common issues related to the physical changes of puberty, as well as emerging identity and autonomy struggles. This allows for an asset-based, rather than a deficit-based approach to the patient.

Especially for females, healthy adolescence involves developing a network of close interpersonal connections that shape emerging identity, autonomy, agency, and the ability to be interdependent with others. A seminal book on longitudinal research findings in adolescent female development by Gilligan, Lyons, and Hanmer (1990) focused on two key issues: "making connections" and the "the relational world of adolescent girls." Making intra- and interpersonal connections, a defining feature of the relational worlds of adolescent girls, goes awry in those developing eating disorders. Conceptualizing eating disorders as "diseases of disconnection" (Tantillo, 2006) is supported by Steiner-Adair's (1986, 1991) work. She emphasizes that eating disorders often cause girls to "go underground," appearing on the surface to remain in connection with self, peers, and family, while actually disconnecting from these sources of growth and support because of the connection with the more powerfully reinforcing eating disorder.

The establishment of growth-fostering and mutual connections is essential in adolescence because connectedness serves as a critical protective factor in relation to development of psychological distress and psychiatric disorder (Resnick, Harris, & Blum, 1993; Seligman et al., 2005). This is especially true for "quietly disturbed behaviors" such as sustaining a poor body image, disordered eating, bingeing, vomiting as a strategy for weight loss, chronic dieting, fear of loss of control of eating, emotional distress, and suicidal ideation or attempts (Resnick et al., 1993). This same need for connectedness is important when adolescents require intensive treatment for eating disorders. Adolescents with AN describe feeling confused about their illness, experiencing it as a "friend ... a shield to hide behind, and something which [gives] confidence and security," as well as "an enemy—suffocating, frightening, and depriving" (Colton & Pistrang, 2004, p. 310). Their paradoxical desire to remain connected with the eating disorder contradicts the desire to connect with their own "healthy voice" and the voices of others telling them to "let go" of the illness. This internal conflict leads to ambivalence about changing eating behaviors, which is heightened by confusion about what "healthy" means, as well as the realization that connection with health requires disconnection from the eating disorder. Thus, they feel guilty about getting well and betraying their eating disorder *and* about not making healthy choices and disappointing personal and professional carers.

Patients have clearly described successful treatment and full recovery as being possible when they want these things for themselves (Colton & Pistrang, 2004; Taylor, Adams, & Kreipe, 2008). To help adolescents with eating disorders become their own change agents, connectedness with adults at home and in treatment programs should be fostered in ways to increase a sense of belonging, authenticity, self-empathy, empowerment, and motivation for change (Tantillo & Sanftner, 2010a). This experience allows the adolescent to decide to *give up* or *replace* the eating disorder, rather than having it *taken away*. In addition, Resnick and colleagues (1993) proposed that the interventions and relationships for successful treatment and recovery should be as intense as the need for relationships and recovery. Thus, intensive programming—inpatient, residential, partial hospitalization program (PHP) and intensive outpatient programming (IOP)—needs to meet the adolescent's needs for connection and belonging to counteract the eating disorder's continued pull to disconnect and isolate the adolescent from self and others.

Evidence-based interventions are an essential part of intensive treatment, but these interventions are best delivered within the context of strong, mutual connections with us as carers, marked by our ability to (1) understand how we influence adolescents; (2) be open to and moved by their internal experiences and behaviors; and (3) let them know how we have been moved (Miller & Stiver, 1997; Tantillo & Sanftner, 2010a). Adolescent patients have described "good staff" as those who cared for them by being available, willing to listen, and able to see them as unique individuals with different needs (Taylor, Adams, & Kreipe, 2008). These staff members "see behind" the eating disorder and allow the patient to be an active part of the treatment plan (Colton & Pistrang, 2004).

Although an adolescent's attitudes toward intensive treatment are often marked by ambivalence and volatility, an encouraging, warm, and supportive relational approach with a carer acknowledging (but not assuming) the patient's perspective, aligns with the patient's autonomy and agency and increases motivation for change and openness to interventions by staff members. A sense of connectedness with staff members is also important to mitigate an adolescent's *feeling* neglected or rejected by his or her family in relation to hospitalization, even when he or she *knows* this is not the case (Colton, & Pistrang, 2004). Staff members can help strengthen the adolescent's relationships with parents, who must balance the need to help the adolescent improve her or his health status with the need to eventually turn over responsibility for recovery to the adolescent.

This chapter describes a model for a comprehensive care program for eating disorders that promotes connectedness and caring for adolescents and fosters collaboration among professionals working within and across various intensive levels of care. This model is informed by the principles noted earlier, which guide the collaborations and outcomes achieved in the development of the Western New York Comprehensive Care Center for Eating Disorders (WNYCCCED), one of three New York State Department of Health–funded Comprehensive Care Centers for Eating Disorders (CCCEDs). Dr. Tantillo is the director of the WNYCCCED and Dr. Kreipe is the medical director of the WNYCCCED. Following a description of connectedness that can be cultivated with adolescent patients, their families, and loved ones, examples of how such connections can extend to the relationships within and between treatment programs are presented. We conclude the chapter with implications and next steps for those who desire to replicate this work.

The Importance of Mutual Connections in Clinical Practice

The work of the WNYCCCED is grounded in relational–cultural theory (RCT) (Miller and Stiver, 1997; Jordan, 2010) and the adaptation of this work to the treatment of eating disorders (Steiner-Adair, 1991; Tantillo, 2004, 2006; Tantillo & Sanftner, 2010a, 2010b). The use of this model requires a shift from the traditional focus on psychopathology to a focus on the tension between connections and disconnections in relationships. With this relational frame, providers, patients, and families (and often insurers) who interact in this context consider eating disorders as "diseases of disconnection" (Tantillo, 2006; Tantillo & Sanftner, 2010a), with the goal of treatment and recovery being disconnection from the eating disorder and reconnection with the self and others.

In our Center eating disorders are seen as illnesses created by a convergence of biopsychosocial risk factors that increase the patient's vulnerability to disconnection from the self and others. Examples of these disconnections include neurobiological factors, such as the possible disconnection between the *insula* and other brain areas, resulting in difficulties in processing information (Lask, 2010), and *serotonergic* disturbance, which contributes to a disconnection in the patient's ability to tolerate or regulate intense emotion (Kaye, Fudge, & Paulus, 2009). Although it is not clear if these abnormalities are primary or secondary to the biological effects of weight control and eating habits, relational disconnections, especially if repeated and serious (e.g., chronic invalidation, rejection, neglect, abuse, or losses) can interact with the neurobiological effects to promote further disconnection from intense emotion, anxiety, uncertainty, and isolation (Miller & Stiver, 1997; Tantillo & Sanftner, 2010a, 2010b). Sociocultural risk factors such as the glorification of thinness, equating thinness with control, and the socialization of males and, especially, females further reinforce a disconnection from authentic internal experience and a focus on appearance and performance (Smolak & Murnen, 2001).

Finally, the intersection of culture and developmental stage creates further possible disconnection from the self and others as vulnerable adolescents attempt to cope with anxiety related to various developmental stressors and demands (Seligman et al., 2005; Smolak & Murnen, 2001; Walsh et al., 2005). Healthy adolescence requires adjustment to (1) the physical changes of girl-to-woman and boy-to-man pubertal transformations; (2) emerging identity in which the individual develops her or his own self in the context of family, peers, school, and community; (3) increasing expectations for autonomy both by the adolescent and by society; and (4) transition to formal operational thought (Kreipe & Dukarm, 1999). Western culture exerts pressure for adolescents to be independent and separate from parents. This experience can create increased stress for adolescent girls, who are socialized early to grow in relationship with others (Gilligan, 1982, 1991; Steiner-Adair, 1986) and who commonly experience decreased self-esteem after age 12 (Abramowitz, Petersen, & Schulenberg, 1984). During adolescence girls are often faced with conflicting alternatives: to succeed they may perceive the need to be independent, aggressive, and competitive, but to fulfill feminine stereotypes they may be drawn to be gentle, kind, and nice, resulting, as previously noted, in the need to "go underground" with the former traits (Steiner-Adair, 1986).

Adolescent boys may suffer too, as the culture emphasizes that masculinity equals muscularity (Tantillo & Kreipe, 2006). Boys feel the push to be physically strong, nonemotional, and nonrelational (Pollack, 1998; Pope, Phillips, & Olivardia, 2000). This male way of being also contrasts with a more contemporary push for men to be more compassionate, nurturing, and supportive of women (Tantillo & Kreipe, 2006). Eating disorders can emerge in adolescence to regulate intense anxiety and other painful feelings, to establish connections in the absence of empathic, reliable connections with others, and/or to establish control and a separate identity. Thus eating disorders can effect more disconnections, thwarting psychological growth and developmental needs.

In the WNYCCCED treatment and recovery are informed by evidence-based approaches such as cognitive-behavioral therapy (Fairburn, 2008; Garner & Garfinkel, 1997), the Maudsley approach (Le Grange & Lock, 2007; Lock, Le Grange, Agras, & Dare, 2001), stages of change (Prochaska, Norcross, & DiClemente, 1994), and motivational interviewing (Miller & Rollnick, 2002), but are also heavily informed by RCT. Therefore, treatment and recovery in the WNYCCCED involve teaching patients and families to name disconnections and points of tension created by the eating disorder, how to grow in connection with one another, and how to create a life without illness. Treatment providers emphasize that the hallmark of psychological maturation and full recovery is the ability to embrace differences in feelings, thoughts, and needs within strong connections with others (Tantillo, 2006; Tantillo & Sanftner, 2010b). Psychological growth is seen to occur within mutual connections (Miller & Stiver, 1997; Tantillo, 2006) with others, including providers in the WNYCCCED, who help to strengthen the patient's relationship with genuine thoughts, feelings, and needs, and with family, friends, and significant others who are essential to recovery (e.g., coaches, teachers, pastor).

Essential to RCT is the belief that all stakeholders, including professional carers, are transformed through mutual connection based on mutual empathy and empowerment. This is the platform from which all evidence-based and motivational interventions emerge because patient and family motivation for change and a sense of perceived mutuality in relationships go hand in hand (Tantillo & Sanftner, 2010b). It is the bidirectional relational movement of thoughts, feelings, and activity (Genero, Miller, Surrey, & Baldwin, 1992) between patients, families, and therapists that builds the mutual empathy and empowerment needed for patients to release themselves from the eating disorder and deliver themselves back to themselves and to others (Tantillo, 2006; Tantillo & Sanftner, 2010b).

This relational frame is especially helpful in promoting continuity of care within the WNYCCCED. Recognizing the anxiety-provoking nature of transitions for individuals with eating disorders and their families, the relational frame emphasizes that the eating disorder will try to create disconnection during recovery, slowing or reversing the path toward wellness. Externalizing the illness as something foreign to the affected individual's true self, and that wreaks havoc through disconnection (e.g., all-or-none thinking, splitting, and highly expressed emotion), facilitates separation of the disorder from the individuals affected by the eating disorder. For all involved, this understanding strengthens team relationships and reduces blame, fault-finding, and guilt, upon which the eating disorder thrives, as it seems to pit individuals against one another. Likewise, promoting gradual, deliberate, and mindful change from one provider to the next ensures continuity of care, decreases anxiety in transition, and models gradual and thoughtful change from one stage of development in the patient's life to the next. The relational frame emphasizes the continuity of connections that patient and family require to successfully move along in recovery and in life.

The Importance of Mutual Connections in Program Development

Because there can be many levels of disconnection between adolescent patients and their parents, there is a high probability that these will be mirrored in disconnections with members of the treatment team staff. Therefore, intensive treatment programs are best developed in ways that promote comprehensive, integrated, and continuous care, with separate programs ideally functioning as "different but connected" within an overall network of care. The same elements of mutual empathy and empowerment fostered among the patient, family members, and the treatment team staff should be promoted among staff members within, and across, programs that function in a network of care. These principles informed the development of the WNYCCCED, one of three centers constituting an integrated statewide network of specialists that provides a full range of comprehensive services for individuals with eating disorders and their families across New York State. The 2004 legislation creating the three CCCEDs included six legislative mandates for each Center (see Table 11.1) to address not only treatment, but also education and out-

TABLE 11.1. Goals of the New York State Comprehensive Care Centers for Eating Disorders

- Provide comprehensive and coordinated integrated services to all individuals with diagnosed eating disorders and their families.
- Provide or arrange for all required levels of care appropriate for individuals with eating disorders.
- Provide or arrange for the full range of services appropriate for the care of individuals with eating disorders.
- Provide case management services for all individuals served by the Center.
- Within the selected service area, sponsor programs that increase the awareness, early identification, and treatment of eating disorders.
- Conduct and participate in research programs to identify and address gaps in evidence-based prevention and treatment methods.

reach, prevention, early identification and intervention, case management, transitional services, research activities, and communication and collaborations within and among Centers. None of these activities would have been possible without funding, which specifically excluded fee-for-service encounters that were covered by health insurance.

Inherent to the New York State (NYS) CCCEDs is a strong spirit of collaboration and frequent communication between providers within and among all three centers. NYSCCCED leadership and staff regularly communicate through the use of joint (i.e., conference) phone calls at least monthly, and other routinely scheduled leadership, case manager, and staff meetings, inservices, and/or retreats. Insurers are also a part of these monthly calls in the WNYCCCED to promote interdisciplinary collaboration and communication related to program development and treatment delivery. Calls and other communications regarding patient care occur throughout the week if patients and families work with more than one provider within or across the Centers. Potential challenges related to timely and smooth referral or transition from one program to another are communicated to the directors of each center and/or are routinely discussed during Quality Improvement/Clinical Care Review portions of monthly NYSCCCED joint calls. This feedback loop promotes continuous quality improvement and the coordinated, continuous care that is central to the work of the Centers.

All three Centers have collaborated on a number of initiatives promoting evidence-based and cost-effective care, including development of shared standardized assessment forms, state conferences and advocacy, and have worked with the New York State Office of Mental Health (NYSOMH) to write regulations for residential treatment. Each program within a Center retains its own licensure, oversight, and institutional practices, policies, and procedures, but also conforms to the New York State Department of Health–approved center policies and procedures, standards, and admission/discharge criteria developed in partnership with the core sites within each CCCED.

Although there are similarities among all three Centers in meeting the legislative mandates listed in Table 11.1, the WNYCCCED has a number of distinct features that make it effective in providing intensive treatment programming for adolescents and their families, across a range of settings and program intensities. Many of these features are related to the deep and enduring connections that have existed between eating disorder specialists and other professionals at the core site of the WNYCCCED, as well as to the strong partnerships with patients and families that have been cultivated over time in this

30-county service region. For example, the director and medical director have collaborated in providing community-based services for patients and families for more than 25 years, and its leader and staff members located at the core and affiliate sites have provided care for patients and families for many years. In addition, the WNYCCCED leadership and staff members have strong connections with professionals in the community and have been involved with families attending community-based videoconferenced Eating Disorder Network support meetings and educational offerings (*www.rochesteredn.org*). The spirit of strong collaboration among providers, school personnel, recovering individuals, and families is a hallmark of the Center. An example of this collaboration is the work of the WNYCCCED Community Advisory Board, which includes professionals, recovering individuals, and family members who provide feedback about programming, prevention, education, and advocacy.

There are also structural features of the WNYCCCED that facilitate intensive adolescent treatment programming. For example, the core and affiliate sites of the WNYCCCED in Rochester comprise a full continuum of care available to adolescents and their families. Adolescents can be referred to Golisano Children's Hospital (*www. urmc.rochester.edu/childrens-hospital/patient-care/adolescent/eating-disorders.cfm*) for shorter-term inpatient treatment in the only geographically distinct pediatric-based adolescent medicine unit in New York north of New York City, and can be stepped down to Harmony Place at St. Joseph's Villa (a family-based adolescent eating disorders residential treatment program serving all of New York State [*www.stjosephsvilla.org/ ProgramsServices/EatingDisordersProgram*]) and/or to The Healing Connection, LLC (*www.thehealingconnectionllc.com/patients.html*), an eating disorders partial hospitalization program (PHP). All three programs are located within a 17-mile radius and have access to the Ronald McDonald House (*ronaldshouse.com*) that is affiliated with Golisano Children's Hospital in Rochester and provides housing for families of patients 12–19 years old from outside the Rochester area. The Healing Connection also has an apartment that parents/patients can rent for patients >17 years old. In addition, a strong multidisciplinary staff, including practitioners in adolescent medicine, psychiatry, psychology, nursing, social work, nutrition, counseling, and family therapy, is available to patients and families who work with programs in the Rochester-based core and affiliate sites of the WNYCCCED.

The director and medical director of the WNYCCCED at all three of the core facilities, as well as at the affiliate satellites, have trained the staff in the etiology of eating disorders, assessment, motivation for treatment, and use of evidence-based treatments, thereby promoting the effective intensive treatment of adolescents across sites. Guided by our values, this training is developmentally appropriate, health-focused, family-centered, and community-based and emphasizes the application of RCT in all work, including collaboration among professionals. For example, like patients and family members, clinicians are trained to understand eating disorders as diseases of disconnection. They are encouraged to name the points of tension and disconnections that occur among patients, family members, and staff, and are specifically asked to name these experiences during individual staff/case review meetings in their own agencies and at regularly scheduled (three times per year) joint staff inservice/case review meetings offered for staff from all three facilities. This approach helps standardize treatment approaches and promotes coordinated, continuous care. It also helps to reduce shame and blame, reveals the disconnecting work of the eating disorder, effectively resolves conflict, fosters shared understanding, and strengthens staff relationships within and among the agencies. This approach keeps staff honest because it requires them to practice the skills they teach patients and families related to negotiating differences and repairing disconnections. It also reminds them that personal and professional support systems experience parallel points of tension and disconnection created by an eating disorder.

Another structural feature of the WNYCCCED that facilitates access to and delivery of intensive adolescent treatment programming is its emphasis on case management services, community education liaison work, and transitional services such as life coaching. These services play an especially important role because the WNYCCCED serves a large geographic area (from the northeast to the southwest corner is a 7-hour drive) with many small rural towns that do not have adequate treatment resources. WNYCCCED case managers are strategically located at the core and outlying affiliate sites of the center (Binghamton, Buffalo, Syracuse, and Watertown) to provide outreach/education, promote timely referral, and engage and keep patients and families in treatment. Harmony Place specifically provides case management for up to 90 days postdischarge through daily, then weekly, calls to parents and patients at home to prevent relapse and facilitate return to community living.

A Maudsley-trained psychologist serving as the WNYCCCED Community Education Liaison provides and/or coordinates education for professionals, family members, and other laypersons; many offerings emphasize family-based treatment for adolescents and adults, with "family" extended to anyone whom patients consider important in their lives and recovery. The liaison also oversees the publication and distribution of a newsletter for laypersons and professionals and has developed the Parent–Partner Program (*www.edsurvivalguide.com/parentpartner.htm*) that is offered through the year at various locations in the region. In addition, a WNYCCCED life coach who is a vocational counselor, certified life coach, and recovered individual, provides group and individual life coaching to older adolescents and adults to help them create lives of their own making without illness and facilitate their return to community living. All these elements were designed to decrease the uncertainty and anxiety associated with patient and family movement along the path of recovery and to ensure coordinated, comprehensive, and continuous care for adolescents and their families. Before providing an example of how the Rochester-based core and affiliate sites interact in providing treatment and promoting connections among patients, families, and professional staff, we outline the essential features of the intensive programs at these sites.

WNYCCCED Intensive Treatment Programs at Core and Affiliate Sites Based in Rochester, New York

The essential features of the programming at Golisano Children's Hospital, Harmony Place at St. Joseph's Villa, and The Healing Connection, LLC are described in following paragraphs. Criteria were developed for each level of care in the WNYCCCED (see Table 11.2 for an example of the PHP level of care criteria). These criteria were informed by the American Psychiatric Association Practice Guidelines for the treatment of eating disorders (American Psychiatric Association, 2006), InterQual Criteria (InterQual, 2002), the National Institute for Clinical Excellence Guidelines (NICE, 2004), and the Society for Adolescent Medicine position paper regarding eating disorders in adolescents (Golden et al., 2003), and after dialogue with various insurers for several years about medical neces-

TABLE 11.2. WNYCCCED Level of Care Criteria: Eating Disorders Partial Hospitalization Program

Inclusion criteria	Exclusion criteria	Discharge criteria
• Age ≥ 12 and has an eating disorder according to DSM-IV. • Body weight ≤ 80% of average weight for height. In some cases, a patient at 75–79% may enter PHP (e.g., strongly motivated for change, good family/social support, good medical follow-up, not losing weight rapidly, not medically compromised). • Motivated and able to participate in an intensive treatment program with mutually agreed-upon goals for symptom interruption, including weight gain and elimination of binge eating and purging. • Demonstrates an ability to relate in a group setting. • Unable to eat one balanced meal per day. • Bingeing and purging more than twice a day and/or is abusing substances (e.g., diuretics, laxatives, or ipecac) to purge. • Metabolically stable. • Not rapidly losing weight. • No an immediate psychiatric risk (e.g., acute suicide risk). • Not severely abusing drugs or alcohol to the degree that would interfere with normalization of eating and weight. • Has at least a few supports in the community. • Has a stable living situation or one in which cohabitants will support the person's therapeutic work or are willing to engage in treatment with the patient. • Has adequate medical attention to monitor physical status.	• Requires increased structure (> 7 hours programming per day) to gain weight and/ or interrupt frequent bingeing and purging, compulsive exercise, and preoccupation with ego-syntonic eating disorder thoughts that occupy a major portion or most of the day. • Body weight is (generally) ≤ 75%. • Medical instability (e.g., rapidly falling weight, compromised cardiac status, and metabolic instability). • An existing medical condition that will worsen or a new medical complication that will occur if the binge–purge cycle is not quickly interrupted (e.g., uncontrolled diabetes mellitus). • Severe concurrent substance abuse and comorbid psychiatric illness requiring increased level of care to maintain safety. • Few or no supports in community to encourage therapeutic work. • Poor motivation to recover.	• Maintenance of ≥ 90% average body weight for height for adults. The patient should have maintained this weight for at least 1 week. Maintenance of ≥ 95% average body weight for height (preferably 100%) in adolescents. The patient should have maintained this for at least 1 week. • Cessation of binge–purge episodes, including vomiting, use of laxatives, diuretics, and ipecac, for ≥ 2 weeks. • Able to complete three balanced meals per day and indicated snacks. • Patient (and parents of adolescent patients) has developed a clear and realistic after-care/relapse prevention plan that outlines progress thus far and future needs/ goals, and provides direction for how to respond quickly to potential lapses and avoid relapse. The after care plan has been communicated to the after-care therapist in the community. • Community supports and resources to promote continued recovery work have been identified and are in place. • Patient has a stable living situation that promotes his or her therapeutic work and recovery and/or a change in living situation is in progress and will occur in the imminent future during after care (e.g., on wait list for supervised apartment living). • Patient is psychiatrically stable, is not at acute psychiatric risk to harm self or others, and has stabilized other comorbid illnesses. • Patient is abstinent from alcohol and drugs. • Patient is medically stable.

sity criteria and practice guidelines. Programming and protocols developed within each level of care are also informed by the aforementioned criteria and guidelines.

Golisano Children's Hospital Inpatient Eating Disorders Programming

The Child and Adolescent Eating Disorders Program (CAEDP) at Golisano Children's Hospital (GCH) offers inpatient and outpatient treatment for adolescents and their families. The adolescent medicine inpatient unit provides treatment of eating disorders for patients ≤ 21 years old from across New York State and upstate Pennsylvania and is one of four pediatric units of GCH, a 121-bed, quaternary, full-service, not-for-profit pediatric hospital and pediatric referral center for the entire Finger Lakes Region in New York state. The on-site presence of many GCH specialized services (e.g., highly specialized cardiac surgery and cardiology; pulmonary services), along with the GCH regional Pediatric Intensive Care Unit, ensures that patients with eating disorders who have medical or surgical complications receive cutting-edge care.

The CAEDP multidisciplinary staff includes six full-time attending adolescent medicine physician faculty members, a part-time consulting psychiatrist, two nurse practitioners, two part-time dietitians, and two part-time social workers (one acts as a case manager and runs the weekly parenting group, and the other runs a weekly support group for patients). The inpatient team also includes nurses, a part-time music therapist, and child life worker, and the psychiatric-liaison psychiatrist and psychiatric nurse practitioner conduct rounds and meet with patients and families several times per week. The director of the program has more than 30 years of experience in working with adolescents with eating disorders and their families, and a majority of the staff members have worked with patients and families for more than a decade. The WNYCCCED case manager works with the social worker to facilitate disposition planning. In addition, advanced-level, professional, interdisciplinary adolescent health trainees (physicians, nurses, dietitians, psychologists, and social workers) see patients under direct supervision of the faculty.

Inpatients receive care according to a highly detailed, yet individualized, 17-day inpatient treatment protocol. Protocol goals include symptom interruption, medical stabilization, and nutritional rehabilitation. Patients receive individual therapy, mealtime coaching and monitoring, and group therapy, including postmeal processing daily, and participate in psychoeducation and cognitive-behavioral skill-building groups several times per week, as well as yoga and stress reduction–based mindfulness training, music therapy, pet therapy, and constructive leisure time. During the school year an in-hospital tutor assures that academic productivity is maintained. Parents participate in a weekly parenting group grounded in Maudsley methods, in which they devise methods to manage problems that may arise following discharge to home; individualized family therapy is also provided.

Inpatient treatment is multimodal and grounded in the biopsychosocial approach that treats the whole person in the context of her or his developmental stage and environment. By the time the patient is discharged, she or he has either demonstrated the ability to—with the help of a parent(s)—continue to eat adequately to maintain physical health recovery or is stepped down to the next level of care. Discharge planning includes determining (1) the roles of parents and the patient in ensuring adequate caloric intake, (2) caloric needs based on weight gain trends and presumed caloric expenditures during planned time with family outside of the hospital, (3) the level of exercise that is allowed, including playing sports, (4) reentry into peer-group and school activities, (5) weight gain expectations and medical follow-up, and (6) mental health outpatient treatment. Following medical stabilization, some patients require transfer to a psychiatric facility where they can be committed for treatment; the only specialized psychiatric inpatient program in New York State with the capacity to accommodate these young people is part of the New York City/Metro CCCED. Other patients who have completed the protocol, but are still not ready to go home, are referred to either the adolescent residential treatment facility (Harmony Place) or to the PHP (The Healing Connection) in the WNYCCCED, as detailed in the following paragraphs.

Harmony Place at St. Joseph's Villa

Harmony Place, the first and only adolescent eating disorders residential treatment program in New York State, is an eight-bed NYSOMH-licensed program located at St. Joseph's Villa, a nationally accredited agency with a rich 70-year history of helping young people overcome emotional and behavioral health issues. Harmony House is a strong family-based residential treatment program serving adolescents ages 12 to 19. It includes a weekly family day on Saturdays when patients and families in the program participate in a multifamily therapy group, parenting group, lunch, and a snack. Parents participate in lunch preparation and receive coaching and education regarding meal preparation. They also receive assistance and coaching from staff members as needed during lunchtimes while patients and families eat together. The aim of Saturday's groups and the overall programming at Harmony Place is to assist the patient in disconnecting from the illness, strengthen connections between patient and family, and empower parents to provide structure and support to their teens for lasting recovery.

Programming at Harmony Place includes 24/7 supervision, more than 20 hours of group therapy per week (e.g., psychoeducation for eating disorders and substance abuse, skills training, art therapy, and relaxation and mindfulness), therapeutic meals and snacks, individual therapy, family therapy, nutritional assessment/counseling and education, recreational therapy, yoga instruction, 2 hours per day of academic tutoring, psychopharmacological evaluation and medication monitoring, daily medical monitoring by nursing staff, and coordination of medical and dental care in collaboration with the teen's pediatrician. Harmony Place is staffed by a multidisciplinary team of nurses, psychiatrists, psychologists, master's-level therapists, dietitians and cooks, all with expertise in addressing the special needs of adolescents with eating disorders and their families. One of the most distinctive features of Harmony Place is its outreach and case management after discharge. The program director or designated case manager continues to call the family daily, then weekly as needed, for 90 days postdischarge to facilitate reentry into community living and assist with relapse prevention. This ongoing commitment to patients and families after discharge has promoted continuity of care and prevented or lessened the impact of the high anxiety that often accompanies discharge from residential treatment back to everyday life.

The Healing Connection, LLC

The Healing Connection is a free-standing NYSOMH-licensed eating disorders PHP serving individuals with eating disorders ≥ 12 years old and their families. RCT undergirds the programming and is the platform from which all evidence-based treatment is delivered. Programming reduces or eliminates symptoms by increasing the understanding of the patient and family regarding the connections between the patient's relationships with the illness, with self, and with others and helping patients develop and practice alternative coping and self-care strategies. Thus, programming aims to have the patient disconnect from the disorder and reconnect with her or his genuine feelings, thoughts, and needs and with significant others who will help the patient attain full recovery after discharge.

Because the program is based on the assumption that full recovery happens within the context of connections, the Healing Connection is primarily a group therapy–based program operating 7 hours/day Monday through Friday. Group therapies include psychoeducation, cognitive-behavioral, body image, skills training, relaxation/mindfulness, relational, art/movement/dance therapy, and the availability of substance abuse psychoeducation and skills training groups. Patients also participate in yoga instruction, mindfulness meditation, and receive 2 hours of academic tutoring in the morning before the start of the program during the school year. In addition, patients receive individual therapy, nutritional assessment/counseling/ education, meal planning, structured supervised mealtimes (lunch, dinner, and afternoon snack, which are prepared by an on-site chef), psychopharmacological evaluation and medication monitoring, and case management. Adolescents and family members participate in weekly family therapy and in a multifamily therapy group led by the clinical director and program therapists. Parents attend a weekly parenting group led by the clinical coordinator and the dietitian. A Maudsley family-based treatment approach informs all family and parent treatment interventions. There is also access to recovered peers and family members who present or participate in various program groups. The Healing Connection is staffed by a multidisciplinary team of doctorally and master's prepared experienced therapists, psychiatrists, a registered dietitian, a mealtime psychiatric technician, yoga instructor, recovered mindfulness meditation coach, chef, and office manager. Certified teachers provide tutoring, and the WNYCCCED case manager provides case management for patients and families. The clinical director and clinical coordinator have more than 25 years of experience in treating individuals with eating disorders and their families, and several other program staff members have worked at least a decade with patients with eating disorders and their families. The program includes an advisory board composed of professionals, as well as individuals in recovery and family members, all of whom have received PHP services in the past.

Intensive Outpatient Programming

Intensive Outpatient Programming (IOP) commonly includes programming 2–3 days per week for several hours per day and can be used to obviate full PHP care or as a more gradual step down from PHP to outpatient care. It is especially helpful for adolescents who need very gradual changes to outpatient care, have a limited number of community supports, and/or have a history/increased risk of relapse after discharge. In New York State there is no Office of Mental Health regulation for eating disorder intensive outpatient programs. Therefore, there is no way to obtain a license for this kind of program, and insurers are less apt to reimburse unlicensed programs. These issues have contributed to the fact that there are very few eating disorder IOPs in the state. When IOP proposals from NYSCCCED leadership have been submitted to insurers, their response has been that they would rather be creative in their use of PHP days to gradually step patients down to outpatient care. They cite the importance of continuity as the reason, inasmuch as their staff members already know the patient and the family. They believe that the fewest transitions from PHP to outpatient care is best. They may also be skeptical about paying for an additional unlicensed level of care. Therefore, within the WNYCCCED the Healing Connection has the capability to step patients down from 5-day/week programming to 2–3 days per week programming (e.g., between 4 and 7 hours per day). An example of this approach is the transition of adolescents from full PHP to fewer days per week, including return to school in the morning, and then to programming for 4 hours in the afternoon. This scenario provides the patient an ability to review his or her responses to the transition back to school and community, while staff and peers continue to provide support and emphasize relapse prevention skills. It also allows staff members to be in contact with school personnel to get their assessment of the transition in a contemporaneous way and, in response, to fine-tune interventions with the student. This alternative approach to intensive outpatient programming works well for adolescents insured by companies willing to reimburse for step-down days. Unfortunately, it cannot be fully applied to patients on Medicaid because state regulation requires them to be in a program at least 4 hours per day for at least 4 days per week.

The WNYCCCED Model of Care: A Clinical Exemplar

We now demonstrate how the Rochester-based core and affiliate sites of the WNYC-CCED effectively promote comprehensive, integrated, coordinated, and continuous care for adolescent patients and families through discussion of the following clinical case. The case involves the care of a 13-year-old female patient, Debbie, and her family—including her parents, Mr. and Mrs. Smith, and her sister Pam (age 15)—in total representing a composite of the issues requiring services from two or three of the Rochester-based WNYCCCED programs. In this case, Debbie made use of all three programs, inpatient, PHP and residential treatment. This case reveals the junctures during treatment at which the eating disorder does all it can to create disconnection within the patient and among the patient, parents, and treatment program staff members. It emphasizes the need for connection and continuity of care among personal and professional carers to help the adolescent move forward in recovery.

Debbie was stepped down to the Healing Connection by the inpatient staff at Golisano Children's Hospital, following inpatient treatment using the 17-day protocol, with the hope that she would continue to normalize her eating, stabilize her weight and other eating disorder–related symptoms, and that her parents would gain more education and confidence related to refeeding their daughter. She was 4 feet 9 inches, was not making expected gains, and had lost 10 pounds over the past year. She weighed 68 pounds before her inpatient stay and had gained 7 pounds by the day of discharge. The patient's mother suspected that she had purged at least a couple times in the 3 months prior to admission, but the patient denied this and there was no evidence of purging during her hospital stay.

During the PHP intake evaluation Debbie stated that she probably had eating disorder thoughts since she was 11 years old. She began restricting food in the sixth grade, but the severity of this was not recognized until the start of seventh grade. Her mother stated that she took the patient to her pediatrician, but he was not quick to diagnose an eating disorder. Instead, based on the patient's somatic complaints and her stated difficulty in eating dairy products, he spent time ruling out various gastrointestinal diagnoses. In addition, Debbie said she was a vegetarian, citing various philosophical reasons underlying this decision, and she maintained that her vegetarianism had preceded the eating disorder.

Debbie was unable to identify any circumstances that triggered her restrictive eating, increased compulsive exercise, and progressive weight loss over the prior year. However, during the intake, ongoing marital difficulties for several years before her parents' divorce—when she was 9 years old—were revealed. Her father had little contact with Debbie and remarried when she was 10 years old, at about the time she started middle school; she did not have any close friends and spent most of her time at home, without much connection with her sister. She maintained that she did not need anyone and could get along on her own "just fine." She reported a strained relationship with her mother and wanted to go to live with her father because she perceived her mother to "work, come home, spend time with a new male friend, then go to bed." When Debbie was 12 years old, her mother's partner, with whom Debbie had developed a very close connection, left her mother. The eating disorder seemed to follow a series of disconnections, including parental divorce, her father distancing himself from his children, her mother's increased isolation and probable depression after the divorce, the patient's isolated existence since her entry to middle school, and the new partner's breakup with her mother and departure from the home.

During individual parent sessions, Debbie's mother acknowledged becoming more distant and depressed since the divorce and, especially, since her most recent partner left her. She was still angry with Debbie's father about his remarriage so soon after their divorce and did not encourage either of her daughters to have a relationship with him, believing that he would only further disappoint them. According to her mother, Debbie's new stepmother did not seem interested in Debbie until recently, when she was hospitalized for an eating disorder. The stepmother became effusively supportive of Debbie and encouraged her to come to live with her and her father. Debbie saw such a move as the answer to her difficulties, which left her mother feeling even more frustrated, especially because she acknowledged her previous problems in connecting with Debbie and was seeking to correct them through her own therapy. Her mother's strengths included an ability to work with staff members, implement plans regarding what needed to be done in nutritional rehabilitation at home, and consistently manage contingency plans. This effectiveness angered Debbie and seemed to contribute to her wanting to live with her father. By the second week of treatment in the PHP, her mother acquiesced allowing the patient to live with her father and stepmother so that Debbie could experience what would occur in this living situation, which Debbie seemed to idealize. Debbie's mother hoped this approach would preclude the drive to live with her father being a distraction for Debbie during treatment. She planned on seeing her daughter during scheduled evenings during the week and alternate time on the weekends.

During individual sessions with Debbie's father, he noted that her mother was not nurturing and that he and her stepmother could probably provide a better environment for Debbie. He was warm with his daughter in sessions, but was unable to consistently implement nutritional rehabilitation plans outside the program on weekends and weekday evenings. He came to two meetings reporting that he was unclear about why his daughter needed to eat "so much" and disagreed with staff regarding Debbie's needing to complete meals. He was not a consistent contingency manager.

In joint parental meetings the primary therapist emphasized the importance of the parents being united, despite their areas of disagreement related to their daughter. The father reported difficulty in attending the meetings because of his schedule. In these meetings the parents discussed their concerns about Debbie and agreed to follow the treatment plan guidelines they had helped to design in a meeting. They were civil to one another in the joint sessions, but the patient reportedly experienced a high degree of tension when with them outside the program. During week 3 of the program, she went to live with her father, but he was still struggling with implementing the refeeding treatment plan. However, she remained strong in her desire to continue to live with him. Her mother was concerned about his not following the treatment plan they had jointly designed with the team staff members. The primary therapist provided support and repeated information to Debbie's father regarding the rationale for prescribed meals and his taking control of the refeeding at the present time, and repeatedly encouraged the father to attend the parenting group with the other parents, but he was unable to do so because of his schedule. Debbie's mother attended these meetings regularly. Her father attended a few multifamily therapy groups, and her mother attended all of them during the PHP stay.

During the program the patient remained quiet in groups. She denied any problems other than needing to gain weight—"according to the team." When she finally did speak in the relational group, she shared information about all the disconnections she had experienced prior to the eating disorder in an editorial fashion, with her affect split off from the content of her discussion. When other patients and the group leader discussed how moving her disclosure was and how it evoked great sadness for them, she could not understand why they felt this way. She said she did not need relationships, and that isolation was better than relying on others who may not come through for you. Debbie could see how someone might feel bad because of the kinds of losses she had described, but she saw no connection between these events and her AN symptoms and her level of isolation. She acknowledged that the disorder helped "numb her" to a certain extent, but did not see this as related to feelings she might have in regard to the aforementioned disconnections because she was "used to being alone." The group leader asked her if her AN took advantage of this feeling and protected her from any possibility of connection with others that might challenge this experience. The leader validated how scary this might be, given the number of times that she cited the adults in her life had failed her—even if they did so unintentionally. Debbie did not have an answer, but she listened when the leader noted this and others agreed with the hypothesis. Other patients gave examples of similar situations in their own lives. Although she listened, she did not seem fully present emotionally, possibly because of her compromised nutritional status.

Debbie was not completing meals in the program, despite much support from therapists and group members. After 4 weeks of PHP (20 days) and attempts to engage the parents and patient community to assist her with meal completion and emotional work, the team discussed having her return for inpatient treatment because she was not fully completing meals, had lost all the weight that she had gained, and seemed as though she could not make use of group work at her low weight. She also complained about having to eat dairy foods—despite previously normal lactose tolerance—which her mother interpreted as being eating disorder related. Staff members also suspected that she may have been vomiting or exercising and was not completing her weekend meals at home, all of which she denied. When the staff members shared their concerns, she did not seem upset about returning to the inpatient unit, but appeared to be comforted by this idea because she had received a great deal of attention on the unit, as she had been the only patient with an eating disorder for much of her inpatient treatment.

This attitude led the treatment team to deliberately frame the stay as a short *medical* stay with the sole purpose of refeeding her via a nasogastric (NG) tube because of concerns for her physical and mental health. Never used as a punishment or a threat, the NG tube was being used to ensure adequate intake and to determine scientifically exactly how many calories she needed to gain weight–an *in vivo* experiment—inasmuch as she and her father did not agree with the caloric level prescribed in program. NG tube feeding would be the only way to determine her caloric needs *and* make sure that she was gaining weight; both of these factors would be important for continued recovery. The primary therapist discussed the plan with the medical director of the inpatient unit, the nurse practitioner who managed Debbie as an outpatient at Golisano Children's Hospital, and the insurer.

The therapist and nurse practitioner also shared with the insurer their joint concerns about Debbie's parents' difficulty in providing a united front and managing the patient's nutritional rehabilitation at home because of unresolved conflict between the parents and the splitting (i.e., working to keep the parents divided and promoting all or nothing thinking) that the eating disorder created. Although each parent had strengths in working with Debbie, they had difficulty bringing these to bear on the central issue of the refeeding process. Because of these concerns, the possible need to step down to Harmony Place for residential treatment following inpatient treatment, rather than back to the Healing Connection for PHP, was openly discussed. The providers jointly underscored the importance of this alternative step-down because each program in the WNYCCCED sees the staff members of other programs as an extended treatment team that participates in ensuring continuity of care, regardless of where the patient and family are currently treated. This unified approach is helpful in discussion with insurers because it shows consensual agreement across facilities about management of the case and further promotes continuity and coordination of care.

Inpatient and PHP staff members believed that step-down to residential treatment at Harmony Place would give the parents time to practice and increase confidence in refeeding and other parenting skills for recovery. This was facilitated by Debbie's living in a neutral, therapeutic environment in which she would not be at the center of parental conflict, could avoid loyalty struggles in choosing one parent over the other, and could safely experience the tension and strongly expressed anger and disappointment, in healthier ways. The primary therapist contacted Harmony Place regarding the step-down from inpatient to residential treatment, which had been previously mentioned by the PHP. The Harmony Place program director contacted the parents to provide program information and answer any questions raised in the event that the step-down occurred.

The final decision to step down to residential treatment was made by the parents, the staff members of all three treatment programs, and the insurer, who remained connected and consistent in their messages, to minimize the possibility of the eating disorder's creating points of tension, splitting of the team members from one another, and furthering disconnection. Through discussion it became clear that the inpatient and PHP teams had a different view of Debbie's presentation. During her first hospital stay, she was compliant, passive, smiling, and engaging with staff members. She successfully completed the 17-day protocol without needing an NG tube. Her stated vegetarianism and lactose intolerance had not been directly challenged, and she was able to avoid ordering a great deal of dairy menu items. At the PHP her diet restrictions were directly challenged and identified as related to the eating disorder, so her prescribed menus included dairy products and occasional poultry and fish choices, along with other sources of protein.

The inpatient staff members were supportive and utilized a strength-based approach with the parents. Although their impression of the patient's mother was that she was somewhat controlling, angry, intrusive, and more concerned with outcome than with the interactions with her daughter, Debbie's father was deemed more warm and nurturing, and the staff members did not have as much contact with her mother. Debbie perceived that the inpatient staff supported her living with her father, which frustrated her mother and caused her to feel estranged, misunderstood, and disconnected from members of the staff.

The PHP staff members perceived the patient as being very quiet, but quite powerful and reticent to follow treatment recommendations. They also had opportunity to observe her responses in the context of relationships with peers and adults in group-based program work. The staff members saw her as a "steel magnolia." Appearing child-like, small, and fragile, she demonstrated willfulness and perseverance in remaining connected to her eating disorder. The patients in the PHP saw only her fragility and worried that authentic feedback might hurt her. The entire patient group doted on her (she was the youngest), and they had some difficulty in voicing their frustration with her continued inability to complete her meals, but they tolerated her meal noncompletion and at times protected her from disapproving comments. They were relieved that the treatment team and parents decided to have her admitted for inpatient treatment.

The PHP staff perceived Debbie's mother to be in alignment with the treatment plan. She was the parent who consistently followed treatment recommendations related to meal completion. She was highly concerned regarding the consistency and outcomes of the interventions with the patient and admitted she was very skeptical about the patient's complaints and concerns. She worried that most, if not all of them, came from the eating disorder. Therefore, she had difficulty in differentiating normal development-based needs/feelings from those that might be more eating disordered. This difficulty probably added to Debbie's frustration in not being believed by her mother. The staff members also noted that the patient's anger and disappointment with her mother probably prevented her from listening to, or connecting with, her. Members of the PHP staff believed that Debbie's strong desire to live with her father was partially fueled by her mother's consistent efforts to enforce meal completion and her anger with her mother related to the divorce.

Her father was perceived as being warmer, more accepting of the patient's expressed needs and concerns, and less preoccupied with outcome. However, he demonstrated difficulty in following through with treatment plans. His parenting style was more permissive; although this was positive and validating for Debbie, at times it enabled the illness. His inconsistency in ensuring meal completion continued, despite validation and support regarding its importance by staff members and families in the multifamily therapy group.

To promote continuity of care and minimize splitting of the team members from one another and disconnection among the extended treatment team as Debbie and her family moved across levels of care, a joint staff meeting was planned to discuss different viewpoints, prior to her transfer to the inpatient unit. The clinical director, one of this chapter's authors (M. T.), facilitated an honest discussion among staff members from the inpatient unit and the PHP who knew Debbie, as well as the coordinator from Harmony Place. As staff members identified potential points of tension/disconnection created by the eating disorder, these points were named and written on a flip chart. The staff then problem solved various approaches for negotiating their different perceptions, experiences, and approaches related to the patient and family. Identifying the differences enriched the understanding of Debbie and her family and strengthened joint efforts in caring for all members of the family. For example, in sharing perceptions about her parents, the staff

members of all three treatment programs developed a fuller and more integrated understanding of their relationships and interactions with Debbie. This helped them to avoid
a dichotomous view of the parents and to improve their connections with each of them.
From this perspective, the staff members could help the parents understand how and why
Debbie might experience certain feelings and needs—because of the impact of the eating
disorder, rather than because of parental deficiencies. Each staff member received a list of
the points of tension/disconnections and problem solutions for future use.

In joint meetings, as described earlier, there are some instances when staff from
the three programs agree to disagree, but these situations relate more to program structure (e.g., the PHP uses a point system to calculate prescribed meals, and the inpatient
unit uses the exchange system), rather than patient management. We orient patients and
families about these differences and explain how either approach is helpful. In doing so,
we provide parents an opportunity to see that differences can exist within strong connections, and we model an ability to effectively deal with differences in relationships
with others. Treatment team efforts to increase patient and parental ability to tolerate
change and differences helps them feel more confident about making transitions in life
that require negotiation of different feelings, thoughts, needs, and goals.

On the few occasions that treatment team members within and/or across programs
have disagreed about a proposed patient or family intervention during a joint meeting,
even after discussion of their different ideas and rationales, the team decided to try one
intervention at a time. The team decided to go with plan A and then moved to plan B if
the first plan did not produce the desired outcome. Treatment team members have also
been transparent about these differences with parents and share with them how joint
problem solving based on present data is the best we can do as providers and parents.
They show how a problem solution can change with additional data. This approach helps
both staff members and parents to remember that what is important in treatment and
parenting is being "good enough" rather than perfect and all knowing. Parents may then
be able to model this lesson for their perfectionistic daughter or son.

Recommendations for the Future and Conclusion

The WNYCCCED provides a model for delivery of comprehensive, coordinated and
intensive treatment of eating disorders for adolescents and their families. Although the
particular conditions that contributed to the development of the WNYCCCED may not
exist in other areas, such as the long-term relationships among providers in a large geographic region, there are opportunities to create these conditions wherever there is a
small group of committed individuals. For eating disorder specialists, patients, and families seeking to replicate the work of the WNYCCCED, we suggest the action strategies
listed in Table 11.3. We recognize the competitive, fiscally driven nature of service delivery, but the increasing economic constraints in health care, combined with the direct and
indirect medical, psychological, emotional, social, and financial costs associated with
not adequately treating eating disorders in a coordinated, comprehensive, and continuous way, underscore the importance of collaboration in providing intensive treatment to
adolescents with eating disorders and their families.

Strong, trusting, mutual connections between patients, families, and providers
increase the likelihood of successful treatment and full recovery for individuals with eat-

TABLE 11.3. Strategies to Develop a Comprehensive Care Center for Eating Disorders

1. Identify and partner with eating disorder treatment providers, individuals in recovery, family members, and leadership from various organizations who share a common concern for prevention, treatment, and research related to eating disorders. Include community-based partners who can influence the various parts of the ecology that promote body image dissatisfaction and other risks related to development of eating disorders, including: schools, primary care providers, dentists, insurers, the Office of Mental Health, local and state governments, nonprofit consumer groups (e.g., Mental Health Association, foundations), and the business community (e.g., grocers committed to healthy eating and living).

2. Meet with NYSCCCED leadership to learn of the process involved in developing CCCEDs.

3. Meet with possible stakeholders individually and then hold a stakeholders' meeting to explore the needs and wishes of stakeholders in relation to the CCCED concept. Solicit support from stakeholders and explore restraining and driving forces for the CCCED concept.

4. Develop a core workgroup of individuals who can meet regularly, strategize, and provide feedback and direction to others.

5. Discuss how to get the center legislatively mandated and work with sympathetic key state legislators and the National Eating Disorders Association in drafting Center legislation.

6. Simultaneously consider identifying key treatment providers/programs interested in pursuing CCCED designation and speak with them about their programming or willingness to develop eating disorder programming for patients and families.

7. Evaluate whether these individuals/programs provide evidence-based treatment, have credentialed staff, conduct quality improvement activities, produce good outcomes, and partner with patients and families in relation to programming. Discuss financial ability/constraints to develop or extend programming without CCCED state monies for start-up. Brainstorm possibilities for alternative funding before legislation is passed (e.g., discussions with area insurers, foundations, county mental health directors, legislators, and businesses).

8. Identify at least one provider within each level of care to create a continuum of care for adult and adolescent patients and their families. If you successfully get legislation to mandate CCCEDs, then a request for applications will likely be issued and these providers would be prepared to apply.

9. Share responsibility with workgroup members and other professionals with expertise to consult and train the identified practitioners/program staff in provision of evidence-based treatment for eating disorders. Involve recovering individuals and families in this consultation and training.

10. Collaborate with the workgroup and aforementioned providers in advocating for the CCCED concept with state legislators and the National Eating Disorders Association (*http:// nationaleatingdisorders.org*). Have all involved also network with their colleagues, family, and friends to advocate for legislation of CCCEDs.

11. If you cannot get adequate support for legislation of state-designated CCCEDs, then get local support for centers of excellence. Discuss this option with stakeholders and solicit support. For example, meet with area insurers about their willingness to support the center of excellence concept and issue a request for applications. This can be a step toward obtaining legislated CCCEDs or an alternative to them if several centers of excellence also agree to collaborate in a similar fashion in your region.

ing disorders. Although we cannot mandate government officials, insurers, and school personnel to join our collaborative efforts, developing mutual relational partnerships with key stakeholders, including adolescent patients and their families, holds promise in increasing effectiveness and reducing the costs associated with eating disorders. The intensity of interventions and relationships required for successful treatment and ongoing recovery for adolescents with eating disorders does not start and stop with the patients, families, and providers involved in intensive treatment programming. The hard work and connections required to prevent eating disorders or help adolescents break free from them must extend farther out into an ecology that promotes body image dissatisfaction and the disconnections that help breed these disorders.

References

Abramowitz, R., Petersen, A., & Schulenberg, J. (1984). Changes in self-esteem during early adolescence. In D. Offer, E. Ostrov, & K. Howard (Eds.), *Patterns of adolescent self-image* (pp. 19–28). San Francisco: Jossey-Bass.

American Psychiatric Association. (2006). *Practice guidelines for the treatment of patients with eating disorders* (3rd ed.). Washington, DC: Author.

Chavez, M., & Insel, T. R. (2007). Eating disorders: National Institute of Mental Health's Perspective. *American Psychologist, 62*(3), 159–166.

Colton, A., & Pistrang, N. (2004). Adolescents' experiences of inpatient treatment for anorexia nervosa. *European Eating Disorders Review, 12,* 307–316.

Fairburn, C. G. (2008). *Cognitive behavior therapy and eating disorders.* New York: Guilford Press.

Garfinkel, P. E., & Garner, D. M. (1982). *Anorexia nervosa: A multidimensional perspective.* New York: Brunner/Mazel.

Garner, D. M., & Garfinkel, P. E. (Eds.). (1997). *Handbook of treatment for eating disorders* (2nd ed.). New York: Guilford Press.

Genero, N. P., Miller, J. B., Surrey, J., & Baldwin, L. M. (1992). Measuring perceived mutuality in close relationships: Validation of the Mutual Psychological Development Questionnaire. *Journal of Family Psychology, 6,* 36–48.

Gilligan, C. (1982). *In a different voice.* Cambridge, MA: Harvard University Press.

Gilligan, C. (1991). Women's psychological development: Implications for psychotherapy. In C. Gilligan, A. G. Rogers, & D. L. Tolman (Eds.), *Women, girls and psychotherapy* (pp. 5–31. New York: Harrington Park Press.

Gilligan, C., Lyons, N., & Hanmer, T. (Eds.). (1990). *Making connections: The relational worlds of adolescent girls at Emma Willard School.* Cambridge, MA: Harvard University Press.

Golden, N. H., Katzman, D. K., Kreipe, R. E., Stevens, S. L., Sawyer, S. M., Rees, J., et. al. (2003). Eating disorders in adolescents: Position paper of the Society for Adolescent Medicine. *Journal of Adolescent Health, 33,* 496–503.

InterQual. (2002). *InterQual behavioral health criteria.* San Francisco: McKesson Health Solutions.

Jordan, J. (2010). *Relational–Cultural Therapy.* Washington, DC: American Psychological Association.

Kaye, W., Fudge, J. L., & Paulus, M. (2009). New insights into symptoms and neurocircuit function of anorexia nervosa. *Nature Reviews Neuroscience, 10,* 573–584.

Kreipe, R. E., & Dukarm, C. P. (1999). Eating disorders in adolescents and older children. *Pediatrics in Review, 20,* 410–421.

Lask, B. (2010, June). *Early onset eating disorders and their developmental consequences.* Paper presented at the International Conference on Eating Disorders, Salzburg, Austria.

Le Grange, D., & Lock, J. (2007). *Treating bulimia in adolescents: A family-based approach.* New York: Guilford Press.

Lock, J., Le Grange, D., Agras, W. S., & Dare, C. (2001). *Treatment manual for anorexia nervosa: A family-based approach.* New York: Guilford Press.

Miller, J. B., & Stiver, I. P. (1997). *The healing connection: How women form relationships in therapy and in life.* Boston: Beacon Press.

Miller, W. R., & Rollnick, S. (2002). *Motivational interviewing: Preparing people for change* (2nd ed.). New York: Guilford Press.

National Institute for Clinical Excellence. (2004). *Eating disorders: Core interventions in the treatment and management of anorexia nervosa, bulimia nervosa and related eating disorders: Clinical guideline 9.* London: Author.

Pollack, W. (1998). *Real boys*. New York: Random House.

Pope, H. G., Phillips, K. A., & Olivardia, R. (2000). *The Adonis complex*. New York: Free Press.

Prochaska, J. O., Norcross, J. C., & DiClemente, C. C. (1994). *Changing for good*. New York: William Morrow.

Resnick, M. D., Harris, L. J., & Blum, R. W. (1993). The impact of caring and connectedness on adolescent health and well-being, *Journal of Paediatric Child Health, 29*(Suppl. 1), S3–S9.

Seligman, M. E. P., Berkowitz, M. W., Catalano, R. F., Damon, W., Eccles, J. S., Gillham, J. E., et al. (2005). The positive perspective on youth development. In D. L. Evans et al. (Eds.), *Treating and preventing adolescent mental health disorders* (pp. 497–527). New York: Oxford University Press.

Smolak, L., & Murnen, S. K. (2001). Gender and eating problems. In R. Striegel-Moore & L. Smolak (Eds.), *Eating disorders* (pp. 91–110). Washington, DC: American Psychological Association.

Steiner-Adair, C. (1986). The body politic: Normal female adolescent development and the development of eating disorders. *Journal of the American Academy of Psychoanalysis, 14*, 95–114.

Steiner-Adair, C. (1991). New maps of development, new models of therapy: The psychology of women and the treatment of eating disorders. In C. L. Johnson (Ed.), *Psychodynamic treatment of anorexia nervosa and bulimia* (pp. 225–241). New York: Guilford Press.

Tantillo, M. (2004). The therapist's use of self-disclosure in a relational therapy approach for eating disorders. *Eating Disorders: Journal of Treatment and Prevention, 12*, 51–73.

Tantillo, M. (2006). A relational approach to eating disorders multifamily therapy group: Moving from difference and disconnection to mutual connection. *Families, Systems, and Health, 24*(1), 82–102.

Tantillo, M., & Kreipe, R. E. (2006). The impact of gender socialization on group treatment of eating disorders. *Group: The Journal of the Eastern Group Psychotherapy Society, 30*(4), 281–306.

Tantillo, M., & Sanftner, J. (2010a). Measuring perceived mutuality in women with eating disorders: The development of the Connection–Disconnection Scale. *Journal of Nursing Measurement, 18*(2), 100–119.

Tantillo, M., & Sanftner, J. L. (2010b). Mutuality and motivation: Connecting with patients and families for change in the treatment of eating disorders. In M. Maine, D. Bunnell, & B. McGilley (Eds.), *Treatment of eating disorders: Bridging the gap between research and practice* (pp. 319–334). London: Elsevier.

Taylor, M., Adams, H., & Kreipe, R. E. (2008). Recovery from anorexia nervosa: Patients' perspectives. *Journal of Adolescent Health, 42*, S9–S10.

Walsh, T., Bulik, C. M., Fairburn, C. G., Golden, N. H., Halmi, K. A., Herzog, D. B., et al. (2005). Defining eating disorders. In D. L. Evans, E. B. Foa, R. E. Gur, & H. Hardin (Eds.), *Treating and preventing adolescent mental health disorders* (pp. 255–332). New York: Oxford University Press.

OUTPATIENT TREATMENT PROGRAMS FOR ANOREXIA NERVOSA

CHAPTER 12

Family-Based Treatment for Anorexia Nervosa

Evolution, Evidence Base, and Treatment Approach

James Lock

Evolution of Family-Based Treatment

Interest in the role of the family in treatment of anorexia nervosa (AN) dates back to the earliest descriptions of the disorder by Charles Lasègue. He notes, "In view of the undoubted psychological aspects [of the disorder], it would be equally regrettable to ignore or misinterpret the patient's psychological surroundings"—by which he meant the patient's family (Lasègue, 1883). He adds, "None should be surprised to note that I always consider the morbid state of the hysterical patient side by side with the preoccupations of her relatives" (Lasègue, 1883). However, Lasègue took a generally negative view of the families of patients with AN, concerned that their psychopathology contributed to the child's disease. Sir William Gull held a similar view and suggested that families were likely to be unhelpful in treating their children: "The patients should be fed at regular intervals, and surrounded by persons who would have moral control over them; relatives and friends being generally the worst attendants" (Gull, 1874). An even harder line was suggested by Charcot, who flatly recommended that parents be excluded from involvement in the treatment of their children with AN: "It is necessary to separate both children and adults from their father and mother, whose influence, as experience teaches, is particularly pernicious" (Silverman, 1997). Together these views informed much of the treatment paradigm used in AN for much of the last century, whereby parents were excluded from treatment and professionals, generally in inpatient hospital settings, were in charge of treatment.

Exceptions to this negative view of the potential role of families in the treatment of AN began in the 1970s in the context of family therapy for psychiatric disorders more generally. Minuchin and colleagues agreed with Lasègue that families were important, but suggested that they should also be considered in the treatment of AN (Liebman, Minuchin, & Baker, 1974). Using the construct of the "psychosomatic family," structural family therapy for AN became a paradigmatic model for this type of intervention (Minuchin, Rosman, & Baker, 1978). The psychosomatic family was described as enmeshed, overprotective, rigid, and conflict avoidant. These four characteristics were seen as inhibiting the child's development and fostering the evolution and maintenance of psychosomatic symptoms—self-starvation in the case of AN. Although the psychosomatic theoretical construct is not proved, structural family therapy for AN was apparently useful. Minuchin and colleagues published their initial series of 53 cases of children and adolescents with AN using structural family therapy where good outcomes (no longer diagnosed as AN) were found in 80% (Minuchin et al., 1978). This seminal work inspired other family therapists using a range of family therapeutic constructs (e.g., systemic, strategic, narrative) to treat AN involving the family (Haley, 1973; Selvini Palazzoli & Viaro, 1988; White, 1987). Family therapists working with these models were strong proponents of their own theoretical notions about how family therapy might change the symptoms of AN through family work, but none conducted systematic research supporting their claims. As a result, family therapy for AN was seen as a clinically useful intervention by many, whereas others took the perspective that individual therapy aimed at supporting independence from parents and professionally driven weight restoration programs (usually in hospitals) were superior strategies (Bruch, 1973; Crisp, 1980).

Evidence Base for Family-Based Treatment

It was not until the first report of the effectiveness of family therapy for AN was published in 1987 that systematic evidence supported the view of family therapists. Russell and colleagues reported that adolescents with a short duration of AN (less than 3 years) responded better to family therapy than to individual supportive therapy in preventing weight relapse (Russell, Szmukler, Dare, & Eisler, 1987). In that study, 21 adolescents between the ages of 12 and 18 years who had been ill with AN for less than 3 years were hospitalized for about 16 weeks for initial weight restoration. Mean ideal body weight (IBW) at the point of hospitalization was about 65%. At the point of discharge (mean IBW 90%), patients were randomized to receive one year of family therapy or one year of supportive individual therapy. At the end of this treatment period, those patients who received family therapy were at significantly higher weights (family therapy = 93%; supportive therapy = 80%). Although the study sample size was small and therefore subject to distortions because of the outcomes of a few individuals in either treatment arm, this was nonetheless the first systematic study to find a treatment effect difference between two treatments for AN.

It is important to note that the study by Russell and colleagues also compared family therapy with supportive therapy in three other populations: adolescents between the ages of 12 and 18, with duration of AN greater than 3 years, adults with AN, and adults with bulimia nervosa (BN). In none of these other groups was there a suggestion that family therapy provided differential benefit. Indeed, for these other groups, individual treatment appeared to be better, though not statistically significantly so (Russell et al., 1987).

For reasons that are somewhat difficult to explain, the important findings of this seminal study by Russell and colleagues were not generally embraced. It part, this may have been a result of a general disinterest in AN research, as there was very little large-scale research attempted during the decade following publication of the study for this population. In addition, it may be that family therapy was considered too esoteric a treatment as compared with other eating disorder treatments that were being studied for BN, for example, cognitive-behavioral therapy (CBT), interpersonal therapy, and medications. However, perhaps the most compelling reason is that family therapy was seen as applicable to young adolescent patients with AN and the few researchers in the field were focused on adult AN. Several studies of adults with AN were published during the decade or so following Russell and colleagues' study, though none identified differential treatment benefits for the interventions examined (e.g., hospitalization, CBT, cognitive-analytic therapy [CAT], group therapy, combined individual and family therapy, antidepressants, antipsychotics, mood stabilizers) (Crisp et al., 1991; Hall & Crisp, 1987; Kaye et al., 2001; Kaye, Weltzin, Hsu, & Bulik, 1991; Malina et al., 2003; Pike, Walsh, Vitousek, Wilson, & Bauer, 2000; Treasure et al., 1995). It is noteworthy that with the exception of one study by Crisp et al., 1991, these studies were small scale, plagued by high attrition rates, and in the case of psychological treatments, generally not provided in a replicable and manualized format.

It was not until 12 years later that the final results of a new study examining family therapy for adolescents with short duration AN was published. This study by Robin and colleagues used a similar model of family therapy (behavioral family systems therapy [BFST]) (Robin, 2003) as that used by the Russell and colleagues study, though it was augmented by the inclusion of some cognitive therapy (Robin et al., 1999). In addition, the individual therapy used was considered to be a more specific treatment than the supportive treatment used in Russell and colleagues (1987). The individual therapy, called ego-oriented individual therapy (EOIT), targeted adolescent development specifically in the areas of self-efficacy, self-awareness, and autonomy. The study randomized 37 adolescents between 12 and 18 years of age to either BFST or EOIT for a period of 18 months. Results from this study suggested that family therapy was superior to individual therapy in terms of weight gain and menstrual return at the end of treatment and one year follow-up. There were no differences in outcome of eating-related cognitions or more general psychological or emotional functioning between the two treatments. In general, both treatments were helpful to many adolescents with AN, with most adolescents reaching normal body mass index (BMI) ranges of between 19 and 21 by the end of treatment. Furthermore, improvement in weight continued in both groups during the one-year follow-up period, suggesting no difference in relapse rates between the two groups after the end of treatment. The authors concluded that both treatments were helpful for adolescents with AN, though BFST was more efficient in promoting physical recovery. The modest scale of this study and small differences in treatment outcome between groups likely diminished the impact of the results of this study on considering family therapy for adolescent AN. Still, the study was a significant step forward as it almost doubled the number of subjects studied, as compared with the study of Russell and colleagues, and employed manualized interventions.

Meanwhile, there were other investigations undertaken in an attempt to better understand for whom family therapy would be most beneficial. A pilot study by Le Grange, Eisler, Dare, and Russell (1992) examined the possibility that families that were highly critical (a measure of expressed emotion) of their child with AN would do less well when family therapy was delivered to the family as a whole (conjoint family therapy). The idea informing this study was that highly critical families (defined as those making two or more critical comments during the Standardized Clinical Family Interview [SCFI]; Kinston & Loader, 1984) might limit the effectiveness of whole family therapy by allowing the parents to be critical of the adolescent in front of the family, whereas separated family therapy would potentially protect the child from these criticisms during family therapy, thereby increasing the likelihood of response. Thus, the study compared conjoint family therapy with family therapy delivered in a separated format (seeing the parents and the child separately). The study randomized 18 patients (16 females and 2 males) between the ages of 12 and 18 years who had had AN for less than 3 years to receive conjoint or separated family therapy. Patients were treated for 6 months, with an average number of 8 sessions of family therapy provided during this period. The mean IBW of patients starting the study was about 78% IBW. The mean IBW at the end of treatment (32 weeks) was about 94%. There were no differences in weight or other clinical measures of outcome between the two groups. A post hoc secondary analysis suggested that maternal critical comments were possibly related to outcome. Thus, although this study did not suggest overall differential benefit for separated family therapy for more critical families in the main outcomes of the study, it did provide additional case material supporting the model of family therapy used in the seminal study by Russell and colleagues for adolescents who had not been previously weight restored in the hospital.

Because limited data suggested benefit for separated family therapy for adolescents with AN, Eisler and colleagues (2007) conducted a larger-scale version of Le Grange and colleagues' pilot study. The design was similar, except that the study randomized 40 participants (39 females and 1 male). The outcomes were also similar, with patients beginning treatment at a mean IBW of about 74% and ending treatment with a mean IBW of 87%. There were also few significant differences in individual measures of change (weight change, eating psychopathology, general psychopathology) between the two treatments. Those that were found favored conjoint family therapy. However, when Morgan–Russell categorical outcomes were used (Morgan & Russell, 1988), those families with higher levels of criticism did better with separated family therapy, whereas there were no differential treatment effects for those with low levels of criticism. Thus, the results of this study tentatively suggest that for some outcomes, separated family therapy is superior to conjoint family therapy for adolescent AN in highly critical families. The study also added further systematic case data that suggested that outpatient family therapy was effective even without using baseline hospitalization to restore weight in promoting improvements in adolescents with short duration AN. Limitations of this study included the relatively small sample size and failure to use manualized interventions.

In 2001 a manual describing in detail the form of family therapy used in Russell and colleagues (1987), Le Grange and colleagues (1992), and Eisler and colleagues (2000) was published by Lock, Le Grange, Agras, and Dare (Dare & Eisler, 1997; Lock, Le Grange, Agras, & Dare, 2001). This manual systematized the approach, calling it family-based treatment (FBT), and described a case series utilizing the manual wherein 19 adolescents (18 females and 1 male) between the ages of 12 and 18 years received manualized FBT. Patients in this case series received 6 months of treatment (Lock & Le Grange, 2001) Their BMIs increased from a mean of about 17 to mean of about 19 during this period. Furthermore, their Eating Disorder Examination (EDE) scores improved on all subscales, and statistically significantly improved on the Restraint and Shape Concerns subscales. Dropout was low (3 patients = 15%), similar to that found in other studies using this form of family therapy that were published at the time. These data suggested that manualized FBT was feasible and acceptable and that outcomes were similar to those found in previous clinical trials using a nonmanualized version of this form of family therapy.

The first randomized clinical trial (RCT) to use manualized FBT was a study designed to determine the optimal therapeutic dose of family therapy for short duration adolescent AN (Lock, Agras, Bryson, & Kraemer, 2005). The study was designed to formally test manualized FBT. It was the first study using FBT outside the United Kingdom (BFST, though similar, differed from FBT in a number of ways, most importantly by including cognitive interventions). It utilized a sample large enough to provide confidence in the outcomes and included the EDE as the gold standard for eating-related psychopathology. The study was also a feasibility study, in preparation for a larger study using manualized FBT in comparison with another treatment for adolescent AN. The study randomized 86 participants (76 females and 9 males) to a longer-duration/higher-intensity dose of FBT (20 sessions over 1 year) or a shorter-duration/lower-intensity dose of FBT (10 sessions over 6 months). The therapists were master's- or doctoral-level psychologists or psychiatrists with expertise in adolescent AN and subsequently trained in manualized FBT through several workshops. Before beginning to treat randomized patients, the therapists treated three cases successfully under the supervision of an experienced FBT therapist. The design of the study precluded therapists or families from knowing before the 8 week/8 session mark (when the two doses of therapy diverged) to prevent therapists and families from knowing at the outset whether they would receive a high or low dose of FBT, which might have influenced how the therapists delivered and families responded to treatment. Outcomes were assessed at baseline, 6 months, and 12 months. No differences on any measures were found on the basis of allocation by dose. Patients began the study with a mean IBW of approximately 78%. At 6 months they were at a mean IBW of about 96%, and by 12 months at 98% IBW. BMIs changed from a mean of about 16 at baseline to 20 at the 1-year assessment point. Improvements in the subscales of the EDE were significant for all four subscales. Ninety-six percent had a BMI greater than the suggested diagnostic cut point of 17.5 in DSM-IV, whereas 67% had a BMI of 20 or greater and a global EDE score of less than 2 standard deviations from population norms. Dropout in this study was about 15%.

Although there were no differences in main outcomes, exploratory post hoc analyses suggested that there were moderators of outcome that might affect dose–response (Lock et al., 2005). For weight change as assessed by change in BMI, those patients who had higher levels of obsessive–compulsive features related to eating as assessed using the Yale–Brown–Cornell Obsessive Compulsive Scale for Eating Disorders (YBC-ED) did better when they were treated with a higher dose of FBT. For change in eating-related psychopathology, those who had intact families (two parents living in the home, nondivorced or reconstituted families) did better with a higher dose of FBT. In the first instance, it is reasonable to consider patients with higher levels of obsessive–compulsive features related to eating as more severely compromised than their cohorts with lower levels of these concerns, making them possibly more challenging to treat. Similarly, FBT depends on parents working together to bring about behavioral change in their child with AN, so those families in which there are fewer or potentially less aligned parental resources (non-intact families), may take longer to achieve similar outcomes. Nonetheless, the data from this study suggested that FBT in a manualized format, even in a low dose, is effective in promoting weight gain and psychological recovery from AN. Furthermore, manualized treatment appeared to be as acceptable (with a low dropout rate) and as effective as that provided in the United Kingdom where the therapy originated.

The most recent study to examine family therapy utilized manualized FBT and compared FBT to a form of EOIT called adolescent-focused therapy (AFT; Fitzpatrick, Moye,

Hoste, Le Grange, & Lock, 2010; Lock et al., 2010). This study was the first multisite study to examine treatments for adolescent AN. One hundred twenty-one subjects (112 females and 9 males) were randomized at two sites (The University of Chicago and Stanford University) to receive either 24 one-hour sessions of FBT over one year or 32 individual sessions lasting 45 minutes (a total of 24 contact hours) of AFT over one year. Up to 8 of these sessions in AFT could be utilized for collateral parental meetings to support the individual therapy. Although Lock and colleagues had described FBT as effective in a 6-month dose, it was considered unlikely that AFT could be effective in so short a treatment, thus a higher dose of FBT was utilized. At the end of treatment, FBT was found to be superior to AFT in terms of change in percentile BMI change and on global EDE. However, these findings did not significantly differ at 6-month or 12-month follow-up. Full remission (weight >94% IBW and EDE 1 *SD* within population norms) favored FBT, but did not statistically differ (FBT, 43% fully remitted; AFT, 22% fully remitted; $p = 0.055$, number needed to treat [NNT] = 5) at the end of treatment. At 6-month (FBT, 42% fully remitted; AFT, 18% fully remitted, $p = 0.03$, NNT = 4) and 12-month follow-up full remission rates (FBT, 50% fully remitted; AFT, 22% fully remitted, $p = 0.024$, NNT = 4) statistically favored FBT. Dropout was relatively low (23%) and similar to that found in other studies of adolescents with AN.

The study by Lock and colleagues had a number of limitations, including a relatively small sample size for longitudinal studies (although the study is the largest outpatient study of adolescent AN published to date) that may limit power to detect differences on some outcomes, treatments were provided in university settings well known for FBT, and subjects were adolescents with short-duration AN, so the outcomes, like those of similar studies discussed earlier, are not likely generalizable to adult or chronic patients (Lock et al., 2010). Overall, however, the study adds significantly to the database supporting the usefulness of family therapy, especially family therapy like FBT for adolescents with short-duration AN. The study builds specifically on the study by Robin and colleagues (1999) and supports the general superiority of FBT over individual therapy for adolescent AN, although, as in the Robin and colleagues study, subjects who received AFT did relatively well on many measures and improved in terms of weight and psychological functioning.

Studies of long-term outcome in relation to family therapy are few. However, there are three studies that suggest that family therapy using the FBT model leads to sustained improvements. Eisler and colleagues (1997) published a 5-year follow-up study of the original Russell and colleagues (1987) cohort. They found that although those subjects who received individual supportive therapy continued to improve, their improvements took almost five times as long to reach normal weight levels (5 years) and family therapy was still superior to individual therapy even at the 5-year mark. Eisler and colleagues (2007) also reported on a 5-year follow-up on their study, comparing separated and conjoint family therapy. They reported no difference in the percentage of IBW of patients based on treatment assignment, with patients in both groups continuing to progress to a mean of about 95% IBW at 5-year follow-up. These data suggest that in either format, family therapy leads to sustained and continued weight improvement. At the same time, the authors found suggestions that the differential impact of highly expressed emotion (family criticism) moderated the longer-term outcome. In their dose study Lock and colleagues found that BMI and EDE scores were stable an average of 4 years posttreatment (Lock, Couturier, & Agras, 2006). Altogether, it appears that family therapy leads to a generally good and sustained outcome.

In reviewing the literature supporting family therapy for adolescent AN, we now find that four studies suggest that manualized FBT can be effectively disseminated (Couturier, Isserlan, & Lock, 2010; Loeb et al., 2007; Tukiewicz, Pinzon, Lock, & Fleitlich-Bilyk, 2010; Wallis, Rhodes, Kohn, & Madden, 2007). Researchers at Columbia University were trained in manualized FBT and reported on a case series of 20 adolescents between 12 and 17 years of age (Loeb et al., 2007). The authors reported that 75% completed treatment, weight change significantly increased from 81% IBW at baseline to 94% at the end of treatment, and 67% were menstruating at the end of treatment. In addition, significant improvements in eating-related psychopathology were noted on several subscales of the EDE. Westmead Children's Hospital in Sydney, Australia, implemented manualized FBT beginning in 2003. Researchers noted that during the 5-year period since initiating this change, readmissions to the medical inpatient service significantly decreased from an average of 2.8 in 2002 (prior to FBT being systematically implemented) to 1.27 in 2006. Furthermore, in a case series of 44 patients treated with FBT in Westmead's outpatient program, weight increased from an average of 83% to 98% by the end of treatment (Wallis et al., 2007). Couturier and colleagues (2010) reported on a case series of 14 adolescents with AN between 12 and 17 years of age treated with manualized FBT. These authors found that weight, dietary restraint, interoceptive deficits, and maturity fears all significantly improved. Most recently, Turkiewicz and colleagues (2010) reported on 11 adolescents with AN treated in São Paolo, Brazil. The data from this study suggest that manualized FBT was acceptable to parents and clinicians. In addition, patients demonstrated significant improvements in weight both at the end of treatment and at 6-month follow-up. Together these results suggest that manualized FBT can be disseminated across a range of cultures.

The use of FBT for younger patients with AN is described in one case series. Lock and colleagues reported on 32 children between the ages of 9 and 12.9 years (mean age 11.9 years) who received FBT for AN (Lock, Le Grange, Forsberg, & Hewell, 2006). The manual was slightly modified for this younger group because themes of autonomy and adolescent development were not relevant for them. These younger patients demonstrated significant improvements in weight (baseline BMI = 15, end of treatment BMI = 18) and eating-related psychopathology (EDE restraint, eating concerns, and shape concern). Treatment was acceptable (dropout rate was 16%). Treatment lasted on average 9 months and consisted of approximately 15 sessions. Global outcomes suggest that 76% were completely recovered by weight (>94% IBW) and the IBW of only one fell below 85% (this subject dropped out). Thus, with only minor modification, FBT appears to be useful for younger patients with AN.

Recent studies have also focused on therapeutic processes in FBT. As noted earlier in the context of the study of dose by Lock and colleagues, many families appear to respond early to FBT. Le Grange and colleagues recently reported using receiver operating curve analysis (ROC); a good outcome could be predicted as early as one month into treatment if 3 pounds or more of weight gain had been accomplished by this point (Doyle, Le Grange, Loeb, Doyle, & Crosby, 2009). Using this cut point at week 4 of treatment, 79% of responders and 71% of nonresponders could be correctly identified. This metric may be a useful marker in future studies to identify families who will need less treatment, as well as those who may need augmented or alternative treatment to FBT.

Related to the theme of treatment augmentation for FBT, several models have been proposed. The use of multifamily groups (MFG), discussed elsewhere (Fairbairn, Simic,

& Eisler, Chapter 13, this volume), has perhaps received the most attention (Dare & Eisler, 2000). Briefly, the theory behind MFG is that these additional intensive group family therapy sessions provide additional support, motivation, and information to families struggling in FBT alone. Studies are under way to examine if and for whom MFG augmentation of FBT may be useful. Many families appear to find MFG acceptable and helpful (Eisler, 2005). Researchers at Westmead Children's Hospital report on the use of parent-to-parent consultation in the context of FBT (Rhodes, Baillee, Brown, & Madden, 2008). They randomized 20 families to either standard FBT or to FBT plus parent consultation. Although there were no significant differences found between groups on any clinical outcome measure, there was some suggestion that early weight gain was greater in the group that had parent-to-parent consultation at the beginning of FBT (Rhodes et al., 2008). Nonetheless, qualitative data suggest that parents experience the parent-to-parent consultation as a supportive intervention that lessens their experience of isolation, increases their confidence to make behavioral changes, and allows them to better reflect on the changes they are making in their families (Rhodes, Madden, & Brown, 2009). Finally, Zucker and colleagues describe the use of parent skills groups as possible augmentation treatment, as detailed elsewhere (Zucker, Loeb, Patel, & Shafer, Chapter 19, this volume), to help parents better understand their child's illness, support the parents in changing behaviors and learning new ways to support emotional and cognitive development in their children with AN (Zucker, 2005; Zucker, Marcus, & Bulik, 2006).

The FBT Model

FBT is at its core a solution-focused therapy aimed at helping parents to change the maintaining behaviors of AN. The approach has three phases. The first phase focuses predominantly on aligning the parents to work effectively together to challenge undereating, overexercising, and any other behaviors that keep their child from gaining weight. The second phase aims to help the parents transfer control of these same eating-related behaviors back to the adolescent in an age-appropriate fashion. The third and final phase aims to identify any adolescent developmental problems that AN may have engendered and to help the family to address these. FBT tries to achieve in an outpatient setting what many inpatient, day hospital, or residential programs attempt to achieve in these more restrictive settings. FBT usually lasts between 6 and 12 months, for 10–20 1-hour sessions. These sessions are generally held weekly for the first few months, but are titrated to biweekly, and then monthly by the end of Phase 3.

When this model of family treatment was conceived, the approach was seen as an alternative to inpatient care, which had some potentially negative effects—traumatic separation of the child from his or her parents, family, and friends, disempowering of parents as effective agents for their children, deleterious effects of institutionalization on adolescent development, and high cost of inpatient care. Thus, in FBT parents can be seen as functioning in many ways similar to an effective inpatient nursing staff—at least during the first phase of treatment—albeit in the home setting. Parents in this role are seen as having some advantages over a typical nursing staff—they love their children, know them well, and are highly invested in their survival. However, parents usually have limited experience, knowledge, or understanding of AN or the procedures needed to promote weight gain. They also often lack confidence in their ability to change the behaviors that are maintaining AN, as they have been unsuccessful to date in doing so. These real and perceived deficiencies are early targets of FBT. Thus, parents are helped to take appropriate control of the behaviors maintaining AN without resorting to force or undue coercion. This control is a temporary procedure, as it is in the hospital, to arrest weight loss and promote weight restoration, which is ultimately relinquished to the adolescent during phases 2 and 3.

The original model of family therapy used in the study by Russell and colleagues (1987) was developed on primarily practical, as opposed to specific theoretical, grounds and used a range of family interventions. The focus on the potential role of family relational structure in weight restoration was drawn from the work of Minuchin and colleagues (1978). The neutral stance of the therapist was inspired by work in systemic family therapy, whereas the use of externalization was derived from narrative family therapy (Haley, 1973; Selvini Palazzoli & Viaro, 1988; White, 1987; White & Epston, 1990). Although each of these schools of family therapy contributed to the model, specific underlying hypotheses about the role of the family in the origin or maintenance of AN were not initially developed (Dare & Eisler, 1997). More recently, however, Eisler and colleagues (2005) have suggested that this form of family therapy is best considered to address familial accommodation to the development of AN in the family context. Building on the family accommodation model by Steinglass (1998), in which families with a medically ill child change their behaviors in response to caring for the sick child, Eisler describes how family processes are changed similarly in AN (Eisler, 2005). First, eating and food-related processes become the narrow focus of the family. This overfocusing leads to more limited ability for the family to engage in other important interactions (e.g., recreation, travel, etc.). As a result, family roles and relationships change, leading to increased anxiety, denial, and conflict. These changes make it more challenging for the family to manage broader family life cycle needs (e.g., promoting adolescent autonomy, engaging in life as a couple, taking care of other children). The net result of all these processes is a loss of agency and increased feelings of helplessness. Families arrive at treatment having spent months to years absorbed in these accommodations. According to this model, Eisler suggests that family therapy aims to help the family to extricate itself from such processes.

FBT is not a stand-alone treatment. Usually therapists using FBT depend on a medical team to provide the family and therapist with reassurance that the patient is safe for outpatient treatment from a medical perspective. In addition to this medical safety net, many patients with AN may require medication for comorbid conditions. In most instances, the FBT therapist is not a child psychiatrist, so it is imperative that psychiatric expertise is available to the team. In addition, many teams use a registered dietician to provide support to the medical team and to parents during FBT. The role of a dietician on a team that includes such a professional differs greatly from his or her role in treating adults with AN. Instead of working out nutrition plans or directly working with the adolescent with AN, the dietician provides consultations to the pediatrician and therapists when there may be nutritional questions they are unprepared to address. In some cases, parents meet with the dietician to gather information about nutrition; however, even in these cases, prescribing meal plans is not a part of consultation. It is important to note that no systematic studies have utilized dieticians, thus their contributions to outcome are unknown.

FBT begins only after a diagnosis of AN is made and referral for treatment using the approach is completed. There is considerable uncertainty about which families are likely not to respond to FBT. Moderator studies to date have not provided sufficient guidance, although nonintact families and patients with high levels of obsessive–compulsive features appear somewhat less responsive to treatment early on. On clinical grounds, parents who do not want to engage in FBT should not be forced to try it, as it will likely fail. Furthermore, parents with severe psychopathology—severe depression, psychosis, or active substance abuse—are not likely to be ideal candidates for a therapy that depends on parents being able to monitor and challenge fixed behaviors and beliefs. It is less certain whether parents who have a history of or current eating disorders are good candidates for using FBT. In some cases the increased awareness about the disorder helps parents to understand their child and to intervene more effectively, whereas in other cases the opposite is true. A frank discussion with the parents and the treatment team about the role of a parental eating disorder in carrying out FBT is often needed prior to embarking on the treatment. Families in which abuse and neglect of the children are present should be carefully evaluated before beginning FBT, as the treatment should not provide an opportunity for further abuse of the children. Other psychiatric disorders can generally be deferred during Phase 1 of FBT or treated with medications alone, but active suicidal behaviors or other severely dangerous behaviors (assault, running away) may require immediate intervention, precluding beginning or continuing in FBT until these issues are resolved.

There are five fundamental tenets that guide all phases and interventions used in FBT: (1) an agnostic view about the cause of AN, (2) initial symptom focus, (3) nonauthoritarian consultative stance as a therapist, (4) an emphasis on parental symptom management (empowerment), and (5) an ability to separate the disorder of AN from the adolescent (externalization). Each of these tenets has a relationship with each of the others, but taken together form a important theoretical basis of FBT.

The first tenet, about being agnostic concerning the cause of AN, is important for several reasons. First, parents often feel blamed and guilty for causing AN, based on many media and some scientific reports (despite the limited substantive evidence that they are responsible). By taking an agnostic view the therapist is free to explore with the family what can be done, rather than focusing on the supposed causes of AN. It is important to point out to families that the cause of AN is unknown and therapy that attempts to change the root causes of the disorder have uncertain and imprecise targets. It also helps to focus the family on behavioral change—getting the child to eat and stop overexercising—as opposed to focusing on more general family or adolescent processes. Taking an agnostic view, however, can be challenging to many novice therapists who have been schooled in theories about the role of parental "overcontrol" and "overprotectiveness" and "preoccupations about weight" as putative causes of AN. Therapists must challenge themselves to adopt this more neutral agnostic stance if they are to be effective FBT therapists. Families may detect subtle references to blame, and this can diminish their confidence in themselves as agents to help their children.

The initial focus of FBT is almost entirely on disrupting the symptoms that maintain AN. In many ways, this is similar to the initial focus of most inpatient treatment programs in which normalizing food intake, increasing nutrition, and prohibiting exercise are the norm. However, many therapies for eating disorders, particularly for AN, focus more broadly on adolescent or family concerns initially in order to provide a context for understanding the development of the disorder. FBT avoids this broader contextual frame and focuses from the start on the specific development, evolution, and current processes that involve restrictive eating, overexercise, or other eating disorder–specific behaviors (e.g., binge eating or purging). Families sometime struggle with this narrow focus initially because they expect therapy to target more general psychological and family processes. Therapists, too, sometimes find this narrow focus challenging because of their interest in broader psychological dilemmas. However, the narrow focus on symptoms in FBT is designed to mitigate the life-threatening behaviors maintaining the starved state and as such is seen as a crucial element in FBT. As interesting and tempting as it may be to turn to other themes and concerns, until the symptoms of AN are effectively disrupted, they remain a hazard to the child's immediate health.

In order to maintain an agnostic stance and to keep the focus on changing the maintaining behaviors of AN, therapists must adopt an active consultative and collaborative stance in relationship to the parents. This is also important for empowering parents (discussed next) as the therapist defers decision making to them, albeit after providing information needed to make informed choices. Therapists must be experts in adolescent development, in the treatment of AN, and in FBT. As such, they have considerable expertise to share and convey to parents and families. At the same time, the FBT therapist is not responsible for weight restoration or directly interceding with patients to address other needed behavioral changes, the parents are. Thus, the FBT therapist does not direct or prescribe interventions for the parents, but rather provides information about strategies that might work, helps parents think through options, and evaluates the success of parental efforts with an eye to identifying ways to improve results. In this way, the FBT therapist is providing a form of supervision for the parents, who are directly managing behavioral change. Again, many parents initially hope the therapist will tell them what to do and how to do it, and they report frustration at not being given a specific plan that they can implement. However, if a therapist makes the mistake of prescribing a plan and it fails, the parents' confidence in the therapist and FBT diminishes and the effects of treatment potentially lessen. Therapists, too, are sometimes tempted to respond to parental requests to "tell us what to do," but they do so at their peril, as they will certainly be blamed for any failure.

At the heart of FBT is the belief that parents can generally be effective in changing the behavior of their child with AN. In order to help parents achieve this, though, they must be empowered to make the necessary changes in their own thinking, behavior, and environment. Empowering parents means giving parents the knowledge they need to make informed changes in behavior, helping to identify the resources they need to carry out behavioral change, and, most important, encouraging them to take the authority upon themselves to manage these changes. Therapists, as described earlier, must defer their own authority if parents are to be the authorities. Therapists must convince parents that they should not hobble themselves with the belief that they caused the AN, as this will diminish their authority. Other experts, medical or nutritional, who may provide information about AN, dieting, or health must also defer their authority to the extent possible to parents. If the adolescent with AN believes that therapists, pediatricians, or nutritionists are the true authorities, resistance to parental efforts to change behaviors can increase and may result in failure.

The final fundamental tenet—the ability to separate the adolescent from AN— serves several purposes. The first is to remind the entire family that AN is a psychiatric disorder and not a "choice," as it sometimes appears to be. This allows the family, and parents in particular, to challenge their child's behaviors despite the appearance of fragility and physical vulnerability. In addition, this type of externalization helps the therapist to maintain a relationship with the adolescent, who may otherwise feel attacked by the therapist. Even though many patients with AN initially refute the idea that AN is somehow separable from themselves, over time many can recognize that the behaviors and concerns associated with AN are not an essential part of their identity. Parents also sometimes struggle because the willful and contentious battles over eating and exercise appear to be personal, so it is beneficial to help them understand that starvation and obsessive preoccupations about weight distort their child's experience of both themselves and others. To be sure, the symptoms of AN, especially over a more chronic course, become more fully integrated into identity; however, in adolescents, it is usually fairly easy to recall the child before the disorder disrupted identity and development.

Taken together, these five fundamental tenets converge to form a consistent guide for the FBT therapist throughout treatment. As specific phases and interventions are described in the following paragraphs, these tenets underlie the specifics provided in all instances. When in doubt about whether what he or she is about to suggest is consistent with FBT, the FBT therapist should consult these tenets. Any intervention that violates any one of them is likely to take the therapist astray and be unhelpful in maintaining the model. In order to help therapists, especially those who are early in their experience with using FBT, working in pairs may be useful to help them stay on track. Certainly, supervision by experts in FBT is helpful. Training, supervision, and certification in FBT are now available. The following outline of FBT summarizes the main interventions and is particularly focused on the early sessions in Phase 1. More detailed descriptions and clinical examples are available in the published manual of FBT (Lock et al., 2001).

Phase 1 of FBT begins once the referral for FBT had been made. Prior to the first face-to-face meeting, though, therapists should contact the parents to discuss the treatment model and to encourage them to bring all family members to treatment. There is often reluctance to bring the entire family in because parents fear the effects of FBT on other family members, resistance by siblings to coming because of competing demands (school, sports, etc.), work demands of parents (e.g., travel, late hours), and therapeutic nihilism on the part of some family members. The therapist should describe the importance of each family member in FBT and that it is critical that all family members learn about AN and how it is affecting all of the family. Most important, the therapist should convey that all family members are needed to help overcome AN.

During Phase 1, the main aim is to restore the adolescent child's weight to near normal levels and disrupt any other maintaining behaviors associated with the eating disorder (e.g., overexercise, dieting, purging, etc.). Parents are put in charge of weight restoration and disrupting these other behaviors. Siblings are asked to support their brother or sister, who will likely be angry, depressed, and frustrated by these parental interventions. This phase usually consists of 5–10 sessions over 3–6 months.

The first session of the first phase of FBT is designed to (1) engage the entire family in treatment, (2) review the development of AN and its effects on the patient and family, (3) separate the illness of AN from the normal developmental challenges of the child, (4) stimulate anxiety and concern about the long-term impacts AN will have on the child, and (5) charge the parents to take action to address the self-starvation of their child. When the therapist greets the family, the aim is to convey a sense of both gravity and warmth. From the start, the therapist must signal the seriousness of AN, while also wishing to provide a sense of containment and caring. This "paradoxical" stance operates throughout the first phase of treatment as the therapist promotes parental anxiety as a means of motivating parents to take action, at the same time preventing this anxiety from becoming overwhelming through the comforting and containing presence of the therapist (Wynne, 1980). In this way, the therapist aims to generate the possibility of a "therapeutic window" that is open wide enough to allow change, but still not so wide that the family feels unsupported. During the first few minutes of therapy the therapist asks each family member to briefly introduce him- or herself, taking time to ask a few questions about the interests and activities of each one. Although this takes only about 5–10 minutes of the session, it is important to acknowledge each family member, as this reinforces the idea that the therapist believes each of them to be critical to the success of treatment. Therapists should be careful that this introduction also gives them an opportunity to describe their own expertise and experience with AN so that family members are reassured about the ability and competence of the person helping them. Common mistakes therapists make during this intervention include spending too much time with the introductions, not including all family members equally, and forgetting to introduce themselves.

After describing the three phases of FBT to the family, the therapist next uses circular questioning to take a specific and focused history of how AN developed and what the family has done to date to try to combat it (Cecchin, 1987; Palazzoli, Boscolo, Cecchin, & Prata, 1980). Circular questioning involves the therapist's asking each family member to build on the previous perspective or statement of another family member. In this way, a joint family narrative is developed that provides a coherent story of how AN emerged and how it is currently affecting the family. Usually, this is the first time that all family members have shared their perspectives on AN. During this interview, the therapist is also collecting information about how AN has changed the patient and the family, to use later in the session to help the family recognize the seriousness of AN as well as to separate the patient from AN. This intervention usually takes approximately 20 minutes of the first session.

Common mistakes that therapists make during this history-taking intervention include not involving all family members, allowing one family member to dominate the narrative, and focusing on family problems or history unrelated to AN. A common challenge is to help the patient to contribute to this discussion. Patients are often angry, silent, and withdrawn and refuse to participate in the circular questioning procedure. The therapist should gently encourage the patient to contribute at regular intervals, comment on how difficult this may be for the patient, and convey to the patient and family sympathy for the patient's struggle, but never insist on participation. Sometimes during this intervention, parents respond critically to the patient and blame him or her for causing the problems the family is experiencing. Should this happen, the therapist should say that sometimes such comments make it more difficult for the patient to participate. However, parents often blame themselves for having caused AN. This too should be challenged by the therapist by saying to the parents that no one knows the cause of AN and that available studies do not support family responsibility.

Armed with the information gathered from the family's responses to circular questioning about how AN developed in the family, the therapist now takes the opportunity to use this information to highlight the differences between how the patient was behaving, thinking, and interacting prior to the onset of AN as compared with current behaviors, thoughts, and relationships. For example, the therapist may point out that prior to the onset of AN, the patient was focused on school, friends, and was generally in a good mood, but that now the patient appears to think only about food and exercise, is too tired to go to school, has withdrawn from friends, and is irritable and depressed. The therapist points out that these are common problems when AN is present but usually resolve once the patient recovers. Specific examples drawn from the family narrative highlight these general themes and make them salient for the family. When the therapist makes these observations, the patient may protest and claim that he or she is at one with AN. If this happens, the therapist may sympathize with the patient's perspective but not agree with it. The purpose of this separation is twofold. First, it may help parents to recognize better that their child has a psychiatric disorder and is not just misbehaving or being rebellious. Second, the therapist uses this separation to communicate that the patient is not seen as willfully causing the disorder or as in some way deficient, but as having an illness. Although this may be rejected outright by the patient at this point, at a later point in therapy the patient may remember that the therapist held this position, promoting the development of trust. This intervention usually takes between 10 and 15 minutes of the session.

The next intervention used in Session 1 is stimulating increased anxiety in the parents about the seriousness of AN. Again, using information gathered in the first part of the session, the therapist describes in a detailed and compelling fashion the insidious but determined progress of AN. The therapist describes the medical complications of severe starvation, including bone loss, infertility, growth retardation, and death. The therapist relates this information to the history of the patient as appropriate, emphasizing medical hospitalizations, results of laboratory tests, changes in personality, and so forth. The intervention, if successful, leads directly to the therapist's giving an imperative to the parents to take charge of the child's eating so that self-starvation is stopped and other maintaining behaviors are disrupted. The family members may protest that they have tried this before, but were ineffective. The therapist should reassure the family members that though that may have been the case, this time will likely be different because the therapist can help them to be successful. The session ends with the therapist asking the parents to bring a meal to the next session which the two of them (if there are two parents) decide will help to begin restoring weight in their child. This intervention usually takes 10–15 minutes of the session.

Session 2 in the first phase of FBT is a family meal modeled, in some respect, after that described by Minuchin and colleagues (1978). However, the family meal in this instance is first and foremost and an opportunity for the therapist to learn about meal-time processes in the family (who cooks the meals, who is there for various meals, what current intake is like, what types of conflicts the family has around food, etc.). A secondary goal is for the parents to help their child eat a bite more than the patient planned to eat. Families bring a range of foods to the meal, but most bring reasonable amounts and types of food that will help to nourish the child. If the patient brings a separate meal, the family brings too little, or the patient refuses to attend, the therapist takes this session as an opportunity to learn about why these decisions and events occurred. The session is designed to help the therapist learn about the resources the family has to bring to help the child and what impediments may need to be overcome to effectively utilize them. Resources vary from family to family, as do disciplinary roles and styles. Thus, each family must consider how to promote weight restoration within these parameters or develop additional resources. The therapist's job is to help the family consider these options, and the family meal is the first step in this process.

In addition to learning about family mealtime processes, the therapist asks the parents to help their child eat one more bite after the patient has stopped eating. This intervention is stressful for parents, patients, and therapists. However, it should not be viewed as a "test" of the parents' ultimate ability to refeed their child, the child's likely response to treatment, or the therapist's abilities. The therapist begins by asking the parents to agree on something they think their child should eat to help him or her gain weight. The main point is for the parents to agree first on what the patient should eat. Getting parents aligned toward specific goals is a major part of the struggle and is essential in most families if they are to be successful. Once the parents agree on what the child should eat, they should be encouraged to try to get the child to eat it. Usually parents try asking the child to eat, but this seldom works. Next, they may try reasoning, coaxing, or bribing (offering a reward) for compliance. Again, these tactics are seldom successful. The therapist may then step in to directly coach the parents. The therapist may suggest that the parents sit on either side of their child. This is a powerful message—that the parents are acting in concert with one another. The therapist may then advise the parents to tell the child that he or she must eat what they are asking. They are asked to say this injunction together, in one voice, and repeatedly until the child complies. The therapist may explain why asking the child to eat is not effective (it leaves the decision up the patient, who does not want to comply), why reasoning doesn't work (the child is not reasonable about eating, as the history has amply demonstrated), and why bribing doesn't work (the rewards are too little for the cost to the patient). Setting clear, reasonable expectations, and firm but caring insistence on compliance is what is required—and if the parents agree and both are persistent, it is difficult for the patient to get out of eating. In about three-quarters of cases, the patient does eat a bit more. This may be accompanied by tears, screams of protest, or other behavioral manifestations. The therapist must help the parents to understand that despite these protestations, self-starvation cannot continue and they need to save their child's life (Lock & Le Grange, 2005).

The rest of Phase 1 consists of coaching sessions with the patient and family together. At the start of each session, the therapist meets with the patient separately for 5–10 minutes and discusses what the parents have been doing to promote weight gain over the past week. Weight is graphed at this meeting. In the beginning, the patient may be silent or reluctant to share information. However, over time, as the patient begins to recover, this time is better utilized. The therapist shares the graph with the family and discusses with the parents their perspective on weight progress over the past week. The progress or lack of progress as documented on this chart generally sets the tone of the session. Although the therapist always looks for opportunities to compliment family members on their work and efforts, heightened concern over weight loss or failure to gain weight is always expressed when either is identified. The emphasis in the session is on what the parents did to promote weight restoration over the past week, what worked, what did not work so well, and what ideas could be considered to improve these efforts. The therapist is active in deliberating these possibilities and may offer examples of strategies that might be considered (e.g., increased meal monitoring, increasing amount of calorie-dense food, prohibiting exercise), but decisions about what the family will undertake are made by the parents. In this way, the therapist provides expert consultation while not directing treatment decisions. Families sometimes ask for advice and the therapist can provide ideas about possible strategies, but does not prescribe a particular action. Siblings are asked in each session about how they are helping to support their brother or sister with AN and to provide examples of how they helped support their sister or brother during the week. Such examples often include comforting their sibling after a difficult meal, doing a chore for him or her, making a card or drawing for him or her, or going for a walk or to a movie.

The second phase of FBT begins when the patient is mostly weight restored and is eating without difficulty under parental control. The aim of the second phase is to transfer eating-related activities back to the patient in an age-appropriate way. This means that younger adolescents are generally still eating most meals with the family with parental oversight, and that older adolescents are likely to eat with friends sometimes and with less parental involvement in food choices or portions than would be expected with younger children. The first part of Phase 2 focuses on identifying the types of graded steps the parents can take in transferring eating back to their child. Usually, snacks or meals at school are the first to be transferred back as these are more often developmentally managed independently. They also tend to be meals with fewer calories, so if the patient is unable to eat them, little progress is lost. Exercise and sporting activities are another key area that is addressed in Phase 2. As driven exercise is often an important component of AN, care is advised in taking up exercise and sports again. This is especially the case for sports that are done repetitively and in isolation (e.g., distance running, swimming) or in which appearance and weight contribute to performance (e.g., gymnastics, ballet, wrestling, crew). Still, it is important that family members help their child take on the challenge of resuming activities, even if they are different from previous activities, so that the patient can learn to manage eating enough to support healthy exercise levels.

In the latter parts of Phase 2, the therapy may focus more on social processes related to eating and adolescence. For example, the patient may wish to spend the night at a friend's house, go out for meals with friend, or buy new stylish clothes. Each of these activities relates to normal adolescent development (Lock, 2002) but may also retrigger thoughts about weight and shape. Therapists ask family members to find opportunities to help their child take on these normative activities and to support the child when he or she does. Sometimes this may require special arrangements. For example, parents may need to pack a special meal for sleepovers or to avoid shopping at certain stores. At this point, however, members of the family usually feel hopeful about recovery and more confident in their ability to find solutions to the vexations of AN. It is important, though, not to promote overconfidence during this stage, as stalling out or relapse is still possible. Some patients become more resistant to weight gain during this phase as they approach the weight they were at when they initially began developing AN. Thus, parents may find themselves facing a child that has retrenched. This can be demoralizing for parents, but the therapist should help them understand why this may be occurring at this point and that they must persevere. The metaphor of climbing a sand hill is sometimes helpful at this point—it is hard work and you cannot stop until you reach the top or you will slide back down. Helping parents to understand that their goal is not just improvement, but actually recovery from the disorder. Phase 2 usually lasts 2–4 months and consists of 3–5 sessions. Most sessions are held at 2-week intervals.

Phase 3 begins when weight is fully restored and the patient is eating in an age-appropriate independent manner. The patient is no longer preoccupied by weight loss and overexercise, but rather focused on other adolescent developmental tasks (Lock, 1998). The therapist begins this phase by providing a brief overview of the tasks of adolescence. The first task is adjustment to a postpubertal body. The second task is the development of a social identity, and the third task is developing goals for work/school and relationships outside the family. A tool the therapist uses to illustrate these tasks is to ask the parents to describe their own experiences with such tasks. In most cases, parents have not discussed their own adolescence with their children, and this provides an opportunity for them to do so in a structured setting with a therapist present. Parents are often able to describe their own dilemmas about body image, social awkwardness, and attempts to find the right work and more intimate partners. The aim is to help the parents to remember better what it is like to be an adolescent so they can better understand the dilemmas their adolescent child is experiencing. The parents and the patient are asked to identify any adolescent problem or concern they would like to address in the next few sessions. Usually, these dilemmas are related to independence, risk taking, or social relationships. It must be stressed that FBT does not aim to help parents manage all problems of adolescence, but rather to help the parents identify problems that may emerge or that they feel may need additional treatment.

Another task of the third phase of FBT is effective termination. As noted, sessions are held less frequently over the course of treatment, so by Phase 3, sessions are spaced at monthly intervals. This is done intentionally to promote self-sufficiency, self-reliance, and independent management by the family over the treatment course. During the last sessions, the therapist aims to identify any signs of possible relapse, help family members to prepare for how they might respond should signs of AN reappear, and in cases where recovery remains uncertain, identify additional steps that may be taken. Furthermore, as other psychiatric or family problems that might have been present have been deferred in FBT in order to focus full attention on AN, strategies for how these remaining problems may be addressed are often considered. Therapists sometimes find it useful to return to data derived from the first session of therapy at this point to compare and contrast the child with AN to the child at this point. Parents are asked to identify any remaining concerns about AN they see present in their child, and the patient is asked the same question. It is not unusual for parents to see few remaining concerns, but the adolescent may report continuing thoughts about weight and shape. Data suggest that, indeed, in many cases the patient's thoughts and cognitions change about 6–12 months later than weight restoration itself (Couturier & Lock, 2006; Eisler et al., 1997; Lock, Couturier, & Agras, 2006; Lock et al., 2010). Hence, therapists can reassure both the patient and the parents that progress in this area is likely to continue, but if it should not, or if these thoughts worsen or lead to changes in eating or exercise, they should return to treatment. However, data suggest that the chance of relapse after full recovery in terms of thoughts related to weight and eating appears to be small.

Future Directions

Although current studies suggest that FBT is likely the best first-line approach for adolescents with short-duration AN, few studies have actually provided adequate comparisons of active treatments (e.g., other family therapies, cognitive-behavioral therapy [CBT], dialectical behavior therapy [DBT]) (Lock et al., 2010). Such studies are needed not only to clarify whether FBT is the best approach, but also to identify other treatments that are effective. Moreover, FBT is not effective for 15–20% of adolescents with AN. Thus, treatment augmentation studies are needed to build on the framework that FBT has shaped. The form of such augmentation strategies may include multifamily groups, family education groups, incorporation of FBT into other treatment models (CBT, AFT, interpersonal therapy, medications) or settings (partial programs, hospital programs). In addition, studies that examine which patients benefit from FBT (moderators) are needed (Kraemer, Frank, & Kupfer, 2006). Such studies should examine not only patient variables, but family and parental variables as well. Studies examining how FBT works are also needed (mediators) (Kraemer, Wilson, Fairburn, & Agras, 2002). Little guidance is currently available supporting any specific mechanisms. If such mechanisms were identified, strategies to improve the treatment or import similar mechanisms into other treatments could lead to better outcomes or novel treatments.

References

Bruch, H. (1973). *Eating disorders: Obesity, anorexia nervosa, and the person within*. New York: Basic Books.

Cecchin, G. (1987). Hypothesizing, circularity, and neutrality revisited: An invitation to curiosity. *Family Process, 26*, 405–414.

Couturier, J., Isserlan, L., & Lock, J. (2010). Family-based treatment for adolescents with anorexia nervosa: A dissemination study. *International Journal of Eating Disorders, 18*, 199–209.

Couturier, J., & Lock, J. (2006). What constitutes remission in adolescent anorexia nervosa: A review of various conceptualizations and a quantitative analysis. *International Journal of Eating Disorders, 39*, 175–183.

Crisp, A. H. (1980). *Anorexia nervosa: Let me be*. London: Academic Press.

Crisp, A. H., Norton, K., Gowers, S., Halek, C., Bowyer, C., Yeldham, D., et al. (1991). A controlled study of the effect of therapies aimed at adolescent and family psychopathology in anorexia nervosa. *British Journal of Psychiatry, 159*, 325–333.

Dare, C., & Eisler, I. (1997). Family therapy for anorexia nervosa. In D. M. Garner & P. Garfinkel (Eds.), *Handbook of treatment for eating disorders* (pp. 307–324). New York: Guilford Press.

Dare, C., & Eisler, I. (2000). A multi-family group day treatment programme for adolescent eating disorders. *European Eating Disorders Review, 8*, 4–18.

Doyle, P., Le Grange, D., Loeb, K., Doyle, A., & Crosby, R. (2010). Early response to family-based treatment for adolescent anorexia nervosa. *International Journal of Eating Disorders, 43*(7), 659–662.

Eisler, I. (2005). The empirical and theoretical base of family therapy and multiple family day therapy for adolescent anorexia nervosa. *Journal of Family Therapy, 27*, 104–131.

Eisler, I., Dare, C., Hodes, M., Russell, G., Dodge, E., & Le Grange, D. (2000). Family therapy for adolescent anorexia nervosa: The results of a controlled comparison of two family interventions. *Journal of Child Psychology and Psychiatry and Allied Disciplines, 41*(6), 727–736.

Eisler, I., Dare, C., Russell, G. F. M., Szmukler, G. I., Le Grange, D., & Dodge, E. (1997). Family and individual therapy in anorexia nervosa: A five-year follow-up. *Archives of General Psychiatry, 54*, 1025–1030.

Eisler, I., Simic, M., Russell, G., & Dare, C. (2007). A randomized controlled treatment trial of two forms of family therapy in adolescent anorexia nervosa: A five-year follow-up. *Journal of Child Psychology and Psychiatry and Allied Disciplines, 48*, 552–560.

Fitzpatrick, K., Moye, A., Hostee, R., Le Grange, D., & Lock, J. (2010). Adolescent focused therapy for adolescent anorexia nervosa. *Journal of Contemporary Psychotherapy, 40*, 31–39.

Gull, W. (1874). Anorexia nervosa (apepsia hysterica, anorexia hysterica). *Transactions of the Clinical Society of London, 7*, 222–228.

Haley, J. (1973). *Uncommon therapy: The psychiatric techniques of Milton H. Erickson*. New York: Norton.

Hall, A., & Crisp, A. H. (1987). Brief psychotherapy in the treatment of anorexia nervosa: Outcome at one year. *British Journal of Psychiatry, 151*, 185–191.

Kaye, W. H., Nagata, T., Weltzin, T., Hsu, B., Sokol, M., McConaha, C., et al. (2001). Double-blind placebo controlled administration of fluoxetine in restricting and restricting-purging type anorexia nervosa. *Biological Psychiatry, 49*, 644–652.

Kaye, W. H., Weltzin, T., Hsu, B., & Bulik, C. M. (1991). An open trial of fluoxetine in patients with anorexia nervosa. *Journal of Clinical Psychiatry, 52*, 464–471.

Kinston, W., & Loader, P. (1984). Eliciting whole-family interaction with a standardized interview. *Journal of Family Therapy, 6*, 347–363.

Kraemer, H., Frank, E., & Kupfer, D. (2006). Moderators of treatment outcomes: Clinical, research, and policy importance. *Journal of the American Medical Association, 296*, 1286–1289.

Kraemer, H., Wilson, G. T., Fairburn, C. G., & Agras, W. S. (2002). Mediators and moderators of treatment effects in randomized clinical trials. *Archives of General Psychiatry, 59*, 877–884.

Lasègue, E. (1883). De l'anorexie hysterique. *Archives Générales de Médecine, 21*, 384–403.

Le Grange, D., Eisler, I., Dare, C., & Russell, G. (1992). Evaluation of family treatments in adolescent anorexia nervosa: A pilot study. *International Journal of Eating Disorders, 12*(4), 347–357.

Liebman, R., Minuchin, S., & Baker, I. (1974). An integrated treatment program for anorexia nervosa. *American Journal of Psychiatry, 131*, 432–436.

Lock, J. (1998). Psychosexual development in adolescents with chronic illnesses. *Psychosomatics, 39*, 340–349.

Lock, J. (2002). Treating adolescents with eating disorders in the family context: Empirical and theoretical considerations. *Child and Adolescent Psychiatric Clinics of North America, 11*, 331–342.

Lock, J., Agras, W. S., Bryson, S., & Kraemer, H. (2005). A comparison of short- and long-term family therapy for adolescent anorexia nervosa. *Journal of the American Academy of Child and Adolescent Psychiatry, 44*, 632–639.

Lock, J., Couturier, J., & Agras, W. S. (2006). Comparison of long term outcomes in adolescents with anorexia nervosa treated with family therapy. *American Journal of Child and Adolescent Psychiatry, 45*, 666–672.

Lock, J., & Le Grange, D. (2001). Can family-based treatment of anorexia nervosa be manualized? *Journal of Psychotherapy Practice and Research, 10*, 253–261.

Lock, J., & Le Grange, D. (2005). *Help your child beat an eating disorder.* New York: Guilford Press.

Lock, J., Le Grange, D., Agras, W. S., & Dare, C. (2001). *Treatment manual for anorexia nervosa: A family-based approach.* New York: Guilford Press.

Lock, J., Le Grange, D., Agras, W. S., Moye, A., Bryson, S., & Jo, B. (2010). Randomized clinical trial comparing family-based treatment to adolescent focused individual therapy for adolescents with anorexia nervosa. *Archives of General Psychiatry, 67*, 1025–1032.

Lock, J., Le Grange, D., Forsberg, S., & Hewell, K. (2006). Is family therapy useful for children with anorexia nervosa? *Journal of the American Academy of Child and Adolescent Psychiatry, 45*, 1323–1328.

Loeb, K., Walsh, B., Lock, J., Le Grange, D., Jones, J., Marcus, S., et al. (2007). Open trial of family-based treatment for adolescent anorexia nervosa: Evidence of successful dissemination. *Journal of the American Academy of Child and Adolescent Psychiatry, 46*, 792–800.

Malina, A., Gaskill, J., McConaha, C., Frank, G., LaVia, M., Scholar, L., et al. (2003). Olanzapine treatment of anorexia nervosa: A retrospective study. *International Journal of Eating Disorders, 33*, 234–237.

Minuchin, S., Rosman, B., & Baker, I. (1978). *Psychosomatic families: Anorexia nervosa in context.* Cambridge, MA: Harvard University Press.

Morgan, H., & Russell, G. (1988). Clinical assessment of anorexia nervosa: The Morgan–Russell outcome assessment schedule. *British Journal of Psychiatry, 152*, 367–371.

Palazzoli, M., Boscolo, L., Cecchin, G., & Prata, G. (1980). Hypothesizing-circularity-neutrality: Three guidelines for the conductor of the session. *Family Process, 19*, 3–12.

Pike, K., Walsh, B. T., Vitousek, K., Wilson, G. T., & Bauer, J. (2000). *Cognitive-behavioral therapy in the relapse prevention of anorexia nervosa*. Kyoto, Japan: Third International Congress of Neuropsychology.

Rhodes, P., Baillee, A., Brown, J., & Madden, S. (2008). Can parent-to-parent consultation improve the effectiveness of the Maudsley model of family-based treatment for anorexia nervosa?: A randomized control trial. *Journal of Family Therapy, 30,* 96–198.

Rhodes, P., Madden, S., & Brown, J. (2009). Parent to parent consultation in the Maudsley model of family-based treatment of anorexia nervosa: A qualitative study. *Journal of Marital and Family Therapy, 35,* 181–192.

Robin, A. (2003). Behavioral family systems therapy for adolescents with anorexia nervosa. In A. E. Kazdin & J. R. Weisz (Eds.), *Evidence-based psychotherapies for children and adolescents* (pp. 358–373). New York: Guilford Press.

Robin, A., Siegal, P., Moye, A., Gilroy, M., Dennis, A., & Sikand, A. (1999). A controlled comparison of family versus individual therapy for adolescents with anorexia nervosa. *Journal of the American Academy of Child and Adolescent Psychiatry, 38*(12), 1482–1489.

Russell, G. F., Szmukler, G. I., Dare, C., & Eisler, I. (1987). An evaluation of family therapy in anorexia nervosa and bulimia nervosa. *Archives of General Psychiatry, 44*(12), 1047–1056.

Selvini Palazzoli, M., & Viaro, M. (1988). The anorectic process in the family: A six-stage model as a guide for individual therapy. *Family Process, 27,* 129–148.

Silverman, J. (1997). Charcot's comments on the therapeutic role of isolation in the treatment of anorexia nervosa. *International Journal of Eating Disorders, 21,* 295–298.

Steinglass, P. (1998). Multiple family discussion groups for patients with chronic medical illness. *Families, Systems, and Health, 16,* 55–70.

Treasure, J. L., Todd, G., Brolly, M., Tiller, J., Nehmed, A., & Denman, F. (1995). A pilot study of a randomized trial of cognitive-behavioral analytical therapy vs. educational behavioral therapy for adult anorexia nervosa. *Behavior Research and Therapy, 33,* 363–367.

Tukiewicz, G., Pinzon, V., Lock, J., & Fleitlich-Bilyk, B. (2010). Feasibility, acceptability, and effectiveness of family-based treatment for adolescent anorexia nervosa: An observational study conducted in Brazil. *Revista Brasileira de Psiguiatria, 32,* 169–172.

Wallis, A., Rhodes, P., Kohn, M., & Madden, S. (2007). Five-years of family based treatment for anorexia nervosa: The Maudsley model at the Children's Hospital at Westmead. *International Journal of Adolescent Medicine and Health, 19,* 277–283.

White, M. (1987). Anorexia nervosa: A cybernetic perspective. *Family Therapy Collections, 20,* 117–129.

White, M., & Epston, D. (1990). *Narrative means to therapeutic ends.* New York: Norton.

Wynne, L. (1980). Paradoxical interventions: Leverage for therapeutic change in individual and family systems. In T. Strauss, S. Bowers, S. Downey, S. Fleck, & I. Levin (Eds.), *The psychotherapy of schizophrenia.* New York: Plenum Press.

Zucker, N. (2005). *Off the C.U.F.F.* Durham, NC: Duke University Eating Disorders Program.

Zucker, N. L., Marcus, M. D., & Bulik, C. (2006). A group parent training program: A novel approach for eating disorder management. *Eating and Weight Disorders: Studies on Anorexia, Bulimia and Obesity, 11,* 78–82.

CHAPTER 13

Multifamily Therapy
for Adolescent Anorexia Nervosa

Pennie Fairbairn
Mima Simic
Ivan Eisler

O ver the last 50 years there has been a growing interest in treating several families together, using a range of different treatment models and across a range of psychiatric conditions. One of the early pioneers of this model was Laqueur and his colleagues, who used multifamily therapy processes and techniques with psychotic patients and their families (Laqueur, 1972, 1973; Laqueur, La Burt, & Morong, 1964). In an era of restricted resources multifamily therapy was almost accidental in formation, offering a solution to staff shortages. However, clinicians quickly observed that there were positive therapeutic advantages (Laqueur, 1972). What transpired was the potential of seeing several families together to create a different context in which alternative behaviors and different relationship patterns could emerge.

The focus for this chapter is on a specific form of multifamily therapy (MFT) for young people with anorexia nervosa (AN), first described by Dare and Eisler (2000), which emphasizes a specific conceptual approach and a high intensity of treatment delivery (Eisler, Lock, & Le Grange, 2010). A detailed account is presented about how a decade of running groups at the Maudsley Child and Adolescent Eating Disorders Service has enabled a coherent model of MFT to evolve.

Brief Overview

The emergence of groups as a model of psychological therapy in the 1920s and 1930s (Bion, 1961) marked a shift in focus from behavioral therapy and individual psychoanalysis and, among others, contributed to the emergence of family therapy as a new treatment (Ackerman, 1938; Jackson, 1957; Jackson & Weakland, 1961; Satir, 1964). A few decades later, the convergence of family systems ideas and the notions of group therapy led to the development of the multifamily treatment model (Detre, Sayers, Norton, & Lewis, 1961;

Hess & Handler, 1961; Ross, 1948), particularly with psychotic patients and their fami-lies (Anderson, 1983; Laqueur, 1972, 1973; McFarlane, 1982). An understanding of the therapeutic benefits of groups (Yalom, 1970) influenced these pioneers of MFT, above all the importance of openness and constructive dialogue in enabling participants to learn from shared experiences (Scholz, Rix, Scholz, & Thomke, 2005).

Laqueur's early focus in MFT was on strengthening family communication in order to help individuals understand that the patient's challenging behavior could be attrib-uted to misunderstood interpretation of situations and unhelpful relational patterns. This early work assumed that the root of the problem that therapy needed to address was some form of family dysfunction, which could be effectively addressed by bringing together several families. The effect of bringing families together, however, very soon highlighted the positive aspects of the multifamily group process as a means of developing collabora-tive and supportive interactions, encouraging nonblaming, empirically informed discus-sions about the nature of the patient's illness, thus reducing shame and stigma (Anderson, 1983; Asen & Scholz, 2010; McFarlane, 1982, 2004).

Combating the sense of isolation and avoiding some of the negative effects encoun-tered in single-family therapy, families started to report on their positive experiences of the multifamily approach (Asen et al., 1981). Clinicians working with other problems followed suit and started applying MFT in their practices. These included substance mis-use (Kaufman & Kaufman, 1979), depression (Anderson et al., 1986; Fristad, Goldberg-Arnold, & Gavazzi, 2003; Lemmens, Eisler, Buysse, Heene, & Demyttenaere, 2009; Lemmens, Eisler, Migerode, Heireman, & Demyttenaere, 2007), bipolar disorder (Bren-nan, 1995), obsessive–compulsive disorder (OCD) (Barrett, Healey-Farrell, & March, 2004), school problems (Dawson & McHugh, 1994; McHugh, Dawson, Scrafton, & Asen, 2010), chronic illness (Gonzalez, Steinglass, & Reiss, 1989; Steinglass, 1998), and eating disorders (Colahan & Robinson, 2002; Dare & Eisler, 2000; Scholz & Asen, 2001; Slagerman & Yager, 1989; Wooley & Lewis, 1987).

The most common format for MFT until the 1970s relied on regular (weekly or biweekly) short meetings, typically 1½ to 2 hours in length. In the late 1970s the Lon-don-based Marlborough Family Day Unit developed a new, more intensive format by introducing MFT concepts and treatment techniques to a therapeutic community setting, targeting multiproblem families in which more than one member had different psychiat-ric and socially challenging issues (Asen et al., 1981; Asen, Dawson, & McHugh, 2001; Cooklin, Dawson, McHugh, & Oakley, 2003; Cooklin, Miller, & McHugh, 1983). Since then the intensive MFT model has been applied to a variety of other problems, including school problems, attention-deficit/hyperactivity disorder (ADHD), Asperger's syndrome, and eating disorders (Asen et al., 2001; Asen & Scholz, 2010; Dare & Eisler, 2000; Daw-son & McHugh, 2005; Scholz, Asen, Gantchev, Schell, & Süß, 2002).

Theories and Concepts Informing MFT

Historically, MFT has drawn on a range of conceptual and theoretical ideas from group therapy, family systems therapy, psychodynamic psychotherapy, attachment theory, and cognitive and behavioral therapies (Asen, 2002; Asen & Scholz, 2010; Behr, 1996; Laqueur, 1972; Lemmens et al., 2007; McFarlane, 2002; Steinglass, 1998; Strelnick,

1977). Psychoeducation and learning and generalizing and strengthening skills have also been an important part of some models of multifamily work, especially with schizophrenia, OCD, and self-harm (Barrett et al., 2004; McFarlane et al., 1995; Miller, Rathus, & Linehan, 2007). Increasingly, MFT approaches are adopting an integrative theoretical frame that brings together both a range of techniques and conceptual ideas from various theoretical models (Eisler & Lask, 2008).

What is common to all forms of MFT is the relatively straightforward idea that by bringing people together, the sharing of complex and stressful experiences can be therapeutically beneficial for potential change and recovery (Asen & Scholz, 2010; Steinglass, Gonzales, Dosovitz, & Reiss, 1982). Families offer each other mutual support, and the power structures between families and therapists are less visible than they appear in single-family therapy. The group context of the therapist working openly with different families offers transparency in regard to the aims and practice of the treatment.

Therapeutic Context

The therapeutic context for MFT focuses on establishing, from the outset, open and collaborative relationships between therapists and families and between families with one another. Working across several families demands that therapeutic relationships are more variable than is usual in individual therapy or single-family therapy. To engage a larger group, therapists change focus from one family to another, facilitating opportunities for wider observation of group and individual interaction. The MFT therapist takes an active and, at times, even quite a directive role but primarily aims to act as a catalyst to encourage interaction between families.

With the introduction of simple ground rules, interpersonal safety and group engagement starts to build (Yalom, 1970). A key ground rule that we have found useful for MFT groups is that each participant (child, adolescent, or adult) decides for him- or herself how actively that person wants to take part in any exercise or discussion. We emphasize that observing and listening are as important as doing and talking. The rule can be introduced playfully as the "Fifth Amendment Rule," but it is important that therapists take it seriously and offer or invoke it themselves from time to time ("I want to ask you a really difficult question, so you may want to plead the fifth amendment on this one"; "I don't think you should answer this question, you better plead the fifth").

Families and their individual members become consultants to each other through observing various interactions that are both similar to and different from their own (Asen & Scholtz, 2010). As facilitators, therapists encourage the families to own their expertise and strengths in fighting the illness. Gradually, the families become proactive in exploring avenues for change within a group atmosphere that is predominantly informal but also draws on the professional expertise of the therapists when apposite. Appropriate use of humor plays an important role in lifting group spirit and dispelling tension. This is often an organic process led by the families and/or clinicians.

Therapeutic intensity is generated quickly by bringing together a number of families and is further increased when MFT meetings continue over several consecutive days. Such an impact creates an immediacy of therapeutic contact, which brings about expectations of rapid yet achievable aims: injecting hope and fostering an expectation that deeper, longer-term change can be in the hands of the family members.

Interventions and Therapeutic Techniques

The MFT program makes use of a wide range of therapeutic techniques derived from family and group therapies, and families soon become accustomed to respond with comparative ease to a number of tasks and exercises. These include circular questioning (Eisler & Lask, 2008; Tomm, 1987a, 1987b) to encourage family members to develop varying perspectives of meaning; externalization (Tomm, 1989; Weber, Davis, & McPhie, 2006; White, 1989) to mobilize individual and family resources to challenge the problem and reduce feelings of guilt and blame; and enactment and intensification (Minuchin & Fishman, 1981), which make specific aspects of problems more visible and can interrupt mechanisms that maintain problems.

Andersen's (1987) exercise, *reflecting team ideas*, can be used in a number of ways in family group settings; both clinicians and families can offer reflections, observed by other members of the group, who then change places in order to reflect their own thoughts. Such reflective processes may include the use of a one-way screen, video recordings, or simple moment-to-moment reflections in the room. Many other techniques and exercises are used to reinforce reflective processes and mentalization (i.e., ability to understand mental states, in oneself and in others) (Fonagy, Gergely, Jurist, & Target, 2002), such as role reversal interviews, conversations in shifted time frames (e.g., asking adolescents to imagine themselves meeting 20 years later and reminiscing about the time when they used to attend the MFT group).

Information giving, in the form of both psychoeducational talks and informal explanations as part of ongoing group discussion, is important, not just as a way of increasing knowledge about eating disorders and challenging myths and disabling beliefs but also as part of the ongoing process of offering expertise to reinforce a sense of safety of the therapeutic environment (Byng-Hall, 1995).

The group context lends itself to the use of a range of other interventions, including nonverbal therapy techniques (drawing, modeling, collage), action techniques (psychodrama, role play and role reversal, family sculpting) or visualization and relaxation techniques. Motivational interventions, including discussions of advantages and disadvantages of change, and letter writing (letters to anorexia my friend, anorexia my enemy; letters from my body, etc.) are useful techniques that can be used in adolescent groups early on to help the young people engage with the group.

Intensive MFT and Eating Disorders

Although there is good evidence that outpatient family therapy is an effective treatment for the majority of adolescents suffering from an eating disorder (Keel, 2008), some do not respond and may therefore require a different or more intensive therapeutic treatment. Most commonly, this is inpatient or residential treatment, but because of concerns about the possible negative effects of hospitalization (Gowers, Weetman, Shore, Hossain, & Elvins, 2000) and the lack of evidence of its efficacy (Meads, Gold, & Burls, 2001), alternative approaches have been suggested. One such alternative is intensive multifamily therapy, developed in the late 1990s in Dresden (Scholz & Asen, 2001) and London (Dare & Eisler, 2000). Building on the efficacy of single-family therapy, a more intensive treatment, whereby families learned directly from each other to generate different possibilities to tackle the eating disorder, started to produce some positive changes toward recovery.

The cornerstone of influence for this new treatment approach to eating disorders was the Marlborough multifamily approach (Asen et al., 2001; Asen & Scholz, 2010), which combines relatively brief intensive work with groups of families, with follow-up treatment over an extended period of time.

When there are specific and often crisis-inducing issues to address, such as AN, increasing the level of intensity of MFT sessions to several consecutive days is a powerful way of mobilizing families (Dare & Eisler, 2000; Scholz et al., 2005). Using a tightly structured 3- to 4-day program, in which common problems can be explored in the safety of a controlled environment, offers families a "live" opportunity to address existing difficulties in order to find new solutions. Often described as creating a hothouse effect (Asen & Scholz, 2010; Eisler, Le Grange, & Asen, 2003; Fairbairn & Eisler, 2007) the group setting is therefore intense enough for mutual observation and learning. Families learn to manage crises in different ways and at times independently of professional interventions. Even though families are often somewhat skeptical when invited to take part in the program, as soon as they come together, they very quickly gain a sense of shared purpose and a feeling of hope.

Evidence Base

Although the clinical experience of using intensive MFT for adolescent AN has been extremely positive (Eisler et al., 2010; Scholz et al., 2005), as has been the feedback from the families themselves, empirical data supporting the efficacy of the treatment is limited as yet. A small open follow-up study (Salaminiou, Campbell, Simic, Kuipers, & Eisler, 2005) in which 30 young people and their families were followed for 6 months has shown significant improvements in the adolescents' weight, eating attitudes, self-esteem, and mood. The young person's weight on average increased from a low of just over 75% at the start of treatment to within the lower level of the normal weight range by 6 months, with most of the weight gain taking place in the first 3 months of treatment. The study also found significant reductions in self-reported depressive symptoms in the parents. Also of note were the high levels of satisfaction with treatment, assessed through both self-report and qualitative interviews, and a very low treatment attrition rate (2/30).

Although these early results are promising, any conclusions about the effectiveness of the treatment await the results of a recently completed multicenter RCT comparing single-family therapy and MFT by the third author (I. E.).

Intensive MFT at the Maudsley

Over the last decade the Maudsley MFT approach has been shaped by a number of factors: the parallel developments of MFT for eating disorders in Dresden (Asen & Scholz, 2010; Scholz & Asen, 2001; Scholz et al., 2005), informal as well as formal feedback from the families who have participated in MFT (Salaminiou, 2005), and our experience in providing MFT multiteam training to clinicians in a range of different contexts in the

United Kingdom, Scandinavia, Canada, United States, Czech Republic, Hong Kong, and elsewhere (Fairbairn & Eisler, 2007).

It is important to note that the model presented in the following discussion is combined with single outpatient family-based therapy (FBT) sessions (see Eisler, 2005; Eisler et al., 2010; Lock, Le Grange, Agras, & Dare, 2001). The shared conceptual focus of MFT and single FBT is on mobilizing family strengths and resources in order to overcome the eating disorder in the young person. The additional aim of MFT is to bring together families with shared experiences, allowing them to explore the impact the problem has had on family life, enabling parents to learn from each other how to tackle the eating problems, creating new and multiple perspectives, and helping families to take an observational stance that makes it easier to address problematic family interactions that have developed around the eating problems. The knowledge and expertise of the clinicians in regard to eating disorders is offered in the context of a highly collaborative therapeutic relationship that typically develops in the multifamily context.

On a practical level, the MFT group is run by two lead therapists/facilitators, who may be joined by other members of the multidisciplinary team, including trainees. It consists of five to seven families, all with a young person suffering with AN or an eating disorder not otherwise specified (EDNOS; restrictive subtype). Families attend an introductory evening, a 4-day intensive workshop, and 6–8 one-day follow-up workshops over approximately 9 months. This is a closed group, with the expectation that families attend both the intensive 4-day workshop and subsequent one-day follow-up meetings. Individual family sessions continue between follow-ups, depending on need.

Assessment for MFT and Composition of the Group

In addition to the general assessment of adolescent eating disorders (see Eddy, Herzog, & Zucker, Chapter 8, and Katzman & Findlay, Chapter 9, this volume), there is an assessment of the patient's and his or her family's suitability for MFT. MFT can be offered to most families with a young person diagnosed with AN or EDNOS (restrictive subtype) as an important part of treatment. There are only a few exclusion criteria for participation in MFT (e.g., child protection concerns, the young person is currently in care, and the presence of severe learning disability and/or autistic spectrum disorder in the child). In addition, some attention to the composition of the group is needed.

Typically our groups include an age range from 13 to 18 years, but we have positive experience of extending the age range in either direction as long as the group remains reasonably homogenous in age (e.g., 11–16 or 13–20). It is generally preferable not to include those with a diagnosis of bulimia nervosa (BN) in the same group as those with AN. This is not an absolute contraindication, of course, as there can be occasions when an individual young person's eating problems shift from a restrictive toward a BN pattern only after the group has started.

Families invited to take part in MFT reflect the full range of family forms, including single-parent families, same-sex parents, and reconstituted families, as well as differences in social and cultural backgrounds. Where parents are divorced or separated a discussion is needed with the family as to which parent should attend. When the family breakup has happened some time ago and the parents have worked out how to share their parental responsibilities, this decision is usually straightforward. With more recent splits, the negotiations can sometimes be quite difficult and may need to be revisited several times even after the group has started, particularly if ongoing differences between the couple are played out in the group.

Given the number of families in a group, the young persons are most likely to be in different phases of treatment and at different stages of the illness and motivation toward recovery can vary. However, this has certain advantages and allows families and young people in initial phases to perceive that change is possible; insight about the eating problem can develop and denial can lessen, and for families and young people in later phases, this reinforces motivation not to go back into the claws/grip of AN and builds further on the changes they have already achieved.

Phases of Treatment

The phases of treatment of the MFT are similar to those described in single-outpatient FBT for adolescent AN (Dare, Eisler, Russell, & Szmukler, 1990; Eisler et al., 2010; Lock et al., 2001). However, progress through these phases tends to be less linear than it is in single-family therapy, as it has to accommodate the unique differences that every group presents. The intensity of the initial 4-day workshop also means that there are opportunities to address a wider range of issues even at an early stage of treatment without distracting from the main, problem-focused task to support parents in finding ways of helping their children overcome their weight and food fears and begin to return to more regular eating. Rather than describing the phases of treatment in detail, we briefly outline some of the specific ways in which MFT differs from single-family therapy at different stages.

Engagement and Development of the Therapeutic Contract

Each family is seen at least once on its own before the group starts and has developed a working relationship with a therapist. The process of developing an engagement with the group builds on this relationship, but also requires the creation of a safe group environment for therapy that allows families to share the various ways they have accommodated to the illness and encourages them to think about alternative ways of managing their child's eating. In the group the families quickly develop a sense of a shared experience, particularly in the case of the parents, although the young people are sometimes more guarded and in some groups may take slightly longer before connecting with each other.

Helping the Family to Challenge AN

During the initial meetings with the family, as well as in the early stages of the group, AN is consistently discussed as an external force affecting the young people, which the parents are invited to join forces to overcome. This externalization of AN (White, 1989) is reinforced by providing psychoeducation about the physiological effects of starvation and by various group exercises (drawing or modeling AN by the young people or role plays, which may include a member of the staff representing the voice of AN, etc.) as described later in the chapter.

Parents are encouraged to exchange ideas about what has worked for them and to challenge each other's beliefs about how impossible it is to fight this illness. Observing other families at mealtimes gives an opportunity to consider alternatives that may have seemed impossible before and allows parents to challenge anorexic behaviors without the usual feelings of guilt and blame. This is discussed in detail in the later section on managing mealtimes in the context of the MFT group.

Exploring Issues of Current and Future Individual and Family Development

During the later stages of the work with the group, the focus increasingly moves toward helping the parents and young people to develop their own strategies and skills in managing AN and working toward their living life to the fullest. This may include less parental supervision of meals and food management as the young people begin to take back responsibility for eating. Family strengths, resilience, and mutual empathy are in many cases rediscovered and reidentified. Parents and other family members review their roles while considering the pros and cons of change. Group exercises at this stage focus on a much broader range of issues, aimed at helping the family and the young person identify and develop further strategies and skills for personal and family growth. These include exercises on relationship issues, exploring the notion of safe uncertainty (Mason, 1993), future-oriented tasks about life without AN, "de-externalizing" conversations (Eisler et al., 2010) about how to differentiate between AN and ordinary adolescent behavior and about taking responsibility for one's own behaviors and actions.

The Structure of the MFT Program

Introductory Evening

The families meet each other for the first time at a relatively formal introductory session, held during the week prior to the 4-day workshop. The MFT team members give information about the workshop and follow-up meetings, the structure of the days, and the range of activities that will take place. This is followed by a psychoeducational presentation on the effects of starvation and the prognosis of AN (usually provided by a medical member of the team).

   In describing the multifamily workshop, it is emphasized that a key aspect is joint meals, and parents are requested to bring food for snacks and lunches they are expecting their child to have. It is important at this point to acknowledge that this is the aspect of the therapy that families are likely to find most challenging, but that they are to be supported by staff members to manage the meals in a safe way. The manner in which this information is given has to convey the therapists' confidence that the goal of helping the young person to eat is achievable.

   The young people and their families are then given an opportunity to talk to members of a "graduate family" who have previously completed the MFT. Sharing their experiences and being able to reflect on how things were for them at their introductory evening offers a potent ingredient, especially to parents who often express feelings of hopelessness and helplessness. In smaller groups (usually separate groups for mothers, fathers, and young people) the families introduce themselves to each other and members of the graduate family. The opportunity to ask questions and hear from someone who has been through the MFT experience is often mentioned in feedback from families as a key moment in acquiring a new sense of hope.

The 4-Day Intensive Workshop

The young people and their families come together again during the week after the introductory session. They have a few days in between to prepare in their own minds what expectations they have about participating in the workshop. In most cases the positive expectations set up by the introductory meeting persist, and the group quickly develops a cohesive and highly supportive style of working. A few families find the time in the runup to the main workshop more stressful and may require additional support from the clinical team via phone discussions to encourage attendance at the intensive workshop.

Over the 4 days families participate in a range of large- and smaller-group tasks and activities (see Figure 13.1 for an example of the first day). The major focus of the work at this stage is challenging the grip of AN: exploration of food management difficulties; trying out different approaches to mealtimes (parent group) and attitudes to change (young people). However, there is also a broader focus on the experiences of living with AN, how this influences family relationships, and how it might change over the coming months as the young person (with the help of his or her family) begins the process of recovery from the illness.

Families adapt to the creative and open approach in the group, which enables them to consider their respective strengths and difficulties in front of one another. Various ways of communicating are introduced, including nonverbal techniques such as family sculpts and trust-building exercises. Using role play to understand a range of perspectives held by various family members fosters the possibility of learning from others. Family meals play a central role in MFT.

Managing Mealtimes as Part of MFT

When we first meet with the family, especially with patients with AN, we generally offer to provide the family with a meal plan to emphasize the need for a clear structure, to deal with potential medical risks such as refeeding syndrome, and the paramount need to make outpatient treatment a safe alternative to inpatient treatment. A metaphor often referred to by clinicians at the beginning and during treatment is "food is medicine and

10:00 A.M. Multifamily introductions—expectations, hopes, and fears.

10:30 A.M. Morning snack: Parents bring food according to agreed-upon meal plan.

11:00 A.M. Parents: What happens at mealtimes.

Young people: "Portrayals of anorexia" (draw, model, or write something that symbolizes anorexia for you/your family), gains and losses of having anorexia.

12:30 P.M. The multifamily lunch: Parents bring food according to agreed-upon meal plan.

1:45 P.M. Break.

2:00 P.M. Feedback about lunch. Young people observed by parents through one-way screen. Swap with young people, who then observe parents' feedback.

3:00 P.M. Afternoon snack.

3:30 P.M. Reflections on the "portrayals of anorexia"/gains and losses of having anorexia. Close with relaxation exercises.

FIGURE 13.1. Outline of a first day of a new group.

the meal plan is a prescription of how you take the medicine." This can give new meaning to parents and place them in a metaposition when faced with persuading their young person to relinquish control over the eating disorder. A prescriptive meal plan may also help parents to refrain from embarking on constant battles with their child about what and how much he or she should eat.

It is important to stress that the use of meal plans is not appropriate for all. The meal plan is presented to families as a guide for adequate food intake toward recovery, which previously some families in treatment found helpful. The family members decide whether they will use it or, if they are confident in what constitutes adequate food intake for recovery, they may opt to plan meals themselves. As a general rule, the more intractable the illness, the more important it is for the team initially to take an expert role in providing dietetic advice, both to avoid medical complications and to reassure the family and contain anxiety. As treatment progresses (as in the phased approach in single-family therapy) meal plans become more flexible and are negotiated between the therapist, patient, and family members, with the goal that they be completely replaced by what the parents and young person agree on as an appropriate food intake and control of eating eventually handed back to the young person.

Both snack and lunchtime meals are central to the MFT program and are supported by the MFT team. Meals take place in a structured environment, with two to three families sitting together at a table and a time boundary given for finishing the meals—15 minutes for snacks and 45 minutes for lunch. The two lead facilitators circulate to support the young people and their parents and therefore do not eat with them.

It is requested that families bring their respective "meal-planned" foods for snacks and lunch. Both these mealtimes provide opportunity for parents, young people, and clinicians to identify unhelpful eating patterns, which can be observed, explored, and gradually replaced with regular and adequate eating patterns. Therapists initially observe the way each family interacts, encouraging and reinforcing any attempt to introduce new behaviors that could lead to change ("That was really good the way you supported each other; keep going"); when appropriate, expressing sympathy with the young person's predicament ("I know this must be really tough for you, but it is important that your parents don't back off right now"), and making suggestions for doing things differently ("Some families have found that it works better if Mom and Dad sit on either side of their daughter during the meal so that they can support each other—why don't you try it?"). The therapists have to be mindful not to take over from the parents—this can be achieved, for instance, by making a brief suggestion and then moving away from the table.

A helpful way of interrupting the patterns of interaction that families have developed around meals is to use the "foster family meal," in which the families are mixed together and each young person eats with a father and a mother from a different family. It is a good idea to introduce this exercise early on in the life of the group, usually at lunch on day 2, before the group itself develops its routines and expectations of how meals progress.

Joint meals in MFT have two aims: (1) to provide a context in which the parents are helped to get their young person to start eating in healthier ways and (2) even more important, to interrupt the fixed patterns that have developed around food and that have usually become part of the maintaining mechanism of the eating disorder. The first aim requires confidence on the part of the therapists and a belief that the parents can succeed in this task. Therapists gain such confidence from having experienced other families overcome their difficulties, and therefore do not assume that the early struggles or setbacks a family may experience during the group meetings are necessarily an indication that the family will not find a way forward. To achieve the second aim it is important that there is plenty of opportunity for feedback both from parents and from the young people about their different experiences during the meals. Listening to and acknowledging the voice of the young people is of paramount importance at this point. This means not assuming automatically that anything they found difficult during the meal is simply "the voice of anorexia," but hearing them out about what was helpful and what was unhelpful. When discussing these issues the young people often support one another, but the group context also frequently allows them to acknowledge more openly the difficulties their parents face.

One-Day Follow-Up Workshops

Over the next 9 months, young people and their families attend one-day workshops in order to monitor and build on their experience and progress from the 4 intensive days. The first follow-up is 2 weeks after these days—the gap between subsequent workshops widens as time progresses. Between the workshop meetings, individual family therapy sessions continue with the key therapist—these meetings become less frequent as the treatment phases unfold.

Ending the Group

Ending the group is not coterminus with ending therapy. Therapy ends as it started, with an individual family session with the key therapist. Each family, therefore, has at least a good-bye session with the therapist but may continue some further individual family work after the group has ended if this is needed. The final work with the group echoes some of the themes from the ending phase of single-family therapy: reflecting on endings in general and how people deal with them, reviewing the progress achieved thus far, considering any further work that needs to be done and by whom, thinking about relapse prevention and discussing where responsibility lies, if problems reemerge, to seek future help.

In addition, there are specific issues around the ending of the group itself. Above all, they include the need to highlight the handing back of responsibility to the families. At the penultimate follow-up, family members are, therefore, invited by the MFT team to think about how they may want to end the 9-month life cycle of their group. Endings can vary from an inclusive event such as a group meal together, often marking public eating as no longer the utmost challenge it was, to a quieter parting when individual families share reflections on progress and change in the room where the group began. Families often develop ending rituals (sometimes devised by individual families, in other groups separately, by mothers, fathers, and adolescents). These are often very creative and moving exercises led and managed by the families themselves and not by the MFT staff.

Case Example: The N Family

The following is a composite case example that illustrates how a family's participation in MFT kept their two adopted anorexic daughters out of the hospital.

The N Family at Outpatient Assessment

Jo (17) was referred to the Child and Adolescent Eating Disorders Service by her general practitioners (GP). She lives with her biological sister Jasmine (15) and their adoptive parents, who also had a daughter together—Anna (23). Jo was severely underweight, having developed entrenched restrictive eating patterns over 12 months.

Following initial assessment Jo was given a clear diagnosis of AN. A treatment plan including MFT was agreed upon. Given Jo's poor physical health and the level of risk, with consequences of starvation, her parents were advised to keep her out of school until she was physically more stable.

At the same meeting, her parents reported their increasing concerns that Jasmine (15) was significantly influenced by her older sister's restrictive food behaviors. Recently, Jasmine had been hiding food after evening meals and making herself sick, which she strongly denied. Her mother described the sisters' relationship as close, but in recent years a competitiveness over their adoptive status, school achievements, and sport successes had developed between them. She was fearful that the eating disorder was another issue over which they could compete. Their older sister Anna had moved to Thailand 2 years earlier after finishing her degree. She has since married and had twins just before Jasmine came to the service. Anna has a strong bond with both sisters, particularly Jo.

Over the last few months their mother had noticed that Jasmine was becoming "increasingly skinny." We recommended that Jasmine be referred to the service so we could assess her current presentation. Her mother was anxious that Jasmine wouldn't agree to any appointments, as every time she tried to talk to her youngest daughter she became aggressive and hostile. Jo was very much affected by her sister's outbursts and had started to self-harm with superficial cutting on her upper arms.

A Month Later

Both sisters were receiving outpatient treatment with different therapists and were in the first treatment phase—both Mom and Dad had taken time off from work and with support from the team had set up a "hospital at home" as a way of taking back control so that both sisters could start to eat. The parents were attending each separate family therapy session. Jo was 4 weeks into treatment and struggling with better food management; Jasmine had been assessed, despite intense opposition about coming to the service, and was starting to eat better but always in a separate room. Like her sister she clearly met the diagnostic criteria for AN and had a similar weight for height as Jo, even though she was 3 centimeters shorter. An MFT group was due to start in 2 weeks. Both parents were keen to participate as AN at home was "reveling in the competition as to who could eat less and get thinner faster"—they were desperate to meet with other families for support and new ideas. Their enthusiasm was not echoed by either of their daughters.

Two Weeks Later

Jo and Jasmine attended the introductory evening with both their parents and five other families. They sat separately and had no verbal communication with each other or with their parents. In the young people's group both sisters engaged well with listening to the "graduate" who had recently ended with her group: "I went to the group because my parents forced me to go—but looking back, I'm glad I did."

Both parents connected well with others and were surprised and reassured to hear that the graduate family had also set up a hospital at home 2 years earlier. Their main concern that evening was whether their two daughters would agree to attend the 4 intensive days.

The Following Week

The weekend after the introductory session was "fraught with arguments about food and unbearable" for the N family. Both sisters argued with each other and blamed their mother for not being the perfect mother and for even going near a psychiatric hospital, let alone agreeing to their treatment at "such a place"—they stuck to their meal plans, but meals took up to 3 hours. Dad was anxious about how they would manage until the group began, and Mom held onto normality by spending a hour an evening with her close friend.

On the first morning of the group both sisters attended with their parents. One of the first things Dad said in the opening exercise was that neither daughter wanted to come. Quite quickly another dad echoed a similar sentiment. As the families connected with each other, the parents joined in commonality while the six young people did the opposite, by sitting in still silence. This started to change after the young people had worked together on an exercise, "what anorexia means to me." Jo, as the eldest in the group, assumed a more authoritative role, and rather than fighting with her sister listened quite actively when Jasmine started talking about her relationship with AN, which was quite different from Jo's. A key difference for the sisters was that Jo saw being thin as socially acceptable, equaling more friends and more fun, but things had gotten out of control. Jasmine believed that being a successful anorexic would open doors for her and there was no way she was going to stop.

During group mealtimes Jo struggled, but after longer sittings ate what her parents brought. Jasmine stuck by her mantra that she wouldn't give up on AN and so refused lunch and snacks on the first day. This stance shifted when she had meals with different parents the next day. That evening she ate dinner with her mother in 45 minutes—the first time since the introductory evening. The sisters continued to fight over who owned AN and who was better at fooling Mom and Dad.

As the 4 days came to an end, although exhausted and running on empty, Mom and Dad expressed renewed vigor, with maintaining the "hospital at home" arrangement monitored and reviewed by their continuing family-based sessions. They were disappointed that both Jo and Jasmine had lost weight by the end of the intensive days, but were leaving with greater insight about the illness, its unpredictability, and the time needed to move on from it.

Mom—"Important to hear other families' experiences, try things that have worked for them and not feel so alone."

Dad—"Had no idea we all needed to be as brave as we have been to fight this illness."

Jo—"Saw a side to my dad that I didn't know was there. ... I want to see if we can stop arguing over food—Jasmine has to try too."

Jasmine—"I can't bear the thought of having to talk about all this for months to come. I wish Anna was here, I want to see the twins. ..."

Six Months Later

The group finished shortly afterwards. Both sisters returned to school a few weeks after the intensive days—Dad went back to work and Mom negotiated a part-time contract. They are still in treatment with individual family therapy and have joint sessions with both therapists.

Jo had just finished high school and despite the stress of exams had managed to reach a nearly normal weight. Jo's relationship with Jasmine remained tense, as she heard her railing against her older sister's recovery. Jasmine was gradually accepting that her life could be bigger than AN was allowing. She was glad to be back at school but angry with her parents for not trusting her more. Her physical health was more stable, but her weight remained below the normal range for her age and height.

Example of a Theme Explored in the First Phase of Treatment

The following is an example of an exercise— interviewing the "grip" of anorexia using role reversal—that we used to introduce the process of externalizing anorexia in the N family's group. This was used during the first phase of treatment and therefore applied to the intensive days of MFT.

Preparation

Subgroups of young people, mothers, and fathers are formed. Each group works on its own for 15 minutes.

Young People Thinking as Parents

The therapist facilitates the young people's group to explore what they would imagine their parents think the grip of AN is and the effect it would be having on the young people during mealtimes and nonfood periods. How does the grip behave: Does it speak, move in a particular way, get angry, or otherwise? The young people consider what strategies their parents have used to help dampen the control of this grip of AN on their lives. Catch phrases, slogans, and thoughts aloud for both tasks are captured on paper.

Parents Thinking as Young People

For parents to gain greater insight about the grip of AN, one therapist each facilitates a separate mothers' and fathers' group (if there are only two therapists running the MFT group, one therapist moves between the mothers' and fathers' groups). They explore different perspectives about what they think/experience/imagine the voice of anorexia to be saying to their young people during mealtimes and nonfood times. What strategies have they used to help dampen the control of AN over their lives? Catch phrases, slogans, thoughts aloud are captured on paper.

Role Reversal

The whole group re-forms. Two young people in the role of parents interview the grips of AN (mothers) with remaining group members observing through either a one-way screen or an imaginary one-way screen. The therapist sits in as a silent observer.

To the grips of AN: "As a parent group we really want to understand what we're up against when you are constantly persuading our children not to eat or gain weight or stop exercising." "What gets you most agitated?" "What do you like to happen?" "What do you not like to happen?" "What or who manages to stop you from 'holding on'?" "When you are tired, where do you go?" "What do you like to call yourself?"

When the interview is over, the therapist invites the group to stay in role and say what it is like to be interviewed by "parents" as the voices of anorexia.

Feedback

Following a "deroling" exercise, group members reflect on what they learned, noticed, and felt.

Points to Consider

This task has added power when it has been preceded by exercise(s) in which the grip/voice of AN has been enacted. This can be either a family sculpt or a role-play exercise when the grip/voice of AN is invited to join (a member of staff voicing AN thoughts during the exercise).

Preparation time is important so that each subgroup has enough time to absorb instructions and meaning. Equally, enough time needs to be given to getting in and out of roles; this would help to build and deflate the appropriate use of tension and intensity.

Therapists need to rely on the caveat "It may be like this for some but not for all" an/or "Taking part in this exercise helps us to imagine what the experience might be like for the young people."

With potentially powerful exercises such as this one, it is effective to call a break period after the feedback and give some processing time once members of the group have realigned with each other.

Future Directions

Although MFT is not a new treatment approach, its specific use in the treatment of adolescent AN is still relatively new and there is a great deal that we still have to learn about it. Future developments will be guided in part by the findings of the multicenter RCT that has recently been completed as well as new research currently being developed. A prospective longitudinal mediator/moderator study is due to start shortly, which should provide information about factors determining which families are most likely to benefit from the treatment and, perhaps more important, what might be the mechanisms of change underpinning the treatment.

There are now a growing number of centers around the world utilizing MFT in the treatment of adolescent AN, and the different service contexts in which this is happening are leading to variations in the MFT programs. This has included the integration of MFT days into inpatient and day programs to promote shorter admissions, earlier discharge, and better preparation for postdischarge family life and reduction of relapse rates. MFT programs are also being utilized in geographical contexts where travel time makes regular attendance at therapy sessions difficult for many families, for whom a greater number of 1- to 2-day group follow-up meetings are easier to organize than weekly or twice weekly outpatient sessions. The MFT program in Dresden, for instance, very seldom includes single-family sessions but has up to 20 follow-up days for the group over 12 months (Asen & Scholz, 2010).

There have been several positive reports of the use of MFT in the treatment of BN (Asen & Scholz, 2010; Slagerman & Yager, 1989; Wooley & Lewis, 1987). These MFT groups have generally been less intensive than those described in this chapter, and more work is needed to determine the type of group that might work best for young people with this disorder.

Conclusion

Although MFT for adolescent AN is still in its infancy, it is showing good outcomes and receiving positive feedback. Work is still needed to continue to empirically examine MFT in adolescent AN and the impact of MFT on clinical outcomes and recovery as well as the cost-effectiveness of such treatment.

References

Ackerman, N. (1938). The unity of the family. *Archives of Pediatrics, 55*, 51–62.

Andersen, T. (1987). The reflecting team: Dialogues and meta-dialogues in clinical work. *Family Process, 26*, 415–428.

Anderson, C. M. (1983). A psycho-educational program for families of patients with schizophrenia. In W. R. McFarlane (Ed.), *Family therapy in schizophrenia* (pp. 99–116). New York: Guilford Press.

Anderson, C. M., Griffin, S., Rossi, A., Pagonis, I., Holder, D. P., & Treiber, R. (1986). A comparative study of the impact of education vs. process groups for families of patients with affective disorders. *Family Process, 25*, 185–205.

Asen, E. (2002). Multiple family therapy: An overview. *Journal of Family Therapy, 24*(1), 3–16.

Asen, E., Dawson, N., & McHugh, B. (2001). *Multiple family therapy. The Marlborough model and its wider applications*. London: Karnac Books.

Asen, E., & Scholz, M. (2010). *Multifamily therapy concepts and techniques*. London: Routledge.

Asen, E., Stein, R., Stevens, A., McHugh, B., Greenwood, J., & Cooklin, A. (1981). A day unit for families. *Journal of Family Therapy, 4*, 345–358.

Barrett, P., Healey-Farrell, L., & March, J. S. (2004). Cognitive-behavioral family treatment of childhood obsessive–compulsive disorder: A controlled trial. *Journal of the American Academy of Child and Adolescent Psychiatry, 4*, 46–62.

Behr, H. (1996). Multiple family group therapy: A group analytic perspective. *Group Analysis, 29*, 9–22.

Bion, W. R. (1961). *Experiences in groups and other papers*. New York: Routledge.

Brennan, J. W. (1995). A short-term psychoeducational multiple-family group for bipolar patients and their families. *Social Work, 40*, 737–743.

Byng-Hall, J. (1995). Creating a secure base: Some implications of attachment theory for family therapy. *Family Relations, 34*, 45–58.

Colahan, M., & Robinson, P. H. (2002). Multifamily groups in the treatment of young adults with eating disorders. *Journal of Family Therapy, 24*, 17–30.

Cooklin, A., Dawson, N., McHugh, B., & Oakley, M. (2003). *Marlborough family therapy basics*. London: Marlborough Family Service.

Cooklin, A., Miller, A., & McHugh, B. (1983). An institution for change: Developing a family day unit. *Family Process, 22*, 453–468.

Dare, C., & Eisler, I. (2000). A multi-family group day treatment programme for adolescent eating disorder. *European Eating Disorders Review, 8*, 4–18.

Dare, C., Eisler, I., Russell, G. F. M., & Szmukler, G. I. (1990). The clinical and theoretical impact of a controlled trial of family therapy in anorexia nervosa. *Journal of Marital and Family Therapy, 16*, 39–57.

Dawson, N., & McHugh, B. (1994). Parents and children: Participants in change. In E. Dowling & E. Osbourne (Eds.), *The family and the school: A joint systems approach to problems with children*. London: Routledge.

Dawson, N., & McHugh, B. (2005). Multifamily groups in schools: The Marlborough model. *Context, 79*, 10–12.

Detre, T., Sayers, J., Norton, N., & Lewis, H. (1961). An experimental approach to the treatment of the acutely ill psychiatric patient in the general hospital. *Connecticut Medicine, 25*, 613–619.

Eisler, I. (2005). The empirical and theoretical base of family therapy and multiple family day therapy for adolescent anorexia nervosa. *Journal of Family Therapy, 27*, 104–131.

Eisler, I., & Lask, J. (2008). Family interviewing and family therapy. In M. Rutter, D. Bishop, D. Pine, S. Scott, J. Stevenson, E. Taylor, et al. (Eds.), *Rutter's child and adolescent psychiatry* (5th ed.). Oxford, UK: Blackwell-Wiley.

Eisler, I., Le Grange, D., & Asen, E. (2003). Family interventions. In J. Treasure, U. Schmidt, & E. van Furth (Eds.), *Handbook of eating disorders: Theory, treatment and research* (2nd ed.). London: Wiley.

Eisler, I., Lock, J., & Le Grange, D. (2010). Family-based treatments for adolescents with anorexia nervosa. In C. M. Grilo & J. E. Mitchell (Eds.), *The treatment of eating disorders: A clinical handbook* (pp. 150–174). New York: Guilford Press.

Fairbairn, P., & Eisler, I. (2007). Intensive multiple family day treatment: Clinical and training perspectives. In S. Cook & A. Almosino (Eds.), *Therapies multifamilales des groupes commes agents therapeutiques* [Multiple family therapy: Groups as therapeutic agents]. Paris: Eres.

Fonagy, P., Gergely, G., Jurist, E., & Target, M. (2002). *Affect regulation, mentalization, and the development of the self*. New York: Other Press.

Fristad, M. A., Goldberg-Arnold, J. S., & Gavazzi, S. M. (2003). Multi-family psychoeducation groups in the treatment of children with mood disorders. *Journal of Marital and Family Therapy, 29*, 491–504.

Gonzalez, S., Steinglass, P., & Reiss, D. (1989). Putting the illness in its place: Discussion groups for families with chronic medical illnesses. *Family Process, 28*, 69–87.

Gowers, S. G., Weetman, J., Shore, A., Hossain, F., & Elvins, R. (2000). Impact of hospitalisation on the outcome of adolescents' anorexia nervosa. *British Journal of Psychiatry, 176*(2), 138–141.

Hess, J., & Handler, S. (1961). Multidimensional group psychotherapy. *Archives of General Psychiatry, 5*, 92–97.

Jackson, D. (1957). The question of family homeostasis. *Psychiatric Quarterly Supplement, 31*, 79–90.

Jackson, D., & Weakland, J. (1961). Conjoint family therapy: Some considerations on theory, technique and results. *Psychiatry, 24*, 30–45.

Kaufman, E., & Kaufman, P. (1979). Multiple family therapy with drug abusers. In E. Kaufman & P. Kaufman (Eds.), *Family therapy of drug and alcohol abuse*. New York: Gardner.

Keel, P. (2008). Evidence-based psychosocial treatments for eating problems and eating disorders. *Journal of Clinical Child and Adolescent Psychology, 37*, 39–61.

Laqueur, H. P. (1972). Mechanisms of change in multiple family therapy. In C. J. Sager & H. S. Kaplan (Eds.), *Progress in group and family therapy*. New York: Brunner/Mazel.

Laqueur, H. P. (1973). Multiple family therapy: Questions and answers. In D. Bloch (Ed.), *Techniques of family psychotherapy*. New York: Gardner.

Laqueur, H. P., La Burt, H. A., & Morong, E. (1964). Multiple family therapy: Further developments. *Current Psychiatric Therapies, 4*, 150–154.

Lemmens, G. M., Eisler, I., Buysse, A., Heene, E., & Demyttenaere, K. (2009). The effects on mood of adjunctive single family and multi-family group therapy in the treatment of hospitalised patients with major depression: An RCT and 15 months follow-up study. *Psychotherapy and Psychosomatics, 78*, 98–105.

Lemmens, G. M., Eisler, I., Migerode, L., Heireman, M., & Demyttenaere, K. (2007). Family discussion group therapy for major depression: A brief systemic multi-family group intervention for hospitalized patients and their family members. *Journal of Family Therapy, 29*, 49–68.

Lock, J., Le Grange, D., Agras, W. S., & Dare, C. (2001). *Treatment manual for anorexia nervosa: A family-based approach*. New York: Guilford Press.

Mason, B. (1993). Towards positions of safe uncertainty. *Human Systems, 4*, 189–200.

McFarlane, W. R. (1982). Multiple family therapy in the psychiatric hospital. In H. Harbin (Ed.), *The psychiatric hospital and the family*. New York: Spectrum.

McFarlane, W. R. (2002). *Multifamily groups in the treatment of severe psychiatric disorder*. New York: Guilford Press.

McFarlane, W. R., Lukens, E., Link, B., Dushay, R., Deakins, S. A., Newmark, M., et al. (1995). Multiple-family groups and psychoeducation in the treatment of schizophrenia. *Archives of General Psychiatry, 52*, 679–687.

McFarlane, W. R. (2004). Family intervention in first episode psychosis. In T. Ehmann, G. W. MacEwan, & W. G. Hone (Eds.), *Best care in early psychosis intervention: Global perspective*. Oxford, UK: Oxon.

McHugh, B., Dawson, N., Scrafton, A., & Asen, E. (2010). "Hearts on their sleeves": The use of systemic biofeedback in school settings. *Journal of Family Therapy, 32*, 58–72.

Meads, C., Gold, L., & Burls, A. (2001). How effective is outpatient care compared to inpatient care for the treatment of anorexia nervosa? A systemic review. *European Eating Disorders Review, 9*, 229–241.

Miller, A. L., Rathus, J. H., & Linehan, M. M. (2007). *Dialectical behavior therapy with suicidal adolescents*. New York: Guilford Press.

Minuchin, S., & Fishman, H. C. (1981). *Family therapy techniques*. Cambridge, MA: Harvard University Press.

Ross, W. D. (1948). Group psychotherapy with psychotic patients and their relatives. *American Journal of Psychiatry, 105*, 383–386.

Salaminiou, E. (2005). *Families in multiple family therapy for adolescent anorexia nervosa. Response to treatment, treatment experience and family and individual change*. Unpublished doctoral thesis, Kings College, University of London.

Salaminiou, E., Campbell, M., Simic, M., Kuipers, E., & Eisler, I. (2005). *Multi family therapy for adolescent anorexia nervosa: A pilot study*. Manuscript submitted for publication.

Satir, V. (1964). *Conjoint family therapy: A guide to theory and technique*. Palo Alto, CA: Science and Behavior Books.

Scholz, M., & Asen, E. (2001). Multiple family therapy with eating disordered adolescents: Concepts and preliminary results. *European Eating Disorders Review, 9*, 33–42.

Scholz, M., Asen, E., Gantchev, K., Schell, B., & Süß, U. (2002). Familientagesklinik in der Kinderpsychiatrie: Das Dresdner Modell—Konzept und erste Erfahrungen. *Psychiatrische Praxis 29*, 125–129.

Scholz, M., Rix, M., Scholz, K., & Thomke, V. (2005). Multiple family therapy for anorexia nervosa: Concepts, experiences and results. *Journal of Family Therapy, 27*, 132–141.

Slagerman, M., & Yager, J. (1989). Multiple family group treatment for eating disorders: A short term program. *Psychiatric Medicine, 7*, 269–284.

Steinglass, P. (1998). Multiple family discussion groups for patients with chronic medical illness. *Families, Systems and Health, 16*, 55–70.

Steinglass, P., Gonzales, S., Dosovitz, L., & Reiss, D. (1982). Discussion groups for chronic hemodialysis patients and their families. *General Hospital Psychiatry, 4*, 7–14.

Strelnick, A. H. (1977). Multiple family group therapy: A review of the literature. *Family Process, 16*, 307–325.

Tomm, K. (1987a). Interventive interviewing:

Part 1. Strategising as a fourth guideline for the therapist. *Family Process, 26,* 3–13.

Tomm, K. (1987b). Interventive interviewing: Part II. Reflexive questioning as a means to enable self-healing. *Family Process, 26,* 153–183.

Tomm, K. (1989). Externalising the problem and internalising personal agency. *Journal of Strategic and Systemic Therapies, 8,* 1–5.

Weber, M., Davis, K., & McPhie, L. (2006). Narrative therapy, eating disorders and groups: Enhancing outcomes in rural New South Wales. *Australian Social Work, 59*(4), 391–405.

White, M. (1989). Anorexia nervosa: A cybernetic perspective. *Family Therapy Collections, 20,* 117–129.

Wooley, S., & Lewis, K. (1987). Multi-family therapy within an intensive treatment program for bulimia. In J. Harkaway (Ed.), *Eating disorders: The family therapy collections.* Rockville: Aspen.

Yalom, I. (1970). *The theory and practice of group psychotherapy.* New York: Basic Books.

CHAPTER 14

Adolescent-Focused Psychotherapy for Anorexia Nervosa

Ann Moye
Kara Fitzpatrick
Renee Rienecke Hoste

This chapter examines the application and structure of adolescent-focused psychotherapy (AFP), a manualized approach to the treatment of adolescents with anorexia nervosa (AN) in which the identified patient is seen individually and parents or parental figures are seen separately in sessions referred to as collateral sessions. Although individual psychotherapy approaches have had a long history in clinical practice, manualized treatment protocols with this population are sparse and not well represented in the scientific literature. The purpose of this chapter is to introduce the reader to the theory and basic tenets of this treatment approach (see also Fitzpatrick, Moye, Hoste, Lock, & Le Grange, 2010). AFP for AN is an approach developed for use with older children, adolescents, and young adults with AN or eating disorder not otherwise specified (EDNOS) who have restrictive eating symptoms and weight loss, with or without purging behaviors. We consider this approach appropriate for those who are medically stable for outpatient treatment, regardless of prior hospitalization status, and for those who can commit to weekly psychotherapy sessions.

AFP is based on the assumption that eating disorders represent a maladaptive strategy for managing the transitions and demands of adolescence. The primary goal of this treatment, along with weight restoration, is to define issues that have overwhelmed the patient's ability to cope with specific developmental conflicts, such as self-evaluation, identity formation, friendship or family conflicts, and/or sexuality issues. The long-term goal is to help patients learn healthier coping skills, then restricting food by defining a healthier sense of self and by basing self-esteem on qualities other than the physical self. This chapter provides further evaluation of the techniques and skills necessary to implement this approach while also providing case material to assist the reader in understanding the implementation of the approach.

Background of Individual Approaches to AN

Individual treatments for adolescents with AN form the majority of the approaches used in clinical practice. However, research on treatment modalities has largely focused on family treatment approaches (Le Grange & Lock, 2005). Despite the growing literature on family-based approaches and their ongoing use, there remains a need for individual approaches to eating disorder treatment. This need exists because not all families are willing or able to participate in family therapy, and 15–30% of patients appear not to benefit from family therapy (Krautter & Lock, 2004). Furthermore, such approaches are important for older adolescents/young adults for whom a family modality may be at odds with their living situations and developmental levels, such as those who live at boarding schools away from families or in families with significant language or cultural barriers to treatment. Finally, individual approaches are also warranted to assist patients and families who identify the need for additional individual support in their efforts toward recovery. Practical examples of families for whom individual treatment options may be of particular importance include those with specific family issues, including the death of a parent, when the remaining parent may be immobilized with grief and/or overwhelmed with additional responsibilities; those in which parents are in marital crisis with a high level of conflict and unable to form a parental coalition of support for their adolescent; those in which there is remarriage and/or emotional issues between the parents and children, such as a history of abuse or neglect or parental psychopathology, including parental eating and substance abuse disorders, which may not have been sufficiently addressed.

Despite the sparse research literature on individual treatments for AN, there is a long history of individual approaches in clinical practice: traditional psychodynamic formulations (Levenkron, 2000; Thoma, 1967), neoanalytic techniques that address both development and ego formation (Robin, Siegal, Koepke, Moye, & Tice, 1994), interpersonal psychotherapy techniques (McIntosh et al., 2005), and cognitive-behavioral and cognitive-analytic techniques (Gowers et al., 2007; Pike, Walsh, Vitousek, Wilson, & Bauer, 2004; Treasure et al., 1995). The goal of most individual therapy approaches for adolescent AN is the development of self-efficacy and self-care in the management of weight, body image, and shape concerns (Crisp, 1980; Robin et al., 1994), and these goals are also relevant for AFP.

Work with adolescents requires an understanding of the nesting of adolescents within families, and newer approaches often no longer carry the pejorative view of families that dominated in early clinical work, but instead seek to create support from the family to assist in the adolescent's recovery (Bryant-Waugh, 2006; Robin et al., 1999). Furthermore, individual therapies with a pediatric population have a strong focus on development, independence, and maturation as fundamental tenets guiding interventions (Crisp, 1997). Thus, the advancement of developmentally focused, targeted interventions for AN in children and adolescents remains an important goal for scientist-practitioners, and such work should include individual as well as family-based approaches.

Research Support for AFP

The initial version of the treatment referred to here as AFP was called ego-oriented individual therapy (EOIT) and was manualized for a study to examine the efficacy of the approach (Robin et al., 1994). In this study, 22 adolescents with AN were randomly assigned to behavioral family systems therapy (BFST) or AFP (Robin et al., 1994, 1999; Robin, Siegel, & Moye, 1995). In BFST, which combined behavioral, cognitive, and family systems components to encourage weight gain, the therapist met with the patient and his or her parents together. In AFP, which focused on strengthening the patient's ego functioning, the therapist met with the patient alone and had bimonthly collateral sessions with the parents. The study found that both treatments were effective in producing weight gain, although patients in the BFST group gained more weight and had greater rates of menstrual return than patients in the AFP group. Both treatments resulted in similar improvements on measures of eating pathology, interoceptive awareness, depression, internalizing behaviors, and eating-related family conflict. Similar results were found with a full sample of 37 adolescents with AN (Robin et al., 1999). These studies provided the basis for a larger multisite study at Stanford University and the University of Chicago (Lock et al., in press). In this study, 121 adolescents with AN were randomly assigned to 12 months of either AFP or family-based treatment (FBT) (Lock, Le Grange, Agras, & Dare, 2001). FBT was superior to AFP in terms of weight gain and changes in eating-related psychopathology at the end of treatment, but these did not differ at 12 month follow-up. However, FBT was superior to AFP in terms of rates of recovery (normal weight and normal eating-related concerns) and lower rates of relapse at 6- and 12-month follow-up. Nonetheless, subjects treated with AFP did well and there were clear benefits to the approach.

Basic Principles of AFP

AFP is derived from self psychology. As noted previously, early manualized versions of this treatment modality used the name EOIT (Robin et al., 1994), but the name to was changed to AFP to reflect the importance of an adolescent-driven, focused means to address core deficits in development associated with AN. Within this model adolescents with AN are viewed as using issues of food and weight to avoid negative mood states and developmental challenges with which they are having difficulty negotiating successfully. The overarching treatment goal for this modality is to teach adolescents with AN to identify and cope effectively with emotional states and to navigate the multiple challenges of adolescence in a successful and healthy manner. This is done by assisting patients in learning to identify emotions, tolerate negative emotions, and begin to adaptively address difficulties without resorting to self-starvation and abnegation.

Although weight gain is the immediate treatment goal, the first premise of the AFP modality is that weight gain, in itself, does not resolve AN, which consists of a set of cognitive beliefs and behaviors that must also change in order to sustain long-term recovery, prevent relapse, and allow the adolescent to return to a normal lifestyle, appropriate to his or her age. The second premise is that a strong therapeutic relationship between the therapist and the patient is necessary and is best defined and treated by what Levenkron (2000) called a "nurturing/authoritative" relationship with the patient. The third premise of AFP is based on the presumption that the foundation of the disorder stems from the patient's maladaptive coping with stresses normal to the life stage of adolescence, when developmental changes have an impact on every aspect of his or her life as well as an individual life crisis (e.g., death of parent, divorce). As adolescents begin experiencing dramatic shifts in their bodies, including brain and cognitive development, they often feel thrown into a disturbing process of change that is both physical and psychosocial.

The young adolescent is usually transitioning from elementary school to middle or high school and thus is often separated from and/or redefining friendships and social identity. In addition, he or she begins to individualize, disengaging from the family and seeking more time with peers, which may create challenges in the family as renegotiation of rules and roles are often in order. This stage of adolescent development, referred to as separation and individuation, represents the transition from childhood that begins roughly at age 13 and typically ends at about 19 years of age. In Western culture, the push toward independence and autonomy are core adolescent goals, and this is manifested in thinking styles, opinions, and most areas of self-expression. In addition, with greater independent interaction, the world of the adolescent becomes rich with more relationships, with both peers and adults, with whom they interact and need to manage potentially competing goals. Finally, in this stage adolescents also experience increased responsibility and self-motivation, which creates the need for the development of skills to regulate emotions, attention, and resources. Adolescents begin to experience peer pressures, and the need to fit in sometimes becomes an overwhelming and driving force. When feelings of inadequacy result in a focus on the physical self, and other aspects of identity formation and self-esteem are not strong, the seeds of an eating disorder can be planted. This is often manifested as a belief that being thin will "cure everything." The adolescent's control over the intake of food may offer some false comfort and sense of empowerment, thus circumventing learning these skills from more natural and sustainable experiences.

The Role of the Therapist

AFP strongly emphasizes the role of the therapist as an agent for change and as an authority figure who assists the patient in developing a sense of self and connection with family and peers, while insisting on behavioral changes that lead to weight restoration and health. As such, it is vital that therapists employing this model have specific characteristics and operating models that we view as critical to overcoming eating pathology. First and foremost, therapists must have a strong background in child and adolescent development and experience in working with families (Lock, 2005). As developmental issues set the stage for this targeted treatment, therapists must have a solid understanding of these issues, as well as a finger on the pulse of the adolescent culture in which they practice. Adolescents continuously seek role models outside the family during this time of development, and society often gives them mixed and confusing messages. Most adolescents work through this confusion successfully, but the adolescent with AN may not. The therapist who has a working knowledge of what adolescents experience has better insight into what has overwhelmed the patient, which facilitates the designing and development of a treatment plan.

Development of a supportive and nurturing relationship with the adolescent helps the patient to think about and respond to areas of developmental impairment and facilitates recovery by providing a nonjudgmental connection and support in navigating (or renavigating) challenges that have been inappropriately resolved in the past. The relationship itself is essential because it is through the creation of a dependable, solid, and well-boundaried relationship that self-exploration and development of insight take place.

Simultaneously, the therapist uses an authoritative approach to emphasize the need for weight gain, healthy behaviors, and adherence to medical recommendations. This may be thought of as a "re-parenting" relationship, although this is not meant to suggest any specific deficits or difficulties with parents of patients, as families are in fact seen as key elements to treatment, but rather that the nature of the parenting role may best describe the balance between firm and focused guidance coupled with enduring respect and caring for the patient. The therapist must never collude with the eating disorder, such as by keeping secrets or enabling an avoidant stance in which issues of food, eating, shape, and weight/weighing are not addressed in treatment. Rather, the therapist must take a stance that encourages growth and supports autonomy. This is often a significant challenge, as the desires of the patient may be directly at odds with the medical recommendations and strategies that support recovery. The ability to maintain a firm stance, in which expectations can be clearly and nonjudgmentally related, can be quite challenging. This is particularly true for novice therapists, who often feel that to create a relationship, one must be supportive of the patient's goals and desires. In a case of AN, however, the therapist must always remain committed to the healthy aspects of the patient, while directly and compassionately addressing the ways in which symptoms interfere with healthy adjustment, even when the patient may have difficulty accepting this information.

The Treatment Team

AFP relies on a team of clinicians to support the therapist. The therapist is the leader of the team and coordinates the team. A physician typically provides ongoing medical feedback, including cardiac assessment and bloodwork evaluations, if indicated. The physician's role is to monitor the patient to ensure that the patient is safe for continued outpatient care, as well as to provide information on the patient's medical progress in recovering from malnutrition and starvation. If possible, this physician should have a thorough knowledge of the medical problems associated with malnutrition and should appreciate the difficulties associated with AN during adolescence. A misplaced statement by a physician can inadvertently encourage continuation of the eating disorder thinking, and many of our patients and families report physicians telling them that they "don't look so bad" or they will "gain weight naturally." Unfortunately, such statements may lead to complacency in the face of disease and/or redoubled efforts at restriction to avoid predictions of weight gain. Physicians are vital in helping patients and families to see the medical consequences of starvation. This is often most necessary when patients have recovered sufficient weight to no longer be visibly or catastrophically medically unstable, but continue to require weight gain to address the long-term consequences of malnourishment.

In addition, teams also utilize a dietician to set weight restoration goals and monitor the progress of the patient. Ideally, the dietician has expertise in understanding how patients with eating disorders struggle with eating normally. In conjunction with the physician, the dietician may be responsible for setting weight goals and meeting with both the patient and the parents. This professional may plan the details of the process of weight gain and educate both the patient and his or her parents in how the body uses food and, particularly, the change in caloric and energy needs as the body recovers from starvation. The rationale for this role's being separate from those of the therapist and physician is that the parents have already struggled to refeed their child and this effort has often become an area filled with conflict and anxiety. The adolescent who has refused to cooperate may increase the feelings of powerlessness and frustration in the parents. The dietician may also recommend meal plans. When no dietician is available, the functions described here often fall to the monitoring physician and the therapist. Usually, parents are responsible for providing the food and the adolescent is responsible for eating it. The team must be consistent in seeing AN as a serious disorder that requires treatment. In general, parents take a supportive role while the patient has the role of learner in order to become responsible for his or her own well-being.

Phases of Treatment

AFP consists of three phases of treatment (see Table 14.1). The goal of the first phase is to establish rapport and begin a formulation of the patient's psychological issues and the ways in which AN serves as a coping strategy for managing or avoiding other challenging developmental issues. In addition, the patient is encouraged to begin to integrate responsibility for food-related issues and self-care into his or her concept of self. The second phase encourages exploration of individuation issues of adolescence (self-efficacy, school and work goals, social identity) with an emphasis on establishing developmentally appropriate independence from the family of origin and self-directed emotion regulation. The third phase focuses on preparing the patient for adolescent problems (sex, drugs, school stress, etc.) and encouraging initiation of behaviors or strategies that continue to lead to independence.

It is important for the therapist to establish a trusting, supportive, and educational relationship with the patient. Patients rarely seek treatment on their own, and they may think of their eating disorder as a friend or a solution instead of a problem, leading to defensiveness in the early stage of treatment. The initial sessions are designed to assess and formulate a hypothesis of the triggering events, either external or internal, that contributed to the development of the AN. No matter how knowledgeable the therapist is about the complexities of AN, the greatest challenge at this early stage of treatment is to create a trusting relationship. The therapist's knowledge must be presented in a language that the adolescent can understand and accept. Because the therapist is often dealing with highly intellectual and verbal adolescents, most patients are good candidates for therapy, yet it is important to remember that they are still adolescents in their thinking. As such, they may struggle with future orientation and abstract reasoning and may be attracted to or drawn into ideas that are not as relevant to the adults around them. An adolescent female, for example, may be more interested in the fact that she may experience hair loss as a result of AN than she is about the longer-term implications of prolonged starvation (e.g., infertility, bone loss, death), as these seem to lie too far in the future to be concerned about. Some symptoms may seem irrelevant to the patient, so it is important to focus on those that impact what most adolescents cherish, such as physical appearance. For young males with AN, it may be the potential loss of height or loss of muscle mass that is most motivating. The therapist should be perceptive to and aware of the challenges, interests, and issues facing adolescents with AN and utilize these to address their unique concerns.

Sometimes adolescents with AN are more comfortable sharing aspects of their lives and emotions more indirectly, and in these cases a journal can be suggested for recording feelings with words and/or pictures. The patient can bring this to each session to share, leading to further discussion. Although it may be important to define parental

TABLE 14.1. The Three Phases of AFP

With patients	With parents
Phase 1	
• Set boundaries, including those for confidentiality and sharing of information.	• Set boundaries, including those for confidentiality and sharing of information.
• Set a framework and expectations for therapy, including timing and frequency of sessions.	• Set a framework and expectations for therapy, including timing and frequency of sessions.
• Set expectations for therapeutic change, including expectations for weight gain.	• Set expectations for therapeutic change, including helping family members understand the nonlinear progression of treatment.
• Psychoeducation on food, nutrition, weight and shape issues.	• Psychoeducation on food, nutrition, weight and shape issues.
• Review of eating behaviors.	• Review of eating behaviors for the patient and other family members.
• Development of a nonjudgmental, supportive relationship with patient.	• Development of a nonjudgmental, supportive relationship with parents.
• Thorough history related to food and eating.	• Family history, including medical and developmental history of the patient.
• Thorough history of family and peer relationships.	• Thorough history related to food and eating of patient.
• Exploration of adolescent culture/themes and activities relevant to the patient.	• Thorough history of family and peer relationships of patient.
• Exploration of cognitive, behavioral, and emotional responses to pivotal events in the patient's history.	• Exploration of adolescent culture/themes and activities according to parents.
• Identification of methods of self-expression (art, music, language, writing).	• Exploration of parental responses to pivotal events in patient's history.
• Separation of the patient from the eating disorder (e.g., "Sounds like AN was really in charge in that situation").	• Assess parents' ability to support refeeding in a nurturing, authoritative stance.
• *For the therapist*: Development of a case formulation identifying patient strengths and the developmental areas in which the patient needs the most support to move toward recovery.	• Coach parents in refeeding.
Phase 2	
• Continued exploration of history, as well as recent events and responses, to begin to create a personal narrative.	• Continued exploration of history, as well as recent events and responses, to begin to help parents see patterns and identify areas of strength and growth.
• Identification of patterns of emotional and behavioral responses to challenges, including continued return to issues of eating, shape, and weight as necessary.	• Normalization of process of recovery (e.g., addressing increases in depression or anxiety, even in the face of decreasing eating disorder symptoms).
• Exploration of emotional expressiveness: ability to identify and express emotions. May include discussions of self-expressive techniques not previously utilized or utilized in other contexts (see Phase 1), such as art, music, and journaling.	• Identification of family patterns of emotional and behavioral responses to challenges.
• Exploration of coping skills/emotion regulation strategies—how the patient manages emotions and various situations, particularly those that trigger certain behaviors.	• Continued psychoeducation on eating disorder symptoms. Coach parents on refeeding challenges.
• Facilitate the development of new strategies, encourage patients to identify strategies used by others, or generalize from strategies used in other situations. Draw from skills such as diaphragmatic breathing, behavioral experiments, grief work, and so forth, as directed by case formulation.	• Education regarding normal adolescent development and local adolescent culture.
	• Assisting with communication patterns that support healthy adolescent development.
	• Encourage family focus on values and emotional development and a move away from performance behaviors.
	• Reinforce skills taught in individual patient sessions.
• Develop insight by exploration and questioning in areas of challenge or behavior patterns.	• Encourage identification of outside resources and supports for the patient and family.

(cont.)

TABLE 14.1. *(cont.)*

With patients	With parents

Phase 2 *(cont.)*

- Appropriate self-disclosure of emotions ("That would have made me feel sad, but I'm not sure ... how did you feel?").
- Appropriate self-disclosure of coping strategies ("We all have things we do to help us manage our feelings, such as listening to particular music when we are feeling a certain way").
- Exploration of patient's intimacy and interpersonal relatedness—what it means to be close to someone, how we know when and how to let people into our inner world.
- Management of ambiguity, learning to accept uncertainty.
- Discussion of values and separation of values and self-evaluation from performance.
- Assertiveness and communication skills.
- Identification of possible resources and supports for patient to facilitate recovery or development or to address concerns.
- Exploration of grief and loss, if warranted by case formulation.

Phase 3

With patients	With parents
• Continued exploration of normal adolescent behaviors. • Problem solving of anticipated difficulties, changes, and potential losses (e.g., moving away from home, change in friendships, termination of treatment; particularly important for those who have experienced previous losses). • Discussion/problem solving and addressing issues of sexuality, intimacy, and risk-taking behaviors. • Fostering continued adjustment in social, academic, and health-related behavior. • Addressing concerns related to relapses. • If comorbidity is present and requires additional intervention, a discussion of means to address these difficulties.	• Parents' exploration of their own adolescence and how this impacts parenting styles and expectations. • Fostering continued adjustment of the patient in social, academic and health-related behaviors. • Addressing concerns related to lapses, relapses, and need for ongoing treatment. • If comorbidity is present and requires additional intervention, a discussion of means to address these difficulties.

issues that cause stress (e.g., feelings about a divorce, drug or alcohol use), a nonblaming attitude toward both the patient and the parents is imperative in order to build a solid foundation. Furthermore, by not resting blame on others, the patient is encouraged to take responsibility for learning better coping skills. As many patients with AN express responsibility for areas clearly outside the realm of their control (e.g., making "everyone else feel happy"), self-exploration into apportioning blame, responsibility, and control may become grist for the therapeutic mill. The goal is typically to assist patients in seeing that they often have less control over situations than they might believe and, in situations in which they have not caused their present difficulties, it is still their responsibility to develop better coping mechanisms to help manage these concerns.

During this first phase of therapy, it is pertinent to educate the patient and parents about the effects of starvation and unhealthy weight loss behaviors and to establish clear expectations for recovery. The patient must understand that food is necessary in order to live and that, once recovered, he or she will enjoy food and not be afraid of it. Goals are set in regard to expectations for intake and weight gain, and fears are directly addressed. Clear, consistent language that directly confronts the adolescent's concerns is essential. For example, patients are reminded that "fat" is not a feeling. Weight restoration is non-negotiable, hence the *authoritative* stance; however, the therapist remains compassionate about the emotional issues presented by the adolescent, hence the *nurturing* stance. The therapist must continuously work on the patient–therapist relationship and agree on the goal of understanding the emotions and conflicts that led to the eating disorder. This relationship does not usually develop smoothly or quickly, as the patient may express fears of getting fat if he or she eats, expressing that he or she likes being thin and may think the therapist wants him or her to get fat. Consequently, the therapist must be patient and calmly continue educating the patient. This education should not be solely focused on cognitions about eating and weight, but can also begin to explore the ways in which certain behaviors may have an impact on relationships with those closest to the adolescent or on the patient's emotional expression.

An important way in which the therapist can support relationship development is by taking an active interest in, and dedicating full attention to, areas of the patient's life in which he or she may express interest, passion, or desires that are separate from the eating disorder. Therapists engaging in AFP often find that they can disentangle patients from AN preoccupations by focusing on specific areas of expressed interest, which allows patients to teach the therapist about areas of their lives that they hold dear. Therapists using this modality often find it important to read the books that patients are reading, or to explore music, art, or sports that are relevant to their patients. This interest is not only a useful tool for engagement, but also allows excellent modeling for the very skills we hope patients will develop in their relationships with others. In addition, therapists may find that modeling emotional language and recognition is important at this stage. Therapists should pay close attention to times when there are changes in affect, then explore these or question the change in mood, to help patients better identify triggers for affective change. Therapists may also find it useful to engage in emotional self-disclosure during Phase I and may suggest ways in which a particular situation, event, or interaction may have made them feel, and wonder if the patients' feelings may be similar or different, as well as why this is the case. Key goals of Phase I are to help patients learn a richer language of emotional expression, identify their own shifts and changes in feelings, and begin to uncouple these from the relationship with food and eating.

In the early phase of treatment, the therapist must pay particular attention to the ways in which the adolescent patient reacts and responds to him or her. For example, a patient may react in ways that seem evocative of other core relationships, or may express fears or expectations in subtle ways. One of us (A. M.) had such an experience with a patient with whom she had been working for some time. The patient's parents were divorced and her father was infrequently involved in parent collateral sessions, but both the patient and her mother believed that including the father in an upcoming collateral session would be critical. The therapist agreed to speak with the girl's father, but then fell ill and did not call him in a timely fashion. At the next session the therapist apologized for not having scheduled the session, and the patient noted, "I know, everyone else is afraid of him too, and everyone avoids him." The therapist noted the subtle implication that both the patient and her mother were afraid of the father, as well as the patient's belief that the therapist would have the same feelings, which led the patient to interpret failure to set up an appointment as evidence that the father was also scary to the therapist. This provided a rich area of discussion about how to approach people whom one is "afraid of," whether avoidance meant fear or if there were other feelings as well, and ways that the therapist could have managed this situation differently. In AFP, even subtle statements and dilemmas can provide a rich tapestry for the exploration of self and others.

During Phase II, dialogue between the therapist and patient and therapist and parents puts emphasis on the development of positive self-esteem, issues of conflict, family dynamics, and behavioral change. Together, the therapist and the patient define and explore issues of separation and individuation. Exploration of ways in which individuals build a healthy self-esteem should continue and are an ongoing focus during this phase of treatment. Because the goal is to develop a healthy self-esteem, discussions should center on supporting the development of relationships that are supportive of the patient. In addition, differentiating between intellectual activities (e.g., curiosity and exploration) and intellectual performance (i.e., getting good grades) is often important at this point. The objective is to help the patient find and define his or her personal passions in life; to discover broader emotions from which a healthy self-esteem evolves, including the capacity for joy, fun, and giving of oneself; and to examine the ways in which one balances the often competing demands of these areas. In some cases, the patient can also use journal writing to enhance this process, which should be encouraged along with other forms of self-expression.

As the patient begins more active self-exploration, this is typically accompanied by behavioral activation, with enhanced steps to manage difficulties outside the session or in response to issues raised in previous therapy appointments. Although in Phase I suggestions for change or exploration may be initiated by the therapist, it is common in Phase II to have patients come to a session having identified and tackled a problematic area or concern. This greater independence and self-motivation to manage conflicts and challenges is the hallmark of the move toward recovery. For example, a patient had been working on developing stronger peer relationships following a move to a new school. In Phase 1, these issues were largely discussed in the context of how she perceived herself and her social skills. However, with greater insight and understanding, she began to take more active steps in the initiation and development of friendships. Between sessions she independently set herself the task of identifying and talking to two people with whom she felt she might be able to have a friendship. When such activation occurs, the tenor of the sessions often shifts from insight development and self-exploration to more active evaluation of the ways in which patients are now acting on their world, their responses to others, and the responses of others toward them. Therapists should be supportive of self-initiated changes and explorations, particularly those that address areas of typical adolescent functioning. It has been the experience of therapists working with this model that some adolescents begin to explore adolescent developmental issues related to sexuality, identity, spirituality, and rule-breaking behavior during this phase of therapy. Most often this is within the realm of normal adolescent exploration, but some adolescents appear to run headlong into adolescent exploration and "make up for lost time" with such behavior, which can be challenging for patients, parents, and therapists alike. As always, the safety of the patient is paramount and must be considered in terms of clinical management.

In addition, the therapist can provide continued assistance in developing a sense of personal narrative. Such a narrative, or understanding of the ways in which AN has served a purpose for the patient in managing specific difficulties, should begin to incorporate new ideas, interests and passions. The narrative may be thought of as a personal tapestry that patients might weave to tell a story about themselves, and this can and should change significantly over the course of adolescence, in general, and in treatment more specifically. Patients often have limited capacity to view themselves and their illness. They may view their worth and their goals as being tied to weight or other performance areas (e.g., grade point average). Through questioning and focused interest on other domains, patients can be encouraged to develop a richer sense of themselves, with more complexity in self-definition and self-esteem. The shift from a narrow focus on eating/ shape and weight as measures of self-worth toward a broader conception of self necessitates a focus on the ways in which eating disorder symptoms interact with other aspects of their lives and relationships with others. Initially, many patients want to reject AN—to act as though they do not have the disorder or to deny that it is relevant to their sense of self as they recover. However, a true and balanced conception of self should include both strengths and weaknesses, areas in which they have successfully navigated challenges as well as those areas in which they may continue to struggle or need to watch to make certain they are not "derailed" from their tasks and goals in the future.

One young patient entered treatment with a very narrow view of herself. She was able to describe herself only in terms of being "thinner than my porky self before and really good at math, which makes other people jealous. Routine is good, change is bad." As treatment progressed, she was able to expand the horizon of values, relationships, and interactions that described her world, such that she was able to describe herself as someone who was intellectual, but not necessarily driven, an animal lover, and a person who wanted to help others. Furthermore, her view of her disorder went from seeing it as a preoccupation with a sense of balance, routine, and rigid ideas regarding weight, to an understanding that these concepts helped her feel more secure when she was faced with uncertainty, but were not necessarily issues "under [her] control" as she had seen them before. She began to enjoy, and even seek out, spontaneity and areas of change, recognizing that change, by itself, could be directed by her, rather than experienced as incongruous or painful. Throughout this process, not only did her sense of self change, her AN and the purpose of her weight loss and dietary restriction became understood in a larger context. Rather than viewing others as "jealous" of her low weight, she began to acknowledge that she was the only one who valued such stringent dietary practices and that her rigid adherence to her goals interfered with her ability to have the comfortable social interactions she longed for. She also began to describe AN as a "state of control" to which she would retreat so as to help her make sense of more challenging emotional or social demands. This expansion of self and insight helped her to see the ways in which she used her eating to cope with social isolation, and the ways in which her eating kept her socially isolated, such that she could begin to explore new ways of approaching these challenges.

During Phase II, patients may be expressing new issues to the therapist with strong emotions, or they may have difficulty managing stronger emotions that arise as they confront problems with eating or in other domains. For example, a patient may express feeling unloved by a parent because the parent may be an alcoholic or may have divorced. A fear of attending school may be expressed as well, believing that he or she does not have friends or that he or she is not accepted. These issues should not be subject to platitudes or simple encouragements, but should be explored for the opportunity to develop insight into the self (e.g., what would make someone want to chose me as a friend or a partner?), understanding of relationship development (e.g., who am I attracted to?), and skill building (e.g., how do I approach, invite, or connect with others?). These issues can be explored in depth, and relevant themes, concerns, or insights that arise can form "touchstones" for anchoring the therapy and providing continuity in the therapeutic process. These also are opportunities to examine how preoccupation with food and other ways of thinking characteristic of AN make it more difficult to achieve self-understanding by distracting attention and focus away from other important developmental areas. For example, the therapist may assist the patient in noticing the ways in which he or she may turn to restriction when frustrated or angry. This self-knowledge can then be used to begin to develop coping skills or strategies or to guide the practice of new behaviors in the face of these emotions. For patients struggling with emotional identification and expression, Phase 2 typically involves increased depth of emotional expression and a broadening of the language to describe feelings, reflecting an increased appreciation for the subtleties of emotions.

In Phase 3 of treatment, the therapist remains supportive of the patient while encouraging the patient to understand his or her emotions and experiences. AFP posits that a critical goal of adolescence is the development of independence and autonomy. Independence skills are those that represent emotional and cognitive individuation while establishing personal values, ideals, and morals. Autonomy, though related to independence, refers to more general behaviors expected of those who are independent, such as self-motivation, self-care, and responsibility behaviors (e.g., doing laundry, paying bills, etc.). Expectations of more independence and self-reliance should be conveyed, both to the patient as well as to the parents, during this stage of treatment. If the parents have been less active in treatment, the therapist should also strive to transfer support of the patient from the therapist to the parents or other social supports. This may occur through the identification of other resources (e.g., peers, extended family, teachers, group therapies, coaches, or sports teams) as well as assisting parents in developing communication skills and strategies (discussed in more detail on the next page in the section "Parent Collateral Sessions"). In this Phase, it is hoped that the parents will experience their child as expressing him- or herself more and as becoming more effective in problem solving. Parents usually begin to understand that all adolescents disagree at times with their parents, typically seek privacy, and often want to be with their friends more than with family, and can accept that these are part of normal adolescent development and a critical part of moving beyond the eating disorder.

Because Phase 3 is the final phase, termination becomes the focus of treatment. In AFP termination is of particular importance, given that the relationship with the therapist is considered the critical change agent. The therapist should broach the topic of termination as patients begin to exhibit normalized behaviors in the realm of food/eating and in relationship development. Even when termination is agreed upon, the patient may begin to fear termination or become afraid of a relapse, which can lead to the need for reassurance that the therapist will be available. The patient may express an ongoing struggle with eating disorder thoughts and a fear of not being healthy. The therapist should respond to the patient's fears by providing education about relapse and praising him or her on the successful learning and identifying of his or her emotions and the ability to separate them from food and body image issues. A genuine satisfaction with the work the patient has completed and the confidence and trust that the therapist now has for the patient's future can be very advantageous for the patient's moving forward. However, the therapist should also reassure the patient that he or she will be available, if needed, and perhaps identify some support systems for wherever the patient may be in the future. It is important to note that many patients terminate treatment, not at a point at which they are thoroughly adjusted, but rather when they have achieved significant goals in relation to health and self-esteem. Therefore, another important part of termination is to anticipate areas that may challenge the patient in the future. This reminds patients and families that self-development continues across the lifespan and is an important focus for patients long after the termination of treatment. For many therapists practicing AFP, contact with patients following termination provides opportunities to view their continued adjustment and development after treatment ends. In addition, many therapists have had the experience of receiving strong positive messages long after termination from even patients who had been the most resistant, which speaks to the enduring importance of the therapeutic relationship formed in AFP.

Parent Collateral Sessions

Recognizing that adolescents with AN have a profound impact on the functioning of the entire family, parent collateral sessions form an essential part of AFP. These sessions engage parents, without the patient present, at critical junctures in treatment. Although we call these sessions "parent" collaterals, the therapist may meet with any members of the family, provided the patient and parents have identified these individuals as support elements. Collateral sessions can involve older siblings who may have a caretaking role, significant others of young adults, grandparents, and family friends who may have an important role in the family or provide support to the family in managing issues related to AN.

Within the collateral sessions, the therapist serves as a resource in helping the family to transfer therapeutic gains to the home environment. This most often begins through psychoeducation on the nature and idiosyncrasies of AN. Parents are often confused by the hold the illness has on their child and find it mystifying that their child might be tremendously successful in many areas other than the eating disorder, but struggles so mightily with AN. Helping families understand the ego-syntonic nature of the disorder is often critical to helping the support system recognize and respond appropriately to eating disorder symptoms.

The separation of these sessions from those of the patient serves two purposes: first, it allows the therapist to develop distinct relationships with the patient and with his or her family members, and second, it allows for communication that is relevant to each group in a clear and consistent manner. In other words, the patient's time is not spent discussing or arguing with parents, and concerns can be voiced and responded to freely by all parties. Sometimes, for example, parents seek treatment after lengthy battles with their adolescent resulting in frustration and/or anger. The emotions of the parents are often so intense that is more appropriate to see them without the patient. The sessions with the parents are designed to provide both education and support in regard to the eating disorder and the delayed development that the eating disorder causes. Because adolescents often start to separate from their parents as they strive to become individuals,

AFP maintains the need to establish a family dynamic that is open to discussing strong emotions of all family members and that can work through areas of potential mixed messages, development of differing value systems, and support for individuation, while continuously supporting development within the context of the family. These sessions are not meant to mimic some types of family therapy sessions in which family process and communication are key targets for intervention, but rather to assist parents in developing an understanding of specific concerns related to AN, their child's development in particular, and adolescent development more generally. Although specific situations may be discussed or problem solved in collateral sessions, in general the focus of these sessions is a better understanding of family support for the patient and assisting parents in identifying resources, challenges, and ways in which they can facilitate recovery for their adolescent.

Goals for the initial collateral sessions include not only psychoeducation on the nature of the illness, but also instruction on the physiological/medical sequelae of the illness. In addition, the therapist serves as the central communicator for the treatment team to ensure that there is clear, consistent communication between the patient, family members, and the treatment team. Parents are considered "co-therapists," to the extent possible; however, the responsibility of recovery rests significantly with the patient. In the initial phase of treatment, collateral sessions focus mainly on refeeding issues. Parents are coached to present a united front with the same nurturing/authoritarian stance as the therapist uses in regard to food issues. The overriding message is that food is medicine and the parents provide the medicine and see that the medicine is taken. In the case where a parent or parental figure is not available, the therapist and the dietician increase their role in this critical aspect of treatment. In this sense, it is also vital that parents and other caregivers understand the nature of therapy. This begins with an understanding of informed consent and the limits of confidentiality. Although these vary across locations, therapists should be clear in discussing how and when they will transmit information to family members and to other team members. In addition, the therapist bears the responsibility for making the boundaries of information sharing clear to family members, discussing steps that will be taken if the patient is no longer considered safe for outpatient treatment (e.g., is medically unstable), and clarifying the role of each team member.

AFP can also be framed by discussing with the family the expected progression in treatment. Many families hope to see immediate progress in weight and associated symptoms, and, although this goal is often shared by clinicians, helping patients and families understand that the therapeutic process is often not a linear one, with clear progression toward goals, is useful in helping them weather early challenges or perceived setbacks. Furthermore, it is important for families to understand that patients may initially make progress on goals that do not appear to be directly related to food, eating, or shape/weight, such as developing stronger relationships and attachments, and that this progress should be viewed as valuable to the overall process of health restoration.

Families may have any number of particular concerns or challenges in initiating treatment. Parents may be terrified or skeptical of the severity of the disorder. They may want to wait for treatment until the adolescent is finished with a seasonal sport, the semester, or finals or until their child wants to pursue treatment. They may even deny that there is a disorder, stating that she or he is too smart for this and has always been the perfect child. The parents may be feeling anger because of their child's constant refusal to eat and ongoing fights over food. Consequently, the therapist needs to develop a nurturing, but less authoritative, relationship with the patient while being supportive and encouraging of the parents and incorporating education on adolescent psychology. The parents need to be reminded that the goal is to have their child return to "normal" adolescent challenges, which may be a marked deviation from previous behaviors, particularly when adolescents begin to explore more challenging behaviors or begin to experiment with sexuality or other previously rejected activities. In addition, parents can be coached in how to communicate more effectively with their adolescent through the understanding of techniques such as focused attention, giving rewards, ignoring, and the setting of limits and consequences. Modeling for parents the nurturing–authoritative relationship style that is effective in establishing more open interactions is a critical strategy for setting up parents to assume a stronger role in helping their adolescent navigate new challenges. When parents have their own challenges in assisting their adolescent with managing ongoing developmental concerns, the therapist may work with the parents to develop necessary skills or address specific family challenges within the parent collateral sessions. The goal is always to shore up the strengths of families, reduce criticism of the patient, and encourage the family to reorient toward stronger coping behaviors in the adolescent.

In later collateral sessions, the therapist and family members may set goals around any number of issues, including understanding and supporting continued efforts toward normalized eating and health, and understanding social and emotional changes in the adolescent. As the AFP therapist should be knowledgeable in adolescent development, this knowledge can be leveraged to assist parents in understanding the nature of adolescent development and to clarify the goals and milestones of development across the age span and in their adolescent, in particular. Parents often benefit from specific guidance in ways to support their adolescent in exploring issues related to independence, autonomy, emotion regulation/expression, and intimacy. This is particularly true for families in which the identified patient is the eldest or only child, or there are cultural differences between the adolescent and his or her family, where the family may lack experience or context for understanding (or remembering) the climate of adolescent change in the realm of cognition, behavior, and relationships. For many parents, AN presents additional frustration inasmuch as, prior to the onset of the illness, the patient may have been viewed as a compliant child, often a perfectionist, with success in both academic and extracurricular activities. To both the adolescent and the parents, success often has come easily, and both are surprised by the disruption in functioning. Assisting families in attenuation of criticism and creating an atmosphere for open communication and introspection may also be relevant goals at this stage of treatment. In addition, assisting parents in setting boundaries in other adolescent behaviors or in broaching the discussion of these topics, including sexuality/intimacy, substance use, and rule-breaking behavior, may also be relevant for discussion at this stage of treatment, particularly for families who may find changing behavior patterns and adolescent exploration to be confusing and even upsetting.

As the sessions proceed, the therapist should have discussions with the parents about the various aspects of treatment. Because the therapist has encouraged the patient to share feelings with the parents, it is appropriate for the therapist to ask the parents how those dialogues went. For example, the patient may have shared a concern, such as a pending divorce, with the therapist, who may then have encouraged the patient to share those concerns with his or her parents. With the patient's permission, the therapist should ask the parents about those discussions. Sometimes it is helpful to talk to a parent about a difficult childhood that he or she may have experienced to determine if that parent developed healthy coping skills that could be shared with the patient. Because the parental sessions are intended to be supportive and educational, it is helpful to check on goals set at previous sessions and to assure parents that although there may be setbacks, their child is developing the ability to identify his or her needs and ask for help in getting these needs met. Parents should be encouraged to continue communicating with their adolescent about how they can support his or her growth and development. Other parents may have difficulty adjusting to a patient who is fighting less about food, but showing increased resistance to rules and expressing a desire to spend less time with the family and more time on the phone or with peers. The therapist can assure parents that this is "normal" adolescent change and can guide them in setting rules and boundaries. Most important, the therapist should stress that the patient's problems may not be completely resolved, but that the patient realizes it is his or her responsibility to address these issues. The patient should, however, be encouraged to continue seeking the parents' support and guidance.

Case Examples

To highlight the ways in which the treatment phases may coalesce in the treatment of an individual with AN, two case studies are presented, utilizing the paradigms to guide treatment application described in this chapter.

Case 1: Identity Conflict, Loss, and AN

A significant move served as the key trigger for the development of AN in C.S., a young mixed-race (African Korean) 14-year-old male. His parents were missionaries with an extended history of travel, which began prior to his birth and lasting until he was 5 years old. During C.S.'s early school years, his parents had been stationed in the United States at a teaching college in the Midwest. After he had graduated from elementary school, C.S.'s parents requested a transfer to work on a missionary project in South Africa. C.S. was excited by this opportunity and described his time in Africa as a time of "richness, friendship, and discovering roots," as he was able to meet his father's extended family that had remained in Africa. After 2 years, however, C.S.'s maternal grandmother became ill, requiring his parents to move to assist in her care. Shortly after C.S.'s 13th birthday, the family made a significant transition to Korea, which was described as challenging for the entire family—not only did it mean a significant move and associated language barrier, but C.S.'s mother was also caught up in caring for her ill and aging mother. C.S.'s grandmother passed away within 6 months, and the family agreed to leave Korea to return to the United States where C.S. could finish his high school education.

Phase 1: Building Therapeutic Alliance and Initial Formulation

In Phase 1, C.S. worked with a therapist in developing a relationship to explore issues of loss, change, and acculturation. The predominant therapeutic techniques utilized in these early sessions focused on gathering the elements of a rich history and in developing a relationship that allowed C.S. to explore different ideas about spirituality and identity. The use of a journal as a complementary therapeutic tool allowed C.S. to formulate possible ways of solving problems, reimagining various scenarios, and developing a language for expressing emotions.

At the intake session, both parents expressed significant guilt for the onset of the eating disorder. They reported that they had believed that each decision had been the best for the family at the time it had been made, but C.S. expressed that, upon returning to the States, he was unhappy and felt left out and unusual in his peer groups. After months of working to establish relationships, his parents noticed his increased weight loss and significant social withdrawal. Most notably, C.S. rejected their spiritual values and retreated from church-based social gatherings, which had been his primary social arena until that point. They were alarmed at his rapid emaciation and took him to see several specialists. Because of the extensive family travels, C.S. was evaluated for numerous travel-related illnesses and viral infections and, not until he had reached 67% of his ideal body weight (IBW), was AN considered as a diagnosis. C.S. reported that he had been a willing participant in all of his family's travels, but realized that he had "no place that was home." Even with his sadness and withdrawal, he demonstrated a wonderful sense of humor, indicating that even though he knew he had to struggle with AN, at least he did not have malaria—a nod to his many medical tests.

Therapy was initiated after hospitalization, which returned C.S. to medical stability and resulted in a discharge weight that was 78% of his IBW. C.S. was initially quiet and somewhat withdrawn in his interactions with the therapist. He could relate activities and adventures from his past, but he did so with relatively little emotion, connection, or passion. Yet he was often tearful in sessions and had difficulty articulating the cause of his sadness. His parents, feeling guilty, attempted to supply him with a variety of foods and activities, but would retreat in frustration when he suggested to them that their choices had led him to this illness. When the therapist pointed out that he seemed to enjoy this power over his parents—the ability to make them do things for him, provide favored foods, and reject any or all of these things on a whim—he agreed and burst into tears. The therapist suggested that this was a hollow victory for him because he had a strong relationship with his parents despite their increasing frustration with his failure to gain weight. He reported feeling that he had moved far from who he had been and did not know what he wanted any more.

From this information, the therapist developed a formulation that involved a predominant theme of grief and loss. In his many moves, C.S. had lost contact with friends and social settings. Each time he had moved, he had immersed himself in a new culture, and sometimes a new language, and had done so successfully. As he aged, however, these social transitions became increasingly difficult. The most recent two moves, to Korea and then back to the United States, had been unique. Previous moves had been well considered and met with significant social support, in the form of church and spiritual structure, that had made it easy for C.S. to assimilate. The move to Korea was the result of a sudden loss and involved an additional challenge, in that C.S.'s mother was suddenly thrust into a new role as caregiver to her ill mother. The combined lack of social structure, financial burden on the family, and C.S.'s mother's own grief had made this a particularly stressful transition.

The return to the United States resulted in C.S. beginning a new high school where he had few of the normative experiences that his peers had shared; he did not know their games, music, activities, or hobbies and felt that he had lost sight of who he had become. Although issues of race and culture were raised and explored in therapy, C.S. rejected these as central to his challenges: however, the therapist continued to hold to these issues as a potential area for future exploration and identity development. Key elements of the case formulation included identification of segments from his past that he had to grieve (as they could not be replicated in his current setting), assistance with expressing his feelings toward his unusual childhood experiences, and developing an identity that would allow him to thrive in his current setting. It should be noted that in integrating his past experiences, the expectation was not that these would be universally negative, as is so often thought of with grief, but rather acknowledging the powerful positive and enjoyable experiences, as well as the difficulties of his past.

C.S. used a journal to write stories about his experiences, often told as tales in the third person, which he entitled "The Story of My Life." He was remarkably talented in his writing abilities and found writing helpful in therapy sessions. His sense of humor and irony provided an avenue to discuss embarrassing emotions or to relate his discomfort in a manner that felt acceptable to him. In this way, he was able to provide the therapist with a view of his isolation, but also his strengths. In retelling these stories, the therapist worked with C.S. to make effective connections to these experiences, modeling emotional expression or encouraging him to relate a tale with and without humor. The therapist also identified themes in these stories and tales that were reflected back to C.S. as unifying elements to his "story of life." For example, C.S. often provided copies of his journal writings for the therapist prior to a session. These were read, even annotated, with ideas related to discussions from previous therapy sessions, questions, and even just highlighting a particularly gifted turn of phrase. C.S. always began a session with a review of his week and an introduction of his new writing. He was capable of providing responses to direct questions, which often focused on the choice of a topic, the use of humor, or an undercurrent of emotion, but he was rarely spontaneous in his responsiveness. During this stage of therapy, weight gain was slow and halting, with minimal progress.

In addition to individual sessions, collateral sessions with C.S.'s parents were of particular importance. In the initial sessions the therapist provided psychoeducation on AN and explained the groundwork of treatment. An effort was made to assist the parents in managing their own grief over their child's illness and the loss of a beloved parent. Furthermore, both parents expressed incapacitating guilt, which prevented them from providing structure and enforcing age-appropriate demands on C.S., allowing him to withdraw and disengage further from the family and social activities. The therapist encouraged the parents to maintain and continue to strengthen their own social structure as well as building consistent, expected social activities into C.S.'s life. For example, as missionaries and ministers, the family was active in the church, and C.S.'s withdrawal from church life was viewed by the parents as a significant rejection of the family. The parents were encouraged to allow C.S. to contemplate issues of faith, but they did require participation in secular family activities and social events.

Phase 2: Exploring Identity and Alternatives to AN

Throughout Phase 2, the focus was on assisting C.S. in developing a fuller notion of himself and his role both in his family and in his community. Although he had stated that he rejected most of his parents' values, he continued to engage with them in neutral activities and began to express feelings and opinions, rather than retreating into silence. Simultaneously, he and the therapist worked to identify peers and activities that would support

C.S. in his evolving conception of self. Specific anxiety-reducing skills were taught, but treatment focused on helping C.S. identify realms in which he could confidently explore relationships with others.

As C.S. became more comfortable in identifying parts of himself that he valued, he and the therapist worked to develop ways of strengthening these behaviors in his new setting. He indicated intense social anxiety at the thought of meeting new people and, as a result, he had been at his local high school for 2 months and had spoken "about four words." He noted that he was the "shy, skinny kid in the back corner," and although he knew he could talk to people, his anxiety prevented him from doing so. He achieved great benefit from relaxation training, including diaphragmatic breathing and imagery. Indeed, without prompting, he reported applying these steps in situations in which he needed to eat and thought that this resulted in greater intake at meals. He was also able to use therapy to practice conversations, allowing him to identify negative thoughts about himself that made him more likely to withdraw. Underlying these discussions was an emphasis on how these behaviors were tied into his disordered eating patterns. For example, his social withdrawal made him more likely to view AN as his "friend," and his continuous self-criticism gave greater strength to his belief that being thinner would allow him to compensate for his perceived personality flaws. He continued to deny any potential challenges of race or cultural identity, although it was evident that many of his perceived weaknesses were related directly to his difficulty in understanding elements of American culture. He had challenges in identifying popular movies, music, and cultural references and often looked at these with some disdain. The therapist recommended that C.S. explore some of the issues he rejected through his writing, such as writing a review of a popular film for the school paper. In this way, he was encouraged to approach cultural issues from his own perspective while not abandoning his beliefs. Thus, an effort was made to integrate these two perspectives utilizing the best of his strengths.

C.S. continued to make positive progress in managing his anxiety and reaching out to others. His writing ability was noticed by his English teacher, who urged him to join the school newspaper and take a journalism course. Although he did so reluctantly, this proved to be a wonderful opportunity, as it provided small-group social interactions around specific ideas and themes in an arena in which C.S.'s skills and talents were praised. He began writing a column, entitled "My Life," in which he detailed the life perspectives of various students, teachers, and school staff members. He found this work tremendously rewarding, as it allowed him to meet and understand others in a personal way through the means of writing. By interviewing, observing, and integrating his knowledge of the lives of his peers and classmates, he gained greater appreciation for the similarities between his own struggles and those of his "normal" peers. His writing became a key way in which he could express his own frustrations, pointing out injustices and finding ways to share common experiences with others. His greater confidence was reflected in his increasing social network and his increased weight. He made steady weight progress over the course of several months and reached his ideal body weight after approximately 7 months of treatment.

Unfortunately, C.S. experienced a significant setback. A popular football player at his school, who had been chronicled by C.S. in his school newspaper column and who had befriended C.S., was killed in a car accident. C.S. was strongly affected by his friend's death, and this intensified when the boy's parents requested that C.S. read the column he had written about their son at his eulogy. C.S. experienced this as another profound loss and was struck by the ways in which he had touched the life of this family and the extent to which the loss brought back his own feelings of isolation and loneliness. C.S. began to isolate himself socially, and to restrict meals, resulting in a slow weight loss. His parents were quick to react and noted that they realized he had been set back by this loss. They responded with a spiritual approach, which C.S. rejected outright. He announced that he did not believe in their faith or their values, which was deeply upsetting to the family. With guidance from the therapist, the parents were able to develop a neutral language for the discussion of this loss for C.S. They acknowledged that their son's dismissal of their core values was painful, but tolerable, and they expressed the need to "fight for his life before his soul." On his part, C.S. expressed a desire to consider several issues in his family. Therapy began to address his disappointment in what he perceived to be his parents' desire to put "all of God's family before our own" and in the way his mother had handled her own grief. He expressed great anger with his parents, himself, and spirituality. This provided an opportunity to discuss ways to express and manage intense emotions of anger and sadness with C.S. while encouraging his family to allow him developmentally appropriate expression of these emotions. He was able to identify a great fear in getting close to others for fear of losing them and related this to his history of moving. He began to weave a story of his own experiences that helped him make sense of his feelings and reactions.

After a month, C.S.'s mood began to improve and he was more receptive to social requests by peers. He won a local journalism contest and several of his columns were reprinted by a national publication, to which he responded with great pride. He noted that he was beginning to take pleasure in the way his mind worked and the way he was able to touch people's lives with his writing. His family relationships also improved. C.S. told his parents that he wanted to pursue a career in journalism, rather than the ministry, as they had hoped. Instead of responding with disappointment, as he had expected, his parents reacted with joy and pride in his talent. They noted that part of what they had loved about missionary work had been travel, meeting new people, and the experiences they had had with other cultures, and they felt that C.S.'s career aspirations embodied many of their own values and matched their son's talents. They also noted that his increased independence and social relatedness helped them feel more secure in supporting his efforts at separation from them.

During this phase, he was able to manage meals and eating independently. Decreased conflict among family members about meals led to stronger ties and improved their relationships with one another. C.S. steadily gained weight throughout Phase 2, and although he began by increasing quantities of "safe" foods, he was later able to tolerate greater flexibility. This issue was addressed in sessions by noting his greater flexibility in spending time with peers and in exploring new activities, which was a natural parallel to his restrictive eating patterns.

Phase 3: Termination

Termination occurred naturally for C.S. He was largely weight restored, achieving approximately 97% of his IBW, with much of this occurring during Phase 2. As he completed his junior year of high school, he opted to participate in a study abroad program that would take him on a tour of Asia for the summer. C.S. had researched this program, applied for it, and chosen to participate after lengthy discussions with his parents.

Although his parents expressed some concern around his ability to maintain his weight, the larger issue was that C.S.'s new girlfriend was also going to be attending the same program and the family was concerned about sexual improprieties. C.S. and his parents struggled with notions of sexuality, values, and problem solving. The family ultimately had frank discussions related to parental expectations of behavior, C.S.'s own value system concerning sexuality, and expected levels of adult monitoring for C.S. The family was able to identify goals across physical, social, and psychological domains that needed to be met prior to departure, and all agreed on these. Physically, C.S. was to maintain his weight and do so with little interference or monitoring by the family. He was expected to prepare his own lunches, though he and his parents continued to eat together as a family at dinnertime. Encouraged to explore physical activity, C.S. joined a capoeira group (an Afro-Brazilian martial art/dance mix) that he felt "fit [his] funky looks and background." Psychologically, the family wanted to see C.S. manage day-to-day chores with less stress and procrastination, and laundry became a "hot topic" in treatment. Socially, it was expected that C.S. continue to behave responsibly in terms of curfew and friendships, but also that he identify and participate in activities of shared value to himself and his family. Surprisingly, C.S. chose one church-based activity (working in a church's homeless shelter) despite his continued assertions that he was not a "man of faith."

C.S. himself reflected on the termination of therapy, seeing it as very important. He expressed his feeling that therapy had been useful for him in terms of thinking about his role in his family, which was surprising, given the nature of his social strides relative to family relationships. He described therapy as "the opportunity to put myself under a microscope that I usually reserved for other people and found that I actually liked what I saw." C.S. wrote a "column" for the therapist as a termination gift—a story of his own life, integrating the key experiences in his life and mapping this out as a journey of discovery that would continue into the future. He cast the therapist as an oracle, "who could be consulted, but usually told the seeker something that he already knew about himself." He noted that he felt much the same way, in that therapy helped him uncover aspects of himself that he knew continued to exist.

Case 2: Identity Conflict and Emotional Neglect

A.S. was an 18-year-old female, living with her mother and 25-year-old sister. Her biological parents divorced when she was 8 years old. Her mother remarried, but at the time of treatment her mother and stepfather were separated. A.S. came for treatment after being discharged from an inpatient eating disorder treatment program. At her first appointment she weighed 112.5 pounds, putting her at 80% of IBW. According to A.S., she began restricting her eating in sixth grade, at which time she also began feeling depressed. She alternated between restricting and overeating for several years, before developing AN as a freshman in high school. At the time of her assessment she was taking Prozac (20 mg).

Phase 1: Building a Therapeutic Alliance and Initial Formulation

In Phase 1, the focus was primarily on developing rapport with A.S. and learning more about her history. Before beginning treatment with the therapist, she had seen another therapist for several months with whom she thought she had developed a good relationship. According to A.S., this relationship was abruptly terminated when her insurance ran out. She felt abandoned by the previous therapist, was angry at therapists in general, and was disinclined to talk to a new person. Thus, it was important for the new therapist to communicate patience with A.S.'s reluctance to open up and a genuine desire to get to know her better. A.S.'s weight stayed fairly stable during the first phase of treatment.

A.S. had had a difficult childhood. When she was a teenager, her stepfather encouraged her to drink alcohol and smoke marijuana with him. He often made derogatory remarks about her weight and made fun of her if she ate a large meal. For several years he weighed A.S. and her sister weekly and ridiculed them if their weight increased. He was regularly emotionally abusive and was physically abusive on a number of occasions, but A.S. denied any history of sexual abuse. Her mother denied any knowledge of the abuse and said that her daughters did not tell her at the time the abuse was occurring because they were protective of her. A.S.'s mother was an attorney who worked long hours and was emotionally quite cold. When she did show emotion, it was usually anger. During a collateral session at the beginning of treatment, it became clear that she was extremely critical of A.S. and believed that many of her behaviors were driven by a desire for attention. She reasoned that her other daughter had also suffered abuse at the hands of their stepfather, but believed that she was functioning better than A.S because A.S. was not a strong enough person. Whereas A.S. was quiet and withdrawn, her sister was very talkative and outgoing. According to A.S., she was also very controlling. As they were growing up, A.S.'s sister always told her what to do, and because her sister had a bad temper, A.S. found it easier to go along with her demands rather than stand up to her. Unfortunately, A.S. became used to other people making decisions for her. As she got older she became very uncomfortable with the increased independence and autonomy that was expected of an 18-year-old.

A.S. grew up in a family that was focused on food, weight, appearance, and exercise. In addition to weighing her regularly, A.S.'s stepfather complained about her appearance and regularly encouraged her to get plastic surgery. These attitudes continued in her current living environment. Her mother and sister were often on diets and were critical of people who were overweight or unattractive or who dressed poorly. A.S. found these views superficial but received little reinforcement for her desire to treat people well or to focus on more meaningful characteristics. Nor did she receive much reinforcement outside her family. Socially, she was shy and awkward, easily overshadowed by others, and never had many friends.

A.S.'s case formulation centered on her regressive needs and her lack of a stable sense of self. A.S. received a great deal of attention from her mother when she lost weight— her mother would do nice things for her and treat her like a child, which A.S. enjoyed. Although she had not had a very loving childhood, she equated acting like a child with feelings of security and love and tried to create a child-like environment for herself in an attempt to capture what she felt she had missed when she was growing up. For example, she regularly played with dolls and enjoyed watching children's television shows. A.S. had some insight into her fear that she would lose her mother's love and attention if she were to recover or become a responsible adult. Although the nurturing aspects of the therapeutic relationship were invaluable in helping A.S. to feel safe and accepted, the authoritative aspect allowed the therapist to communicate that she had expectations of A.S. that were consistent with those one would have of an 18-year-old, including getting to know herself better and developing the ability to manage negative emotions without restricting her eating.

A.S.'s history of abuse and invalidation had contributed to low self-esteem, extreme self-doubt, and the lack of a stable sense of self, which was manifested in her tendency to second-guess her own beliefs and experiences, to value others' beliefs and opinions above her own, and to lack confidence in her ability to accomplish things. She accepted a great deal of unnecessary guilt because she always thought she was wrong. This also made it difficult for her to stand up for herself in situations that impeded her recovery process. For example, A.S. believed that her mother's comments about food and weight triggered a desire to restrict her eating. However, she was unable to effectively communicate to her mother that she wanted her to stop making these comments, and instead would start to cry, isolate herself, or restrict her eating. A.S.'s mother knew such comments bothered her but thought that A.S. just needed to stop being so sensitive. This invalidation happened often, and A.S. described feeling trapped by this toxic environment.

The therapist did not spend a great deal of time addressing A.S.'s regressive needs in the early part of treatment because A.S. was quite protective of her mother. She did come to recognize, however, that being at home was stressful for her. Even this recognition was an accomplishment for A.S. because she tended to disregard her own needs and just concern herself with meeting other people's needs. Thus, in the early sessions A.S. was encouraged to identify her needs and be more assertive in meeting them. A.S. was in her first semester of college and found studying to be a nice escape from home, so she spent a great deal of time at the library. She also joined a basketball team at school, became involved in an environmental club, and began going out of her way to meet people. Having some social contact helped her feel like a "more normal person." However, socializing was new for her, so some time was spent in therapy developing her social skills through role playing and helping her raise her awareness of how certain actions, behaviors, or comments might come across to other people. For example, A.S. was often up-front about her eating disorder, which seemed to make some of her classmates uncomfortable. The therapist agreed with A.S. that she should not be embarrassed about the eating disorder, and at the same time encouraged her to consider how others might respond to her frank discussion of her eating behaviors.

Phase 2: Developing a Voice

The middle phase of treatment continued to focus on developing A.S.'s sense of self, and near the end of this phase the focus shifted from the therapist doing most of the validating to A.S. beginning to do more of it herself, and feeling more comfortable in doing so. The focus also shifted from changing social behaviors (e.g., getting out of the house, practicing social skills) to deepening her understanding of, and developing a more objective view of, herself and her family. For example, A.S. often described her mother as a wonderful, loving person. At one point she described her mother this way immediately after discussing her mother's tendency to be emotionally absent and her belief that her mother really did not care about her. She then went on to say that she hoped her mother and stepfather would get back together because then her mother would be happy, and that she deserved to be happy because she was such a wonderful person. The therapist gently challenged her by pointing out this discrepancy and asking what A.S. believed was actually wonderful about her mother. The following week A.S. came to the session saying that she had been giving this a great deal of thought and believed that her eyes had been opened to the reality of her relationship with her mother. A.S. found it hard to accept that her image of her mother did not reflect reality, and felt that this was a significant loss. However, she also believed that it was preferable to see things realistically. This thought, in turn, had a profound impact on her interactions with her mother. For example, prior to this revelation, when her mother was in a bad mood, A.S. always believed that it was her fault (in part because her mother occasionally blamed her bad moods on A.S.'s eating disorder) and then felt guilty and depressed. After realizing that her mother was not perfect and had her own shortcomings, A.S. could see that her mother's anger had much more to do with her mother than it did with her. Although it was still upsetting to see her mother angry, A.S. no longer felt responsible and paralyzed with guilt.

Therapy continued to support A.S.'s efforts to identify and stand up for her needs, which included setting limits with her mother and sister. Role-playing these new ways of interacting with people was helpful. One day her mother was complaining that she had gained a few pounds. Instead of crying, isolating herself, or restricting her eating, A.S. was able to calmly say that she found comments such as these upsetting because they triggered a desire to restrict her own eating, and she asked her mother to stop. In this situation her mother did stop discussing her weight, but made a similar comment several days later. A.S. was very proud of the way she handled the situation but was still upset that her mother continued to make such comments, even after A.S. had repeatedly asked her not to. This was explored in session. Did her mother say these things in an attempt to be helpful and "immunize" A.S. to the comments? Did she do it because she *didn't* want A.S. to get better? A.S.'s conclusion was that her mother was not trying to make her better or worse, but that she simply did not respect A.S.'s request and did not really care about anyone other than herself. Whether or not this conclusion was accurate, it was another example of A.S. being able to see her mother as her own person with her own problems, rather than blaming herself.

Throughout treatment, A.S. continued to work actively on changing her environment, rather than passively letting it act on her. This was particularly important because her mother attended only two collateral sessions, so there was little opportunity for the therapist to discuss these issues or make suggestions directly to the mother. This change in A.S.'s level of assertiveness seemed to stem in large part from the therapist's validation of her thoughts and feelings. She often expressed surprise when the therapist agreed with her, even about things that were seemingly difficult to disagree with (e.g., "Yes, that must hurt your feelings when your mother blames her unhappiness on your eating disorder"). A.S. stated that her family "always thinks I'm wrong about everything because I have an eating disorder and am on meds." She was used to living in an invalidating environment, and validation from the therapist helped build her self-confidence and enabled her to believe that her thoughts, feelings, and needs were valid and deserved to be recognized.

The therapeutic relationship was central to strengthening A.S.'s sense of self, as she had had so few positive relationships in her life. It was important for the therapist to be patient with her while also reflecting on and validating her feelings, opinions, and reactions to things, as well as reinforcing any positive steps she took and appreciating her unique qualities. For example, the therapist commented on A.S.'s sense of humor, which A.S. claimed no one had ever recognized before. The therapist's acknowledgement and appreciation of A.S.'s positive qualities allowed a trusting, positive relationship to be built, which proved to be invaluable in laying the groundwork for her to feel confident in trying new ways of doing things and thinking about things.

Journaling and art also proved to be helpful for A.S. They enabled her to reflect on her experiences and helped A.S. to conceptualize the eating disorder as a separate entity. Journaling also enabled her to build her personal narrative. She realized that some of her early childhood experiences were quite difficult and that she did not develop an eating disorder because there was something fundamentally wrong with her. Writing gave her an opportunity to develop empathy for herself and get to know herself better.

Throughout this phase A.S. managed her eating independently. She gained weight fairly steadily during the middle phase of treatment.

Phase 3: Termination

During the last phase of treatment, a great deal of time was spent processing A.S.'s feelings about termination. Given her lack of positive relationships in the past, she had become attached to the therapist. The therapist encouraged A.S. to express her feelings about the ending of the relationship, while also encouraging her to continue to develop relationships with peers, thereby transferring A.S.'s support system from her therapist to a more age-appropriate network.

In addition to the interventions already described, therapist self-disclosure was used regularly during this phase, as it was important for A.S. to know that the therapist also valued the relationship and regretted its coming to an end. A.S.'s new sense of self was still fragile and the changes she was making were being met with a great deal of resistance at home, so much of the third phase of therapy focused on how to help her maintain the gains she had made in treatment. A maintenance plan was developed that included looking for supportive relationships outside her family, including further developing her peer relationships, staying busy outside the house, and spending less time with her sister and mother; and further developing and pursuing her own interests, including art and writing. By the end of treatment, A.S. was at a normal weight and had started menstruating again for the first time in several years (see Figure 14.1).

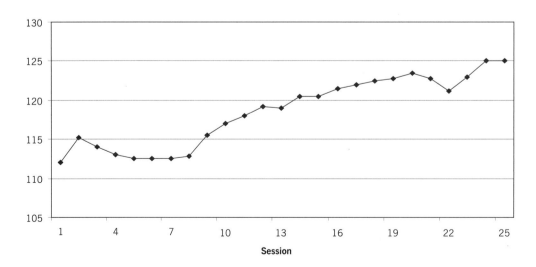

FIGURE 14.1. A.S.'s weight chart.

A.S. seemed to flourish in AFP. She was insightful, regularly reflected on topics discussed in therapy, and responded well to the nurturing and authoritative aspects of the therapeutic relationship, which allowed her to feel validated and valued, while also encouraged to challenge herself and strive to work toward recovery.

Summary

These case studies highlight the relationship between the therapist and the patient as the foundation on which the case specifics are formulated. Both cases illustrate how the therapist and patient together set goals to help the adolescent to challenge emotional fears and separate them from food/eating/shape/weight concerns. They also illustrate how two sets of parents can contrast so dramatically in their ability to be engaged as co-therapists in the treatment of their adolescent with AN. These cases illustrate that in either condition, the responsibility lies with the patient, regardless of the level of social and familial support. In one case, the parents are engaged in learning more about their son's conflicts and are able to support his individuation and encourage more normal developmental explorations. In the other case, a parent is unable to participate as a co-therapist, but the patient continues through recovery with the support of the therapist. Future research will continue to unravel the multidimensional causes of eating disorders in adolescents. Because both family therapies and AFP have been shown to have efficacy in the treatment of adolescents with eating disorders, ongoing challenges will include identifying the treatment model that is the best fit for a particular patient, and continuing to train clinicians to provide treatments that have shown efficacy in clinical trials. Another challenge for further study is to explore the ability of younger patients with AN to utilize and respond to AFP in the manner in which older patients appear to, and to determine whether significant developmental modifications are necessary to assist younger patients in using an individual collateral parental therapy format.

References

Bryant-Waugh, R. (2006). Pathways to recovery: Promoting change within a developmental-systemic framework. *Clinical Child Psychology and Psychiatry, 11*, 213–224.

Crisp, A. H. (1980). *Anorexia nervosa: Let me be.* London: Academic Press.

Crisp, A. H. (1997). Anorexia nervosa as flight from growth: Assessment and treatment based on the model. In D. M. Garner & P. E. Garfinkel (Eds.), *Handbook of treatment for eating disorders* (pp. 248–277). New York: Guilford Press.

Fitzpatrick, K., Moye, A., Hoste, R., Lock, J., & Le Grange, D. (2010). Adolescent focused psychotherapy for adolescents with anorexia nervosa. *Journal of Contemporary Psychotherapy, 40*, 31–39.

Gowers, S., Clark, A., Roberts, C., Griffiths, A., Edwards, V., Bryan, C., et al. (2007). Clinical effectiveness of treatments for anorexia nervosa in adolescents. *British Journal of Psychiatry, 191*, 427–435.

Krautter, T., & Lock, J. (2004). Is manualized family-based treatment for adolescent anorexia nervosa acceptable to patients? Patient satisfaction at end of treatment. *Journal of Family Therapy, 26*, 65–81.

Le Grange, D., & Lock, J. (2005). The dearth of psychological treatment studies for anorexia nervosa. *International Journal of Eating Disorders, 37*, 79–81.

Levenkron, S. (2000). *Anatomy of anorexia.* New York: Norton.

Lock, J. (2005). Adjusting cognitive behavioral

therapy for adolescent bulimia nervosa: Results of a case series. *American Journal of Psychotherapy, 59*, 267–281.

Lock, J., Le Grange, D., Agras, W. S., & Dare, C. (2001). *Treatment manual for anorexia nervosa: A family-based approach.* New York: Guilford Press.

Lock, J., Le Grange, D., Agras, W. S., Moye, A., Bryson, S. W., & Jo, B. (in press). Randomized clinical trial comparing family-based treatment to adolescent focused individual therapy for adolescents with anorexia nervosa. *Archives of General Psychiatry.*

McIntosh, V. W., Jordan, J., Carter, F. A., Luty, S. E., McKenzie, J. M., Bulik, C. M., et al. (2005). Three psychotherapies for anorexia nervosa: A randomized, controlled trial. *American Journal of Psychiatry, 162*, 741–747.

Pike, K., Walsh, B. T., Vitousek, K., Wilson, G. T., & Bauer, J. (2004). Cognitive-behavioral therapy in the posthospitalization treatment of anorexia nervosa. *American Journal of Psychiatry, 160*, 2046–2049.

Robin, A., Siegal, P., Koepke, T., Moye, A., &

Tice, S. (1994). Family therapy versus individual therapy for adolescent families with anorexia nervosa. *Journal of Developmental and Behavioral Pediatrics, 15*, 111–116.

Robin, A., Siegal, P., Moye, A., Gilroy, M., Dennis, A., & Sikand, A. (1999). A controlled comparison of family versus individual therapy for adolescents with anorexia nervosa. *Journal of the American Academy of Child and Adolescent Psychiatry, 38*, 1482–1489.

Robin, A. L., Siegal, P. T., & Moye, A. (1995). Family versus individual therapy for anorexia: Impact on family conflict. *International Journal of Eating Disorders, 17*, 313–322.

Thoma, H. (1967). *Anorexia nervosa.* New York: International Universities.

Treasure, J. L., Todd, G., Brolly, M., Tiller, J., Nehmed, A., & Denman, F. (1995). A pilot study of a randomized trial of cognitive-behavioral analytical therapy vs. educational behavioral therapy for adult anorexia nervosa. *Behaviour Research and Therapy, 33*, 363–367.

OUTPATIENT TREATMENTS FOR BULIMIA NERVOSA AND BINGE-EATING DISORDER

■ CHAPTER 15 ■

Family-Based Treatment for Bulimia Nervosa

Theoretical Model, Key Tenets, and Evidence Base

Daniel Le Grange

Although family-based treatment (FBT) has come to be seen as the treatment of choice for adolescents with anorexia nervosa (AN), the benefit of parental participation in the treatment for adolescents with bulimia nervosa (BN) remains mostly unexplored. This chapter focuses on the theoretical model that underpins manualized FBT for adolescent BN (FBT-BN), highlights the key tenets of this treatment, briefly describes the three treatment phases, summarizes the main differences of this model in its application to BN as opposed to AN (see Lock, Chapter 12, this volume), and reviews the only two published randomized controlled trials of FBT-BN showing preliminary support for the parents' involvement in the treatment of adolescent BN.

Background

The lifetime prevalence of DSM-IV BN among adolescents is 0.9% (Swanson, Crow, Le Grange & Merikangas, in press), and an additional 3% engage in binge eating and purging (Stice & Agras, 1998). Despite such alarmingly high levels of bulimic symptoms among adolescents, the overwhelming preponderance of a now substantial literature on the treatment of BN has focused on adults with this disorder. Most of these treatment studies have focused on three treatments—that is, cognitive-behavioral therapy (CBT), interpersonal therapy (IPT), and antidepressant medications—in which the average age of participants is ~30 years with a duration of illness ~10 years (Wilson, Grilo, & Vitousek, 2007). In contrast, significantly less is known about the treatment of adolescents with BN. A small number of case series have described treatment efforts (Dodge, Hodes, Eisler, & Dare, 1995; Le Grange, Lock, & Dymek, 2003; Lock, 2005; Schapman-Williams, Lock, & Couturier, 2006), and only two randomized controlled trials (RCTs) for adolescent BN have been published (Le Grange, Crosby, Rathouz, & Leventhal, 2007; Schmidt et al., 2007). These RCTs have utilized family-based treatment for this patient population (FBT-BN) (the subject of this chapter), CBT (see Campbell & Schmidt, Chapter 16, this volume), and supportive psychotherapy (see Hoste & Celio Doyle, Chapter 17, this volume).

Early Support for Family Involvement in the Treatment of BN

The first study to provide preliminary support for parental involvement in the treatment of adolescents with BN was conducted at the Maudsley Hospital in London. In a series of five cases, Dodge and her colleagues (1995) utilized family therapy and demonstrated that it was possible to bring about significant reductions in bulimic behaviors through educating the parents about this disorder and providing them with support to disrupt and curtail binge eating and purging. At about the same time, early treatment studies at the Maudsley Hospital utilizing FBT for AN provided indirect support for family involvement in addressing bulimic symptomatology. Commenting on the effectiveness of this treatment for adolescents with AN binge–purge subtype, Eisler and his colleagues (2000) found parents to be as effective in curtailing binge and purge episodes as they were in supporting weight gain.

Following this original work, and based on this family therapy, we presented a detailed description of an adolescent completing a course of what is now known as FBT-BN (Le Grange et al., 2003). Taken together these reports show that family involvement in the recovery of adolescents with BN is a promising route to pursue, and prepared the groundwork for a more formal investigation of the efficacy of FBT-BN.

Theoretical Model of FBT-BN

Following early reports supportive of family involvement, a clinician's manual of family-based treatment for adolescents with bulimia nervosa (FBT-BN) was developed (Le Grange & Lock, 2007). FBT-BN was developed to represent a close approximation of its precursor for adolescents with AN (FBT-AN) (see Lock, Chapter 12, this volume). We often assume that involving the parents in the treatment of their children and adolescents is a prerequisite for successful outcomes. In eating disorders this assumption is convincingly argued from both a theoretical and clinical perspective and is perhaps best illustrated in FBT-AN. In this treatment, the parents' dedication to their child and family is mobilized in order to bring about change in the adolescent's eating behaviors and to support rapid weight restoration. In fact, both clinicians and researchers would agree that it is exactly the steps taken in mobilizing parents to be in charge of weight restoration that are at the heart of the effectiveness of FBT in the treatment of adolescent AN (Le Grange & Eisler, 2009).

Parental involvement in the treatment of adolescents with BN does not readily resonate in the same way as for AN despite considerable overlap in symptomatology between these two eating disorders. There are significant ways in which adolescents with BN differ from their counterparts with AN. For instance, adolescents with bulimic symptoms often express considerable feelings of shame and guilt associated with the eating-disordered behavior. Such feelings can lead to the adolescent's increased isolation from his or her parents, which leaves parents unable to provide the necessary support and often serves to further reinforce the symptomatic behavior. However, there is also substantial overlap between AN and BN. One example is that similar to those with AN, adolescents with BN are inclined to deny the severity of their symptoms and, as a consequence, appear unable to appreciate the seriousness of their eating disorder.

FBT-BN is based on the assumption that AN and BN are more similar than different. Consequently, and as is the case with FBT-AN, this treatment in its format for adolescents with BN does not probe possible causes of the eating disorder but remains *symptom focused*. FBT-BN therefore concentrates on the behavioral steps that ought to be taken to curtail binge eating and purging. Second, disordered eating behavior and its associated secrecy and shame negatively impact adolescent development, which leaves the parents confused and disempowered. This state of affairs is further compounded by inevitable parental guilt about having possibly caused the disorder as well as anxiety about how best to resolve this dilemma. These circumstances further add to the parents' sense of being disempowered. As a consequence, this treatment aims to promote a *collaborative effort* between the parents and their child. This stance serves to empower parents and acknowledges the adolescent as an active participant in the joint effort to disrupt restrictive dieting, binge eating and purging, or any other pathological weight control behaviors. Third, FBT-BN aims to *externalize* the illness, that is, to separate the affected adolescent from his or her disordered eating behaviors in order to promote parental action and at the same time to reduce the adolescent's opposition to his or her parents' assistance.

Even though FBT-BN encourages the parents' active involvement in helping their child restore healthy eating habits, this intervention is time limited. The goal is for the parents to return full control over eating to the adolescent once he or she approaches abstinence from the eating-disordered behavior. Once this change in stance has been negotiated successfully, the parents assist the adolescent in navigating more predictable adolescent development tasks. Although the therapist supports the parents in playing an active role in addressing the eating disorder symptoms, the siblings are protected from the job assigned to the parents and are encouraged to be supportive of their affected sibling in domains other than mealtimes.

FBT-BN is closely modeled on the approach employed with adolescent AN (FBT-AN). Most important among the characteristics shared with FBT-AN is that in this treatment for BN parents are regarded as a *resource*. As a result, attempts are made to alleviate misperceptions of blame that are either held by the parents or commonly directed to the parents. Similarly, the adolescent is not to be blamed for his or her predicament. Removing blame does not absolve the family from the responsibility to restore healthy eating in their offspring. Despite the behavioral focus of FBT-BN, the therapist does not direct the parents and adolescent in terms of the necessary steps to take in the treatment process. Rather, the therapist takes an authoritative stance and serves as an educator, consultant, and sounding board for the family, but leaves decision making to the parents. This therapeutic stance is critical, as it facilitates parental ownership of the decisions made in treatment and, as a result, increases the parents' sense of efficiency or empowerment.

Although FBT-BN is similar to its counterpart for AN in several ways, it is a distinct therapy and uniquely accounts for the differences between these two eating disorders. As is the case in AN, the adolescent with BN is often unable to recognize or effectively manage his or her disordered eating patterns. In FBT-AN, the parents are supported and encouraged to take charge of the adolescent's eating in order to bring about rapid weight gain and recovery. The adolescent's distress is recognized, but he or she is not consulted in how to achieve weight recovery. In contrast, it is recognized that most adolescents with BN are developmentally more "on track" than the average adolescent with AN. Consequently, the parents as well as the affected adolescent are coached to work collaboratively to develop ways to restore healthy eating. It is unique to FBT-BN that the adolescent is an active participant in the attempts to curtail binge eating and purging, and the therapist encourages the adolescent to express his or her point of view and experience in lieu of arriving at a solution to the eating disorder symptoms. In other words, struggles around mealtimes, unhealthy eating at other times, and the impact of these disordered eating behaviors on family relationships are explored, and possible solutions are jointly planned and implemented.

To summarize, the key tenets of FBT-BN are as follows:

- Agnostic view of cause of illness (neither adolescent nor parents are to blame).
- Initial focus on symptoms (pragmatic approach to treatment).
- Parents *and* the adolescent are responsible for normalizing eating (collaboration).
- Nonauthoritarian therapeutic stance by the therapist (joining).
- Separation of adolescent and the disorder (respect for adolescent).

Three Phases of FBT-BN

The manual of FBT-BN (Le Grange & Lock, 2007) guides the clinician to proceed through three phases of treatment, which is typically conducted over a period of 6 months and utilizes about 20 treatment sessions. Most patients spend between 2 and 3 months in Phase 1, with sessions held at weekly intervals. For Phase 2, sessions are scheduled every second week over a period of 1–2 months, and Phase 3 lasts about 6 weeks, with sessions scheduled every 2–3 weeks. The next section of this chapter briefly summarizes these three treatment phases.

Phase 1: Reestablishing Healthy Eating for the Adolescent (Sessions 1–10)

In Phase 1 of FBT-BN the primary focus of treatment is to support the parents *and* their affected adolescent to develop strategies to confront the eating disorder symptoms and curtail the destructive impact of these symptoms on the adolescent and his or her development. This endeavor can be successful only if the therapist succeeds in uniting the parents in their effort, and this effort is delivered in a persistent and consistent way. At the same time, every attempt should be made to invite and support the adolescent in collaborating with the parents in this process.

Every meeting throughout this treatment starts with a brief 10- to 15-minute check-in between the therapist and the patient. This brief one-on-one moment provides the therapist with an opportunity to monitor the adolescent's weight and gather data on weekly binge and purge frequencies. The therapist reminds the adolescent that it is critical to track the bulimic behavior and that it will be helpful if he or she can monitor and report weekly binge and purge episodes. These weekly reports are to be recorded in the *Patient Binge–Purge Log* (to be handed to the adolescent at the start of each session and collected the following week; cf. Le Grange & Lock, 2007). This brief meeting between the therapist and the adolescent also provides the patient an opportunity to share his or her thoughts and feelings about the prior week without the parents being present. This meeting should not exceed the 10- to 15-minute window, at which time the rest of the family is asked to join.

Once the family is convened, the therapist explains that the information gathered from the log will be shared with the parents. The parents' task is to reconcile their account of events over the past week, especially in terms of binge–purge frequency, with the account that the adolescent provided the therapist. It is these reconciled frequencies that are collaboratively gathered in a joint effort between the parents, patient, and therapist and finally recorded on the *Therapist's Binge–Purge Chart* (cf. Le Grange & Lock, 2007).

Each session starts with the therapist first meeting the adolescent. However, the greater part of the sessions is spent with the entire family present. In these meetings the therapist cautiously directs discussions in such a way to both facilitate and bolster a strong *parental alliance* in the parents' efforts to bring about healthy eating in the affected adolescent. Yet this task is not entirely in the parental sphere of influence, as the therapist attempts to facilitate a *collaborative effort* between the adolescent and his or her parents about decisions on how best to address the eating disorder symptoms. It is this maneuver on the part of the FBT-BN therapist that most clearly differentiates this treatment from its counterpart for AN. A reminder: The therapist in FBT-AN supports the parents in their efforts to restore the adolescent's weight and does not consult the adolescent in this domain. Instead, the therapist empathizes with the adolescent about the dilemma he or she is facing.

In addition to facilitating a strong parental alliance, while at the same time fostering a collaborative effort between the parents and their adolescent, another key intervention early in treatment is for the therapist to make an effort to remind the parents that they have not caused their child's predicament. The therapist undertakes this strategy for several reasons, such as there is no evidence to suggest that parents are to blame for eating disorders, and *diminishing parental guilt* helps to mobilize parents to take effective action in the battle against their child's disorder. This therapist achieves this treatment goal by assuming a caring and concerned stance—that is, the role of *consultant* to the family rather than an authoritarian force. In so doing, the therapist seeks out every opportunity to compliment the parents on the positive aspects of their parenting.

Another critical therapeutic maneuver to undertake early on in treatment is for the therapist to *separate* or *externalize* the adolescent from the eating disorder. This maneuver by the therapist is both respectful of the adolescent in affirming that he or she did not "bring this upon (him- or) herself," and helpful in allowing the parents to understand the distressing and confusing symptoms as separate from the adolescent. It is this capacity to separate the illness from their offspring on the part of the parents that renders them more capable of intervening. At the same time, this maneuver also underscores that no one in the family is to blame for the eating disorder, demonstrates empathy toward the parents in their plight, and reduces shame in the adolescent.

Several steps on the part of the therapist are often required in order to achieve this goal. To mobilize parents to play an active role in curtailing bulimic symptoms, it is often necessary for the therapist to increase parental anxiety about the severity of the disorder. The therapist has to carefully calibrate this intervention so as to raise parents' concern to help facilitate their best capacity to seek out a resolution for the eating disorder, and simultaneously not become critical or angry with their adolescent for his or her behavior. Several strategies can be helpful here. Through a process of psychoeducation the therapist can help the parents understand and appreciate the various and serious medical, as well as psychiatric, symptoms that can develop as a result of the eating disorder, such as electrolyte imbalances and dehydration, esophageal tears, mood and anxiety disorders, and so on. There are instances in which parents have already separated the illness from their adolescent prior to embarking on a course of treatment. For the most part, though, the therapist has to labor quite hard to reinforce the distinction between the illness and the adolescent. In doing so, the therapist can chose from a number of metaphors that suit his or her own style or fit with the family he or she is working with in order to help everyone understand this concept. In using one such metaphor, which is often helpful in achieving this treatment goal, the therapist equates the eating disorder with a malignant tumor. As is the case with cancer, the adolescent did not bring the BN upon him- or herself, nor is the adolescent in control of how this disorder exerts influence over his or her body or mind, and outside help is almost always a requirement. In practice, the therapist encourages the parents to attribute symptomatic behaviors to the eating disorder, rather than viewing them as being within the adolescent's domain of control and, as a result, blaming the adolescent.

The background for treatment has now been set, and it provides a new framework for the family in which the eating disorder is seen as separate from the adolescent. If this goal has been achieved, the therapist can help shift the focus toward resolving the bulimic behavior. To challenge the bulimic behavior or symptoms, it is important that the therapist allows the members of each family to work out for themselves how they should proceed in their effort to help their adolescent with BN. Allowing each family some space in which to figure out what steps to take to address the eating disorder symptoms may make the family's task easier and serves to *empower the parents* in this challenging endeavor. Taking a step away and allowing parents to come up with the solutions that can work in their family does not imply that the therapist will withhold guidance or suggestions should the family be floundering. However, the therapist refrains from giving the family direct instructions, as that might not achieve the goal of empowering the parents. Instead, the therapist sketches several scenarios of the presented problem, accompanied by solutions that other families have arrived at, and invite the parents to consider whether any of these prospects may work for them. The therapist refrains from giving the parents direct instructions, and instead may say:

> "Many families that I work with struggle with this issue and some have approached this particular issue (in this way), and yet others have resolved the same issue (in that way). Hearing about these different solutions, do you think any of them might work for you?"

The therapist convenes a family meal at the second treatment session. This is an important therapeutic maneuver in FBT-BN but uses quite a different rationale and format than its counterpart in FBT-AN. At least three functions are served by convening the family: first, the therapist is provided with an opportunity for direct observation of the family's interactions around eating; second, the therapist utilizes this opportunity to initiate the parents' direct involvement in their adolescent's recovery; and third, it provides the therapist with an opportunity to support the adolescent in finding the words to express some of his or her internal turmoil and shame about his or her weight concerns and eating behavior. Adolescents with BN usually come to therapy at a healthy weight, and the purpose of the family meal and the parents' efforts going forward are therefore centered on reestablishing healthy eating—that is, adhering to regular and healthy meal consumption without binge eating or purging. This maneuver is in stark contrast to the use of the "typical" meal in FBT-AN, with its focus on weight restoration. However, as in FBT-AN, the parents and the adolescent are requested to bring along a meal that is in keeping with their regular lunch or dinner habits. The content of the meal will differ, depending on the time of day the meal is scheduled for. In addition to this meal, the adolescent is instructed to let his or her parents know of a typical "forbidden" or "trigger" food to accompany the meal. If the adolescent is not ready to collaborate in this way at this early stage of treatment, the parents have to make this decision on their own. The goal here is for the parents to support their adolescent so that he or she can consume a healthy and appropriate amount of food. An additional goal is for the parents to persuade the adolescent to eat some of the "forbidden" food.

There are several reasons why the therapist undertakes these steps. First, it is important to establish early on that a healthy diet includes a variety of foods and that none of these foods should be on a "forbidden" list. Second, the family meal provides the parents with an opportunity to succeed in helping their adolescent eat some of these feared foods. Third, and perhaps most important, this session offers the adolescent an opportunity to let his or her parents know, perhaps with the help of the therapist, just how much inner torment accompanies any transgression of the narrowly defined food rules. We make the assumption that the secrecy around binge eating and purging will have kept most adolescents from voicing these inner struggles, at least not to their parents. The therapist should seize on this opportunity to encourage the adolescent to "educate" his or her parents and let them know just how distraught their child feels when there is any transgression in these rigidly adhered-to food rules. Moreover, the therapist should encourage the adolescent to let his or her parents know how such a "slipup" is usually followed by a desire to "give up" and "eat the entire bag of chips." Once the adolescent has stepped over this line, the only "solution" is to purge this transgression. It is not always possible for the adolescent to express his or her feelings or thoughts about this delicate matter. When the adolescent is reluctant or perhaps ashamed to talk about binge eating and purging, the therapist may say something along these lines:

> "Young people, such as your son/daughter, who struggle with issues about weight, shape, and eating, usually do not like to talk about these behaviors or thoughts and feelings. At times, this may be so because they feel embarrassed about what they have eaten or how much they have eaten, and certainly don't want to tell anyone that they are then overcome with incredible urges to rid themselves of the food they have eaten. These are both intense and embarrassing struggles, and the adolescent often feels overwhelmed and would rather not share these issues with anyone."

If the therapist succeeds in helping the adolescent disclose some of these struggles during the family meal, then at least two goals have been achieved; first, this may provide the adolescent with his or her first opportunity to be less secretive about the bulimic symptoms, and second, the parents may be able to gain a greater understanding of how much the eating disorder occupies and torments their adolescent's mind, and come to appreciate how much shame is felt as a result of the eating disorder symptoms and how much effort must have been invested in keeping these symptoms a secret. The most important reason for the family meal session is to cement the parents' role as a resource for their adolescent in his or her struggle to figure out healthy portion sizes that also include forbidden or feared food. This session also begins the formulation of essential ground rules about issues such as mealtimes, food quantities, and how much or for how long parents may have to supervise the adolescent post-mealtimes in order to prevent purging behavior. One way in which these ground rules can be tested early in treatment is to allow about 20 minutes post–family meal when the adolescent cannot leave the therapist's office, in order to prevent purging. At home, this supervision ideally lasts closer to an hour; however, this office "test" provides parents with perhaps their first opportunity to begin to talk with the adolescent about how best to structure these post-mealtimes at home. In practice, the family should aim to have these "supervision" times feel more like quality family time, when the adolescent and his or her parent may go for a leisurely walk, watch their favorite movie or television program, and so on. Parents are advised to make sure that these times are not experienced by the adolescent as "being watched over."

To summarize, one of the key treatment features that differentiates FBT-BN from FBT-AN is that the former encourages the parents and the adolescents to seek out collaboration in their efforts to challenge the bulimic symptoms. An important step in achieving this goal is for the therapist to help diminish the shame and guilt experienced by most adolescents with BN, and to sympathize with the adolescent for the predicament the eating disorder has created. The therapist acknowledges and reminds everyone, the adolescent in particular, that allowing parents to be so involved in the eating behaviors and weight concerns of the adolescent is out of sync with what parents of teenagers ordinarily do *and* a time-limited intervention. For example, the therapist can say:

> "What I am asking of everyone is different from the way you would ordinarily go about managing parenting. However, helping your teenager overcome an eating disorder often requires a different set of guidelines and strategies than regular circumstances would. I really want to make sure that everyone understands that helping your teenager with her (or his) eating in this way is a temporary intervention. Under the circumstances, I am suggesting that you change the way you ordinarily go about parenting your adolescent when he or she is healthy."

The degree of parental involvement prescribed by the therapist in this treatment is restricted to the eating domain and is time-limited. Therefore, the FBT-BN therapist makes every effort to be respectful of the adolescent and his or her developmental status and to emphasize to the family that intervening in regard to the eating behaviors is only a temporary intrusion. The therapist tries to reassure the adolescent that the parents' involvement is mostly required to help change the course of the eating disorder symptoms during the early part of treatment. It is also at this stage of treatment that the therapist can guide the parents in how to demonstrate their understanding of the adolescent's struggle, and how to help him or her manage confusing feelings at a difficult time like this. Although FBT-BN does not directly address issues of core self-worth and/or body image, offering parental support and understanding of the dilemma in which the adolescent finds him- or herself, allows the parents to guide and help their adolescent to feel supported and comforted in treatment.

As shown in studies of FBT-AN, this treatment in its format for BN also assumes that healthy eating will lead to reduced concerns about eating, weight, and shape (Le Grange, Crosby, Rathouz, & Leventhal, 2007). For the most part, however, the therapist's stance in FBT-BN is quite similar to that in FBT-AN. The similarity of the two treatments are most in evidence in that the therapist consistently and resolutely holds the parents and their family in positive regard. In practice, this means that the therapist looks for every opportunity to provide the parents with positive feedback for their efforts and supports these efforts by complimenting them as much as possible on the positive aspects of their parenting.

Phase 2: Returning Control of Eating to the Adolescent (Sessions 11–16)

This phase of treatment aims to restore the adolescent's autonomy in regard to eating; that is, the therapist helps the parents navigate a return of control over problematic eating that until this time was still under the parents' watchful eyes. A transition to the second phase of treatment is usually signaled when the adolescent's eating behavior begins to return to normal. A significant reduction in binge eating and purging usually brings about a change in the mood of the family. Up to this point in treatment, the family may have experienced frustration and anxiety with the continuing eating disorder symptoms. With a reduction in these symptoms, a sense of relief develops as mastery over eating disorder symptoms has been accomplished. The therapist oversees the return to regular meals that now occur without the tension that earmarked these occasions for most of Phase 1. However, this is done without diminishing the continuing focus on the symptoms of disordered eating. At each session the therapist achieves this goal through a detailed inquiry, directed at the parents and the adolescent, into what a typical day during the prior week "looked like." Gathering an idea of how the family now organizes itself around mealtimes allows the therapist to make a clinical judgment as to whether these occasions are now largely occurring without the tensions and anxieties that were typical of earlier mealtimes.

At this point in the treatment process the goal is for the adolescent to take charge of these challenges on his or her own, but not to shy away from parental support when it is indicated. What this means in day-to-day management of the eating disorder is for the adolescent to make his or her own food choices, but for the parents to retain some oversight that allows them to assist the adolescent when it is clear that some choices are still influenced by the eating disorder. This degree of independence for the adolescent in regard to these choices is not only age appropriate but also possible, as the parents and the adolescent have worked together in Phase 1 to interrupt the hold that excessive weight concern, dieting, and binge eating and purging have had on the teenager.

In addition to returning control of eating to the adolescent, in Phase 2 the parents also attempt to reinforce healthy adolescent peer relationships. Total independence in regard to friendships may initially be tempered, as the parents are encouraged to remain vigilant should they suspect that social engagements may allow for the ongoing reinforcement of the stranglehold of the eating disorder on their adolescent. What this means in practice is that the parents are to encourage the adolescent to join his or her friends for an outing (e.g., going to the mall or cinema). However, the adolescent should be required to have a healthy meal with his or her parents either before or after such an outing. The goal is for the adolescent to reestablished age-appropriate independence in both peer relationships and eating behavior. Once this goal has been achieved, the therapist will signal that treatment can transition to the third and final phase.

Phase 3: Adolescent Developmental Issues and Termination (Sessions 17–20)

Once abstinence of binge eating and purging has been achieved, treatment turns to focus more on specific issues pertaining to adolescent development. The third phase serves as a review of adolescent developmental issues rather than an in-depth discussion and attempt to resolve such challenges. It is more typical that meetings are scheduled for every second or third week for this stage of treatment. The main goal of these meetings is to assist the adolescent and the parents in developing a healthy relationship between them. More specifically, the therapist works to help the adolescent to establish greater autonomy, underlines the need for healthy intergenerational boundaries, and reinforces a relationship between the adolescent and the parents in which the eating disorder no longer interferes with nor constitutes the basis of their relationship. Phase 3 focuses almost exclusively on adolescent developmental issues; however, the therapist also touches base with the parents in terms of their own relationship, recognizing their lives together, given that their child is about to embark on his or her own next challenge outside the family home (e.g., at college or work). Although both the family's and the therapist's focus is on the adolescent's pending departure from his or her family, parents are often more concerned about a possible relapse of the eating disorder, whereas the adolescent shows more interest in his or her pending freedom from parental oversight. Time is limited in this phase of treatment. Consequently, the therapist has a difficult task in addressing both the adolescent's independence and the parents' own relationship once the adolescent leaves home, all before bringing treatment to its conclusion.

Specific Challenges in FBT-BN

Although FBT-BN was adapted from its counterpart for AN and therefore the two have much in common, some specific features of BN among adolescents highlight several clinical challenges that separate FBT-BN from FBT-AN.

Developmental Stage of Adolescents with BN

In FBT-AN only, the parents are mobilized to take charge of restoring the adolescent's weight. Although the adolescent is comforted for being in such a predicament, input in this aspect of his or her treatment is deliberately not sought. In FBT-BN, in contrast, the eating disorder symptoms are addressed in a collaborative effort between the adolescent and his or her parents. Several reasons can be put forth to explain this important component of FBT-BN. First, most adolescents with BN are typically somewhat older when they are seen for treatment, as compared with adolescents with AN. Second, many adolescents with BN are not developmentally delayed, as is the case with so many adolescents with AN. Adolescents with BN are therefore more autonomous, which serves to underscore why it is therapeutically more viable for the therapist to encourage collaboration between the adolescent and his or her parents in this treatment. There is some anecdotal evidence to suggest that most adolescents with BN are typically more interactive and talkative in treatment as compared with their counterparts with AN. This ability of the adolescent with BN allows for a more interactive quality in the therapy, which is often not the case with a typically quieter and/or more withdrawn adolescent with AN. Although patients with BN do attempt to "protect" their symptoms, the associated guilt and shame brought on by binge eating and purging symptoms lead many patients to report significant discomfort with these symptoms. It is this discomfort that gives BN a more ego-dystonic quality as compared with the typical ego-syntonic nature of AN. Consequently, and relative to AN, more adolescents with BN are prepared to engage in treatment and work on their symptoms.

Emphasis on Regulating Food Intake, and Curtailing Binge–Purge Behavior

In FBT-BN the emphasis is on regulating eating and curtailing purging, and not on weight restoration, notwithstanding a few patients who may be first seen when they are at relatively low weights. Consequently, the family meal (Session 2) focuses on supporting the adolescent in eating a regular meal in terms of caloric value, but includes food that would typically trigger a binge. This scenario provides the therapist with an opportunity to explore the adolescent's feelings about urges to binge and purge.

Secretiveness (Shame and Guilt) of BN

The person who suffers with BN is usually quite secretive about his or her illness behavior. Although there are several possible explanations for this guarded quality, it can in part be explained because of the considerable guilt and shame that are brought on by symptoms such as binge eating and purging. This secretiveness on the part of the sufferer results in the parents not being fully aware of the symptoms or their severity. In contrast, the emaciated patient with AN more obviously looks unwell. This visual image is a stark reminder of how unwell the sufferer with AN is, thereby making it relatively less complicated for the therapist to convince the parents of the seriousness of the disorder and to keep them focused on the task at hand. This is clearly not the case for most adolescents with BN, who are typically first seen at healthy weights and, as alluded to, inclined to hide their symptoms. Consequently, in FBT-BN the task of convincing the parents of the seriousness of the disorder is much more arduous.

Heterogeneity and Comorbidity of BN

Given the greater prevalence of comorbid psychiatric diagnoses among adolescent with BN, as opposed to their counterparts with AN (cf. Fischer & Le Grange, 2007), FBT-BN can often be more challenging. More specifically, it becomes difficult for the therapist to maintain treatment focus on the bulimic symptoms when other concerns such academic struggles, drug use, or risky sexual behavior rival the former in intensity and perceived importance. The difference between AN and BN is that for the former, only acute suicidality can trump self-starvation, thereby reducing the challenge for the clinician engaged in FBT-AN to maintain focus on weight restoration. FBT-BN is also a focused therapy; however, at times comorbid psychiatric illnesses, developmental challenges, or family dilemmas can require equal or even more attention than the bulimic symptoms. Such "rival" concerns are not only causes of great distress, but stand to dilute the therapist's focus on the eating disorder. In such cases, additional therapy to address these coexisting concerns needs to follow the focused work of FBT-BN.

To summarize the challenges specific to FBT-BN:

- Developmental stage of the adolescent (treatment is more collaborative).
- Emphasis on regulating food intake rather than on starvation.
- Secretiveness of BN (challenges parents to appreciate the full spectrum of symptoms).
- Heterogeneity of BN (challenges parents to remain focused on bulimic symptoms).

Evidence for the Effectiveness of FBT-BN

There is but limited evidence available in support of FBT-BN, as only two RCTs for adolescents with BN have been published (Le Grange et al., 2007; Schmidt et al., 2007). Both these studies utilized forms of family treatment, thereby extending the findings from the case series data discussed earlier in this chapter.

In our own study (Le Grange et al., 2007), 80 adolescents (M = 16.1 years, SD = 1.6) with DSM-IV BN or partial BN were randomly assigned to either FBT-BN (n = 41) or individual supportive psychotherapy (SPT) (n = 39). Both treatments were manualized, and participants received 20 therapy sessions over a period of 6 months (M = 17.5, SD = 4.6). Assessments were conducted at baseline, midtreatment, end of treatment, and 6-month follow-up. Treatment adherence (only 11% of patients dropped out of therapy prematurely) as well as therapeutic alliance were high and did not differ between FBT-BN and SPT (Zaitsoff, Celio Doyle, Hoste, & Le Grange, 2008).

FBT-BN was statistically and clinically superior to SPT at both the posttreatment and the 6-month follow-up marks. At posttreatment, significantly more patients in FBT-BN (39%) than in SPT (18%) were free of binge eating or purge episodes for the preceding 28 days. Whereas abstinence rates at 6-month follow-up were reduced for both treatments, FBT-BN maintained its advantage over SPT. Almost 30% of patients in FBT-BN versus 10% of patients in SPT were binge and purge free for the preceding 28 days. Secondary analyses showed that patients in FBT-BN showed significantly greater improvements over patients in SPT on measures of behavioral and attitudinal features of eating disorder psychopathology. Moreover, FBT-BN showed a more rapid rate of improvement in core bulimic symptoms with patients in FBT-BN demonstrating significant treatment gains over SPT by the 10th treatment session (halfway mark). Taken together, these results suggest that FBT-BN is superior to SPT for both behavioral and attitudinal aspects of BN (Le Grange et al., 2007).

In the only other RCT to date, Schmidt and colleagues (2007) randomly assigned 85 adolescents and young adults (M = 17.6 years, SD = 0.3) with DSM-IV BN or EDNOS to either family therapy (n = 41) or cognitive-behavioral therapy guided self-care (n = 44) (CBT-GSC). There were no discernable differences in achieved abstinence rates between these two treatments. At posttreatment, 12.5% of patients in family therapy versus 19.4% in CBT-GSC were abstinent from binge eating and purging, and at 6-month follow-up, these rates rose to 41.4% versus 36%, respectively. The only difference between the two treatments to emerge was in terms of direct cost. This was lower for CBT-GSC, although there were no differences in other cost categories. Schmidt and colleagues provide some suggestions to explain why their two treatments delivered similar outcomes. First, the study may have been underpowered to detect statistically significant differences between two active treatments for some of their outcomes. Second, the absence of either a wait-list condition or a control group rules out that improvement was due to nonspecific effects or the passage of time.

Family therapy as described by Schmidt and colleagues (2007) and FBT-BN utilized in the 2007 study of Le Grange and colleagues largely overlap, although no published manual for the former is available. A key difference between family therapy provided by Schmidt and colleagues and FBT-BN is the much broader definition of "family" allowed for in the former. Here, "family" was defined as any "close other," rather than requiring the availability of a parent or legal guardian as was the case for FBT-BN. Schmidt and colleagues recruited a somewhat older sample of late adolescents and young adults in which the mean age of participants was 17.6 years ($SD = 0.3$). This is an age quite close to adulthood, especially in the United Kingdom, where the age of consent is 16 years, which led to one-quarter of their cases utilizing a "close other" rather than a parent in their treatment. Defining family as a "close other" probably fits well with this older age group; however, using this definition of family may not be the most effective way to approach FBT-BN with younger adolescents who live with their parents and are dependent on parents in several ways (e.g., economically, emotionally, etc.). Notwithstanding this difference between these two studies, the abstinence rates for family therapy and FBT-BN were quite comparable.

Some important questions regarding the implementation and dissemination of family-based treatments for BN need to be considered. In the study by Schmidt and colleagues (2007), a substantial number of eligible subjects (28%) refused participation because they did not want their families involved in treatment. CBT-GSC in this study, as well as FBT-BN in the study by Le Grange and colleagues (2007), appeared to have fewer barriers to participation. Moreover, CBT-GSC delivered similar results to those of family therapy in Schmidt's study or FBT-BN in Le Grange's study. An apparent advantage of CBT-GSC over family therapy was in terms of cost of delivery, with the former being more cost-effective. These findings remain preliminary and serve to underscore the fact that treatment studies for adolescents with BN are still in their infancy and further evaluation of effective treatments is needed (see also Campbell & Schmidt, Chapter 16, and Hoste & Celio Doyle, Chapter 17, this volume).

Conclusions and Future Directions

Until recently few if any systematic studies of the treatment of adolescents with BN were available. Although known efficacious treatments for this patient population remain uncertain, we now have the benefit of at least two published RCTs (Le Grange et al., 2007; Schmidt et al., 2007). A clinician's manual of FBT-BN is also available (Le Grange & Lock, 2007), which is succinctly summarized in this chapter. FBT-BN is closely modeled on the better established FBT-AN, although it remains largely untested. It is fair to say that investigations into the efficacy of this treatment are in their infancy. That said,

results from the available two RCTs are encouraging and provide at least some preliminary support to the conclusion that parental involvement in the treatment of adolescents
with BN can be beneficial.

It remains clear, though, that the best avenues to pursue in regard to treatment for
adolescents with BN are not known, which underscores our need for more systematic
studies into the treatment of this patient population. To this end, a multicenter comparison of FBT-BN, CBT, and supportive psychotherapy is currently in progress at the
University of Chicago and Stanford University.

References

Dodge, E., Hodes, M., Eisler, I., & Dare, C. (1995). Family therapy for bulimia nervosa in adolescents: An exploratory study. *Journal of Family Therapy, 17,* 59–77.

Eisler, I., Dare, C., Hodes, M., Russell, G., Dodge, E., & Le Grange, D. (2000). Family therapy for adolescent anorexia nervosa: The results of a controlled comparison of two family interventions. *Journal of Child Psychology and Psychiatry, 41,* 727–736.

Fischer, S., & Le Grange, D. (2007). Comorbidity and high-risk behaviors in treatment seeking adolescents with bulimia nervosa. *International Journal of Eating Disorders, 40,* 751–753.

Le Grange, D., Crosby, R., Rathouz, P., & Leventhal, B. (2007). A controlled comparison of family-based treatment and supportive psychotherapy for adolescent bulimia nervosa. *Archives of General Psychiatry, 64,* 1049–1056.

Le Grange, D., & Eisler, I. 2009. Family interventions in adolescent anorexia nervosa. *Child and Adolescent Psychiatric Clinics of North America, 18,* 159–173.

Le Grange D., & Lock, J. (2007). *Treating bulimia in adolescents: A family-based approach.* New York: Guilford Press.

Le Grange, D., Lock, J., & Dymek, M. 2003. Family-based therapy for adolescents with bulimia nervosa. *American Journal of Psychotherapy, 67,* 237–251.

Lock, J. (2005). Adjusting cognitive behavior therapy for adolescents with bulimia ner-

vosa: Results of case series. *American Journal of Psychotherapy, 59,* 267–281.

Schapman-Williams, A., Lock, J., & Couturier, J. (2006). Cognitive-behavioral therapy for adolescents with binge eating syndromes: A case series. *International Journal of Eating Disorders, 39,* 252–255.

Schmidt, U., Lee, S., Beecham, J., Perkins, S., Treasure, J., Yi, I., et al. (2007). A randomized controlled trial of family therapy and cognitive behavioral guided self-help for adolescents with bulimia nervosa and related conditions. *American Journal of Psychiatry, 164,* 591–598.

Swanson, S., Crow, S., Le Grange, D., & Merikangas, K. (in press). Prevalence and correlates of eating disorders in adolescents: Results from the National Comorbidity Survey Replication Adolescent Supplement. *Archives of General Psychiatry.*

Stice, E., & Agras, W. S. (1998). Predicting onset and cessation of bulimic behaviors during adolescence. *Behavior Therapy, 29,* 257–276.

Wilson, G. T., Grilo, C. M., & Vitousek, K. (2007). Psychological treatments for eating disorders. *American Psychologist, 62,* 199–216.

Zaitsoff, S., Celio Doyle, A., Hoste, R., & Le Grange, D. (2008). Therapeutic alliance and treatment acceptability with adolescents with bulimia nervosa: A comparison between individual and family based treatments. *International Journal of Eating Disorders, 41,* 390–398.

CHAPTER 16

Cognitive-Behavioral Therapy for Adolescent Bulimia Nervosa and Binge-Eating Disorder

Mari Campbell
Ulrike Schmidt

Bulimia nervosa (BN) and binge-eating disorder (BED) used to be thought of as disorders mainly occurring or presenting in adulthood. However, recent studies have shown that binge eating, a key symptom for both BN and BED, affects about 6% of preadolescent children (Hilbert, Rief, Tuschen-Caffier, de Zwaan, & Czaja, 2009; Tanofsky-Kraff et al., 2004). The peak incidence of BN occurs in the 10- to 19-year-old age bracket (Currin, Schmidt, Treasure, & Jick, 2005), and there is evidence that age of onset of BN is decreasing (Favaro, Caregaro, Tenconi, Bosello, & Santonastaso, 2009). Early onset of BN is linked with early menarche, which in turn is related to childhood obesity (Day et al., 2011). BN impacts on the young person's psychological and physical well-being, and his or her quality of life (Keilen, Treasure, Schmidt, & Treasure, 1994). It also imposes substantial medical and economic burdens (Crow & Peterson, 2003; Striegel-Moore, Leslie, Petrill, Garvin, & Rosenheck, 2000).

In contrast, much less is known about the incidence and prevalence of BED in adolescence. Two different patterns of onset of BED have been highlighted (Marcus & Kalarchian, 2003): the first, in which the onset of binge eating follows a period of dieting behavior, seems to be linked to adult onset (mean age of onset = 28.0 years), and a second in which binge eating precedes any dieting behaviors, which appears to be linked to adolescent onset (mean age of onset = 12.8 years) (Marcus, Moulton & Greeno, 1995). A recent large-scale epidemiological study of eating disorders prevalence in Portuguese adolescents found the prevalence of BED to be in the region of 0.1%, that is, significantly lower than that typically found in adult cohorts (Machado, Machado, Gonçalves & Hoek, 2007).

Unsurprisingly, most of the research on treatment of BN and BED has been conducted in adults, suggesting that cognitive-behavioral therapy (CBT) is the treatment of choice for both of these disorders (National Institute of Clinical Excellence [NICE], 2004). In this chapter we review the limited research literature on the use of CBT in adolescents with BN and BED. We outline why CBT is a viable approach for use with adolescents and consider how the model can be adapted when working with this population.

Overview of Research to Date

Cognitive-behavioral approaches to the treatment of BN in adults have been developing since the early 1980s (Fairburn, 1981) and have been adapted and expanded upon with clinical experience and through the results of experimental, efficacy, and effectiveness studies (Fairburn, Cooper, & Shafran, 2003; Ghaderi, 2006). Empirical research shows good short- and long-term outcomes and acceptability (for review, see Hay, Bacaltchuk, Stefano, & Kashyap, 2009), and CBT is being recommended as the treatment of choice for this population (Hay et al., 2009; NICE, 2004; Shapiro et al., 2007). A small study by Ghaderi (2006) supports the use of a more flexible individualized approach, over the strict manualized form of treatment. More recently a transdiagnostic cognitive-behavioral program that treats all eating disorder psychopathology has been suggested (CBT-E; Fairburn 2008). This treatment can be delivered in either a focused form (CBT-Ef) that targets eating disorder psychopathology alone or a broader form (CBT-Eb) that targets common maintenance factors (e.g., clinical perfectionism, low self-esteem, and interpersonal difficulties) in addition to eating disorder psychopathology. Recent empirical investigation of the two models suggests that CBT-Ef should be used as a first-line treatment (Fairburn et al., 2009), with the broader treatment being used in more complex cases.

A sizable number of studies have investigated CBT in adults with BED. In a systematic review and meta-analysis of treatments of BED, psychological therapy and structured self-help based on cognitive-behavioral interventions were found to have large effects on the reduction of binge eating but not on weight (see Vocks et al., 2010).

As yet, very little is known about effective and acceptable treatments and routes for accessing treatment for adolescents with BN or BED. Of note, there typically appears to be a delay (about 4–5 years after onset) in patients with BN before they seek treatment (Turnbull, Ward, Treasure, Hershel, & Derby, 1996). Fear of stigma and feelings of shame and embarrassment have been suggested as possible reasons (Hepworth & Paxton, 2007), and ways of reducing this delay through facilitating earlier access to treatment need to be thought about. In what follows we mainly focus on adolescent BN, given the lack of available evidence in BED; however, much of what is said is applicable to BED too.

Lock (2005) conducted a case series, examining the use of CBT to treat 12- to 18-year-olds with BN. He highlighted the need to adapt the model in relation to developmental factors associated with adolescence (e.g., biological, cognitive, psychological, and social changes). Results show an overall reduction in rates of binge eating and purging, abstinence rates of 56%, and good adherence to treatment (dropout = 18%). More recently, Pretorius, Rowlans, Ringwood, and Schmidt (2010) investigated the use of a CBT guided self-care program (BT-GSC), adapted from the Overcoming Bulimia Online Program (Williams, Aubin, Cottrell, & Harkin, 1998), in 101 young people aged 13 to 20 suffering from BN (or eating disorder not otherwise specified–BN [EDNOS-BN]). Recruitment was partly via specialist eating disorder services and partly via an advertisement on the website of *beat*, the United Kingdom's charity for patients with eating disorders and their carers (*www.beat.co.uk*), as *beat* is often the first port of call for advice and support for people with eating disorders. Results showed significant decreases in eating-disordered behaviors and attitudes, which remained 6 months after treatment. The treatment also showed good acceptability (with good uptake and positive reports from participants) (Pretorius et al., 2009; Pretorius et al., 2010).

To date, there is only one randomized controlled trial (RCT) investigating the efficacy of cognitive-behavioral guided self-care in adolescents with BN. Schmidt and colleagues (2007) compared CBT guided self-care and family therapy. The CBT guided self-care approach was adapted from a manual used with adults with BN (Perkins & Schmidt, 2005; Schmidt & Treasure, 1997). Patients allocated to the guided self-care group received 10 weekly sessions and three follow-up sessions at monthly intervals. They also had the option of two sessions with a close other, in order to improve mechanisms of support. Patients in the guided self-care group showed a quicker reduction in binge eating than those in the family therapy group, although there was no difference in outcome at 12-month follow-up. The acceptability of the guided self-care approach also appeared to be greater, with more patients declining family therapy because of a wish for their families not to be involved in treatment.

Why Adapt CBT for Use with Adolescents with BN?

Although there is limited empirical evidence to date supporting the use of CBT in treating adolescents with eating disorders, Wilson and Sysko (2006) outlined three reasons why CBT should be considered as a treatment choice for adolescents suffering from BN. First, the model's efficacy has already been established for treating BN in adults (NICE, 2004) and research shows little difference in relation to risk factors and presentation between early- and late-onset cases (Day et al., 2011; Schmidt, Hodes, & Treasure, 1992). Second, there is evidence supporting the use of CBT in treating other adolescent clinical disorders, including anxiety and mood disorders (Brent & Weersing, 2008; Pine & Klein, 2008; Walkup et al., 2008). Finally, there is a conceptual fit between a cognitive-behavioral approach and the clinical presentation of adolescents with BN. In addition, as BN generally develops postpubertally, this may suggest that adolescents usually have the cognitive ability to use CBT, and possibly respond better, as they may be more "malleable" and responsive to change and cognitive challenging than adults (Schmidt, 2009).

Treatment

The cognitive-behavioral model of treatment used with adolescents with BN closely resembles the model used with adults who have the illness. There is literature available that can provide further detail on using CBT in treating eating disorders (Fairburn, 2008; Lock, 2005; Waller et al., 2007), but because of space constraints this section focuses on potential adaptations to the model and specific areas to consider in working with young people. Weisz and Hawley (2002) identified three general areas for consideration in adapting cognitive-behavioral approaches for use with adolescents. These include levels of motivation for change and cognitive and social development. More specifically, in using a cognitive-behavioral approach in the treatment of adolescent BN, Gowers and Bryant-Waugh (2004) identify the need for an increased focus on motivation and family involvement. The NICE (2004) guidelines for the treatment of BN also stress the need to make adjustments to CBT for age, circumstances, and level of development of the adolescent, as well as including family members in treatment, as appropriate. These adaptations are discussed in turn in the following sections. It is also important to be aware of the medical complications associated with the disorder and to ensure that physical health and risk are continually monitored throughout treatment (see Katzman & Findlay, Chapter 9, this volume, for further details).

Engagement and Motivation to Change

Like adults with eating disorders, adolescents with BN can often be ambivalent to change. Such ambivalence may be exacerbated by young people not presenting for treatment themselves, but instead responding to the concerns raised by other people in their lives (e.g., parents, friends, and professionals). In addition, they may not have experienced many of the negative physical and psychological consequences of the illness. However, Perkins and colleagues (2007) found no difference in levels of motivation between older and younger, earlier-onset patients with BN. Lock (2005) notes that adolescents have poorer abstracting, executive functioning, goal-setting, and planning abilities than adults, which can limit their understanding of the hazards of their behaviors and decrease motivation for treatment. Wilson and Sysko (2006) and Schmidt (2009) emphasize the importance of the development of a collaborative relationship and suggest the use of specific techniques, such as a motivational stance and techniques (Geller, Williams, & Srikameswaran, 2001; Treasure & Schmidt, 2001), and Socratic questioning (Wells, 1997) to support personal autonomy and enhance motivation, as well as allowing the development of treatment goals that are focused on a desire for personal change rather than the wishes of parents or professionals (Schmidt, 2005). Techniques and activities, such as examining the pros and cons of the illness, employing timelines, and so forth, can be used to enhance motivation (Serpell & Treasure, 2002; Waller et al., 2007). Adaptations for the younger population can include shortening time frames to match adolescents' more "here and now" thinking style, using a more structured approach to eliciting concerns, writing tasks, the use of creative activities (e.g., art, writing, role play, etc.), and externalization techniques (Schmidt, 2005). Externalization techniques may also be helpful in engaging parental support during this stage, as they allow the separation of the child from the disorder (White, 1988; White & Epston, 1990). In addition, a specific motivation for young people may be to get their parents (and professionals) "off their backs." Lock suggests that adolescents may benefit from increased intensity of contact early in treatment in order to build an alliance. Psychoeducation is also important during this stage of treatment, as young people may not be aware of the risks and consequences associated with the illness. Psychoeducation can take place with the young person and family members, both in session and through the use of age-appropriate worksheets. The information can also convey the message that young people and their parents are not alone in fighting the illness.

Case Formulation and Treatment Planning

Adolescence is a stage of development in which individuals are working to become more autonomous. Therefore it is important that the development of a formulation and treatment plan is a collaborative process that is driven by the young person. A joint formulation can aid understanding of the therapeutic process and the relationship between physiology, thoughts, feelings, and behaviors. Patients can also use the formulation to consider and agree on areas for change. It is important that it is kept simple and that the adolescent's own language is used where possible. A diagrammatic or pictorial representation of the formulation may be beneficial in working with younger adolescents, as well as a rewording of the key elements of the formulations—for example, using questions such as "Why me?" "Why now?" "Why still?" to establish predisposing, precipitating, and maintaining factors. Because adolescents often still reside with, and are dependent on, their families, it may be useful to build the impact of the illness on the family into the formulation (Dummett, 2006).

Regulating Eating and Reducing Eating Disorder Symptomatology

Explaining the importance of regular eating is a requisite from the start of treatment, and it may be helpful to request dietetic input from the whole family. It is important to think with the young person, and his or her parents, about how he or she can integrate a regular eating pattern into his or her lifestyle and how the young person can be supported by family and friends during or after meals. For example, adolescents may find it helpful to eat meals with family and friends around to normalize the process, or they may prefer to take prepacked lunches that include "safe" foods, to school at first. The implementation may have to be staggered, with the young person starting with "easier" meals and snacks in the beginning.

Behavioral experiments can be helpful in testing adolescents' beliefs about what would happen to their weight if they follow a regular eating pattern. Young people are particularly primed to understanding the concept of a behavioral experiment, as they are still actively, or were recently, involved in science lessons at school. They are aware of how to develop hypotheses and experiments and how to perform a "fair test" and can apply this knowledge to the eating disorders work.

Exploration of Other Salient Issues

Adolescence is a time of change and turbulence, when young people are developing their own personalities and belief systems. They may also be trying to manage or understand other difficult situations, which can act as maintaining factors for the eating disorder. It is therefore important to be flexible in the use of treatment time to examine other issues that are important, but less directly related to the eating disorder psychopathology. This may include addressing comorbid problems, such as managing anxiety or low mood, addressing some of the underlying issues associated with the development of the eating disorder, such as feelings associated with early menarche (Day et al., 2011), or thinking about other areas of development and moving forward, including discussions about relationships with others and developing body acceptance, self-confidence, and assertiveness skills. These areas may be included in the original formulation or added as treatment progresses. When addressing these areas, young people can build on some of the skills learned earlier in therapy. Recent empirical investigation comparing an eating disorder–focused model of CBT with a broader model that also addressed common maintenance factors suggests that both treatments are useful in treating eating disorders in adults, but that the simpler treatment should be used as a default approach (Fairburn et al., 2009). There does not appear to be any reason why a similar approach cannot be taken with adolescents.

Relapse Prevention and Endings

The final stage of treatment is focused on maintaining the changes made during therapy and planning for discharge. It involves reviewing the progress made since the start of treatment, with the adolescent being able to take ownership of the changes. It is also important to work with the adolescent, and his or her parents, to set realistic expectations for the future. Highlighting the difference between a lapse and a relapse and developing a "blueprint" that identifies potential triggers, signs, and strategies to manage both is important. Discussion about the process of ending, hopes and fears, and so forth, with both the young person and his or her family, is important, as well as thinking about how they may manage some of the differences in viewpoints in this area.

Additional Areas of Consideration in Working with Adolescents

Other areas that need to be considered throughout treatment, and adapted to, include the young person's level of cognitive and emotional development, social factors and interpersonal functioning, and family involvement. These are discussed, in turn, in the following sections. It is also vital that clinicians remain flexible in their approach to treatment and in addressing developmental needs (Weisz & Hawley, 2002; Wilson & Sysko, 2006), both in terms of the structure of treatment and the specific approaches and techniques used. Lock (2005) highlights the importance of being flexible about the tasks of therapy (e.g., homework, food logs, etc.). The requirements of homework can also be particularly difficult for young people, who already have other demands on their time from school, friends, parents, and so forth, and they may find completing these tasks difficult (Christie, 2000). In order to establish a strong therapeutic alliance, clinicians need to be clear in regard to the rationale for the work and may need to start by having the tasks completed in session, recruiting outside support, or using more focused, time-limited activities (Lock, 2005; Waller et al., 2007).

Cognitive, Emotional, and Physical Development

To be able to use CBT effectively, young people need skills in abstraction, hypothetical reasoning, and consequential thinking (Weisz & Hawley, 2002). These skills should be evaluated during the assessment sessions. However, it has been suggested that from early adolescence (e.g., 11–13 years of age) young people develop the ability to reason logically, articulate their thoughts in an abstract manner, and have metacognitions (Forehand & Weirson, 1993). Throughout therapy attention must be paid to the language and communication style used by the therapist, and some simplification of both language and concepts may be necessary. However, our own experience suggests that some young people can be very sensitive to feeling patronized or treated like younger children, so it is important to strike a balance here.

Verbal and visual aids can be used to support the session. Wilson and Sysko (2006) suggest using more behavioral approaches with young people who find cognitive restructuring difficult. However, behaviors and cognitions may be less entrenched in this younger population, and therefore more malleable to change. Changes in cognitive abilities may also be the focus of some of the additional work young people want to address, and specific techniques and tasks may be better suited to different age groups (Forehand & Weirson, 1993).

Social Factors, Interpersonal Functioning, and Family Involvement

Research evidence supports the use of family-based treatment as the treatment of choice for adolescent anorexia nervosa (AN) (NICE, 2004). Lessons learned in this area may be transferred to working with adolescents with BN (Eisler, 2005), especially as there is evidence from two trials suggesting that family therapy can be effective in treating adolescent BN (Le Grange, Crosby, Rathouz & Leventhal, 2007; Schmidt et al., 2007).

Young people are still practically and emotionally dependent on their families (Lock, 2005) and often come for treatment in response to concerns raised by family members, rather than a strong desire for change themselves. Moreover, the impact of caring for a person with BN is significant, with carers often highly distressed and with many unmet needs (Perkins, Winn, Murray, Murphy, & Schmidt, 2004; Winn et al., 2007; Winn, Perkins, Murray, Murphy, & Schmidt, 2004). Given these factors, it is important to think about how family members can be involved in treatment (Wilson & Sysko, 2006). The involvement of parents can take many forms, including psychoeducation about the illness and model of treatment, Web-based support for carers (Grover et al., in press), equipping them with skills and strategies for helping their child or responding to his or her needs, and/or assessing conflict or patterns of behavior that are maintaining the problem. Parents can help facilitate individual treatment but there must be a balance between parental control and adolescent autonomy. It is important that clinicians be flexible in involving the family and close others, responding to both the parents' and the adolescent's requests and needs. Initial sessions can be used to develop a contract in regard to family involvement, considering the limits of confidentiality, as well as making the adolescent the gatekeeper for highlighting areas that he or she wishes to remain confidential. Depending on the stage of treatment, age and stage of the young person, and level of concern or risk, family involvement can take the form of joint sessions, separate sessions, or a mixture of the two.

Some young people, especially those who have chosen to come for treatment by themselves, may find the idea of involving their parents difficult. Our group previously investigated the reasons why adolescents choose not to involve their parents in treatment (Perkins et al., 2005). Patients who did not involve their parents were significantly older, had a longer duration of eating disorder symptomatology, and were less likely to live with their parents. They were also more likely to have a history of obesity, current depression, more comorbid behaviors (e.g., impulsivity, self-harm, shoplifting) and perceive their mothers to display higher levels of expressed emotion. There was no difference in current levels of eating disorder symptomatology between the patients who involved their parents and those who did not. The most common reasons given for noninclusion were discomfort in discussing personal issues in front of their parents, feeling that the illness was their own problem, and other personal reasons. The main reasons why patients chose to include their parents were that they saw them as supportive, interested, and having time for them, and the parents' wishing to be involved and learn more. Discussion about parental involvement may include thinking about the adolescent's independence, less practical parental involvement, and the possibility that the desire to separate may be motivated by poor relationships. Clinicians may need to address the young person's concerns about parental involvement and support the parents in becoming more accepting and less blaming, possibly through psychoeducation about the illness.

Pressures to be thin can come from a variety of sources and in a number of different forms (Stice, Maxfield, & Wells, 2003). The "thin ideal" is often promoted in the media, and young people tend to read magazines and to watch television programs and films that give both direct and indirect messages that they should conform to the current standards. These messages and their impact can be discussed in treatment. Peer involvement in treatment should also be considered. Schmidt (2009) highlights the importance of being aware of the young person's social context, including the parents' parenting style and the importance of peer relationships. Adolescence is associated with a move away from the family of origin, toward closer and stronger relationships with peers (Forehand & Weirson, 1993). Young women's self-esteem is strongly influenced by their relationships with and perceptions of others, and difficulties in interpersonal relationships can be addressed using social skills training, strengthening communication and negotiation skills, and teaching conflict resolution strategies (Wilson & Sysko, 2006). It has been noted that friendship groups tend to be similar in levels of concern about body image and the use of behaviors to manage weight and shape, and that peer beliefs influence individuals' eating habits and concern about body image (Paxton, Schutz, Wertheim, & Muir, 1999; Stice et al., 2003). Yet, peers can still be useful in challenging beliefs and identifying new strategies for change. For example, they can be involved in answering surveys, giving positive feedback, or eliciting different patterns of thinking and behaviors. Older adolescents may come for treatment with a friend or partner, rather than parents, and their ongoing involvement in therapy may have to be considered. It may also be important to discuss the young person's use of "pro" websites that advocate the disorder as a lifestyle choice, as well as the evidence for and against this viewpoint. It is also important to alert parents of such websites (Royal College of Psychiatrists, 2009).

Case Example

Jane is a 17-year-old young woman who lives with her parents and younger brother. She is currently studying for her final school exams and hopes to study at the university in the next academic year. The onset of her BN was 2 years prior to presentation for assessment, following a period of turbulence in her relationships with her peers and increased anxiety about school performance in the runup to some important exams. Jane disclosed the illness to her parents after they had raised concerns about her fluctuating mood, avoiding family meals and large amounts of food going missing. With their encouragement she approached her medical doctor for advice in regard to treatment.

On her first visit to a specialist eating disorders service, Jane reported alternating between periods of restriction, often not eating until the evening meal, and binge eating (three to four times a week). Jane reported self-inducing vomiting following binges, after meals when she felt she had eaten too much and at times when she was feeling low in mood. She reported a high level of preoccupation with thoughts of eating, weight, and shape and fears of fatness. Her weight was at the lower end of the healthy weight range for someone of her age and height, and she was menstruating regularly. Jane and her parents reported an increasingly conflictual relationship, with Jane becoming more secretive as her parents became more intrusive as a result of their increasing worry.

Initially, treatment focused on helping Jane to understand the role and impact of BN on her life, as well as supporting her parents to understand the nature of the illness. Psychoeducation about the effects of starvation, irregular eating, and self-induced vomiting was given to both Jane and her parents. Jane was able to write letters to bulimia as a friend and an enemy (see Serpell & Treasure, 2002); these worked to enhance her motivation and provided the clinician with a greater understanding of the role the eating disorder was playing in her life.

An individual formulation (see Figure 16.1) was developed through discussion with Jane, which included outlining the impact of the illness on other family members' thoughts, feelings, and behaviors. As the sessions developed, Jane was able to share bits of the formulation with her parents and to think of support strategies and exits out of

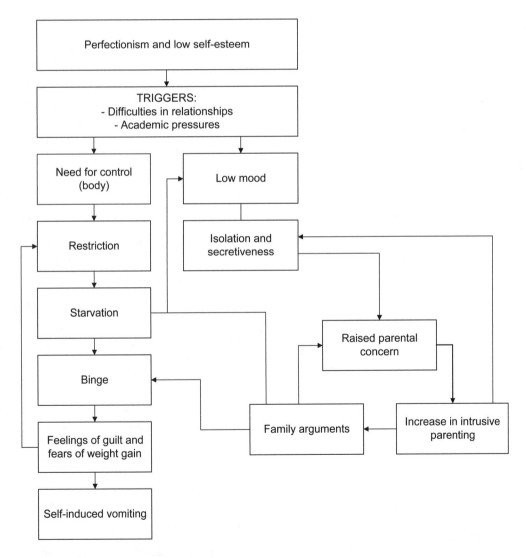

FIGURE 16.1. Formulation developed with Jane and her family.

the vicious cycles. Jane's belief that following a regular meal plan would substantially increase her weight was tested with the use of a behavioral experiment involving food diaries and regular weighing.

As treatment progressed, Jane was able to develop techniques to manage her low mood (including thought monitoring, cognitive challenging, and activity scheduling). She also started to talk about her relationships with her friends and family, including her concerns about being able to meet their expectations and her low sense of self-worth. Discussions with the important people in her life and the use of surveys to test her beliefs aided in cognitive challenging of these perfectionist traits. As Jane's eating became more regular and she developed more strategies to manage times of high anxiety, the frequency of her binge eating and vomiting decreased. The frequency of sessions also decreased over the course of treatment and as Jane found ways in which she could feel supported outside therapy.

Jane and her parents found the prospect of ending treatment unsettling, and they reflected on how their worries were contained by the ongoing support from her therapist. We discussed their concerns, hopes, and fears for the future and how these differed between family members. A comprehensive relapse prevention plan, detailing potential triggers, signs, and strategies to manage both lapses and relapse, was developed in collaboration between Jane and her parents. Jane also exchanged "good-bye" letters with her therapist, which offered an opportunity to highlight the skills she had developed and the progresses she had made over the course of therapy. By the end of treatment she had been symptom free for 3 weeks.

Summary and Future Directions

Overall, it appears that CBT is a valuable resource in treating adolescents with bulimic eating disorders. However, adaptations must be made to address the developmental needs of this population. Given our knowledge that adolescents are strongly reliant on their families, and considering the results of research studies showing good outcomes using family approaches in the treatment of adolescent AN (Eisler et al., 2000; Eisler, Simic, Russell, & Dare, 2007; Le Grange, Binford, & Loeb, 2005; Le Grange, Eisler, Dare, & Russell, 1992; Lock, Agras, Bryson, & Kraemer, 2005; Lock, Couturier, & Agras, 2006; Lock, Le Grange, Forsberg, & Hewell, 2006; Paulson-Karlsson, Engstrom, & Nevonen, 2009) and BN (Dodge, Hodes, Eisler, & Dare, 1995; Le Grange et al., 2007; Schmidt et al., 2007), we suggest that it is essential to build in a systemic element to current cognitive-behavioral models that involves thinking about the influence of and impact on the family and close others. Further research into the efficacy and effectiveness of CBT (rather than guided self-help) for adolescents with BN or BED is urgently needed. This effort should also include investigation of the mediators and moderators of treatment.

Acknowledgments

This work was supported by the National Institute for Health Research (NIHR) Biomedical Research Centre for Mental Health, South London, and Maudsley NHS Foundation Trust and Institute of Psychiatry, King's College London, and by a NIHR Programme Grant for Applied

Research (Reference No. RP-PG-0606-1043). The views expressed herein are those of the authors and not necessarily those of the NHS, the NIHR, or the Department of Health.

References

Brent, D., & Weersing, V. R. (2008). Depressive disorders in childhood and adolescence. In M. Rutter, D. Bishop, D. S. Pine, S. Scott, J. Stevenson, E. Taylor, et al. (Eds.), *Rutter's child and adolescent psychiatry* (5th ed., pp. 628–647). Oxford, UK: Blackwell.

Christie, D. (2000). Cognitive-behavioural therapeutic techniques for children with eating disorders. In B. Lask & R. Bryant-Waugh (Eds.), *Anorexia nervosa and related eating disorders in childhood and adolescence* (2nd ed., pp. 205–226). New York: Psychology Press.

Crow, S. J., & Peterson, C. B. (2003). The economic and social burden of eating disorders: A review. In M. Maj, K. Halmi, J. J. Lopez-Ibor, & N. Sartorius (Eds.), *Eating disorders* (pp. 385–398). Chichester, UK: Wiley.

Currin, L., Schmidt, U., Treasure, J., & Jick, H. (2005). Time trends in eating disorder incidence. *British Journal of Psychiatry, 186*, 132–135.

Day, J., Schmidt, U., Collier, D., Perkins, S., Van den Eynde, F., Treasure, J., et al. (2011). Risk factors, correlates and markers in early-onset bulimia nervosa and EDNOS. *International Journal of Eating Disorders, 44*, 287–294.

Dodge, E., Hodes, M., Eisler, I., & Dare, C. (1995). Family therapy for bulimia nervosa in adolescents: An exploratory study. *Journal of Family Therapy, 17*, 59–77.

Dummett, N. (2006). Processes for systemic cognitive-behavioural therapy with children, young people and families. *Behavioural and Cognitive Psychotherapy, 34*, 179–189.

Eisler, I. (2005). The empirical and theoretical base of family therapy and multiple family day therapy for adolescent anorexia nervosa. *Journal of Family Therapy, 27*, 104–131.

Eisler, I., Dare, C., Hodes, M., Russell, R., Dodge, E., & Le Grange, D. (2000). Family therapy for adolescent anorexia nervosa: The results of a controlled comparison of two family interventions. *Journal of Child Psychology and Psychiatry, 41*, 727–736.

Eisler, I., Simic, M., Russell, G. F. M., & Dare, C. (2007). A randomised controlled treatment trial of two forms of family therapy in adolescent anorexia nervosa: A five-year follow-up. *Journal of Child Psychology and Psychiatry, 48*, 552–560.

Fairburn, C. (1981). A cognitive-behavioural approach to the treatment of bulimia. *Psychological Medicine, 11*, 707–711.

Fairburn, C. G. (2008). *Cognitive behavior therapy and eating disorders*. New York: Guilford Press.

Fairburn, C. G., Cooper, Z., Doll, H. A., O'Connor, M. E., Bohn, K., Hawker, D. M., et al. (2009). Transdiagnostic cognitive-behavioral therapy for patients with eating disorders: A two-site trial with 60-week follow-up. *American Journal of Psychiatry, 166*, 311–319.

Fairburn, C. G., Cooper, Z., & Shafran, R. (2003). Cognitive behaviour therapy for eating disorders: A "transdiagnostic" theory and treatment. *Behaviour, Research and Therapy, 41*, 509–528.

Favaro, A., Caregaro, L., Tenconi, E., Bosello, R., & Santonastaso, P. (2009). Time trends in age at onset of anorexia nervosa and bulimia nervosa. *Journal of Clinical Psychiatry, 70*, 1715–1721.

Forehand, R., & Weirson, M. (1993). The role of developmental factors in planning behavioural interventions for children: Disruptive behaviour as an example. *Behavior Therapy, 24*, 117–141.

Geller, J., Williams, K., & Srikameswaran, S. (2001). Clinician stance in the treatment of chronic eating disorders. *European Eating Disorders Review, 9*, 1–9.

Ghaderi, A. (2006). Does individualization matter?: A randomized trial of manual-based versus individualized cognitive behavior therapy for bulimia nervosa. *Behaviour Research and Therapy, 44*, 273–288.

Gowers, S., & Bryant-Waugh, R. (2004). Management of child and adolescent eating disorders: The current evidence base and future directions. *Journal of Child Psychology and Psychiatry, 45,* 63–83.

Grover, M., Williams, C., Eisler, I., Fairbairn, P., McCloskey, C., Smith, G., et al. (in press). An off-line pilot evaluation of a Web-based systemic cognitive-behavioral intervention for carers of people with anorexia nervosa. *International Journal of Eating Disorders.*

Hay, P. P., Bacaltchuk, J., Stefano, S., & Kashyap, P. (2009). Psychological treatments for bulimia nervosa and binging. *Cochrane Database of Systematic Reviews,* Issue 4 (Article No. CD000562), DOI: 10.1002/14651858. CD000562.pub3.

Hepworth, N., & Paxton, S. J. (2007). Pathways to help-seeking in bulimia nervosa and binge eating problems: A concept mapping approach. *International Journal of Eating Disorders, 40,* 493–504.

Hilbert, A., Rief, W., Tuschen-Caffier, B., de Zwaan, M., & Czaja, J. (2009). Loss of control eating and psychological maintenance in children: An ecological momentary assessment study. *Behaviour, Research and Therapy, 47,* 26–33.

Keilen, M., Treasure, T., Schmidt, U., & Treasure, J. (1994). Quality of life measurements in eating disorders, angina and transplant candidates: Are they comparable? *Journal of the Royal Society of Medicine, 87,* 441–444.

Le Grange, D., Binford, R., & Loeb, K. L. (2005). Manualized family-based treatment for anorexia nervosa: A case series. *Journal of the American Academy of Child and Adolescent Psychiatry, 44,* 41–46.

Le Grange, D., Crosby, R. D., Rathouz, P. J., & Leventhal, B. L. (2007). A randomized controlled comparison of family-based treatment and supportive psychotherapy for adolescent bulimia nervosa. *Archives of General Psychiatry, 64,* 1049–1056.

Le Grange, D., Eisler, I., Dare, C., & Russell, G. F. M. (1992). Evaluation of family treatments in adolescent anorexia nervosa: A pilot study. *International Journal of Eating Disorders, 12,* 347–357.

Lock, J. (2005). Adjusting cognitive-behavior therapy for adolescents with bulimia nervosa: Results of case series. *American Journal of Psychotherapy, 59,* 267–281.

Lock, J., Agras, W. S., Bryson, S., & Kraemer, H. C. (2005). A comparison of short- and long-term family therapy for adolescent anorexia nervosa. *Journal of the American Academy of Child and Adolescent Psychiatry, 44,* 632–639.

Lock, J., Couturier, J., & Agras, W. S. (2006). Comparison of long-term outcomes in adolescents with anorexia nervosa treated with family therapy. *Journal of the American Academy of Child and Adolescent Psychiatry, 45,* 666–672.

Lock, J., Le Grange, D., Forsberg, S., & Hewell, K. (2006). Is family therapy useful for treating children with anorexia nervosa?: Results of a case series. *Journal of the American Academy of Child and Adolescent Psychiatry, 45,* 1323–1328.

Machado, P. P., Machado, B. C., Gonçalves, S., & Hoek, H. W. (2007). The prevalence of eating disorders not otherwise specified. *International Journal of Eating Disorders, 40,* 212–217.

Marcus, M. D., & Kalarchian, M. A. (2003). Binge eating in children and adolescents. *International Journal of Eating Disorders, 34*(Supp.), S47–S57.

Marcus, M. D., Mouton, M. M., & Greeno, C. G. (1995). Binge eating onset in obese patients with binge eating disorder. *Addictive Behaviors, 20,* 747–755.

National Institute of Clinical Excellence. (2004). *Eating disorders: Core interventions in the treatment and management of anorexia nervosa, bulimia nervosa and related eating disorders.* London: British Psychological Society.

Paulson-Karlsson, G., Engstrom, I., & Nevonen, L. (2009). A pilot study of family-based treatment for adolescent anorexia nervosa: 18- and 36-month follow-ups. *Eating Disorders, 17,* 72–88.

Paxton, S. J., Schutz, H. K., Wertheim, E. H., & Muir, S. L. (1999). Friendship clique and peer influences on body image attitudes, dietary restraint, extreme weight loss behaviours and binge eating in adolescent girls. *Journal of Abnormal Psychology, 108*, 255–266.

Perkins, S., & Schmidt, U. (2005). Self-help for eating disorders. In S. Wonderlich, J. Mitchell, M. de Zwann, & H. Steiger (Eds.), *Eating disorders review: Part 1. Academy for Eating Disorders* (pp. 87–104). Oxford, UK: Radcliffe.

Perkins, S., Schmidt, U., Eisler, I., Treasure, J., Berelowitz, M., Dodge, E., et al. (2007). Motivation to change in recent onset and long-standing bulimia nervosa: Are there differences? *Eating and Weight Disorders, 12*, 61–69.

Perkins, S., Schmidt, U., Eisler, I., Treasure, J., Yi, I., Winn, S., et al. (2005). Why do adolescents with bulimia nervosa choose not to involve their parents in treatment? *European Child and Adolescent Psychiatry, 14*, 376–385.

Perkins, S., Winn, S., Murray, J., Murphy, R., & Schmidt, U. (2004). A qualitative study of the experience of caring for a person with bulimia nervosa: Part 1. The emotional impact of caring. *International Journal of Eating Disorders, 36*, 256–268.

Pine, D. S., & Klein, R. G. (2008). Anxiety disorders. In M. Rutter, D. Bishop, D. S. Pine, S. Scott, J. Stevenson, E. Taylor, et al. (Eds.), *Rutter's child and adolescent psychiatry* (5th ed., pp. 628–647). Oxford, UK: Blackwell.

Pretorius, N., Arcelus, J., Beecham, J., Dawson, H., Doherty, F., Eisler, I., et al. (2009). Cognitive-behavioural therapy for adolescents with bulimic symptomatology: The acceptability and effectiveness of Internet-based delivery. *Behaviour Research and Therapy, 47*, 729–736.

Pretorius, N., Rowlans, L., Ringwood, S., & Schmidt, U. (2010). Young people's perceptions of and reasons for accessing a Web-based cognitive behavioural intervention for bulimia nervosa. *European Eating Disorders Review, 18*, 197–206.

Royal College of Psychiatrists. (2009). Position paper on pro-anorexia and pro-bulimia websites. Retrieved March 30, 2010, from *www.rcpsych.ac.uk/docs/Pro-ANa%20 2ndof%20June2009[2].doc.*

Serpell, L., & Treasure, J. (2002). Bulimia nervosa: Friend or foe?: The pros and cons of bulimia nervosa. *International Journal of Eating Disorders, 32*, 164–170.

Schmidt, U. (2005). Engagement and motivational interviewing. In P. Graham (Ed.), *Cognitive behaviour therapy for children and families* (pp. 67–83). Cambridge, UK: Cambridge University Press.

Schmidt, U. (2009). Cognitive behavioural approaches in adolescent anorexia and bulimia nervosa. *Child and Adolescent Psychiatric Clinics of North America, 18*, 147–158.

Schmidt, U., Hodes, M., & Treasure, J. (1992). Early onset bulimia nervosa: Who is at risk? A retrospective case-control study. *Psychological Medicine, 22*, 623–628.

Schmidt, U., Lee, S., Beecham, J., Perkins, S., Treasure, J., Yi, I., et al. (2007). A randomized controlled trial of family therapy and cognitive-behavior therapy guided self-care for adolescents with bulimia nervosa and related disorders. *American Journal of Psychiatry, 164*, 591–598.

Schmidt, U., & Treasure, J. (1997). *Getting better bit(e) by bit(e): A treatment manual for sufferers of bulimia nervosa.* Hove, East Sussex, UK: Psychological Press.

Shapiro, J. R., Berkman, N. D., Brownley, K. A., Sedway, J. A., Lohr, K. N., & Bulik, C. M. (2007). Bulimia nervosa treatment: A systematic review of randomized controlled trials. *International Journal of Eating Disorders, 40*, 321–336.

Stice, E., Maxfield, J., & Wells, T. (2003). Adverse effects of social pressure to be thin on young women: An experimental investigation of "fat talk." *International Journal of Eating Disorders, 34*, 108–117.

Striegel-Moore, R. H., Leslie, D., Petrill, S. A., Garvin, V., & Rosenheck, R. A. (2000). One-year use and cost of inpatient and outpatient services among female and male patients with an eating disorder: Evidence from a national database of health insurance claims. *International Journal of Eating Disorders, 27*, 381–389.

Tanofsky-Kraff, M., Yanovski, S. Z., Wilfley, D. E., Marmarosh, C., Morgan, C. M., & Yanovski, J. A. (2004). Eating-disordered behaviors, body fat, and psychopathology in overweight and normal-weight children. *Journal of Consulting and Clinical Psychology, 72*, 53–61.

Treasure, J., & Schmidt, U. (2001). Ready, willing and able to change: Motivational aspects of the assessment and treatment of eating disorders. *European Eating Disorders Review, 9*, 4–18.

Turnbull, S., Ward, A., Treasure, J., Hershel, J., & Derby, L. (1996). The demand for eating disorder care: An epidemiological study using the General Practice Research Database. *British Journal of Psychiatry, 169*, 705–712.

Vocks, S., Tuschen-Caffier, B., Pietrowsky, R., Rustenbach, S. J., Kersting, A., & Herpertz, S. (2010). Meta-analysis of the effectiveness of psychological and pharmacological treatments for binge eating disorder. *International Journal of Eating Disorders, 43*, 205–217.

Walkup, J. T., Albano, A. M., Piacentini, J., Birmaher, B., Compton, S. N., Sherrill, J. T., et al. (2008). Cognitive behavioral therapy, sertraline or a combination in childhood anxiety. *New England Journal of Medicine, 359*, 2753–2766.

Waller, G., Cordery, H., Corstorphine, E., Hinrichsen, H., Lawson, R., Mountford, V., et al. (2007). *Cognitive behaviour therapy for eating disorders: A comprehensive treatment guide.* Cambridge, UK: Cambridge University Press.

Weisz, J. R., & Hawley, K. R. (2002). Devel-
opmental factors in the treatment of adolescents. *Journal of Consulting and Clinical Psychology, 70*, 21–43.

Wells, A. (1997). *Cognitive therapy of anxiety disorders: A practice manual and conceptual guide.* Chichester, UK: Wiley.

White, M. (1988, Summer). The externalizing of the problem and the re-authoring of lives and relationships. *Dulwich Centre Newsletter.*

White, M., & Epston, D. (1990). *Narrative means to therapeutic ends.* New York: Norton.

Williams, C. J., Aubin, S. D., Cottrell, D., & Harkin, P. J. R. (1998). *Overcoming bulimia: A self-help package.* Leeds, UK: University of Leeds.

Wilson, G. T., & Sysko, R. (2006). Cognitive-behavioural therapy for adolescent bulimia nervosa. *European Eating Disorder Review, 14*, 8–16.

Winn, S., Perkins, S., Murray, J., Murphy, R., & Schmidt, U. (2004). A qualitative study of the experience of caring for a person with bulimia nervosa: Part 2. Carers' needs and experiences of services and other support. *International Journal of Eating Disorders, 36*, 269–279.

Winn, S., Perkins, S., Walwyn, R., Schmidt, U., Eisler, I., Treasure, J., et al. (2007). Predictors of mental health problems and negative caregiving experiences in carers of adolescents with bulimia nervosa. *International Journal of Eating Disorders, 40*, 171–178.

CHAPTER 17

Supportive Psychotherapy for Bulimia Nervosa in Adolescents

Renee Rienecke Hoste
Angela Celio Doyle

M any treatment studies have contributed to the recognition of cognitive-behavioral therapy (CBT) as the gold standard treatment for adults with bulimia nervosa (BN) (Wilson & Shafran, 2005). In contrast, very few randomized controlled trials (RCTs) have been conducted for adolescents with BN, and there is currently no clear recommendation as to a preferred form of treatment for this population. Recent studies indicate that family-based treatments are promising, as are cognitive-behavioral approaches adapted for use with adolescents (Le Grange, Crosby, Rathouz, & Leventhal, 2007; Lock, 2005; Schapman, Lock, & Couturier, 2006; Schmidt et al., 2007). Unlike family-based treatment and CBT, however, supportive psychotherapy (SPT), a manual-based, short-term individual psychotherapy, puts adolescents in charge of their recovery and allows them to explore the possible origins of their disorder, which may provide them with a sense of empowerment and increased insight into their problems. Furthermore, SPT provides a less structured environment in which to examine these issues. Many parents and adolescents may prefer an approach such as this, with the expectation that SPT can help patients effectively address underlying problems for longlasting change, with more focus on general mental health and development than a treatment like CBT, which focuses primarily on the symptoms of BN.

The overall rationale for SPT is similar to that of many psychologically oriented therapies based on psychodynamic and developmental principles (Shedler, 2010). SPT makes use of the therapeutic alliance, focuses on expression of affect and emotion, identifies recurring themes and patterns, especially from the past, and encourages and respects the developing autonomy of the adolescent by being nonjudgmental and nondirective. Many of these principles are found in other effective treatments for eating disorders, such as specialist treatment (McIntosh et al., 2005), ego-oriented individual therapy (EOIT; Robin et al., 1999), and interpersonal psychotherapy (IPT; Agras, Walsh, Fairburn, Wilson, & Kraemer, 2000; Fairburn et al., 1991). However, SPT has the advantage of being a therapy that most clinicians can deliver without additional specific training beyond that mastered in most clinical mental health training programs. After a review of the relevant empirical literature, a detailed description of the treatment is provided here, followed by a case study that serves to illustrate SPT in practice.

SPT was initially developed by Fairburn, Kirk, O'Connor, and Cooper (1986) for use in the treatment of adult women with BN. The therapy was later modified by Walsh and colleagues (1997) to remove any therapeutic elements that would overlap with CBT, such as self-monitoring of eating or triggering situations, and implicit advice from the therapist on changes in eating patterns. This therapy was designed to be a credible comparison treatment to CBT and was meant to approximate the type of treatment one might receive from a psychodynamically informed therapist providing short-term individual psychotherapy. In Walsh and colleagues' study, 120 adult women meeting *Diagnostic and Statistical Manual of Mental Disorders* (3rd ed., rev.) (DSM-III-R) criteria for BN were randomized to one of five groups: CBT + medication, CBT + placebo, SPT + medication, SPT + placebo, or medication. Treatment consisted of approximately 17 sessions over 17 weeks. The authors found that the number of episodes of binge eating and vomiting from baseline to end of treatment was significantly reduced in all treatment groups. Patients in the CBT group had higher rates of reduction and cessation of binge eating and vomiting than did patients in the SPT group, but there were no differences between the two treatment groups in improvement in mood as measured by the Beck Depression Inventory (BDI; Beck, 1987) or the Symptom Checklist–90 (SCL-90; Derogatis, Lipman, & Covi, 1973). Thus, SPT, although somewhat less effective than CBT, was nonetheless a helpful treatment for many adults with BN.

The empirical support for the use of SPT with adolescents is also limited, with only one RCT examining SPT in this population. In order to use SPT with adolescents, Walsh et al.'s manual was modified slightly to allow for collateral sessions, in which the therapist meets separately with the patient's parents (Le Grange et al., 2007). Le Grange and colleagues compared SPT with family-based treatment (FBT) in a sample of 80 adolescent patients between the ages of 12 and 19 (mean age 16.1 years) who met DSM-IV (American Psychiatric Association, 1994) criteria for BN or partial BN (defined as meeting all DSM-IV criteria except for binge and purge frequency, which was reduced to once per week for the past 6 months, consistent with presentation of early BN in adolescents). Treatment consisted of approximately 18 sessions over 6 months.

Assessments were conducted at pretreatment, midtreatment, posttreatment, and 6-month follow-up. To assess eating-disordered behavior and cognitions, the Eating Disorder Examination (EDE; Cooper & Fairburn, 1987) was administered at pretreatment, posttreatment, and 6-month follow-up, and the Eating Disorder Examination–Questionnaire (EDE-Q; Fairburn & Beglin, 1994) was administered at midtreatment. The Schedule for Affective Disorders and Schizophrenia for School-Age Children (KSADS; Kaufman et al., 1997) was administered at pretreatment, and the BDI (Beck, 1987) and the Rosenberg Self-Esteem Scale (RSE; Rosenberg, 1979) were administered at all four assessment points. Patients rated their perceptions of the suitability of treatment and how well they thought they would respond to treatment after Sessions 1 and 2, at midtreatment, and at posttreatment. Patients and parents also completed the Helping Relationship Questionnaire (HRQ; Luborsky, 1984), which assessed their perceptions of the therapeutic relationship, at midtreatment and posttreatment.

At posttreatment significantly more participants in FBT (39%) than in SPT (18%) had reached full remission (defined as no binge eating or purging over the previous 4 weeks), and these differences remained significant at 6-month follow-up, with 29% of

FBT participants reporting full remission versus 10% of SPT patients. However, a more general measure of outcome, partial remission rates (defined as no longer meeting the adjusted DSM-IV diagnostic criteria for the study), did not differ significantly between the groups at either posttreatment or follow-up. FBT was superior to SPT at midtreatment and at posttreatment on several measures of eating-disordered behavior and cognitions. However, participants in SPT continued to improve after treatment ended, and by 6-month follow-up no significant differences were found between the two treatment groups on these measures, or on measures of self-esteem and depression. There were also no differences between SPT and FBT in patients' perception of the suitability of treatment, their expectation of their response to treatment, or their assessment of the therapeutic relationship. Thus, although more research support is required, SPT may be a suitable treatment for adolescent patients with BN.

Treatment Structure and Philosophy

Supportive psychotherapy consists of 18 sessions over 5–6 months. Although the majority of sessions are individual sessions with the adolescent patient, three collateral sessions can be used for the therapist to meet with the patient's parents. The treatment philosophy is explained to patients and parents at the beginning of treatment. They are told that eating disorders are viewed as solutions, albeit maladaptive ones, to underlying psychological conflicts, past traumas, or relationship difficulties. The overarching goals of SPT are to help the patient identify these underlying problems, understand how the eating disorder has masked and perhaps perpetuated the problems, and then to seek effective solutions to these problems. As opposed to the specific therapeutic techniques implemented by CBT (e.g., self-monitoring, maintaining thought logs), SPT is designed to encourage self-mastery and improve self-esteem and self-confidence through focusing on the patient's exploration of past and current events and problems as they relate to the development of the eating disorder.

Because of the medical complications that can accompany BN, SPT is not intended to be a "stand-alone" treatment. In addition to having regular meetings with the therapist, the patient should be monitored by a physician for medical stability and by a psychiatrist for medication management when needed. Some treatment teams also include members who give dietary advice for adolescents with eating disorders, though none of the published studies of SPT utilized dieticians.

Therapeutic Style

The SPT therapist is supportive and nondirective and does a great deal of active and reflective listening. It must be communicated to patients that what they feel is important and will be heard. The therapist helps the patient to identify problems and solutions, but at no point does the therapist direct the patient in how to solve these problems. It is up to the patient to take responsibility for changing his or her circumstances. This nondirective approach is based on Bruch's fact-finding style of psychotherapy: "For effective treatment, it is decisive that a patient experience himself as an active participant in the therapeutic process. If there are things to be uncovered and interpreted, it is important that the patient makes the discovery on his own and has a chance to say it first. ... Such a patient needs help and encouragement in becoming aware of impulses, thoughts and feelings that originate within himself" (Bruch, 1973, p. 338).

This nondirective style is perhaps one of the more challenging aspects of this treatment, particularly for those who are trained in the more directive style of CBT or other behavioral therapies. It is particularly challenging when patients ask the therapist, as they almost inevitably do at some point in therapy: "What should I do?" The SPT therapist should not tell the patient what to do, but should have responses at the ready for this kind of question. Appropriate responses may include, "What have you thought about so far?" "What have you tried in the past?" "Let's take some time to think about what you can do about this." It is important to keep in mind that the therapist is helping the adolescent find solutions. It is helpful for the therapist to believe that being able to find and develop solutions to problems can be beneficial to the patient by increasing an internal sense of self-efficacy and confidence, and that this is possible with some guidance and support by the therapist. Although this does not include giving specific advice to the patient, the therapist can encourage the patient to consider various options using carefully timed questions and observations. The therapist should avoid making explicit connections between, for example, stressful events and the patient's binge eating, but can ask the patient to notice patterns that connect events and eating behavior. More elaborate clarifications are used by the therapist only to highlight discrepancies and inconsistencies and to suggest ways in which connections might be made between past events and the present circumstances. Thus, the therapy uses a subtle approach to encourage self-understanding.

At each session the therapist weighs the patient and collects information about binge eating and purging over the previous week. This information can be used to provide an overall picture of the patient's progress, as well as to identify any significant changes in symptoms that might warrant medical attention. It is not used, as in CBT, to identify triggers for disordered eating, and in fact is not discussed in session unless initiated by the patient. An exception to this may be made if the therapist notices a significant degree of weight loss between sessions, or a significant worsening of binge eating and purging symptoms. These circumstances can put the adolescent's physical health at risk and should be addressed immediately by assessing them with the patient and by contacting the treating physician.

The rationale for not discussing weight or eating disordered behaviors is that focusing on symptoms distracts from the more important work of identifying and working through the underlying issues that may have led to the development of the eating disorder. If the patient wishes to discuss weight or eating-disorder symptoms, the therapist may encourage exploring thoughts and feelings about the behavior while avoiding giving advice to the patient. For example, if the patient notices a connection between mood and a tendency to binge eat, the therapist might ask, "Is this pattern typical for you?" "When do you think this first started?" "How have you tried to deal with this?" or "Do you want to do something about it?" If the patient identifies an alternative coping strategy, the therapist would likely encourage this independent thought by saying, "That sounds like a great idea!" or "What might get in the way of your trying this?" The therapist facilitates exploration on the part of the patient and encourages him or her to try new ways of coping, but does not suggest a specific course of action. Changes in patients' behavior should be the result of their own efforts (Bruch, 1973).

Stage 1: Building the Therapeutic Alliance and Identifying Key Issues in Therapy

SPT consists of three stages. The goals of the first stage (Sessions 1–6, at weekly intervals) are as follows: (1) to develop therapeutic rapport, (2) to obtain a detailed history of the eating disorder and its development, (3) to obtain a detailed personal and family history, (4) to identify up to four "underlying issues," and (5) to inform the patient of the dangers of eating-disordered behavior.

In the first session the therapist begins by explaining the structure of SPT and the treatment philosophy to both the parents and the patient. The therapist explains that although people often think that their lives would be fine if it were not for the eating disorder, this is rarely the case, as eating disorders often mask underlying problems and can serve to perpetuate these problems. For example, a young woman treated in our clinic suffered from social anxiety and had a particular fear of eating in front of friends at school. Her eating disorder motivated her mother to have the patient eat lunch at home in a monitored environment, thereby maintaining her anxiety. In this situation the patient benefited from the isolation that accompanied her eating disorder by avoiding the challenge of confronting her social anxiety head-on. Thus, the eating disorder can serve as a distraction that keeps patients from facing and confronting the underlying problem.

The purpose of SPT is to help patients identify the underlying problem and then take steps to change it. Patients are told that if they participate in treatment and make it a priority, they can expect to see an improvement in their symptoms by the time treatment ends. This is especially important to impress upon adolescents, who are often brought to treatment by their parents and may not be particularly motivated to engage in therapy. However, it is also important for the patient and parents to have realistic expectations of therapy. The therapist explains that although the patient can expect to benefit from therapy, a cure may not be possible by the time therapy is finished, in that eating-disordered behaviors and/or cognitions may remain. The patient should be reassured that this is not unusual and that patients often continue to improve after treatment has ended (Le Grange et al., 2007). For example, a 16-year-old patient found herself at the end of treatment still reluctant to leave behind a strict low-calorie vegan diet, despite some weight gain and progress toward a more normal pattern of eating. However, the patient continued to work on identification and expression of thoughts and feelings through journaling and art after treatment ended, and continued to gain weight and gradually let go of strict dietary rules.

After this introduction, the therapist meets with the adolescent alone and begins the process of history taking. The patient is told that the purpose of history taking is to identify several underlying issues, or themes, that may be related to the eating disorder and that will form the basis for the work in the second stage of treatment. The therapist explains that in order to figure out what led the patient to develop the eating disorder in the first place, it is necessary to retrace his or her steps and recreate the story of what led to where the patient is today. To put the adolescent patient at ease, it is often easiest to begin by talking about the course and development of the eating disorder, including previous treatment attempts and the adolescent's family's reaction to the illness. Other topics to cover during history taking include information about the patient's family and relationships with all family members, peer relationships, school performance and activities, likes and dislikes, significant or stressful events, perceptions of childhood, early memories, and future plans and aspirations.

The patient is asked in the first session, and throughout therapy, to reflect on the issues discussed in treatment outside the treatment sessions. The patient is encouraged to consider the past, to contemplate ways in which past experiences may be related to the current situation, and to bring ideas into therapy for discussion. In this way, therapeutic work can occur outside the treatment sessions and may allow for more ground to be covered in therapy. Adolescents vary a great deal in the extent to which they comply with this request. Gentle reminders throughout therapy can reinforce the message that the topics discussed in treatment are important and that contemplating them on the patient's own time can facilitate progress. Some patients find it helpful to keep a journal of their thoughts and bring it to treatment sessions. However, in keeping with the style of SPT, the decision to do this should be left up to the patient and should not be suggested by the therapist.

It is important for the patient to be aware of the adverse physical and psychological consequences of binge eating and purging, so psychoeducation regarding the patient's weight and disordered-eating behavior is provided in the second session. The patient is told that it is best to keep weight above 90% of ideal body weight (IBW), and that it is difficult to maintain weights below 90% of one's IBW without resorting to disordered eating. In addition, the patient is told that maintaining a weight below 90% IBW is unlikely to reduce feelings of fatness because these feelings tend to occur in response to unpleasant emotions and not necessarily in response to actually being overweight. The patient is provided with a handout that outlines the dangers of binge eating and purging and offers ideas for controlling eating-disordered behavior. The therapist reviews this handout with the patient but presents the material in an informational manner. It is hoped that the patient will use this information to change eating behavior or to increase motivation to change, but the decision to do so is left up to the patient. Although all patients are given this information, the level of detail with which it is discussed may differ, depending on the age of the patient. For example, a therapist may give a more in-depth explanation of the ineffectiveness of purging to a 17-year-old than to an 11-year-old. The rest of Session 2 is spent continuing the history taking that began in the first session.

The history-taking process continues over the next several sessions. During this process, the therapist forms a tentative list of underlying issues, or themes, that may have led to the development of the eating disorder. This can usually be accomplished by the sixth session, at which time the therapist presents the patient with the list of underlying issues and the rationale for choosing them, and asks the patient's opinion on the themes. Common themes that are identified in SPT include low self-esteem, perfectionism, difficulties with parents, black-and-white thinking, significant or stressful life events, problems with assertiveness, inability to correctly identify feelings, difficulty in developing appropriate autonomy or assertiveness, and problems with romantic relationships or friendships. The therapist and patient agree on as many as four themes that will form the basis for the second stage of treatment. For example, a certain 16-year-old girl often felt that she needed to impress people by having the "popular kids" over to her house for parties. However, this left her feeling uncomfortable because of the disrespect these "friends" showed to her and her house. She was also persuaded by two boys to become sexually active with them during the same time period because she wanted to be liked, but these experiences made her feel bad about herself. In this situation, the theme chosen by the therapist and patient was the patient's desire to be liked by others and the consequent tendency to put herself in situations that lessened her self-esteem.

Although there may be occasions when the therapist and patient differ on how to conceptualize a problem they are working on together, it is important for the therapist to allow the patient to manage the themes in therapy. For example, the therapist may believe that a parents' divorce seemed to coincide with the development of the eating disorder and that it is an important issue to discuss. The patient may believe that he or she has coped well with the divorce and would rather discuss current difficult relationships with friends and romantic partners. Although the divorce can still be discussed in treatment, the therapist should allow the patient to choose his or her own themes, thereby helping the patient feel that the issues discussed in therapy are relevant.

A challenging aspect of this first phase of treatment is to keep the exchange from turning into a question-and-answer session; that is, the therapist must avoid falling into a pattern of asking questions and having the patient answer them. This can set the expectation that the therapist will lead the sessions and the patient will take on a more passive role. This can make the second phase, in which the patient is encouraged to take a more active role in directing therapy sessions, much more difficult. Instead, the therapist should allow patients as much room as possible to tell their own stories. Patients will almost certainly need guidance from the therapist in developing their histories, but it should be given only as needed. The therapist should avoid unnecessary interruptions and should encourage the patient to take the lead as much as possible. This can be quite difficult with uncooperative or shy patients. In these cases the therapist may have to take a more active role in directing the questioning and history taking. For example, a 12-year-old patient who was quite shy needed a fair bit of prompting from the therapist, particularly at the beginning of the sessions: "Last time, we talked about your relationships with your friends, and you mentioned that you haven't been feeling as close to them as you usually do. Can you tell me more about this? What has that been like for you?" However, in these cases the therapist should be sure to emphasize that this style of conversing will not continue throughout the rest of therapy. Often, by the end of the first phase, the patient is feeling more comfortable with the therapist and therapeutic rapport has developed sufficiently that the patient is more able and willing to talk with less guidance from the therapist.

Stage 2: Encouraging Self-Exploration and Self-Efficacy

The second stage of treatment includes Sessions 7–14, which are held at weekly intervals. The goals of Stage 2 are as follows: (1) to encourage the patient to examine and address the underlying issues that led to or are maintaining the eating disorder, (2) to help the patient identify and express feelings and thoughts, (3) to encourage assertiveness and autonomous functioning where appropriate, and (4) to raise the issue of termination near the end of Stage 2.

The therapist uses several techniques to achieve these goals. First, the therapist encourages the patient to take the lead in discussing personally relevant topics. These concerns do not necessarily have to be those that were identified at the end of the first stage of treatment, but can be those that are important to the patient at the time. However, the therapist keeps in mind the themes that were agreed upon at the end of Stage 1 and relates these to what the patient is discussing whenever possible. When an opportunity presents itself, the therapist highlights the connection between the topic being discussed and the identified theme. The patient may be asked to consider whether this connection helps improve his or her understanding of the issue or suggests alternative ways of coping. If the patient rejects these suggestions, however, the therapist does not push the issue further. It is possible that the patient is not ready or willing to explore the connection, and the therapist should respect this. Although it is not discussed further at this point, the therapist continues to look for ways to draw such connections in the future as the patient is better prepared to consider them.

The SPT therapist also helps patients develop more confidence in their own opinions and respect for their own ideas and feelings. Ambiguous feelings (e.g., feeling fat, or saying that everything is "fine") are pointed out by the therapist, and the patient is encouraged to explore and clarify what he or she is feeling. Signs of increasing independence, assertiveness, and autonomy are to be encouraged to whatever extent is age-appropriate. Over the course of treatment, confidence and self-esteem should increase. The therapist should be alert to small signs of change and should reinforce patients' efforts and highlight their developing strengths.

Near the end of the second stage of treatment, the issue of termination is raised with the patient. Although some patients may be troubled by the prospect of ending therapy, they should be told that a necessary part of treatment is no treatment at all. Patients are encouraged to see themselves as effective agents who will likely be able to manage present and future dilemmas without the guidance of the therapist. To ease patients into this transition, sessions begin to occur less frequently in Stage 3.

Stage 3: Review of Treatment Progress and Termination

The third stage of treatment includes Sessions 15–18, which occur biweekly. The goals of the third stage are as follows: (1) to review the underlying issues identified in Stage 1, (2) to instill hope in the patient, and (3) to discuss termination issues (e.g., feelings of loss, abandonment, or fear of being on one's own).

By Stage 3 the therapist and patient will have spent much of their time discussing the underlying issues that may have contributed to the development and maintenance of the eating problem. A thorough review of the underlying issues should occur toward the end of treatment. The patient is encouraged to consider to what extent these issues have been resolved and to what extent they remain problematic. If challenging issues remain, the patient is encouraged to consider how these issues will be tackled after treatment ends.

The issue of termination will have been broached near the end of Stage 2. Some adolescents are not particularly concerned about the ending of treatment and are eager to return to their normal activities without the "inconvenience" of going to therapy. Others are more distraught and need reassurance that they will be able to maintain the progress they have made without the help of the therapist. Patients should be reminded that they have identified the issues that contributed to their disordered eating and have learned how to better cope with these issues. Finishing therapy can give them an opportunity to practice these skills on their own. Although patients are often concerned about their ability to manage without therapy, they should be reminded that such concerns are normal and do not necessarily indicate an inability to continue to be successful. Thus, it is important to instill hope in the patient. The therapist may tell patients that they can expect to continue to improve after treatment has ended, and should express confidence in their ability to do so.

Some patients may experience termination as a form of rejection or loss. It is important that the therapist explore this with the patient, particularly if loss is one of the patient's underlying issues. The patient is encouraged to consider differences between the termination of the therapeutic relationship and earlier experiences of loss or abandonment, and to view the termination of treatment objectively. For example, patients who experience termination as abandonment by the therapist may be encouraged to consider whether they are in reality being abandoned and what they can gain from the ending of the therapeutic relationship (e.g., increased independence or self-confidence).

Collateral Sessions

Collateral sessions with the patient's parents can be initiated by the patient, therapist, or parents. It is often helpful to have a collateral session near the beginning of treatment, as parents are often eager to learn more about the treatment approach and would like to share their thoughts and observations with the therapist. In keeping with the nondirective spirit of SPT, these sessions are generally for information gathering and for educating the parents about eating disorders. Just as the therapist avoids giving advice to the patient, he or she also refrains from giving advice to the parents. Because the responsibility for change lies heavily with the patient, parents are encouraged to support their child through the recovery process but are not told to take a particular course of action. However, there are certain circumstances in which the therapist must intervene and make specific recommendations. An example is the presence of a parent's unmanaged psychopathology (e.g., active drug or alcohol abuse, severe depression, psychosis, neglect or child abuse) that contributes to a conflictual or unstable home environment for the adolescent and may be impeding recovery.

The following case study illustrates the treatment of an adolescent girl and offers an example of family circumstances that indicate a need for the therapist to take a more directive role in SPT.

Case Example

History of Presenting Illness

E.K., a 16-year-old white female, was a junior in a large public school. She lived with her mother and 15-year-old sister. Her parents had divorced when she was approximately 5 years old and her father lived in a nearby state. When E.K. came for treatment she was 110 pounds and 63 inches tall, putting her at 95.2% of IBW with a BMI of 19.5. According to E.K., she first became quite concerned about her weight and shape during the seventh grade, at which time she was 12 years old. During the eighth grade, she began engaging in compensatory behaviors, exercising more often and fasting for a couple of days each week in order to lose weight. When explaining how she got the idea to induce vomiting, she said, "I learned about it in health class." She binged for the first time when in the eighth grade. Over the previous 3 years, E.K. binged and purged regularly (an average of 2–3 times/week) and fasted approximately 2 days/month. She engaged in driven exercise approximately 2 days/month (jogging intensely for 45 minutes). E.K.'s mother found out that she had been purging about 8 weeks prior to the time they came for treatment. E.K.'s boyfriend of almost 2 years was the first to learn about it, when E.K. confided in him, and he told E.K.'s mother. Prior to starting SPT, she had been seeing an individual therapist close to her home on a weekly basis and a dietician every few weeks. She had been seen by the therapist and dietician for 5 weeks before she initiated treatment at our clinic, but E.K. and her mother felt that "it wasn't helping."

E.K. reported feeling guilty after she had eaten large or normal quantities of food and stated that she felt better after she purged, both emotionally and physically. E.K. also reported symptoms consistent with depressive disorder not otherwise specified. These included depressed mood (crying daily and feeling down more often than not), being easily annoyed, thinking of suicide (no plan or intent), feeling frequently fatigued, having a negative self-image (body image, but also poor opinion of personality and social skills), and feelings of pessimism regarding the future. She reported that she began feeling depressed about 1.5 years ago. E.K. also reported some symptoms consistent with social phobia, but she did not meet the full criteria. Specifically, she noted that she often avoided interactions with strangers and spoke up in class only if absolutely necessary. She said she had been this way since elementary school and really felt comfortable only around family and friends she knew well.

E.K. reported having a largely uneventful childhood up until the past 3 years, when she entered high school. Since that time, she reported that her mother had been arrested for driving while intoxicated and that her sister had attempted suicide last year after a year of being very depressed. E.K. was "very close" to her sister, who appeared dysphoric when seen in the waiting room. According to their mother, E.K.'s younger sister was also very insecure and jealous of E.K.'s attractiveness and ability to get good grades, although E.K. was unaware of this. E.K. reported being "somewhat" close to her father, whom she saw about four or five times a year.

E.K.'s mother was very attractive and took good care of her appearance. The mother–daughter relationship was close and warm. Although E.K.'s family did not often discuss weight, shape, or eating, physical attractiveness was important and E.K. was given attention for her attractiveness and talent in applying makeup and styling hair.

Stage 1

The first six sessions were spent developing rapport, obtaining a history of the eating disorder and the patient's life experiences, and (in the second session) providing psychoeducation on the dangers of eating disorder symptoms. By Session 6, the goal was to establish as many as four themes related to the onset and maintenance of the eating disorder. Per SPT guidelines this exploration was led largely by E.K., with follow-up questions and clarification by the therapist. By Session 6, the following themes were determined by E.K:

Theme 1: Difficulties with Peer Relationships

E.K. described the onset of her body image concerns as coinciding with a change in friends when she entered junior high. Prior to seventh grade, her friends had been primarily members of her soccer team and had shared her lack of concern with body shape and overall appearance. E.K. identified herself as being "tomboyish" during this time. When she entered seventh grade, E.K. was sought out by a clique of attractive, popular girls who influenced her to become more focused on her clothes, shape, and overall appearance. Although she did not particularly like these girls, she felt good about being "chosen" to be with them. She was not aware of any of the girls in her cohort having a problem with an eating disorder, but it was common for the girls to talk about "feeling fat" and being on a diet. When E.K. entered high school, many of the girls in this group began engaging in more risky behaviors, including sexual activity with male acquaintances and drinking alcohol on a weekly basis. E.K. was intimidated by this behavior and felt that she should not spend time with these girls anymore. She began to reengage in friendships with other "nicer" girls from sixth grade, although this was difficult. At the time of treatment, her female friends consisted of one best friend and several less close friends. Her friendships with these girls appeared rather lopsided in that E.K. always made herself available to them, but they were not always responsive to her needs for support. In particular, each of these girls tended to have boyfriends with whom they spent most of their time.

Theme 2: Problematic Males and Romantic Relationships

E.K. had started a relationship with a boy (J.L.) whom she had met during her freshman year and had been dating for almost 2 years. She described J.L. as "nice," but as having a "bad temper." He was regularly emotionally abusive to E.K., calling her "dumb," telling her she was "crazy," and saying she "wouldn't find anyone better than him." He also criticized the clothes she wore and ordered her to do things, such as get him something to drink. After an argument, he apologized and said that he did not mean what he had said. However, E.K. felt that "the truth comes out when you're mad" and, therefore, what her boyfriend said about her was true. She felt that she was crazy for being with J.L.—"He's so mean and I just take it," but said that they had been together for a long time and when they were not fighting, he was nice. In addition, she noted that she liked his family. Ultimately, E.K. saw J.L. as "the one" and intended to marry him. E.K. had been involved in several short and superficial relationships with boys up until the time she met J.L. (approximately one month each). E.K. tended to enter into a relationship quickly after the last one ended.

E.K.'s overall relationship with males was problematic for her. She expressed extreme discomfort when, frequently, other boys (and occasionally older men) showed an interest in her. She often found herself overwhelmed and almost paralyzed when boys approached her at school. E.K. was relieved that she could tell interested boys that she had a boyfriend, so she could gracefully deflect their advances.

E.K. saw her relationships with males as being related to her eating disorder in two interrelated ways. First, whenever things were not going well with her boyfriend, she felt "devastated," "shocked," and "less of a person." She was unable to moderate these intense negative feelings, and she found it helpful to drastically restrict her eating for a couple of days at a time. E.K. noticed that her fasting would ultimately lead to binge eating and purging when she could no longer continue fasting because of hunger. Second, E.K.'s intense discomfort with males kept her in her relationship with her boyfriend. She saw her boyfriend as a "shield" or protection from the advances of other boys and men. Her lack of confidence in dealing with males reinforced her reliance on her abusive boyfriend for protection.

Theme 3: Low Self-Esteem

In E.K.'s view, the first two themes were associated with the collateral problem, and third theme, of poor self-esteem. She doubted her intellectual abilities, other talents, positive personality traits, and attractiveness. In fact, E.K. achieved mostly As in school, was a varsity tennis player, had a sweet and caring personality, and was very beautiful (evidenced by the attention she got from males and females alike). She was uncertain about the reasons for her low self-esteem, but saw a connection between her relationships with friends and boys and having very little self-confidence.

Although these three themes appeared central from the therapist's standpoint, there were other major events and issues that could have lent support to other themes. Because the patient did not see them as important in the evolution of her eating disorder, they were not addressed. For instance, E.K. did not identify her strained relationship with her sister (perhaps because E.K. was unaware of her sister's ambivalent feelings toward her) or her sister's suicide attempt the previous year as potential factors in the development or maintenance of her eating disorder symptoms. E.K. was asked about her feelings about the suicide attempt, but she denied any relevance of these feelings to her eating disorder and felt that she had dealt with these feelings. Likewise, E.K. denied concerns about her mother's drinking problem or ambivalent feelings toward her father, who was only minimally involved in her life. The therapist believed that E.K.'s denied emotional experiences with her family—if realized—could have resulted in the identification of other themes, but the therapist deferred to E.K.'s self-identified themes.

Stage 2

Stage 2 was used to further explore the role of E.K.'s three themes and to address the underlying issues. E.K. shared her reflections on each of the themes, depending on what had occurred over the previous week(s). It took a couple of sessions for her to understand the way in which she was expected to bring her reflections from the previous week into sessions and to make connections with her themes. Initially, the therapist began the sessions with open-ended prompts (e.g., "Tell me about your week") and when E.K. described events, the therapist further queried, "How does this relate to your themes?" When E.K. was able to make connections with a theme, she was reinforced by the therapist's responses (e.g., "It seems as though you have really given a lot of thought to how your boyfriend makes you feel when he criticizes your appearance, and you have thought of some great ways to deal with these feelings"). Once E.K. understood this process, she actively considered the themes between sessions and, although she did not always have an additional insight every session, progress occurred throughout Stage 2, as evidenced by a number of steps taken toward addressing the themes. For example, in regard to Theme 1 (difficulties with peer relationships), E.K. realized that she had not been verbally expressing her needs for support to her friends. Instead, she would "shut down" after providing requested support to her friends. In addition, E.K. spent much of her free time with J.L., which took away from her efforts at developing positive female friendships. Moreover, when with her female friends, E.K. almost continuously texted her boyfriend. In reaction to hearing this, the therapist asked, "How does this affect your time with friends?" E.K. was able to see the negative impact of the texting on developing her friendships and determined, without direct guidance from the therapist, that she would reduce this texting and overall try to spend more time with girlfriends.

In relation to Theme 2 (problematic males and romantic relationships), E.K. described many different occasions from week to week when she was unable to comfortably turn down boys when they expressed interest in her. The frequency of interest from other boys was alarming to her and came from every direction—strangers in study hall, boys at parties, "friends" on social networking websites—and even male friends frequently expressed a desire to date or otherwise be physically involved with E.K. After E.K. was asked to consider ways in which she could respond to aggressive flirting from boys in an earlier session, she reported that she had successfully "ducked" out of a boy's attempt at putting his arm around her while watching a movie at a friend's house. E.K. felt extremely proud of having done this. However, this act took a tremendous amount of courage for her and she was concerned about how it made him feel.

When E.K. brought up a recent visit with her father and stated that she "didn't connect well" with him, the therapist asked if she felt that her relationship with her father was at all related to her feelings about other males, or whether her relationship with her father was related to her eating disorder symptoms. She denied seeing any connection. As a result, this was not pursued any further. In addition, the therapist attempted during Stage 2 to understand the reasons for E.K.'s discomfort with boys demonstrating interest in her. E.K. denied sexual abuse, but recalled her discomfort beginning in junior high when a 17-year-old male friend of a girl in her social group kissed E.K. against her will at a party. There was no further relationship with the boy, but E.K. was very unhappy about this event.

Notably, E.K. broke up with her abusive boyfriend late during Stage 2 and, although she was very upset about the breakup, was able to avoid turning to bingeing/purging and fasting. As an alternative, E.K. spoke to her best friend and her mother for support. Although she started dating someone else very soon after the breakup (continuing her pattern of relying on a boyfriend to protect her from other boys' interest), E.K. was aware of the potential pitfalls of this strategy and continued to work on her assertiveness with boys.

E.K.'s third theme (low self-esteem) was discussed frequently, as it related to her two other themes. Although no specific suggestions were given, E.K. found that she felt better about herself when she expressed her feelings more clearly to her friends, boyfriend, and family.

Stage 3

E.K. reported feeling sad about termination and said she would miss the therapist because of "getting used to talking" to her each week. However, E.K. was encouraged to see the end of therapy as an opportunity to continue exploring the themes discussed in sessions, and it was pointed out to her that all of her improvements (e.g., reduced need for the eating disorder to help her deal with feelings related to difficulties with friends, boys, and low self-esteem) were due to solutions that she came up with herself. E.K. was comfortable with termination and felt optimistic about the future.

Collateral Sessions

E.K.'s mother was seen three times for collateral sessions, once during each stage of treatment. The first meeting early in Stage 1 was initiated by both the therapist and E.K.'s mother in order to share more information about the treatment and to gather information from the mother about her insights into E.K.'s eating disorder. E.K.'s mother (L.) stated that she felt that E.K. was "missing a father figure" and, as a result, L. felt quite guilty about the divorce and subsequent geographical distance from E.K.'s father. However, when E.K. was a young child, there was open hostility between the parents and, at times, L. left the home with the two children to escape the conflict. There was no physical abuse. L. was glad that her ex-husband was no longer a major part of their lives, but resented his lack of active involvement in their daughter's lives. L. was given information about eating disorders and the way they can be used to deal with other, more fundamental concerns.

In the second collateral meeting during Stage 2, which was initiated by the therapist, L. was given an update on the progress of treatment and was informed generally of E.K.'s themes (with permission from E.K.). L. understood how these themes applied to E.K.'s eating disorder and asked how she could help. L. was asked by the therapist how she thought she might help, and L. was able to suggest that she provide a supportive and nonjudgmental ear to E.K. about her relationships with her friends and her boyfriend. L. noted that she had been very positive about E.K.'s relationship with J.L. because she was unaware of E.K.'s difficulties with him. Also related to the second theme of relationships with boys, L. recalled also feeling quite overwhelmed by attention from boys when she was in high school and college and stated that she could share her experiences and strategies for dealing with aggressive male attention with E.K. Finally, L. wondered aloud how she could help E.K. improve her self-esteem. No suggestions were given by the therapist, but L. was encouraged to think about what she could do to support E.K. in her efforts. However, L. was given specific advice about her alcohol use. Due to L.'s recent arrest for a DUI and additional information provided by E.K. about L.'s daily intake of alcohol, the therapist directly suggested to L. that she seek treatment for alcohol abuse. L. was receptive to this suggestion and began attending Alcoholics Anonymous during the course of E.K.'s treatment.

The final collateral session with L. was called by both the therapist and L. to review progress and to plan for the future. L. noted that E.K. was sad to conclude treatment, but L. was supportive of treatment ending so that E.K. could "work on these issues more on her own." L. stated that she was pleased with the changes she saw in E.K. related to her greater assertiveness and confidence, especially in the contexts of friends and boys.

Eating Disorder Symptoms and Conclusion

During treatment E.K. kept her weight within a healthy range and, although she was bingeing and purging two times a week at the time of the first few sessions, this gradually decreased until she was abstaining from all eating-disordered behaviors (including fasting) by the beginning of Stage 3.

Following the end of treatment, a follow-up assessment was conducted 6 months later and E.K. reported continued abstinence from binge eating, purging, fasting, and other compensatory behaviors. Her weight and shape concerns still existed but had been reduced significantly. E.K. remained in good physical health in regard to her weight.

Future Directions

There is evidence that SPT can be helpful in reducing binge eating and purging behavior, although it may work more slowly than FBT (Le Grange et al., 2007). However, there are several aspects of SPT that may make it particularly appealing for use with adolescents. It has been found that adolescents with BN can be reluctant to involve their parents in treatment (Perkins et al., 2005). The focus on individual work in SPT may be especially attractive to older adolescents who are more independent from their parents and who have a level of cognitive development that may enable them to engage in and benefit from the introspective nature of the therapy. SPT may also be beneficial for families who are unable to participate in FBT. As compared with CBT, adolescents in SPT may find the lack of homework appealing and may enjoy the broader focus allowed in SPT. This less structured approach allows attention to be paid to other issues that are relevant to adolescents, including peer and romantic relationships. Although which specific aspects of SPT are appealing to patients remain a question to be answered empirically, SPT is a potentially useful form of treatment for adolescents with BN.

References

Agras, W. S., Walsh, T., Fairburn, C. G., Wilson, G. T., & Kraemer, H. C. (2000). A multicenter comparison of cognitive-behavioral therapy and interpersonal psychotherapy for bulimia nervosa. *Archives of General Psychiatry, 57,* 459–466.

American Psychiatric Association. (1994). *Diagnostic and statistical manual of mental disorders* (4th ed.). Washington, DC: Author.

Beck, A. T. (1987). *Beck Depression Inventory.* San Antonio, TX: Psychological Corporation.

Bruch, H. (1973). *Eating disorders: Anorexia, obesity, and the person within.* New York: Basic Books.

Cooper, Z., & Fairburn, C. G. (1987). The Eating Disorder Examination: A semistructured interview for the assessment of the specific psychopathology of eating disorders. *International Journal of Eating Disorders, 6,* 1–8.

Derogatis, L. R., Lipman, R. S., & Covi, L. (1973). The SCL-90: An outpatient psychiatric rating scale. *Psychopharmacology Bulletin, 9,* 13–28.

Fairburn, C. G., & Beglin, S. J. (1994). Eating Disorder Examination: Interview or self-report? *International Journal of Eating Disorders, 16,* 363–370.

Fairburn, C. G., Jones, R., Peveler, R. C., Carr, S. J., Solomon, R. A., O'Connor, M. E., et al. (1991). Three psychological treatments for bulimia nervosa: A comparative trial. *Archives of General Psychiatry, 48,* 463–469.

Fairburn, C. G., Kirk, J., O'Connor, M., &

Cooper, P. J. (1986). A comparison of two psychological treatments for bulimia nervosa. *Behaviour Research and Therapy, 24,* 629–643.

Kaufman, J., Birmaher, B., Brent, D., Rao, U., Flynn, C., Moreci, P., et al. (1997). Schedule for Affective Disorders and Schizophrenia for School-Age Children—Present and Lifetime Version (KSADS-PL): Initial reliability and validity data. *Journal of the American Academy of Child and Adolescent Psychiatry, 36,* 980–988.

Le Grange, D., Crosby, R. D., Rathouz, P. J., & Leventhal, B. L. (2007). A randomized controlled comparison of family-based treatment and supportive psychotherapy for adolescent bulimia nervosa. *Archives of General Psychiatry, 64,* 1049–1056.

Lock, J. (2005). Adjusting CBT for adolescent bulimia nervosa: A report of a case series. *American Journal of Psychotherapy, 59,* 267–281.

Luborsky, L. (1984). *Principles of psychoanalytic psychotherapy.* New York: Basic Books.

McIntosh, V. W., Jordan, J., Carter, F. A., Luty, S. E., McKenzie, J. M., Bulik, C. M., et al. (2005). Three psychotherapies for anorexia nervosa: A randomized, controlled trial. *American Journal of Psychiatry, 162,* 741–747.

Perkins, S., Schmidt, U., Eisler, I., Treasure, J., Yi, I., Winn, S., et al. (2005). Why do adolescents with bulimia nervosa choose not to involve their parents in treatment? *Euro-*

pean Child and Adolescent Psychiatry, 14, 376–385.

Robin, A., Siegal, P., Moye, A., Gilroy, M., Dennis, A., & Sikand, A. (1999). A controlled comparison of family versus individual therapy for adolescents with anorexia nervosa. *Journal of the American Academy of Child and Adolescent Psychiatry, 38,* 1482–1489.

Rosenberg, M. (1979). *Conceiving the self.* New York: Basic Books.

Schapman, A. M., Lock, J., & Couturier, J. (2006). Cognitive-behavioral therapy for adolescents with binge eating syndromes: A case series. *International Journal of Eating Disorders, 39,* 252–255.

Schmidt, U., Lee, S., Beecham, J., Perkins, S.,

Treasure, J., Yi, I., et al. (2007). A randomized controlled trial of family therapy and cognitive behavior therapy guided self-care for adolescents with bulimia nervosa and related disorders. *American Journal of Psychiatry, 164,* 591–598.

Shedler, J. (2010). The efficacy of psychodynamic psychotherapy. *American Psychologist, 65,* 98–109.

Walsh, B. T., Wilson, G. T., Loeb, K. L., Devlin, M. J., Pike, K. M., Roose, S. P., et al. (1997). Medication and psychotherapy in the treatment of bulimia nervosa. *American Journal of Psychiatry, 154,* 523–531.

Wilson, G., & Shafran, R. (2005). Eating disorders guidelines from NICE. *Lancet, 365,* 79–81.

OTHER TREATMENTS
OR CLINICAL GROUPS

CHAPTER 18

Early Treatment for Eating Disorders

Katharine L. Loeb
Katherine E. Craigen
Michal Munk Goldstein
James Lock
Daniel Le Grange

The Importance of Early Intervention in Eating Disorders

The onset of eating disorders typically occurs in adolescence (Lewinsohn, Striegel-Moore, & Seeley, 2001; Lucas, Beard, & O'Fallon, 1991), a time of profound developmental change in the physiological, psychosocial, and cognitive domains (Casey, Getz, & Galvan, 2008; Casey, Giedd, & Thomas, 2000; Giedd et al., 1996, 1999). Anorexia nervosa (AN) and bulimia nervosa (BN) introduce delay or insult to each of these aspects of development (Golden, Kreitzer, & Jacobson, 1994; Golden & Shenker, 1992; Le Grange, Loeb, Van Orman, & Jellar, 2004; Mitchell, Specker, & de Zwaan, 1991; Palla & Litt, 1988; Pomery & Mitchell, 2001; Striegel-Moore, Seeley, & Lewinsohn, 2003; Wentz, Gillberg, Gillberg, & Rastam, 2001). Although many of the medical complications associated with eating disorders can improve with recovery, there are some potentially irreversible sequelae, such as deficient bone mass (Biller et al., 1989; Castro, Lazaro, Pons, Halperin, & Toro, 2000), growth retardation (Danzinger, Mukamel, Zeharia, Dinari, & Mimouni, 1994; Lantzouni, Frank, Golden, & Shenker, 2002; Modan-Moses et al., 2003), and loss of dental enamel (Hazelton & Faine, 1996). Eating disorders tend to foster social isolation and family conflict, which are especially detrimental to the adolescent moving through a turbulent phase of development when peer and family supports are essential (Eisler et al., 1997; North, Gowers, & Byram, 1997). The isolating direct effects of the illness, in combination with treatments that often take the adolescent out of his or her normal milieu and into one saturated with other sufferers of these ego-syntonic disorders, can collectively impart a negative impact on autonomy, self-concept, self-esteem, and mastery of skills crucial to functioning as an adult (Eisler et al., 1997; North et al., 1997).

If left untreated, eating disorders typically worsen and become chronic (Kotler, Cohen, Davies, Pine, & Walsh, 2001; Lewinsohn et al., 2001; Newman et al., 1996; Striegel-Moore, Leslie, Petrill, Garvin, & Rosenheck, 2000) and, in turn, yield greater liabilities for a normal course of development. In a subset of cases, eating disorders can result in death over time (Crisp et al., 2006; Crow, Praus, & Thuras, 1999; Herzog et al., 2000; Keel et al., 2003; Sullivan, 1995). With anorexia nervosa (AN) in particular, suicide accounts for a significant portion of mortality (Berkman, Lohr, & Bulik, 2007; Bulik et al., 2008; Franko & Keel, 2006; Herzog et al., 2000; Pompili, Mancinelli, Girardi, Ruberto, & Tatarelli, 2004), presumably in the context of depression (O'Brien & Vincent, 2003) associated with starvation and related serotonin dysfunction (Kaye, Frank, Bailer, & Henry, 2005; Laessle, Kittle, Fichter, Wittchen, & Pirke, 1987; Matsubara, Arora, & Meltzer, 1991; O'Brien & Vincent, 2003; Stockmeier, 2003), whereas the rest result from the direct effects of malnourishment or extreme weight control efforts (Crisp et al., 2006). These dual negative prognostic outcomes of course (of illness and of development) because of delayed intervention have prompted a consensus in the field concerning the need for clinicians to advocate for early case identification and treatment, for aggressive attempts to reverse the course of illness in already diagnosed or clinically identified patients, and for the prevention of conversion from prodromal to diagnostic status in high-risk individuals (Currin & Schmidt, 2005; Le Grange et al., 2004; Le Grange & Loeb, 2007; Schoemaker, 1997), while keeping in mind that a subset of symptomatic cases can spontaneously remit (Chamay-Weber, Narring, & Michaud, 2005). However, the evidence for the positive prognostic influence of early treatment is confounded by covariates such as duration of illness (Reas, Schoemaker, Zipfel, & Williamson, 2001; Schoemaker, 1997). Despite these methodological limitations, the realities of the burden of illness on patient and caregivers alike (Nielsen & Bara-Carril, 2003; Perkins, Winn, Murray, Murphy, & Schmidt, 2004; Treasure et al., 2001; Winn, Perkins, Murray, Murphy, & Schmidt, 2004), coupled with an equal interest in outcome variables not specific to course of illness, such as comorbidity and quality of life (Hay & Mond, 2005; McIntosh et al., 2004; Striegel-Moore et al., 2003), highlight the need for action as soon as the clinical significance of an eating disorder presentation is established.

The Challenges of Early Treatment for Eating Disorders

There are several challenges to case identification of children and adolescents who would be appropriate candidates for early treatment. Clinicians are limited by diagnostic criteria that do not fully appreciate or take into account developmental considerations in the assessment of eating disorders, including the level of cognitive maturation and corresponding ability to articulate and endorse abstract psychological symptoms, physiological developmental stage, and idiosyncratic premorbid growth histories that would inform reference points for underweight status in a younger population (Bravender et al., 2007, 2010; Nicholls, Chater, & Lask, 2000; for more on this topic, see Loeb, Brown, & Goldstein, Chapter 10, this volume). In addition, the ego-syntonic nature of the disorder, coupled with its often socially sanctioned status among adolescents, discourages patients from seeking help. Moreover, many aspects of normal adolescent development can obfuscate parental awareness of the emergence of an eating disorder. Preoccupation with appearance, individuation from parental support systems, expression of strong attitudes, and mood lability are all common markers of the transition to adolescence and are also associated features of eating disorders in youth. Eating disorders are often evidenced by the strong will and affect of typical adolescence, resulting in alienation from family members (Perkins et al., 2004; Treasure et al., 2001; Winn et al., 2004) and increased space for the disorder to intensify.

Research on Early Treatment for Eating Disorders

Long-term outcome data have repeatedly emphasized the benefit of early treatment for eating disorders. Within this literature, the latency between onset of illness and receipt of treatment demonstrates that shorter duration of illness, before treatment, is predictive of and correlated with better outcomes (Deter & Herzog, 1994; Eisler et al., 1997; Katzman, 2005; Ratnasuriya, Eisler, Smuckler, & Russell 1991; Reas et al., 2001; Reas, Williamson, Martin, & Zucker, 2000; Russell, Szmukler, Dare & Eisler, 1987; Schoemaker, 1997; Steinhausen, 2002; Van Son, van Hoeken, van Furth, Donker, & Hoek, 2010; Zipfel, Löwe, Reas, Deter, & Herzog, 2000). Conversely, lower remission rates are associated with longer duration of illness (Eisler, Simic, Russell, & Dare, 2007; Nilsson, & Hagglof, 2005; Richard, Bauer, & Kordy, 2005) and inpatient treatment (Fichter, Quadflieg, & Hedlund, 2006; Wentz, Gillberg, Anckarsäter, Gillberg, & Rastam, 2009). Although these studies do not elucidate the underlying variables that may be represented by early treatment or that may mediate the association with positive prognosis (e.g., level of parental monitoring), they do provide support for the intuitive notion, "the sooner the better."

There is a high prevalence of adolescents who meet partial diagnostic criteria for eating disorders (Stice, Marti, Shaw, & Jaconis, 2009) and a large proportion of adolescents who are diagnosed with eating disorder not otherwise specified (EDNOS) who could be subtyped as meeting partial criteria for AN or bulimia nervosa (BN) (Eddy, Doyle, Hoste, Herzog, & Le Grange, 2008). If left untreated, such a disorder may persist and develop into the full disorder (Ben-Tovim et al., 2001; Herzog, Hopkins, & Burns, 1993; King, 1989; Le Grange & Loeb, 2007; Le Grange et al., 2004; Patton, Johnson-Sabine, Wood, Mann, & Wakeling, 1990; Schmidt et al., 2007; Yager, Landsverk, & Edelstein, 1987). Although there has been little research on the optimal methods for early intervention for this high-risk subset, there are suggestions in the literature that family-based treatment (FBT) reduces extant psychopathology in subthreshold child and adolescent cases; however, whether such intervention will ultimately prevent conversion to the full diagnosis remains unknown. Specifically, treatment studies that have included subthreshold cases indicate that FBT looks promising for adolescents with partial AN (Le Grange, Binford, & Loeb, 2005; Lock, Le Grange, Forsburg, & Hewell, 2006; Loeb et al., 2007) and for those meeting partial criteria for BN (Le Grange, Crosby, Rathouz, & Leventhal, 2007), with one study indicating that patients with subthreshold BN fare better in treatment in certain respects than those who meet full DSM criteria (Schmidt et al., 2008). Other treatment methods have also evidenced success with individuals who meet partial diagnostic criteria, including cognitive-behavioral guided self-help with adolescents (Schmidt et al., 2007) and acceptance and commitment therapy (ACT) with late adolescents (undergraduate students) (Juarascio, Forman, & Herbert, 2010). From the prevention literature, a program based on Festinger's (1957) dissonance theory has demonstrated efficacy in reducing eating disorder pathology in high school and college students at risk for BN by challenging the thin ideal (Stice, Mazzoti, Weibel, & Agras, 2000; Stice, Trost, & Chase, 2003; Stice, Marti, Spoor, Presnell, & Shaw, 2008), and this might have theoretical application in more symptomatic or prodromal cases. Hypotheses regarding the mechanisms that may facilitate the success of early intervention have been posited, which include theories that a shorter duration of illness means that patients are more amenable to treatment (Currin & Schmidt, 2005), that many of these patients are undergoing intervention before reaching a too severe low weight (Currin & Schmidt,

2005; Le Grange & Loeb, 2007), and that increased resources are available to adolescent patients (Le Grange & Loeb, 2007).

Although research on early intervention in eating disorders is in its infancy, such research has demonstrated effective outcomes and improved long-term prognoses with targeted treatment at prodromal stages for other psychiatric disorders, including psychotic disorders (Bhangoo & Carter, 2009) and bipolar spectrum disorders (Luby & Navsaria, 2010). A primary obstacle to this area of research in the eating disorder field is distinguishing between the stage in which specific risk factors are exhibited, for which targeted prevention is appropriate, and the prodrome, for which early treatment is key. It has been suggested that those symptoms diagnostically essential for the full disorder be conceptualized as prodromes, whereas symptoms that lead to a vulnerability for progression to the full disorder be treated as risk factors (Stice, Ng, & Shaw, 2010). Although the field has yet to come to a consensus on this differentiation, it remains clinically warranted to expand on research of effective interventions for those eating disorder symptoms having a current negative effect on the physical, emotional, and psychosocial health of those afflicted.

As part of a clinical trial funded by the National Institutes of Health on the early identification and treatment of AN (No. 5K23MH074506-05; Principal Investigator: Loeb), Mount Sinai School of Medicine is conducting a randomized controlled trial comparing a modified version of FBT for AN with individual supportive psychotherapy for children and adolescents with clinically significant eating disorders that may represent prodromal AN. Although the actuarial data do not yet exist to predict which of these patients' symptom profiles will remit, stabilize, or portend ultimate conversion to full AN (i.e., be truly prodromal), they are sufficiently clinically significant to warrant intervention. Such intervention serves two purposes: acute reduction in extant symptomatology (treatment) and durability of treatment effects in arresting development from a high-risk status to full AN (prophylaxis, or prevention).

The target population of this study consists of children and adolescents who meet two or three of the four DSM-IV criteria for AN without ever having met the criteria for the full disorder. If criterion A (weight below 85% expected) is not met, participants must meet DSM-IV EDNOS, Example 2 ("All of the criteria for Anorexia Nervosa are met except that, despite significant weight loss, the individual's current weight is in the normal range"), *or* have engaged in dietary restriction leading to a below-normal (below 100% of expected) weight, in combination with two or three of criteria B through D for AN, for inclusion in the study. The purpose of the restrictive nature of these exceptions is to *exclude* individuals who are exhibiting only shape and weight concerns and to include higher-risk individuals who are exhibiting inappropriately restrictive dietary habits, the normalization of which is a key goal of treatment, in the context of the AN prodrome.

A Family-Based Model for Early Treatment of AN: Intervening at the Point of High Risk

FBT modified for this high-risk population is based fully on the original FBT-AN model and manual (Lock, Le Grange, Agras, & Dare, 2001), while incorporating some elements of FBT for BN (Le Grange & Lock, 2007) and the shorter course of treatment (14 sessions over 6 months as opposed to 20 sessions over a full year), supported by research on FBT-AN (Le Grange et al., 2007; Le Grange & Lock, 2007; Lock et al., 2006; Lock, Couturier, Agras, 2006; Loeb & Le Grange, 2009). The FBT manual for children and adolescents at high risk for AN by virtue of exhibiting the prodrome (Stice et al., 2010) is designed to be used adjunctively to the original FBT-AN (Lock et al., 2001) and FBT-BN (Le Grange & Lock, 2007) published manuals. FBT was chosen as the foundation approach for prodromal or subsyndromal AN (SAN) in children and adolescents because of its strong efficacy data for adolescent AN (Eisler et al., 2000; Le Grange, Eisler, Dare, & Russell, 1992; Lock, Agras, Bryson, & Kraemer, 2005; Loeb et al., in press) and its early but promising data for childhood AN (Lock et al., 2006) and adolescent EDNOS (Le Grange et al., 2005; Loeb et al., 2007). FBT has a history of controversy in that contrary to some traditional clinical perspectives on AN that focused on the purportedly enmeshed family—with corresponding recommendations that curtailed parental involvement—FBT prescribes constructive parental management of the eating disorder symptoms in the early phase of treatment and views parents as a valuable resource in effecting change. As with the foundation approach, treatment consists of three phases. In Phase 1, parents are asked to manage their child's eating disorder symptoms by providing appropriate quantity and quality of foods, supervising the consumption of meals and snacks, and preventing engagement in behaviors such as excessive exercise and purging. Parents accomplish this with a judicious blend of firmness and empathy and never resort to punitive or harsh measures. Parents' increased level of involvement in their child's eating is temporary and restricted to the domain of eating disorder symptoms, consistent with the patient's regression in his or her ability to adequately self-feed. Developmentally appropriate autonomy is afforded to the patient in all other realms. The therapist externalizes the illness in an effort to reduce blame, especially directed toward the patient, while also actively reducing parental self-blame by explaining the unknown etiology of AN spectrum disorders. Siblings are involved and assigned a purely supportive role. In Phase 2 of treatment, control of food and weight are gradually transferred back to the patient as symptoms abate. Phase 3 is focused on broader concerns of child and adolescent development and family functioning in the absence of the patient's eating disorder.

Sessions are conducted with the entire family present, although a separated version of FBT has been studied relative to the conjoint format, with results suggesting that families with high levels of expressed emotion fare better when parents are seen separately from their child (Eisler et al., 2000; Le Grange, Eisler, Dare, & Hodes, 1992). In Phase 1, sessions are weekly, tapering to biweekly in Phase 2 and monthly in Phase 3. The FBT therapist balances a directive style in providing a framework and mission statement for treatment and functioning as an expert in eating disorders, with a deferential stance in respecting the parents' knowledge of their child and family and decisions regarding the idiosyncratic application of treatment techniques.

In conducting family treatment with this high-risk population, the following important revisions to standard FBT for AN must be kept in mind:

- First, the foundation approach is modified to address a wider range of developmental stages, such as middle-late childhood. The onset of AN typically occurs in mid-late adolescence; prodromal AN by definition precedes this.
- Second, part of the definition of prodromal AN in this study requires either underweight status or significant loss of weight to below that expected for age, gender, height, or weight history. For participants with SAN who have lost weight but

do not yet meet the weight cutoff for AN, regulation of eating patterns and the incorporation of a full range of foods in the child or adolescent's diet may be as important goals as weight gain early in treatment.

- Third, the goals and language of the treatment are modified to incorporate the notion of risk of progression from SAN to AN, at the same time emphasizing the clinical severity of the SAN in and of itself and the need for reduction and resolution of the presenting symptoms.
- Fourth, the revisions for high-risk children and adolescents also stress the importance of regular family meals at home and the modeling of healthy, nonrestrictive eating habits by parents.

Evaluation for Treatment

The evaluation required prior to the selection and initiation of FBT for SAN should be sensitive to the potential for denial and minimization (Couturier & Lock, 2006), intentional obfuscation of symptom presence and severity to avoid intervention efforts, and lack of abstract cognitive skills required to endorse some of the psychological features of AN (Bravender et al., 2007, 2010; Hebebrand, Casper, Treasure, & Schweiger, 2004; Nicholls & Bryant-Waugh, 2008; Nicholls et al., 2000). In addition, interviewing parents is essential for formulating a complete picture of the patient's eating disorder and for ensuring accurate case identification, particularly for those young individuals who might be mistakenly categorized as having EDNOS instead of AN as an artifact of the limitations in the standard diagnostic tools for eating disorders, the majority of which rely exclusively on patient report (Le Grange & Loeb, 2007). (For a complete discussion of these issues, see Loeb et al., Chapter 10, this volume.)

Weighing the Patient

As with the AN and BN FBT protocols, the therapist meets with the patient one-on-one at the start of each session to obtain height and weight and provide an opportunity for the patient to voice any issues or concerns without the family present. The weight is marked on a graph, which is presented each session as soon as the family convenes. The focus on weight, although integral to FBT for AN, may not take center stage in FBT for SAN; however, weight is monitored and tracked for all patients. As noted earlier, not all patients with SAN as defined in this study may be underweight per AN diagnostic criteria. However, patients may have at least lost clinically significant amounts of weight, with the burden of meeting additional criteria increased when a patient falls shy of the diagnostic weight threshold. For the majority of patients with SAN, at least some weight gain will be a goal of treatment, and feeding practices have to be commensurate with a weight gain protocol. At a minimum, the focus is the normalization of eating behavior, the result of which may or may not be weight gain. For example, consider a patient who has lost 115 to 95% expected body weight in 2 months with extreme caloric restriction (500 kcal/day) and food avoidance (consuming only fat-free, carbohydrate-free items) and who exhibits an intense fear of gaining weight and regards several parts of his or her body as "too fat." The parents' primary goal in Phase 1 is to reverse the restriction and provide a range of foods, including "forbidden" foods, in quantities appropriate to the age of the patient, within a regular pattern of eating consisting of three meals plus two or three snacks. As such, Phase 1 will likely yield a degree of reversal of weight loss, but complete weight restoration may not be necessary, assuming the patient is functionally intact below 115% of expected body weight. As discussed in the original FBT-AN manual (Lock et al., 2001), functional improvement is more important than specific weight goals, provided the patient is clearly above a minimally acceptable weight for age, height, and gender. With the patient described here, parents could transition to Phase 2 when resistance to a regular pattern of eating with a full range of foods is significantly reduced and when the intensity of the psychological features of AN has decreased. If this patient had also become oligomenorrheic or amenorrheic in the process of losing weight, return of menses—which may occur with increased fat consumption and minimal weight regain—can also serve as a functional marker of improvement.

Session 1

Parallel to the goals and interventions of the original FBT-AN protocols (Le Grange & Lock, 2007; Lock et al., 2001) there are five aims of the first session: family engagement, history taking, assessing family functioning and structures, blame reduction through externalization of illness, and mobilization of parents to prevent AN in their child by heightening their anxiety about the risks inherent in the disorder. In taking a history of how the eating disorder has affected the family, it is notable that the impact of some variants of SAN may be less dramatic than AN, in both duration and intensity. For example, the family of a patient with recent onset of SAN, as in the preceding example, may have experienced less disruption and distress than the family of a patient with chronic SAN, at 80% of expected body weight, with oligomenorrhea and disturbed experience of shape and weight, and who denies a fear of weight gain but consumes only 400 kcal/day (i.e., the type of case that could arguably be considered an adolescent manifestation of full AN). However, all SAN presentations are clinically significant to the extent they are self- or doctor-referred for treatment, and therefore the therapist should be able to assess the individual and familial levels of functional impairment or distress caused by the eating disorder, regardless of severity.

The task of externalizing the illness may also vary slightly, depending on the severity and chronicity of the eating disorder in a particular family. The depiction of the illness as a pernicious entity beyond the patient's direct control can apply to all cases, with minor modifications as a function of chronicity and severity of the eating disorder. For a patient with recent onset, higher-weight SAN, the illness might be portrayed as an octopus whose tentacles have just taken hold and are squeezing harder and harder over time. For a patient with chronic, low-weight SAN, the typical AN analogies may apply (e.g., cancer). As with AN, the dual goals of externalizing the illness are to provide a clear "enemy" target for the parents and to permit and facilitate rapport with the healthy side of the child or adolescent. It is also helpful to use the Venn diagram depicted in the original AN manual (Lock et al., 2001) to accomplish the task of separating the illness from the patient. Depending on the level of clinical severity, the therapist can depict two circles as not fully overlapped at present, but at risk of complete occlusion if the parents do not take immediate action.

Mobilizing an adaptive level of anxiety for the parents requires the orchestration of an "intense scene" concerning the seriousness of the illness, and, should SAN convert to full AN, the difficulty in recovering. This intervention, as applied to SAN, requires two tasks: first, to convey the seriousness of the subsyndromal variant of AN, and second, to emphasize how difficult recovery will be should the SAN be allowed to progress to full AN. This dual task is the crux of Session 1 and sets the stage for the rest of treatment. The therapist must make a convincing case that SAN is problematic in its own right, that it qualifies as an eating disorder, and that it is worthy of immediate intervention, as well as raise parental anxiety about the challenges in turning back once the threshold to AN is crossed. The therapist is honest with the parents that as members of a scientific field, we cannot predict precisely who will ultimately develop AN, but is clear that their child is at greater risk by virtue of his or her current symptom profile.

In approaching the first message (i.e., that SAN is a clinically severe phenomenon), it is helpful for the therapist to address both the general and the specific—namely, the functional impairment associated with the overall presentation as well as the how each individual symptom is dangerous. For example, the therapist might say:

> "As a family, you have all told me how [the patient] is not herself since this eating disorder took hold. She is not participating in family meals or activities, she is less interested in friends, and she is irritable whenever the subject of food or weight is approached. Nothing is more important to [the patient] these days as losing another pound or going down another clothing size. This is understandably frightening to each of you as worried parents and siblings. A number of other things we've discussed must also be making you [the parents] very anxious. Your daughter is eating only non-fat, carbohydrate-free foods, which is an inadequate diet for a 13-year-old and can significantly affect growth and development. And although you caught this problem before it became full anorexia nervosa, your daughter has lost enough weight and body fat that her periods have stopped. This can lead to osteoporosis, even at a young age."

The second message—how difficult the resolution of full AN can be—may be conveyed as follows:

> "Fortunately, you have come to treatment early, before this eating disorder has a chance of turning into full anorexia nervosa. We cannot know with certainty that this will happen, but your child is at the precipice of a deadly disorder and we must work hard to keep it at bay. This is extremely important because if we let this eating disorder progress, it can become highly resistant to treatment. Someone with anorexia nervosa typically undergoes repeated hospitalizations, each one followed by relapse. As you can imagine, this disrupts an adolescent's academic course and social life and drains families' emotional and financial resources. Anorexia nervosa is also deadly; approximately one in ten patients with anorexia nervosa will die. We must help your daughter before she is at risk of becoming such a statistic."

The therapist should solicit each family member's reaction to hearing this information, maximizing the affective impact of these messages. For example, the therapist can turn to the more stoic parent and ask, "What is your reaction to hearing that your daughter is at risk of developing such a serious illness? What images come to mind when you think about what the future might bring? How do these images contrast with what your daughter was like before developing an eating disorder?"

Session 1 ends by assigning parents the task of helping their child normalize his or her eating and weight, and of representing these efforts during a family meal held at the second visit. Given the variability in SAN presentation, it is not sufficient to universally end the session with the original manual's instructions to bring a picnic meal commensurate with the patient's level of starvation. For SAN patients who are within an AN weight range, this is appropriate. However, for patients at a higher weight, such an assignment may be misleading and miss an opportunity for the parents to shape their daughter's eating in other important ways. Therefore, for the high-risk population, the parting words of the therapist to the parents at the end of Session 1 should be:

> "I would like you to bring a picnic meal for your family to the next session. In deciding what to bring for [the patient] to eat, consider her degree of weight loss and how you want to help her eat normal, healthy amounts of food again. Please include at least one food that she used to like but has stopped eating."

This statement addresses both quantity and quality of food and places the responsibility of deciding what to bring on the parents. It is very important to *not* be more specific or directive than this; observing if and how these instructions were followed is an important part of the assessment that takes place in Session 2.

Session 2: The Family Meal

During the picnic meal the therapist observes the degree to which the parents followed the instructions set forth in the prior session, within a broader assessment of the parents' ability (in terms of family structure and process, particularly around meals (Neumark-Sztainer, Eisenberg, Fulkerson, Story, & Larson, 2008), to facilitate normalization of eating habits and weight restoration, as applicable. An important goal of Session 2 is to provide a simulated context for feeding efforts in the home environment and, *in vivo*, to help the parents improve their child's food consumption. This is accomplished by the therapist coaching the parents to have their child consume at least one more mouthful than he or she is willing to eat. The primary adaptation for high-risk children and adolescents at the family meal is that for some patients, an equal goal to the quantity of food eaten ("one more bite") may be the quality of this bite (i.e., that it contains a forbidden food). Similarly, for some patients, the focus may have to be on the overall normalization of eating habits as opposed to refeeding. Notably, even for severely underweight individuals with SAN, it behooves parents to attack all forms of restriction simultaneously. Parents who try to accomplish weight gain with only "safe" foods may ultimately find themselves with a weight-normalized child who still appears actively ill, with rigid food-related rules and rituals. Ideally, parents target quantity, quality, pattern (three meals plus two to three snacks), rules (e.g., I must not eat after 6:00 A.M.), and rituals (e.g., eating only one mouthful of food per unit of time) aggressively from day one of treatment. The therapist should send this message over the course of Phase 1 of treatment without being unduly directive, as an equally important goal of treatment is to infuse the parents with a sense of agency and power. The therapist might say,

> "Other families have regretted approaching the strategies to overcome this illness incrementally. Early on in treatment, each change you impose is challenging for you

and for your daughter, but families have found that it becomes harder, not easier, to introduce new interventions later on."

However, it is unwise for the therapist to set too many goals for Session 2. It is important for parents to have an experience of success in this family meal, so they can return home more confident in their ability to help their child. Therefore, based on clinical presentation, the therapist should decide in advance whether the goal of Session 2 will be one more bite—period—or a bite of a specific type of food.

The Rest of Phase 1 (Sessions 3–8)

Consistent with the original FBT manuals (Le Grange & Lock, 2007; Lock et al., 2001), the primary goals of the rest of Phase 1 are to keep parents focused on the resolution of their child's eating disorder symptoms, to shape and refine parents' implementation of techniques designed to reverse the high risk for AN status, and to assist the siblings in establishing and maintaining a supportive role. The therapist continues to modify maladaptive perceptions of the illness (e.g., that it is within the patient's capacity to control; that criticism will mobilize change in the patient).

A common sentiment of patients at this age is the importance of weight to social status. If children or adolescents have been the victims of bullying or social isolation, they may attribute this negative experience to their weight. In the following example, a 13-year-old female patient expresses her plea that she not be able to gain any more weight:

> PATIENT: I can't gain weight, I'll be miserable; no one will be friends with me.
>
> PARENT: Your friends don't care what you weigh when they decide to spend time with you.
>
> PATIENT: Yes they do, people only spend time with me because I'm skinny. If I gain weight I'll lose them all. I know I will.
>
> THERAPIST: I'm so sorry that the eating disorder has made you believe that your weight is so important. It's hard to find good friends. Can you think of any other reasons that they might like to spend time with you?

When conducting FBT with patients with SAN, the therapist must be sensitive to the importance of the child's or adolescent's social life. This can be challenging during Phase 1 refeeding because it is strongly recommended that all meals be monitored, including school lunch periods. This requires the therapist to encourage creativity by the parents so that they ensure that their child is fed under supervision, while simultaneously not depriving the adolescent of developmentally appropriate social activities. For example, if parents are concerned, wanting their 12-year-old daughter to be able to attend a fellow classmate's birthday party dinner, they should not trust that she will eat on her own accord at the party. Rather, they should find ways to ensure that she is well nourished before leaving the house by providing dinner before the birthday dinner and a dessert or snack upon her arrival home. This type of flexibility is especially important with adolescents, as peer socialization is an integral part of the adolescent years and has implications for identity formation and the establishment of a strong social support system (Zarbatany, Hartmann, & Rankin, 1990).

There are three main changes to the original manual to address the needs of patients with SAN in the rest of Phase 1:

- Focus on normalization of eating habits, as applicable.
- Implement regular family meals at home and the modeling of healthy, nonrestrictive eating habits by parents.
- Revise criteria for progression to Phase 2.

First, as explained earlier, for some patients the focus will be on discussing, supporting, and helping the parental dyad's efforts at normalizing the eating patterns and habits of their child, as opposed to a pure refeeding emphasis. Regardless of the particular emphasis for each patient, the task for parents in Phase 1 is to address *all* behavioral aspects of the eating disorder including:

- Dietary restriction
  o Overall quantity
  o Types of food
  o Going for long periods of time without eating (fasting)
- Rules about eating
- Rituals associated with eating
- Excessive exercise
- Binge eating
- Purging
- Weight-checking rituals
- Body-checking rituals

The therapist's job is threefold: to highlight the existence of the problem areas and the importance of addressing them aggressively, immediately, and simultaneously; to support the parents' efforts at resolving them and redirect the parents to these issues as necessary; and to use examples from other families or from inpatient protocols when the parents seek advice on how these behavioral problems can be resolved. Essentially, the parents must create a zero-tolerance environment for these behaviors by making it difficult for the patient to engage in them. In the case of refusal behaviors (e.g., restriction), parents set the expectation, with a judicious blend of firmness and kindness, that eating will occur. In the case of active behaviors (e.g., excessive exercise, purging), parents are expected to monitor, supervise, contain, and distract their child to prevent symptom engagement. Most important, parents must convey their resolve, sending a message to the patient/illness that they will prevail. Parents should never be punitive—they would never think of punishing their child if he or she had a tumor that was not shrinking in response to chemotherapy. Instead, they would consider alternative therapies and even experimental interventions until they and the doctors found an effective strategy. Within these broad parameters (firmness, kindness, resolve, and a nonpunitive stance), parents must find their own particular strategies that work via trial and error. The therapist is not prescriptive about the details of these strategies. Strategies for the resolution of binge eating and purging behaviors can be found in the FBT-BN manual (Le Grange & Lock, 2007). The second modification of the original manual to address the needs of a person with SAN is the prescription of regular family meals at home and the modeling of healthy, nonrestrictive eating habits by parents. Recent research has shown that the implementation of regular family dinners that all family members are expected to attend is associated with lower rates of eating disorders (Ackard & Neumark-Sztainer, 2001; Burgess-Champoux, Larson, Neumark-Sztainer, & Hannan, 2009; Fulkerson, Story, et al., 2006; Neumark-Sztainer, Wall, Story, & Fulkerson, 2004), extending prior research demonstrating its negative correlation with a variety of other problematic adolescent behaviors (CASA, 2009; Eisenberg, Neumark-Sztainer, Fulkerson, & Story, 2008; Eisenberg, Olson, Neumark-Sztainer, Story, & Bearinger, 2004; Franko, Thompson, Affenito, Barton, & Striegel-Moore, 2008; Fulkerson, Story, et al., 2006; Sen, 2010). Specifically, family meals have been found in prospective research to predict lower rates of disordered eating among adolescent girls, even after controlling for other family variables for which the frequency of family meals might be a proxy (e.g., family connectedness, parental encouragement to diet) and for baseline levels of extreme weight control behaviors (Larson, Neumark-Sztainer, Hannan, & Story, 2007; Neumark-Sztainer et al., 2008). Conversely, eating alone is associated with the development of eating disorders in longitudinal research (Martinez-Gonzalez et al., 2003). Although further research is needed to tease apart self-selection from effect (e.g., are families who choose to eat together different, or is the establishment of family meals directly protective?), common sense dictates that family meals at least provide the following: (1) an opportunity to observe and correct unhealthy eating patterns in offspring (Burgess-Champoux et al., 2009), (2) an opportunity for parents to model healthy eating patterns (Fulkerson, Neumark-Sztainer, & Story, 2006), and (3) a forum in which to identify and discuss stressors that may predispose a person to the development of an eating disorder (Stice et al., 2010).

It is important that at these meals, and more generally, the parents do not explicitly exhibit behaviors and attitudes consistent with an eating disorder. Ideally, they would model better-than-normative behavior and attitudes. This is not emphasized in the original AN manual, inasmuch as the difference between AN and other presentations (e.g., normative discontent regarding one's shape and weight, fad dieting) is sufficiently stark that the illness offers a clear target. When a child with unequivocal AN complains, "Why can my mother diet and I can't?", it is easy to respond that AN is a disorder that goes vastly beyond dieting, to the point of death in a significant percentage of cases. For a patient receiving FBT-SAN, this answer is adapted to emphasize the danger the child is in if immediate, aggressive action is not taken to reverse the existing eating patterns.

With certain SAN presentations, the boundaries between the eating disorder and nondisordered but still unhealthy behaviors and attitudes may be more diffuse from the family's perspective (whereas professionals can easily draw the distinction). It is therefore essential that parents "practice what they preach." Parents who are overweight may engage in healthy lifestyle-based dieting, and parents of normal weight may preferentially consume lower-fat, balanced meals and snacks, provided that no food is deemed forbidden in the home. In addition, parents may engage in exercise, but not to an excessive level (e.g., to the point that it interferes with role functioning, or exercising vigorously to the point of or despite injury). All parents, regardless of weight, should avoid making comments about their own (or their children's) appearance and instead should link self-evaluation to controllable, effort-based accomplishments and prosocial interpersonal behaviors. For example, it is contraindicated for a mother of normal weight to skip meals or to ask her husband, "Do I look fat?" in front of her ill child. Such remarks can confuse the child and obfuscate the goals of treatment.

Yet parents need not consume the level of nutritional intake required for the reversal of a low-weight eating disorder. Consider the example of a 14-year-old male engaged in Phase 1 who was refusing to eat greater amounts of food as compared with other family members:

PARENT: I have to admit that we have all been eating more lately.

THERAPIST: How do you mean?

PARENT: Well, he is always watching us during meals and never eats faster than we do. If I choose not to eat the bread that came with my soup, he will refuse to eat his bread. So I often end up eating the bread, to make sure that he eats it too.

THERAPIST: It sounds as if you're trying to make sure that your son eats the appropriate amount of food at meals, but he is sick and you can require him to eat the food his body needs without making changes in your own diet. If your son were afflicted with cancer and needed to undergo chemotherapy treatments, you would be harming your body if you underwent the same treatment as he does, whereas the same medicine would be helping his body fight the disease. (*to the patient*) Your body needs lots of energy to make up for the weight you have lost, and you're growing so your body needs even more energy. The eating disorder doesn't care about your growth, but your parents will do whatever they have to to make sure that you get better.

This prescription for positive parental modeling to help reverse the trajectory toward AN is not intended to imply the inverse, namely that parents are necessarily to blame for the development of an eating disorder. In fact, FBT is explicitly atheoretical in regard to etiology, reassuring self-blaming parents that the cause of AN is complex and poorly understood and that parents, rather than being directly and exclusively implicated in the primary origins of the illness, are essential resources in reversing its course. FBT does not fall prey to the seductive, clinically face-valid (Bulik, 2005) mother-blaming attributions that have ultimately been disproven in other cases of severe psychopathology, such as schizophrenia and autism. It is important to note that although genetics may inform our understanding of the literal role of family influence in eating disorders, this body of literature cannot legitimately—and should not—be used in support of blaming parents for their child's AN or BN (Le Grange, Lock, Loeb, & Nicholls, 2010). However, the field must be equally cautious not to throw the proverbial "baby out with the bathwater" and ignore the import of genetics and of passive gene–environment correlations, such as a genetically influenced family environment, in the development of eating disorders (Allen, Byrne, Forbes, & Oddy, 2009; Bulik, Reba, Siega-Riz, & Reichborn-Kjennerud, 2005; Bulik et al., 2006; Mazzeo & Bulik, 2008; Nicholls & Viner, 2009). Family studies, twin studies, and molecular genetic studies (association and linkage studies) have all been conducted with eating disorders with significant and intriguing findings in support of genetic contribution to the variance at each level of investigation (for recent reviews in the context of risk factors for eating disorders, see Bulik, 2005; Jacobi, Hayward, de Zwaan, Krawmer, & Agras, 2004; Mazzeo & Bulik, 2008; Stice at al., 2010; Striegel-Moore & Bulik, 2007). Yet genetic findings alone do not provide nearly sufficient explanatory power for the development of eating disorders. Mazzeo and Bulik (2008) recommend educating patients and their families about the fallacy of genetic determinism and the interplay of multiple variables in producing an eating disorder outcome. Gene–environment interactions are likely at play in the risk of eating disorders, given, for example, the emphasis on the thin ideal (Rodin, Silberstein, & Striegel-Moore, 1985) in cultures and subcultures most vulnerable to developing AN (e.g., Hoek et al., 2005; Hoek, van Harten, van Hoeken, & Susser, 1998; Rogers Wood & Petrie, 2010; Vander Wal, Gibbons, & del Pilar Grazioso, 2007) coupled with the rarity of the disorder even within these environments (Bulik, 2005; Striegel-Moore & Bulik, 2007). The range of potential fully explanatory models for what causes AN and BN is wide, and the field faces significant challenges in uncovering the true mechanisms of risk (Striegel-Moore & Bulik, 2007). Understanding such factors, including the adverse environmental influences that may activate genetic susceptibility, can have significant implications for the development of targeted interventions to prevent the onset of AN and BN (Striegel-Moore & Bulik, 2007). For example, Bulik and colleagues (2005) have outlined a theoretical "cycle of risk" for AN that synthesizes some of the best established prospective genetic and environmental risk factors, including perinatal events, and demonstrates how a mother's history of AN, in combination with genetically influenced "cycle-perpetuating environmental factors" (insufficient nutrition and weight gain during pregnancy, a focus on appearance, and ongoing restrictive eating), might collectively increase the likelihood for the development of AN in her offspring. Longitudinal research on children of mothers with eating disorders relative to controls is consistent with this model (Stein et al., 2006). Bulik and colleagues also depict how the field might use this model to identify buffering factors that can interrupt the cycle. A preliminary study involving focus groups for mothers with eating disorders suggests that such parents are seeking guidance in this regard (Mazzeo, Zucker, Gerke, Mitchell, & Bulik, 2005). (See Racine, Root, Klump, and Bulik, Chapter 3, this volume, for a more extensive review of risk factors for eating disorders.) Some of these potentially buffering factors, such as the prescription for the modeling of healthy, nonrestrictive eating by parents, are included in the adaptation of FBT-SAN, although this intervention does not exclusively target offspring of mothers with AN.

The third modification of the original manual (Lock et al., 2001) pertains to the criteria for moving from Phase 1 to Phase 2. As in the treatment of patients with AN, the first sign of readiness for Phase 2 may be reduced anxiety and tension in non-food-related discussions. In SAN, however, unlike AN, steady weight gain is not the exclusive yardstick by which the therapist assesses the family's readiness to progress to the second phase of treatment. Although this is the most relevant criterion for a subset of patients with SAN, others' readiness for Phase 2 can be better marked by some weight gain followed by weight stabilization, coupled with a significant reduction in resistance to eating regular meals and snacks. Parents must also feel confident in their ability to ensure both a healthy weight and healthy eating patterns in their offspring in order to progress to Phase 2.

Phase 2 (Sessions 9–12)

Sessions in Phase 2 take place biweekly (four sessions over 8 weeks). As with the original FBT-AN and FBT-BN protocols (Le Grange & Lock, 2007; Lock et al., 2001), the primary goals of Phase 2 are to gradually fade parental management of eating disorder symptoms and transfer control over eating and related behaviors back to the patient, at a developmentally appropriate level, and to explore the relationship between child/adolescent developmental issues and the eating disorder. The SAN population, a subset of which represents prodromal AN, encompasses a wider (younger) age range than AN. Therefore, Phases 2 and 3 have to address not only issues of adolescent development but also earlier developmental stages such as middle-late childhood. For preadolescents, the developmental disruptions or arrest caused by the illness are age-specific (e.g., less in psychosexual development and more in the friendship domain). In addition, across developmental stages the insult to development in SAN may be reduced relative to AN, depending on the specific SAN profile (i.e., which AN criteria are met), severity, and chronicity. Note that exploring developmental issues in relation to the eating disorder and its resolution does not imply an etiological relationship between developmental issues and the onset of the eating disorder. For patients in middle-late childhood, the parents should take extra care during this phase of treatment to not assign more autonomy in eating than is developmentally appropriate. The goal is to return or bring the child to the level of autonomy that would be in place had the eating disorder never struck, not to accelerate general autonomy beyond an age-appropriate level.

One means of accomplishing this shift may be to introduce occasional social eating activities without supervised meals prior to the outing. This allows parents an opportunity to test the patient's ability to make good choices as they begin the return to developmentally normative, more independent eating interactions for their child. Parents can be encouraged to have a dialogue with the patient before and after he or she goes out regarding making plans for the meal and a review of the choices the patient made and any difficulties he or she experienced.

Regardless of developmental stage (childhood, adolescence), family meals should remain a priority for families of patients with SAN throughout Phases 2 and 3 and even beyond treatment termination. Prioritizing family meals does not require rigid adherence, and the realities of extracurricular activities and the child's or adolescent's social life will inevitably compromise perfect compliance.

Phase 3 (Sessions 13 and 14)

The goals and interventions in Phase 3 of FBT-SAN are to restore or establish healthy family relationships, particularly parent–child interactions, outside the framework of the eating disorder; to review the developmental issues of childhood or adolescence and model problem solving in areas of concern (e.g., tension over broader themes and manifestations of separation and individuation on the part of the patient as the illness recedes); to plan for the future, including signs of relapse or worsening toward AN; and to terminate treatment. As noted earlier, a primary modification for the population with SAN, relative to the original manuals, is attention to middle childhood, as applicable to a portion of those with SAN, whereas the general theme—a return to normal development—remains the same. However, it is important that adolescent development, in addition to middle childhood development, be reviewed with families with preadolescent children with SAN, as this next stage is imminent and parents must be prepared for the pending changes in their child. A primer on adolescent development is included in the original FBT manuals for AN and BN (Le Grange & Lock, 2007; Lock et al., 2001). In addition, there is a dual emphasis on prevention of relapse in SAN and on continued prevention of the development of full AN. Thus, not only is the fear that the eating disorder will resurface encouraged, but parents are informed that by continuing to keep the SAN at bay, they are by definition preventing AN, a deadly and pernicious disorder. Patients continue to be weighed at each session.

A Primer on Middle Childhood and Its Relationship to the SAN Population

From a cognitive-developmental/Piagetian perspective, middle childhood is characterized by a transition to concrete operational thinking (Piaget & Inhelder, 1969). Examples of this with the greatest relevance to the population with SAN—and to what parents can expect as the illness recedes—include a decline in egocentrism (Damon & Hart, 1988; Rosenberg, 1979) and shifts in social relations (Bigelow, 1977). Specifically, children in this age range can assume the perspective of others (particularly toward themselves) (Selman, 1980), recognize any disconnect between thought or affect and behavior, and factor intent in their appraisal of another's behavior (Harter, 2008). The primary implication for SAN is that a self-consciousness about appearance may develop. A focus on how others perceive the child may be a factor that maintains the illness (when it is distorted and the child believes that others perceive him or her as fat) and, later, can aid in its resolution (with the understanding that friends are uncomfortable with his or her illness and that the public in fact perceives him or her as emaciated). Parents can capitalize on the declining egocentrism by encouraging healthy behaviors (e.g., eating) while acknowledging that their child is resistant to engaging in them. Parents can also be assured that their child is old enough to ultimately understand their positive intent in demanding food consumption in the face of extreme resistance.

From a social-developmental perspective, the later stage of middle childhood is characterized by a continued and growing emphasis on peer relationships (which at this stage, is more child- than parent-directed) (Zarbatany et al., 1990), whereas time spent with parents is correspondingly reduced. The eating disorder may have reversed this trend. Parents must expect and support this development, that as the eating disorder is resolved, peers will increase in importance to their child. At this developmental stage, peer interactions are likely to be sex segregated with an emphasis on same-sex "best friendships" (Graham, Cohen, Zbikowski, & Secrist, 1998), although at the cusp of adolescence, increasing violations of these socially imposed boundaries will occur. By extension, peer-based, unrealistic eating and appearance norms may develop. It is also normal for children of this age to engage in peer interactions without the direct supervision of adults (Zarbatany et al., 1990) and to resolve conflicts independently of adult intervention. Parents of an ill child may have a difficult time narrowing their protective behavior to the appropriate target (SAN). Note that this is not a statement about etiology and does not imply that overprotectiveness has a causal influence on the development of AN. Parents of an ill child—particularly those who participate in an intervention that demands dramatic and heroic efforts to save their child from death—might simply overgeneralize their protective instincts during the acute stages of the illness or of treatment, and this is actively corrected by the treatment model. Middle childhood also marks a time when children develop social identities outside the home environment (Zarbatany et al., 1990) and may behave differently across contexts. Depending on when the eating disorder strikes, parents may be aware of only the child they know at home and the child as influenced by SAN. The resolution of the illness may reveal a range of context-dependent social presentations.

Children in this age range are also acutely aware of social conventions and expectations (Bigelow, 1977), potentially contributing to their internalization of the thin ideal, which has been linked to the development of eating disorders (Thompson & Stice, 2001);

moreover, patients may cite peer dieting and appearance norms in their resistance to treatment. Social status continues to be established in this age range, and physical attractiveness is strongly associated with popularity (Boyatzis, Baloff, & Durieux, 1998). Self-concepts become more abstract and stable and are solidified via social comparison (Pomerantz, Ruble, Frey, & Greulich, 1995; Ruble & Frey, 1991). Appearance-based social comparison is potentially associated with risk for an eating disorder. Self-evaluation becomes more differentiated, with input from multiple domains of competence (cognitive, social, physical), while at the same time children develop overall self-esteem (a general sense of self-worth) (McCarthy & Hoge, 1982). In eating disorders, self-evaluation can narrow to a consideration of shape and weight, rather than becoming more differentiated. Children also develop a self-representation that reflects the discrepancy between actual and ideal selves (Harter, 1999), a concept studied in relation to body image disturbance and eating (Fallon & Rozin, 1985; Strauman, Vookles, Berenstien, Chaiken, & Higgins, 1991; Thompson & Psaltis, 1988; Tiggemann, 1992).

The nature of parent–child interactions also shifts during middle childhood. Parents expect more from their children during this developmental stage, in several domains of competency, including emotional maturity, compliance, politeness, independence, social skills, verbal assertiveness, and self-directed adherence to household and school-based rules (Goodnow, Cashmore, Cotton, & Knight, 1984; Harter, 2008). Although certain of these expectations may be reduced during the acute period of illness, parents should quickly endeavor to bring their expectations in alignment with their child's degree of recovery. Moreover, parents need not entirely eliminate their expectations during the severe stages of the eating disorder. Consistent with the notion that parents should assume more authority only in the eating and associated domains, and not increase control in other aspects of their child's life, parents should similarly be cautious in relaxing general rules and expectations. Although parents need to be understanding if their child yells or curses at them during mealtimes, they should limit this behavior as much as possible both within and across contexts. For example, if a child screams and throws food at the parents during dinner, they can calmly say, "We know that your eating disorder is very angry that we have taken charge and are not going to let you be sick. Nothing it does will deter us. We expect you to eat this food because it is like medicine for your very serious illness. We also know you to be a kind and gentle person who would behave like this only under the influence of an awful disorder. The healthy part of you must feel terrible about this behavior, but don't worry. As that part of you grows and the eating disorder shrinks, this will stop." The parents should set firm limits if such behavior generalizes to other contexts, (e.g., if the child throws a tantrum about being denied a new iPod).

During middle childhood there is an increasing transfer of control from parents to their offspring as children assume more authority over their personal, social, and academic lives (Collins, 1995). However, parental monitoring is positively correlated with positive adjustment during this developmental stage and remains essential (Patterson & Stouthamer-Loeber, 1984). This balance (termed co-regulation; Maccoby, 1984) is dynamic, with a changing ratio as development progresses. This concept is highly relevant to the family contending with SAN, particularly those who are undergoing FBT. FBT introduces what may seem like a radical insult to this process by asking parents to think of their ill child as regressed in self-feeding and to respond accordingly, reimplementing techniques generally more appropriate to early childhood or even infancy. The therapist must emphasize that this is (1) absolutely necessary, (2) limited to the eating realm, and (3) temporary. Parents must also navigate the changes in parenting style required by FBT. During Phase 1, parents are asked to become authoritarian in the eating domain but to avoid an authoritarian stance in other aspects of their child's life. Phase 2 requires an authoritative style in regard to food and eating. Throughout treatment, and especially in Phase 3, an authoritative parental style is encouraged for domains beyond the eating disorder.

References

Ackard, D. M., & Neumark-Sztainer, D. (2001). Family meal time while growing up: Associations with symptoms of bulimia nervosa. *Eating Disorders: The Journal of Treatment and Prevention, 9*, 239–249.

Allen, K. L., Byrne, S. M., Forbes, D., & Oddy, W. H. (2009). Risk factors for full- and partial-syndrome early adolescent eating disorders: A population-based pregnancy cohort study. *Journal of the American Academy of Child and Adolescent Psychiatry, 48*, 800–809.

Ben-Tovim, D. I., Walker, K., Gilchrist, P., Freeman, R., Kalucy, R., & Esterman, A. (2001). Outcome in patients with eating disorders: A 5-year study. *Lancet, 357*, 1254–1257.

Berkman, N. D., Lohr, K. N., & Bulik, C. M. (2007). Outcomes of eating disorders: A systematic review of the literature. *International Journal of Eating Disorders, 40*, 293–309.

Bhangoo, R. K., & Carter, C. S. (2009). Very early interventions in psychotic disorders. *Psychiatric Clinics of North America, 32*, 81–94.

Bigelow, B. J. (1977). Children's friendship expectations: A cognitive developmental study. *Child Development, 48*, 246–253.

Biller, B. M., Saxe, V., Herzog, D. B., Rosenthal, D. I., Holzman, S., & Kiblanski, A. (1989). Mechanisms of osteoporosis in adult and adolescent women with anorexia nervosa. *Journal of Clinical Endocrinology and Metabolism, 68*, 548–554.

Boyatzis, C. J., Baloff, P., & Durieux, C. (1998). Effects of perceived attractiveness and academic success on early adolescent peer popularity. *Journal of Genetic Psychology, 159*, 337–344.

Bravender, T., Bryant-Waugh, R., Herzog, D., Katzman, D., Kreipe, R. D., Lask, B., et al. (2007). Classification of child and adolescent eating disturbances. Workgroup for Classification of Eating Disorders in Children and Adolescents (WCEDCA). *International Journal of Eating Disorders, 40*(Suppl.), S117–S122.

Bravender, T., Bryant-Waugh, R., Herzog, D., Katzman, D., Kreipe, R. D., Lask, B., et al. (2010). Classification of eating disturbance in children and adolescents: Proposed changes for the DSM-V. *European Eating Disorders Review, 18*(2), 79–89.

Bulik, C. M. (2005). Exploring the gene–environment nexus in eating disorders. *Journal of Psychiatry and Neuroscience, 30*, 335–339.

Bulik, C. M., Reba, L., Siega-Riz, A. M., & Reichborn-Kjennerud, T. (2005). Anorexia nervosa: Definition, epidemiology, and cycle of risk. *International Journal of Eating Disorders, 37*, S2–S9.

Bulik, C. M., Sullivan, P. F., Tozzi, F., Furberg, H., Lichtenstein, P., & Pederson, N. L. (2006). Prevalence, heritability, and prospective risk factors for anorexia nervosa. *Archives of General Psychiatry, 63*, 305–312.

Bulik, C. M., Thornton, L., Pinheiro, K., Klump, K. L., Brandt, H., Crawford, S., et al. (2008). Suicide attempts in anorexia nervosa. *Journal of Psychosomatic Medicine, 70*(3), 378–383.

Burgess-Champoux, T. L., Larson, N., Neumark-Sztainer, D., & Hannan, P. J. (2009). Are family meal patterns associated with overall diet quality during the transition from early to middle adolescence? *Journal of Nutrition Education and Behavior, 41*, 79–86.

CASA. (2009). The importance of family dinners V. The National Center on Addiction and Substance Abuse at Columbia University. Retrieved from *www.casacolumbia.org/templates/Publications_Reports.aspx#r81. Accessed May 2010.*

Casey, B. J., Getz, S., & Galvan, A. (2008). The adolescent brain. *Developmental Review, 28*, 62–77.

Casey, B. J., Giedd, J. N., & Thomas, K. N. (2000). Structural and functional brain development and its relation to cognitive development. *Biological Psychology, 54*, 241–257.

Castro, J., Lazaro, L., Pons, F., Halperin, I., & Toro, J. (2000). Predictors of bone mineral density reduction in adolescents with anorexia nervosa. *Journal of the American Academy of Child and Adolescent Psychiatry, 39*, 1365–1370.

Chamay-Weber, C., Narring, F., & Michaud, P. A. (2005). Partial eating disorders among adolescents: A review. *Journal of Adolescent Health, 37*, 417–427.

Collins, W. A. (1995). Relationships and development: Family adaptation to individual change. In S. Shulman (Ed.), *Close relationships and socioemotional development* (pp. 128–154). New York: Ablex.

Couturier, J. L., & Lock, J. (2006). Denial and minimization in adolescents with anorexia nervosa. *International Journal of Eating Disorders, 39*, 212–216.

Crisp, A., Gowers, S. G., Joughin, N., McClelland, L., Rooney, B., Nielsen, S., et al. (2006). Death, survival, and recovery in anorexia nervosa: A thirty-five year study. *European Eating Disorders Review, 14*, 168–175.

Crow, S., Praus, B., & Thuras, P. (1999). Mortality from eating disorders: A 5- to 10-year record linkage study. *International Journal of Eating Disorders, 26*, 97–101.

Currin, L., & Schmidt, U. (2005). A critical analysis of the utility of an early intervention approach in the eating disorders. *Journal of Mental Health, 14*, 1–14.

Damon, W., & Hart, D. (1988). *Self-understanding in childhood and adolescence.* New York: Cambridge University Press.

Danzinger, Y., Mukamel, M., Zeharia, A., Dinari, G., & Mimouni, M. (1994). Stunting of growth in anorexia nervosa during the prepubertal and pubertal period. *Israel Journal of Medical Science, 30*, 581–584.

Deter, H. C., & Herzog, W. (1994). Anorexia nervosa in a long-term perspective: Results of the Heidelberg–Mannheim study. *Psychosomatic Medicine, 56*, 20–22.

Eddy, K. T., Doyle, A. C., Hoste, R. R., Herzog, D. B., & Le Grange, D. (2008). Eating disorder not otherwise specified in adolescents. *Journal of the American Academy of Child and Adolescent Psychiatry, 47*, 2.

Eisenberg, M. E., Neumark-Sztainer, D., Fulkerson, J. A., & Story, M. (2008). Family meals and substance use: Is there a long-term protective association? *Journal of Adolescent Health, 43*, 151–156.

Eisenberg, M. E., Olson, R. E., Neumark-Sztainer, D., Story, M., & Bearinger, L. H. (2004). Correlations between family meals and psychosocial well-being among adolescents. *Archives of Pediatrics and Adolescent Medicine, 158*, 792–796.

Eisler, I., Dare, C., Hodes, M., Russell, G. F. M., Dodge, E., & Le Grange, D. (2000). Family therapy for adolescent anorexia nervosa: The results of a controlled comparison of two family interventions. *Journal of Child Psychology and Psychiatry, 41*, 727–736.

Eisler, I., Dare, C., Russell, G. F. M, Szmukler, G., Le Grange, D., & Dodge, E. (1997). Family and individual therapy in anorexia nervosa: A 5-year follow-up. *Archives of General Psychiatry, 54*, 1025–1030.

Eisler, I., Simic, M., Russell, G. F., & Dare, C. (2007). A randomized controlled treatment trial of two forms of family therapy in adolescent anorexia nervosa: A five-year follow-up. *Journal of Child Psychology and Psychiatry, 48*, 552–560.

Fallon, A., & Rozin, P. (1985). Sex differences in perceptions of desirable body shape. *Journal of Abnormal Psychology, 91*, 102–105.

Festinger, L. (1957). *A theory of cognitive dissonance.* Stanford, CA: Stanford University Press.

Fichter, M. M., Quadflieg, N., & Hedlund, S. (2006). Twelve-year course and outcome predictors of anorexia nervosa. *International Journal of Eating Disorders, 39*, 87–100.

Franko, D. L., & Keel, P. K. (2006). Suicidality in eating disorders: Occurrence, correlates, and clinical implications. *Clinical Psychology Review, 26,* 769–782.

Franko, D. L., Thompson, D., Affenito, S. G., Barton, B. A., & Striegel-Moore, R. H. (2008). What mediates the relationship between family meals and adolescent health issues? *Health Psychology, 27,* S109–S117.

Fulkerson, J. A., Neumark-Sztainer, D., & Story, M. (2006). Adolescent and parent views of family meals. *Journal of the American Dietetic Association, 106,* 526–532.

Fulkerson, J. A., Story, M., Mellin, A., Leffert, N., Neumark-Sztainer, D., & French, S. A. (2006). Family dinner meal frequency and adolescent development: Relationships with developmental assets and high-risk behaviors. *Journal of Adolescent Health, 39,* 337–345.

Giedd, J. N., Blumenthal, J., Jeffries, N. O., Castellanos, F. X., Liu, H., Zijdenbos, A., et al. (1999). Brain development during childhood and adolescence: A longitudinal MRI study. *Nature Neuroscience, 2,* 861–863.

Giedd, J. N., Viatuzis, A. C., Hamburger, S. D., Lange, N., Rajapakse, J. C., Kaysen, D., et al. (1996). Quantitative MRI of the temporal lobe, amygdala, and hippocampus in normal human development. *Journal of Comparative Neurology, 366,* 223–230.

Golden, N., Kreitzer, P., & Jacobson, M. (1994). Disturbances in growth hormone secretion and action in adolescents with anorexia nervosa. *Journal of Pediatrics, 125,* 655–660.

Golden, N., & Shenker, I. (1992). Amenorrhea in anorexia nervosa: Etiology and implications. *Adolescent Medicine, 3,* 503–517.

Goodnow, J. J., Cashmore, J., Cotton, S., & Knight, R. (1984). Mothers' developmental timetables in two cultural groups. *International Journal of Psychology, 19,* 193–205.

Graham, J. A., Cohen, R., Zbikowski, S. M., & Secrist, M. E. (1998). A longitudinal investigation of race and sex as factors in children's classroom friendship choices. *Child Study Journal, 28,* 245–266.

Harter, S. (1999). *The construction of the self.* New York: Guilford Press.

Harter, S. (2008). The developing self. In W. Damin & R. M. Lerner (Eds.), *Child and adolescent development* (pp. 216–260). Hoboken, NJ: Wiley.

Hay, P. J., & Mond, J. (2005). A review of health-related quality of life in people with eating disorders. *Journal of Mental Health, 14,* 539–552.

Hazelton, L. R., & Faine, M. P. (1996). Diagnosis and dental management of eating disorder patients. *International Journal of Prosthodontics, 9,* 65–73.

Hebebrand, J., Casper, R., Treasure, J., & Schweiger, U. (2004). The need to revise the diagnostic criteria for anorexia nervosa. *Journal of Neural Transmission, 111,* 827–840.

Herzog, D. B., Greenwood, D. N., Dorer, D. J., Flores, A. T., Ekeblad, E. R., Richards, A., et al. (2000). Mortality in eating disorders: A descriptive study. *International Journal of Eating Disorders, 28,* 20–26.

Herzog, D. B., Hopkins, J. D., & Burns, C. D. (1993). A follow-up study of 33 subdiagnostic eating disordered women. *International Journal of Eating Disorders, 14,* 261–267.

Hoek, H. W., van Harten, P. N., Hermans, K. M., Katzman, M. A., Matroos, G. E., & Susser, E. S. (2005). The incidence of anorexia nervosa on Curacao. *American Journal of Psychiatry, 162,* 748–752.

Hoek, H. W., van Harten, P. N., van Hoeken, D., & Susser, E. (1998). Lack of relation between culture and anorexia nervosa: Results of an incidence study on Curacao. *New England Journal of Medicine, 338,* 1231–1232.

Jacobi, C., Hayward, C., de Zwaan, M., Krawmer, H. C., & Agras, S. (2004). Coming to terms with risk factors for eating disorders: Application of risk terminology and suggestions for a general taxonomy. *Psychological Bulletin, 130,* 19–65.

Juarascio, A. S., Forman, E. M., & Herbert, J. D. (2010). Acceptance and commitment therapy versus cognitive therapy for the treatment of comorbid eating pathology. *Behavior Modification, 34,* 2.

Katzman, D. K. (2005). Medical complications in adolescent anorexia nervosa: A review of the literature. *International Journal of Eating Disorders, 37,* S52–S59.

Kaye, W. H., Frank, G. K., Bailer, U., & Henry, S. E (2005). Neurobiology of anorexia nervosa: Clinical implications of alterations of the function of serotonin and other neuronal systems. *International Journal of Eating Disorders, 37*, S15–S19.

Keel, P. K., Dorer, D. J., Eddy, K. T., Franko, D., Charatan, D. L., & Herzog, D. B. (2003). Predictors of mortality in eating disorders. *Achives of General Psychiatry, 60*, 179–183.

King, M. B. (1989). Eating disorders in a general practice population: Prevalence, characteristics and follow-up at 12–18 months. *Psychological Medicine: Monograph Supplement, 14*, 1–34.

Kotler, L. A., Cohen, P., Davies, M., Pine, D. S., & Walsh, B. T. (2001). Longitudinal relationships between childhood, adolescent, and adult eating disorders. *Journal of the American Academy of Child and Adolescent Psychiatry, 40*, 1434–1440.

Laessle, R. G., Kittle, S., Fichter, M. M., Wittchen, H-U., & Pirke, K. M. (1987). Major affective disorder in anorexia nervosa and bulimia: A descriptive diagnostic study. *British Journal of Psychiatry, 151*, 785–789.

Lantzouni, E., Frank, G. R., Golden, N. H., & Shenker, R. I. (2002). Reversibility of growth stunting in early onset anorexia nervosa: A prospective study. *Journal of Adolescent Health, 31*, 162–5.

Larson, N. I., Neumark-Sztainer, D., Hannan, P. J., & Story, M. (2007). Family meals during adolescence are associated with higher diet quality and healthful meal patterns during young adulthood. *Journal of the American Dietetic Association, 107*, 1502–1510.

Le Grange, D., Binford, R., & Loeb, K. (2005). Manualized family-based treatment for anorexia nervosa: A case series. *Journal of the American Academy of Child and Adolescent Psychiatry, 44*, 41–46.

Le Grange, D., Crosby, R. D., Rathouz, P. J., & Leventhal, B. L. (2007). A randomized controlled comparison of family-based treatment and supportive psychotherapy for adolescent bulimia nervosa. *Archives of General Psychiatry, 64*, 1049–1056.

Le Grange, D., Eisler, I., Dare, C., & Hodes, M. (1992). Family criticism and self-starvation: A study of expressed emotion. *Journal of Family Therapy, 14*, 177–192.

Le Grange, D., Eisler, I., Dare, C., & Russell, G. F. M. (1992). Evaluation of family therapy in anorexia nervosa: A pilot study. *International Journal of Eating Disorders, 12*, 347–357.

Le Grange, D., & Lock, J. (2007). *Treating bulimia in adolescents: A family-based approach.* New York: Guilford Press.

Le Grange, D., Lock, J., Loeb, K. L., & Nicholls, D. (2010). Academy for Eating Disorders position paper: The role of the family in eating disorders. *International Journal of Eating Disorders, 43*, 1–5.

Le Grange, D., & Loeb, K. L. (2007). Early identification and treatment of eating disorders: Prodrome to syndrome. *Early Intervention in Psychiatry, 1*, 27–39.

Le Grange, D., Loeb, K. L., Van Orman, S., & Jellar, C. (2004). Adolescent bulimia nervosa: A disorder in evolution? *Archives of Pediatrics and Adolescent Medicine, 158*, 478–482.

Lewinsohn, P. M., Striegel-Moore, R. H., & Seeley, J. R. (2001). Epidemiology and natural course of eating disorders in young women from adolescence to young adulthood. *Journal of the American Academy of Child and Adolescent Psychiatry, 39*, 1284–1292.

Lock, J., Agras, W. S., Bryson, S., & Kraemer, H. (2005). A comparison of short- and long-term family therapy for adolescent anorexia nervosa. *Journal of the American Academy of Child and Adolescent Psychiatry, 44*, 632–639.

Lock, J., Couturier, J., & Agras, W. S. (2006). Comparison of long-term outcomes in adolescents with anorexia nervosa treated with family therapy. *Journal of the American Academy of Child and Adolescent Psychiatry, 45*, 666–672.

Lock, J., Le Grange, D., Agras, W. S., & Dare, C. (2001). *Treatment manual for anorexia nervosa: A family-based approach.* New York: Guilford Press.

Lock, J., Le Grange, D., Forsburg, S., & Hewell, K. (2006). Is family therapy effective for children with anorexia nervosa? *Journal of* the American Academy of Child and Adolescent Psychiatry, 45, 1323–1328.

Loeb, K. L., & Le Grange, D. (2009). Family-based treatment for adolescent eating disorders: Current status, new applications and future directions. International Journal of Child and Adolescent Health, 2, 243–254.

Loeb, K. L., Le Grange, D., Hildebrandt, T., Greif, R., Lock, J., & Alfano, L. (in press). Eating disorders in youth: Diagnostic variability and predictive validity. International Journal of Eating Disorders.

Loeb, K. L., Walsh, B. T., Lock, J., Le Grange, D., Jones, J., Marcus, S., et al. (2007). Open trial of family-based treatment for full and partial anorexia nervosa in adolescence: Evidence of successful dissemination. Journal of the American Academy of Child and Adolescent Psychiatry, 46, 792–800.

Luby, J. L., & Navsaria, N. (2010). Pediatric bipolar disorder: Evidence for prodromal states and early markers. Journal of Child Psychology and Psychiatry, 51, 459–471.

Lucas, A. R., Beard, C. M., & O'Fallon, W. M. (1991). 50-year trends in the incidence of anorexia nervosa in Rochester, Minn.: A population-based study. American Journal of Psychiatry, 148, 917–929.

Maccoby, E. E. (1984). Middle childhood in the context of the family. In W. A. Collins (Ed.), Development during middle childhood: The years from six to twelve. Washington, DC: National Academy Press.

Martinez-Gonzalez, M. A., Gual, P., Lahortiga, F., Alonso, Y., de Irala-Estevez, J., & Cervera, S. (2003). Parental factors, mass media influences, and the onset of eating disorders in a prospective population-based cohort. Pediatrics, 111, 315–320.

Matsubara, S., Arora, R. C., & Meltzer, H. Y. (1991). Seratonergic measures in suicide brain: 5-HT$_{1A}$ binding sites in frontal cortex of suicide victims. Journal of Neural Transmission, 85, 181–194.

Mazzeo, S. E., & Bulik, C. M. (2008). Environmental and genetic risk factors for eating disorders: What the clinician needs to know. Child and Adolescent Psychiatric Clinics of North America, 18, 67–82.

Mazzeo, S. E., Zucker, N. L., Gerke, C. K.,

Mitchell, K. S., & Bulik, C. M. (2005). Parenting concerns of women with histories of eating disorders. International Journal of Eating Disorders, 37, S77–S79.

McCarthy, J., & Hoge, D. (1982). Analysis of age effects in longitudinal studies of adolescent self-esteem. Developmental Psychology, 18, 372–379.

McIntosh, V. V., Jordan, J., Carter, F. A. McKenzie, J. M., Luty, S. E., Bulik, C. M., et al. (2004). Strict versus lenient weight criterion in anorexia nervosa. European Eating Disorders Review, 12, 51–60.

Mitchell, J. E., Specker, S. M., & de Zwaan, M. (1991). Comorbidity and medical complications of bulimia nervosa. Journal of Clinical Psychiatry, 52, 13–20.

Modan–Moses, D., Yaroslavsky, A., Novikov, I., Segev, S., Toledano, A., Miterany, E., et al. (2003). Stunting of growth as a major feature of anorexia nervosa in male adolescents. Pediatrics, 111, 270–276.

Neumark-Sztainer, D., Eisenberg, M. E., Fulkerson, J. A., Story, M., & Larson, N. I. (2008). Family meals and disordered eating in adolescents: Longitudinal findings from Project EAT. Archives of Pediatric and Adolescent Medicine, 162, 17–22.

Neumark-Sztainer, D., Wall, M., Story, M., & Fulkerson, J. A. (2004). Are family meal patterns associated with disordered eating behaviors among adolescents? Journal of Adolescent Health, 35, 350–359.

Newman, D. L., Moffitt, T. E., Caspi, A., Magdol, L., Silva, P. A., & Stanton, W. R. (1996). Psychiatric disorder in a birth cohort of young adults: Prevalence, comorbidity, clinical significance, and new case incidence from ages 11 to 21. Journal of Consulting and Clinical Psychology, 64, 552–562.

Nicholls, D., & Bryant-Waugh, R. (2008). Eating disorders of infancy and childhood: Definition, symptomatology, epidemiology, and comorbidity. Child and Adolescent Psychiatric Clinics of North America, 18, 17–30.

Nicholls, D., Chater, R., & Lask, B. (2000). Children into DSM don't go: A comparison of classification systems for eating disorders in childhood and early adolescence. Inter-

national Journal of Eating Disorders, 28, 317–324.

Nicholls, D. E., & Viner, R. M. (2009). Childhood risk factors for lifetime anorexia nervosa by age 30 years in a national birth cohort. *Journal of the American Academy of Child and Adolescent Psychiatry, 48,* 791–799.

Nielsen, S., & Bara-Carril, N. (2003). Family, burden of care and social consequences. In J. Treasure, U. Schmidt, & E. van Furth (Eds.), *Handbook of eating disorders* (pp. 191–207). Chichester, UK: Wiley.

Nilsson, K., & Hagglof, B. (2005). Long-term follow-up of adolescent onset anorexia nervosa in northern Sweden. *European Eating Disorders Review, 13,* 89–100.

North, C., Gowers, S., & Byram, V. (1997). Family functioning and life events in the outcome of adolescent anorexia nervosa. *British Journal of Psychiatry, 171,* 545–549.

O'Brien, K. M., & Vincent, N. K. (2003). Psychiatric comorbidity in anorexia and bulimia nervosa: Nature, prevalence, and causal relationships. *Clinical Psychology Review, 23,* 57–74.

Palla, R., & Litt, I. (1988). Medical complications of eating disorders in adolescents. *Pediatrics, 81,* 613–23.

Patterson, G. R., & Stouthamer-Loeber, M. (1984). The correlation of family management practices and delinquency. *Child Development, 55,* 1299–1307.

Patton, G. C., Johnson-Sabine, E., Wood, K., Mann, A. H., & Wakeling, A. (1990). Abnormal eating attitudes in London schoolgirls: A prospective epidemiological study: Outcome at twelve month follow-up. *Psychological Medicine, 20,* 383–394.

Perkins, S., Winn, S., Murray, J., Murphy, R., & Schmidt, U. (2004). A qualitative study of the experience of caring for a person with bulimia nervosa. Part 1: The emotional impact of caring. *International Journal of Eating Disorders, 36,* 256–268.

Piaget, J., & Inhelder, B. (1969). *The psychology of the child.* New York: Basic Books.

Pomerantz, E. M., Ruble, D. N., Frey, K. S., & Greulich, F. (1995). Meeting goals and confronting conflict: Children's changing perceptions of social comparison. *Child Development, 66,* 723–738.

Pomery, C., & Mitchell, J. E. (2001).Medical complications of anorexia nervosa and bulimia nervosa. In C. G. Fairburn & K. D. Brownell (Eds.), *Eating disorders and obesity: A comprehensive handbook* (2nd ed., pp. 278–285). New York: Guilford Press.

Pompili, M., Mancinelli, I., Girardi, P., Ruberto, A., & Tatarelli, R. (2004). Suicide in anorexia nervosa: A meta-analysis. *International Journal of Eating Disorders, 36,* 1.

Ratnasuriya, R., Eisler, I., Szmukler, G. I., & Russell, G. F. (1991). Anorexia nervosa: outcome and prognostic factors after 20 years. *British Journal of Psychiatry, 156,* 495–456.

Reas, D. L., Schoemaker, C., Zipfel, S., & Williamson, D. A. (2001). Prognostic value of duration of illness and early intervention in bulimia nervosa: A systematic review of the outcome literature. *International Journal of Eating Disorders, 30,* 1–10.

Reas, D. L., Williamson, D. A., Martin, C. K., & Zucker, N. L. (2000). Duration of illness predicts outcome for bulimia nervosa: A long-term follow-up study. *International Journal of Eating Disorders, 27,* 428–434.

Richard, M., Bauer, S., & Kordy, H., (2005). Relapse in anorexia and bulimia nervosa: A 2.5-year follow-up study. *European Eating Disorders Review, 13,* 180–190.

Rodin, J., Silberstein, L., & Striegel-Moore, R. (1985). Women and weight: A normative discontent. In T. B. Sonderegger (Ed.), *Psychology and gender: Nebraska Symposium on Motivation 1984* (pp. 267–307). Lincoln: University of Nebraska Press.

Rogers Wood, N. A., & Petrie, T. A. (2010). Body dissatisfaction, ethnic identity, and disordered eating among African American women. *Journal of Counseling Psychology, 57,* 141–153.

Rosenberg, M. (1979). *Conceiving the self.* New York: Basic Books.

Ruble, D. N., & Frey, K. S. (1991). Changing patterns of comparative behavior as skills are acquired: A functional model of self-evaluation. In J. Suls & T. A. Wills (Eds.), *Social comparison: Contemporary theory and research* (pp. 770–112). Hillsdale, NJ: Erlbaum.

Russell, G. F. M., Szmukler, G. I., Dare, C., & Eisler, I. (1987). An evaluation of family therapy in anorexia nervosa and bulimia nervosa. *Archives of General Psychiatry, 44*, 1047–1056.

Schmidt, U., Lee, S., Beecham, J. Perkins, S., Treasure, J., Yi, I., et al. (2007). A randomized controlled trial of family therapy and cognitive behavior therapy self care for adolescents with bulimia nervosa and related disorders. *American Journal of Psychiatry, 164*, 591–598.

Schmidt, U., Lee, S., Perkins, S., Eisler, I., Treasure, J., Beecham, J., et al. (2008). Do adolescents with eating disorder not otherwise specified or full-syndrome bulimia nervosa differ in clinical severity, comorbidity, risk factors, treatment outcome, or cost? *International Journal of Eating Disorders, 41*, 498–504.

Schoemaker, C. (1997). Does early intervention improve the prognosis in anorexia nervosa?: A systematic review of the treatment–outcome literature. *International Journal of Eating Disorders, 21*, 1–15.

Selman, R. L. (1980). *The growth of interpersonal understanding*. New York: Academic Press.

Sen, B. (2010). The relationship between frequency of family dinner and adolescent problem behaviors after adjusting for other family characteristics. *Journal of Adolescence, 33*, 187–196.

Stein, A., Woolley, H., Cooper, S., Winterbottom, J., Fairburn, C. G., & Cortina-Borja, M. (2006).Eating habits and attitudes among 10-year-old children of mothers with eating disorders: Longitudinal study. *British Journal of Psychiatry, 189*, 324–329.

Steinhausen, C. (2002). The outcome of anorexia nervosa in the 20th century. *American Journal of Psychiatry, 159*, 1284–1293.

Steinhausen, H. C., Rauss-Mason, C., & Seidel, R. (1991). Follow-up studies of anorexia nervosa: A review of four decades of outcome research. *Psychological Medicine, 21*, 447–454.

Stice, E., Marti, C. N., Shaw, H., & Jaconis, M. (2009). An 8-year longitudinal study of the natural history of threshold, subthreshold, and partial eating disorders from a community sample. *Journal of Abnormal Psychology, 118*, 587–597.

Stice, E., Marti, C. N., Spoor, S., Presnell, K., & Shaw, H. (2008). Dissonance and healthy weight eating disorder prevention program: Long term effects from a randomized efficacy trial. *Journal of Consulting and Clinical Psychology, 76*, 2.

Stice, E., Mazzoti, L., Weibel, D., & Agras, W. S. (2000). Dissonance prevention program decreases thin-ideal internalization, body dissatisfaction, dieting, negative affect, and bulimic symptoms. A preliminary experiment. *International Journal of Eating Disorders, 27*, 206–217.

Stice, E., Ng, J., & Shaw, H. (2010). Risk factors and prodromal eating pathology. *Journal of Child Psychology and Psychiatry, 51*, 518–525.

Stice, E., Trost, A., & Chase, A. (2003). Healthy weight control and dissonance-based eating disorder prevention programs: Results from a controlled trial. *International Journal of Eating Disorders, 33*, 10–21.

Stockmeier, C. A. (2003). Involvement of serotonin in depression: Evidence from postmortem and imaging studies of serotonin receptors and the serotonin transporter. *Journal of Psychiatric Research, 37*, 357–373.

Strauman, T., Vookles, J., Berenstien, V., Chaiken, S., & Higgins, T. (1991). Self-discrepancies and vulnerability to body dissatisfaction and disordered eating. *Journal of Personality and Social Psychology, 61*, 946–956.

Striegel-Moore, R. H., & Bulik, C. M. (2007). Risk factors for eating disorders. *American Psychologist, 62*, 181–198.

Striegel-Moore, R. H., Leslie, D., Petrill, S. A., Garvin, V., & Rosenheck, R. A. (2000). One-year use and cost of inpatient and outpatient services among female and male patients with an eating disorder: Evidence from a national database of health insurance claims. *International Journal of Eating Disorders, 27*, 381–389.

Striegel-Moore, R. H., Seeley, J. R., & Lewinsohn, P. M. (2003). Psychosocial adjustment in young adulthood of women who experienced an eating disorder during adolescence. *American Academy of Child and Adolescent Psychiatry, 42,* 587–593.

Sullivan, P. F. (1995). Mortality in anorexia nervosa. *American Journal of Psychiatry, 152,* 1073–1074.

Thompson, J., & Psaltis, K. (1988). Multiple aspects and correlates of body figure ratings: A replication and extension of Fallon and Rozin (1985). *International Journal of Eating Disorders, 7,* 813–817.

Thompson, J. K., & Stice, E. (2001). Thin ideal internalization: Mounting evidence for a new risk factor for body image disturbance and eating pathology. *Current Directions in Psychological Science, 10,* 181–184.

Tiggemann, M. (1992). Body-size dissatisfaction: Individual differences in age and gender, and relationship with self-esteem. *Personality and Individual Differences, 13,* 39–43.

Treasure, J., Murphy, T., Szmukler, T., Todd, G., Gavan, K., & Joyce, J. (2001). The experience of caregiving for severe mental illness: A comparison between anorexia nervosa and psychosis. *Social Psychiatry and Psychiatric Epidemiology, 36,* 343–347.

Vander Wal, J. S., Gibbons, J. L., & del Pilar Grazioso, M. (2007). The sociocultural model of eating disorder development: Application to a Guatemalan sample. *Eating Behaviors, 9,* 277–284.

Van Son, G. E., van Hoeken, D., van Furth, E. F., Donker, G. A., & Hoek, H. W. (2010). Course and outcome of eating disorders in a primary care-based cohort. *International Journal of Eating Disorders, 43,* 130–138.

Wentz, E., Gillberg, C., Gillberg, I., & Rastam, M. (2001). Ten-year follow up of adolescent-onset anorexia nervosa: Psychiatric disorders and overall functioning scales. *Journal of Child Psychology and Psychiatry, 42,* 613–622.

Wentz, E., Gillberg, I. C., Anckarsäter, H., Gillberg, C., & Rastam, M. (2009). Adolescent-onset anorexia nervosa: 18-year outcome. *British Journal of Psychiatry, 194,* 168–174.

Winn, S., Perkins, S., Murray, J., Murphy, R., & Schmidt, U. (2004). A qualitative study of the experience of caring for a person with bulimia nervosa. Part 2: Carers' needs and experiences of services and other support. *International Journal of Eating Disorders, 36,* 269–279.

Yager, J., Landsverk, J., & Edelstein, C. K. (1987). A 20-month follow-up study of 628 women with eating disorders: Course and severity. *American Journal of Psychiatry, 144,* 1172–1177.

Zarbatany, L., Hartmann, D., & Rankin, D. (1990). The psychological functions of preadolescent peer activities. *Child Development, 61,* 1067–1080.

Zipfel, S., Löwe, B., Reas, D. L., Deter, H. C., & Herzog, W. (2000). Long-term prognosis in anorexia nervosa: Lessons from a 21-year follow-up study. *Lancet, 355,* 721–722.

CHAPTER 19

Parent Groups in the Treatment of Eating Disorders

Nancy L. Zucker
Katharine L. Loeb
Sheetal Patel
Autumn Shafer

P arents of children with eating disorders are burdened with a range of difficulties related to the management of their child's disorder (Treasure et al., 2001). In fact, the unique challenges faced by these parents distinguish their experience from that of parents of children with other disorders. For instance, the child has a potentially life-threatening illness, there is a known and 100% effective "cure" for the dangerous effects of the illness due to malnutrition, behaviors of the child perpetuate this illness, and the child often refuses or refutes the treatment plan necessary for survival. Yet, burgeoning evidence supports the importance of involving parents to facilitate successful treatment of eating disorders (Berkman et al., 2006; Lock, Agras, Bryson, & Kraemer, 2005; Lock & Le Grange, 2005). Finding ways to maximize the utility of parents, improve their mental health, and reduce caregiver stress is essential if researchers and clinicians are to address the psychological and economic costs of treatments. This chapter reviews the use of parent groups and other forms of parent support in the treatment of eating disorders. In addition, we outline the development of a health communication program designed to improve parent willingness to obtain the support they need. The word *parent* is used here to signify any adult who is responsible for caring for the child or adolescent with an eating disorder, regardless of whether he or she is a biological parent, legal guardian, extended family member, or another individual.

Rationale for Parent Support

Parents of children with eating disorders (hereafter "parents") face unique challenges that augment their burden. As highlighted by Schmidt and Treasure (2006), stigma, or fear of stigma, about eating disorders may increase a parent's social isolation at a time when he or she is most in need of interpersonal support. In fact, the stigma associated with caring for someone with an eating disorder is likely a contributing factor to the finding that these parents experience greater subjective burden relative to parents of children with other severe psychiatric disorders such as psychosis (Treasure et al.,2001). Indeed, lay misconceptualizations about the nature or seriousness of eating disorders (Holliday, Wall, Treasure, & Weinman, 2005), biased reporting of eating disorders in the entertainment sections of periodicals, rather than in science or health sections (O'Hara & Smith, 2007), and perhaps the ability of children with eating disorders to push themselves through profound levels of impairment to maintain relative success in domains other than health (e.g., academics, sports), obscures the severity of these disorders, leaving parents vulnerable to stigmatizing attitudes about the nature and danger of their experience. Furthermore, unlike severe medical conditions such as cancer or chronic conditions such as type 1 diabetes, eating disorders are often attributed to familial psychopathology and dysfunctional parenting, leading to significant blame (Schmidt & Treasure, 2006). In fact, the early historical literature describing families with a child with an eating disorder was notable for the responsibility given to family dynamics, and maladaptive emotional and behavioral control by parents, for the emergence of the disorder (Pearce, 2004). Although such beliefs have dramatically changed among researchers and providers of eating disorder treatment, the legacy of such sentiments among the general populace is continued stigma and a tendency to blame parents for causing these disorders.

There is often great misunderstanding about the nature of eating disorders among parents as well. Repeated themes of nonacceptance of the child's illness and intimations that eating disorder symptoms are attempts to manipulate and control others are often found in qualitative and quantitative studies of caregivers' burden in regard to these disorders (de la Rie, Noordenbos, & van Furth, 2005; Treasure et al., 2001; Whitney et al., 2005). Such descriptions indicate a failure of the research and clinical community to better educate the public about the nature of eating disorders and highlight needed domains of education for parents and other family members.

The logistical efforts required to manage an eating disorder can tax any family system. The physical and emotional requirements needed to care for someone with an eating disorder likely interferes with other important parental responsibilities (e.g., care of other children, social and recreational activities, care of themselves). However, distress related to the illness goes beyond these logistical constraints. To nourish their child, parents often establish a hospital-like environment in the home, supervising every meal. Many parents may oversee school lunches, as the child's urge to engage in restrictive or purgative behaviors may be too difficult for the child to resist without supervision. Furthermore, children with eating disorders often refuse to "take their medicine," which can result in constant, daily conflict about adherence to nutritional and exercise prescriptions. Such conflict, time demands, and knowledge of the dangerous consequences of nonadherence to nutritional prescriptions impose significant psychological duress on parents.

It may also be difficult for parents to synthesize the conflicting aspects of the emotional and behavioral performance of their child: simultaneously putting forth excessive effort to complete homework assignments, excelling at sports performances, and yet, not sufficiently capable to sustain health. It is understandable that eating disorder behaviors are sometimes perceived to be "oppositional," when parents are not educated in how eating-disordered thinking and behaviors, compounded by the effects of starvation, affect emotion, cognition, and social relationships and augments behavioral rigidity (Keys, 1950). With education about these effects of eating disorders on their children, these seemingly divergent behavioral performances can be quite understandable to parents. Both behavioral patterns reflect rigid perseveration of premorbid tendencies (i.e., achievement-striving and food restriction), patterns that become exacerbated by starvation.

It is also understandable that parents of a child with an eating disorder are sometimes challenged to maintain their own emotional equilibrium and mental health. Some studies suggest that regardless of the biological contributions that increase vulnerability to the onset of a disorder, eating disorders may emerge during times of increased stress (Ruggiero et al., 2008)—stress that may have enveloped the entire family, leaving parents equally vulnerable to stress-related psychopathology. The timing of mental health issues in the caregiver relative to illness onset in the child is unclear. However, regardless of etiology, caregivers report that mental health symptoms significantly impact their quality of life when referenced relative to population norms (de la Rie, Van Furth, De Koning, Noordenbos, & Donker, 2005). There are numerous reports of family histories of psychopathology (Kaye et al., 1996; Lilenfeld et al., 1998; Stein et al., 1999), and hence vulnerability to cope ineffectively with severe life stressors such as the illness of a child. To be sure, family-based treatments have had a remarkable impact on the prognosis of adolescent eating disorders, and the information provided via these treatment modalities tends to decrease burden. Yet, such treatments demand a lot of parents. Developing services to support parents may maximize treatment effectiveness and minimize treatment burden.

Forms of Group-Based Treatment

Before discussing the various modalities that have been used to assist parents, we give a brief description of the formats often used to provide these interventions.

Support Groups

The term "support group" is broadly used to encapsulate an array of group-based treatments. Here support groups are those groups in which the group leader is not a trained health care professional, but rather an individual who has struggled or is still struggling (directly or as caregiver) with the disorder that is the focus of the group. The stated purpose of these groups can vary widely, such as to serve a strictly supportive function for individuals engaged in more structured therapy or, for some, to serve as sole source of treatment. Although any group in which people are gathered together for a common purpose is supportive, these groups are usually distinguished by making *support* the stated purpose of the group. Group members share experiences and use prior experiences to provide advice to other individuals in similar circumstances. Given that a standard psychological treatment often lasts one hour per week, and that individuals struggling with mental health problems must frequently battle persistent urges to engage in maladaptive behaviors, these groups can theoretically provide value by maintaining behavior changes (Kaskutas, Subbaraman, Witbrodt, & Zemore, 2009). In the case of such groups for caregivers, the analogous value may be in helping maintain the stamina needed to support the ill relative.

Group Psychoeducation

Group psychoeducation is usually conducted like a seminar. Often led by health care professionals, such groups are intended to provide *information*. Although there may be opportunity for questions related to the content being discussed, there is not a focus on the exchange of personal narratives as found in more support-based formats.

Skills Groups

Skills groups use a combination of supportive and psychoeducation formats. Unlike psychoeducation groups, in which the composition of the audience may vary greatly from lecture to lecture, skills groups are often conducted like any manualized or structured treatment in that a specific cohort of individuals are expected to attend the group for a prescribed period of time. Although relationships usually develop among participants as individuals share an emotionally evocative experience (the treatment of their child's disorder), this is not the overt purpose; instead, the purpose is often the dissemination of information regarding management of the disorder. Nevertheless, such groups often have the added benefit of facilitating adherence to a treatment plan as there is accountability inherent in the need to report progress to the group. Unlike psychoeducation seminars, which may include the entire family, parent skills groups usually include only parents.

Family-Based Groups

Family-based groups involve the entire family in a group format, combining education with experiential activities as if a family were participating in family therapy, but in the company of other families undergoing similar experiences. This group can thus be considered a combination of the other modalities described earlier, with the added benefit that each family may also learn by directly observing other families , who can serve as positive role models or provide opportunities for mirroring behavior that a particular family seeks to change (Dare & Eisler, 2000).

Peer Mentors

A model related to family-based groups found, for example, in treatment models for addiction, is the use of peer mentors, or "sponsors" (Kaskutas, 2009). These individuals are considered senior in terms of experience and prior success in managing symptoms and thus offer advice and availability to help individuals new to the treatment process to maintain sobriety or other desired treatment outcomes. Such mentors potentially extend the impact of group meetings by providing coaching and support outside the group meeting context.

Group-Based Curricula

There are common themes among the topics discussed across the various intervention formats. For instance, a frequent topic is education regarding the biological nature of eating disorders and the related impact of starvation on cognition and behavior (Geist, Heinmaa, Stephens, Davis, & Katzman, 2000; Uehara, Kawashima, Goto, Tasaki, & Someya, 2001). Parents learn that biological changes associated with starvation may augment long-standing trait features in their child (e.g., starvation potentiates and exacerbates premorbid behavioral and cognitive rigidity in the child). Consider a typical experience of a parent of a child with anorexia nervosa (AN). The child breaks the food into tiny pieces, chews incredibly slowly, and makes a typical 30-minute meal last for hours. Imagine the different experience of a parent knowing that this is a biological adaptation to starvation: her starving child is attempting to ration food rather than displaying stubbornness or defiance (Uehara et al., 2001).

The importance of communicating such information may have prognostic significance. There is preliminary evidence that psychoeducation groups may decrease expressed emotion in parents (Uehara et al., 2001). Expressed emotion was originally operationalized in the context of families with a child diagnosed with schizophrenia as the number of critical comments a parent made about his or her child when interviewed alone (Vaughn & Leff, 1976). In the context of eating disorders, families with increases in expressed emotion have poorer outcomes in family-based treatments in which members of the whole family are seen together (Eisler et al., 2000; Eisler, Simic, Russell, & Dare, 2007) and are more likely to drop out of treatment (Szmukler, Eisler, Russell, & Dare, 1985). Such findings highlight the imperative need for education regarding the nature of eating disorders and, in turn, the putative value of psychoeducation approaches (see the sample curricula that follow for further discussion of expressed emotion).

The educational content of group-based curricula often encompasses both illness-specific information as well as general knowledge about adolescent development. Parents often feel stymied by the timing of their child's eating disorder. During a developmental window in which their child is supposed to be attaining increased autonomy in opinions, preferences, and so forth, parents are faced with the conflicting challenge of restricting autonomy and narrowing options in the service of managing their child's illness. Parents require information about how managing an eating disorder fits into this developmental context. Related issues include nutrition and the related nutritional needs of developing adolescents, adolescent growth, the multidetermined etiology of eating disorders, the multidetermined nature of eating disorders, the medical and psychological sequelae of eating disorders, the multidetermined nature of body image and self-esteem, and relapse prevention. Although not established empirically, content depicting the complexity of the onset and maintenance of a disorder has potential to decrease an oft-cited theme in qualitative research with caregivers, namely guilt about their roles in contributing to the disorder's development.

Process issues such as communication are also common topics in a psychoeducation curriculum. There is usually a need for parents to understand patterns of interaction between family members and others who may inadvertently reinforce eating disorder symptoms (e.g., spending time with the adolescent only during mealtimes and not at other times). As articulated by Schmidt and Treasure (2006), AN is a visually provocative disorder. The sight of the emaciated frame of one's child would test any parent's capacity to regulate her or his emotions, and when paired with seemingly defiant food refusal can result in the protective tendencies of any parent to defend the life of the child at any cost. Of course, the irresolvable dilemma for parents is that both the perpetrator and the victim is their child, and the resulting competing urges to defend and attack immobilizes the most competent of caregivers. Added to this dilemma is that symptoms of disordered eating may be negatively reinforced as they reduce anxiety and numb emotional experience (Wildes, Ringham, & Marcus, 2010). Thus, symptoms may be exacerbated when parents most need them not to be—when the family system is stressed. Alerting families to these processes by presenting educational topics pertaining to starvation and behavior management can make what otherwise might seem like manipulative behavior understandable as a learned adaptation to increased stress and facilitate adaptive communication.

Furthermore, it is helpful for parents to understand the experience of their children with eating disorders so they can appreciate the conflicting motivations that complicate their treatment. Several curricula described in the literature include discussions about the transtheoretical model of change (Geist et al., 2000; Wilson & Schlam, 2004). This model stages the experiential processes of change so parents can better adapt their mode of responding to match the state of their child. For example, *precontemplation* is a state in which the child questions whether she or he warrants an eating disorder diagnosis, despite robust clinical indicators. Helping parents understand that such appraisals are both a function of poor risk appraisal due to the child's stage of cognitive development, and part of the presentation of the illness, can assist parents in proceeding with illness management—even though their child does not acknowledge the presence of a problem. In addition, complex etiological factors that lead to the eating disorder pathology (e.g., temperamental factors, such as elevation in neuroticism; Bulik et al., 2006), differ in important respects from the diverse factors that maintain eating disorders (e.g., increased attention from parents related to illness management; Schmidt & Treasure, 2006). Helping parents distinguish etiological factors and maintaining factors may not only decrease the burden of caregivers by relieving them of guilt and responsibility, but may also increase the effectiveness of their management of the disorder by helping them focus on the things they can change (i.e., maintaining factors).

While psychoeducational groups are used widely, there is little systematic evidence of their effectiveness. Still, some components of psychoeducational group interventions are part of most empirically supported treatments for eating disorders (Garner, Rockert, Olmsted, Johnson, & Coscina, 1985). In addition, consumers demand to know more about the illnesses and the treatments for eating disorders. This is especially the case as parents are seen as critical components of treatment. Parents' need for information has been undeniable, as evidenced by the rapid increase in websites and lay publications devoted to this topic (an approximately 10-fold increase since 1989, when there was only one book specifically addressing the psychoeducational need of parents; Siegel, Brisman, & Weinshel, 1989). Despite the increased use of psychoeducation for parents with children who have eating disorders, little specific research has been conducted to identify the best approach. New research should focus on determining the most efficacious manner to educate and support parents. At this point, the case examples described in the following sections provide the best available evidence about how to conduct psychoeducation groups for parents.

Psychoeducation Groups

A prototypical intervention is described by Holtkamp, Herpertz-Dahlmann, Vloet, and Hagenah (2005), who report on a five-session program delivered to family members whose adolescent child was in either inpatient or outpatient specialized treatment for an eating disorder. The group was described to parents as neither self-help nor therapy but rather as a vehicle to communicate information, a format that was reinforced by having highly structured initial sessions, with questions regarding individual family challenges deferred to individual therapy sessions. The remaining sessions were more permissive in terms of questions and answers. The intervention was highly regarded by parents, with

98% willing to recommend it to other parents and 88% perceiving the group as helpful in coping with their child's illness.

Support Groups

Pasold, Boateng, and Portilla (2010) noted that makeshift parent support groups develop in the waiting rooms of their specialized eating disorders programs. While waiting for their child, parents exchanged tips and personal narratives about the management of their children's illness. The researchers organized an ongoing weekly support group in which all individuals concerned about the person with an eating disorder could attend (e.g., friends of the family, siblings, grandparents). The group was supervised by health professionals in the program; however, the agenda was dictated by the needs of the group members. Researchers obtained a 21% response rate to a mailed survey of program satisfaction. Mean satisfaction ratings of the parent group ranged from 4.51 (±.70) to 4.67 (±.70) on a 5-point Likert scale on ratings of illness knowledge, helpful information from other parents, understanding the complexity of eating disorders, and general helpfulness. Finally, the authors noted that participation in the parent group was positively correlated with treatment satisfaction ($r = .50$, $p < .01$). Whether parent groups can facilitate the retention of families in treatment for their child's eating disorder is an area in need of inquiry.

Combined Education and Therapy Groups

Whereas education can certainly have therapeutic effects, other group models are explicit in their therapeutic focus.

Uehara and colleagues (2001) describe a combination psychoeducation/multifamily group designed specifically to *decrease expressed emotion in families*. As introduced earlier, expressed emotion is one of the few robust prognostic indicators in a family of a child with an eating disorder (Eisler et al., 2007; Szmukler et al., 1985). In a seminal investigation of family-based treatment for AN, families described as having elevations in expressed emotion had better treatment outcomes in separated versus combined family therapy (i.e., parents seen separately from the child; Eisler et al., 2007).

Expressed emotion is a multifaceted construct containing components of critical comments about the child, emotional overinvolvement (expressions of self-sacrifice or overt emotional displays), and hostility (van Furth et al., 1996). This construct is not unique to families of children with eating disorders. Expressed emotion has prognostic significance across a variety of psychiatric disorders, including schizophrenia, the disorder for which the construct was first operationalized (Vaughn & Leff, 1976), and mood disorders (Butzlaff & Hooley, 1998). In fact, the malignancy of this feature in predicting outcome is rather unique in psychiatry where the search for variables that can assist in tailoring treatments is challenging (Butzlaff & Hooley, 1998). Yet, despite the predictive validity of this feature, the essence of the construct of expressed emotion is poorly specified and may relate to a variety of deficits in emotional functioning and social cognition. Zucker and colleagues (2007) posit that elevations in expressed emotion reflect deficits in empathic capacities (e.g., relative inability of parents to take on the perspective of their child), irrespective of the parents' love and strong motivation to help their child. Thus, information may be a key strategy in assisting with expressed emotion as it helps parents appreciate the complex etiological and maintenance factors that complicate the course of an illness.

To address this feature, Uehara and colleagues (2001) combined 1 hour of psychoeducation with an hour of family discussion. These researchers described changes in family members' perceptions of their child's illness following a five-session protocol conducted over 5 months. Using the Five-Minute Speech sample and the Family Adaptability and Cohesion Measure of family function, Uehara and colleagues described significant changes in the proportion of 28 families rated as high in expressed emotion as well as positive changes in family cohesion and adaptability. Notably, the child was admitted to a comprehensive and specialized inpatient eating disorder program, making it unclear whether changes in parental attitudes were due to the intervention or to clinical signs of improvement in the child. Nonetheless, such findings highlight that it is feasible to target expressed emotion.

Geist and colleagues (2000) examined the efficacy of a multifamily group (MFG) therapy as compared with a generic form of family therapy. The authors postulated that MFG because of the group format, would be more *cost-effective*. Twenty-five families were randomized to receive eight sessions of either family therapy or MFG during the adolescent's inpatient hospitalization for eating disorder treatment. In this MFG model, psychoeduation was provided for 45 minutes, and adolescents and parents broke into separate groups during the second 45 minutes to discuss the information presented. Between-group comparisons demonstrated a main effect of time, but no effect of group by time. The researchers concluded the small sample size precluded sensitivity to detect between-group differences and no change in psychological measures of the adolescent was reported. Given insufficient power to detect group differences (15–30% in most analyses), it is difficult to assert that MFG is a more cost-effective alternative to family therapy. However, it is notable that the degree of weight gain between the two groups was of similar effect and was maintained for 4 months posttreatment, with equivalent lengths of stay. Such findings justify further investigation of the viability of MFG approaches to treatment.

In fact, Dare and Eisler (2000) have designed an MFG to be delivered on an outpatient basis (see Fairbairn, Simic, & Eisler, Chapter 13, this volume). Their model combines the intensity of a day hospitalization program with an MFG format. The dosage is gradually diluted, beginning with a 4-day program (8 hours per day), a 1-day program one week later, and a 1-day program 1 month later. Half-day programs are scheduled at 4-week and 6-week intervals. Between the initial move from the weekly to once-monthly frequency, individual family sessions may be scheduled. Although Dare and Eisler do not delineate specific criteria to warrant admission to this model, they require all inpatients to participate and, intriguingly, have families who have failed to make progress in outpatient family therapy attend.

The program itself combines strategies from a variety of therapeutic models. Parents also learn via role-modeling by other parents, by witnessing the interactions of other families, and by engaging in behavioral strategies such a role plays. For example, the families engage in an exercise designed to enhance *theory of mind*, the ability to take on the perspective of another person. In this exercise, a child with AN designs a meal for her or his "child" with AN and feeds this meal to her or his parent (i.e., the "child"). The treatment is organized around three emphases: (1) learning or discovering ways in which to manage symptoms, (2) helping the adolescent child build the life she or he desires, while respecting family values and traditions, and (3) emphasizing change, that is, parental involvement as a temporary solution.

Although data for this approach remain limited, the authors note several surprising findings, based on a combination of qualitative observation and quantitative surveys. First, in contrast to their experiences with family therapy, the authors report via case examples that families were enthusiastic about the model. The authors posit that this may be due to reductions in shame and guilt, given the opportunity to witness other families undergoing similar experiences. Such a sense of community may have extended to the adolescents, as the authors express surprise at the extent to which the adolescents supported each other throughout the intervention. Finally, the authors note the positive experience of the health professional delivering the treatment. In a clinical population marked by high therapist burnout, the positive experience of working with multiple families in a very intense and evocative therapeutic experience is a qualitative outcome deserving further exploration. Future work in this area requires the investigation of pragmatic ways in which to explore this model.

Leichner, Hall, and Calderon (2005) describe the use of a manualized program and video used to help parents with the task of *meal support* to facilitate discharge from an inpatient program for eating disorders. The program emphasized family process as opposed to behavioral management per se. Parents were guided in fostering a collaborative relationship with their child to ensure successful nourishment. The program demonstrated face acceptability and feasibility, but data as to its effectiveness in improving eating and promoting weight gain have not been reported.

Parent Skills Groups in Adolescent Eating Disorder Treatment

Modeling group format after the structure of parent skills groups that have been utilized for the treatment of attention-deficit/hyperactivity disorder, Zucker and colleagues have developed a group parent-training program (GPT) designed to treat adolescent AN. The content of this model is influenced by extant models of cognitive-behavioral and emotion-focused therapies (Greenberg & Paivio, 2003; Linehan, 1993). Not only is this treatment model designed to help parents manage their child's eating disorder symptoms, but the intervention was also created to address trait modes of responding in the child and parent that may increase vulnerability to symptom relapse. Broadly, this treatment is designed to enhance adaptive self-regulation in adolescents diagnosed with AN by using parents as role models of responsivity to their own basic biological needs and being mindful of their emotional experience to decipher the intrapersonal and interpersonal needs and guide adaptive behavior. We reasoned that adolescents would not be motivated to change maladaptive patterns of self-regulation if their parents were not also willing to change such patterns in themselves (e.g., neglecting basic needs to achieve performance deadlines, modeling extreme self-loathing in response to error, etc.). In the sections that follow, we describe the theoretical model that guided the development of this intervention and delineate the core skills that serve as the bedrock of all intervention content.

Theoretical Model Guiding Intervention Content in GPT

Responsive parenting may be a pivotal construct to guide the development of eating disorder interventions. Propper and Moore (2006) define responsive parenting in relation to caregiver behaviors that may influence infant emotionality: "Caregivers facilitate the establishment of physiological homeostasis as they assist in attaining a balance between endogenous needs and exogenous stimuli" (p. 435). Although this parenting style is usually considered in the classical context of parenting (i.e., between a parent and child), we co-opt this definition to consider and teach the construct of "self-parenting," the capacity to be attuned and adaptively responsive to one's own emotional and related motivational drives (e.g., hunger, fatigue, fear). To be sure, whatever the complex array and combination of influences that impact the emergence of AN, in essence, individuals with AN have failed to incorporate the task of responsively "parenting" themselves, they neglect many basic needs (e.g., basic sustenance, need for rest, social and familial relationships, or the motivations expressed by emotional experience—such as the need to seek nurturance when in a depressed mood). Instead, they are at war with their bodies by trying to manipulate and control what should be a seamless connection between bodily needs and adaptive response.

Using this approach, parents aim to teach their children to be their own "self-parents" by using themselves as examples. Parents attempt to attune deliberately to their own emotional experiences at the same time they are validating the emotional experiences of their children. As they do so, they very concretely teach the very abstract notion of responsive parenting, much like the "motherese" of parents of toddlers who try to label their own emotional experiences so that their children learn emotional descriptors for the complex motivated states that constitute affective experience. Parents learn to know their children, in part, via pattern recognition: by repeatedly deciphering and associating their affective signals and nonverbal gestures in certain contexts and following certain events (e.g., when Jamie cries like that, it means that she is tired, when she whimpers like that, she needs to be held). It is not unreasonable to assume that the same process happens with the development of "self-parenting"—attunement and response help to develop a sense of identity, the "I" who is needing something. AN has long been conceptualized as a disorder of the self, and thus the construct of "self-parenting" and related constructs such as "self-compassion" warrant further exploration in the treatment of AN.

Core Skill: Emotion Regulation in GPT

The elaboration of emotional experience and the development of emotion regulatory skills assist parents in disorder management and may enhance adaptive self-regulation in themselves more generally. Given prior work on the maladaptive effects of expressed emotion on eating disorder management (see the earlier section "Group Curricula"), a core skill in GPT is helping parents become more adept at perceiving, deciphering, and utilizing emotional experience in the service of goal-directed actions rather than merely reacting to intense emotions (Lewinsohn, Sullivan, & Grosscup, 1980). For example, a parent may notice he is too angry to think clearly, goes outside to clear his head and lower his emotional intensity, and then returns to the dinner table to help his child (vs. the same dad feeling angry and immediately expressing his rage via verbal explicatives).

Capitalizing on topographies of emotion that categorize affect based on arousal and valence, we provide parents with a simplified framework for organizing their emotional experience (e.g., depression—low arousal, negative valence; anxiety—high arousal, negative valence) (Brosch, Pourtois, & Sander, 2010; Rainville, Bechara, Naqvi, & Damasio, 2006; Zachar, 2010). We use the metaphor of a wave to help parents identity their current level of emotional arousal (i.e., being on "top of the wave" is the peak period of emotional intensity). The wave metaphor also helps to illustrate the interplay between the intensity of affective experience and access to cognitively mediated actions (i.e., the more intense our feelings, the more challenging it is to think things through rationally; see Figure 19.1). When parents cross the "logic line," the ability to consider solutions rationally may be compromised. The choice of regulatory strategy should thus match their level of emotional intensity (e.g., blaring loud music and taking a hot shower may be more appropriate when on "top of the wave"). Thus, parents are first taught to position themselves on the wave so that they become adept at recognizing their levels of emotional intensity. This emotion-focused work, in particular, is heavily influenced by the theoretical writings and intervention strategies of Linehan (1993) and Greenberg and Paivio (2003).

The next stage is to use emotions to facilitate goal-directed actions—not to interfere with them. Thus, parents match their choice of emotion regulatory strategy to their level of subjective emotional intensity so that actions are guided by the integration of rational thought and emotional experience rather than by cold rationality or sheer passion (see Figure 19.2).

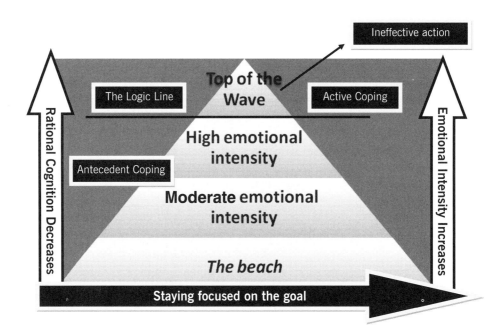

FIGURE 19.1. Illustration of the concept of the "emotional wave" introduced in GPT. In Phase 1, parents work on not allowing their level of emotional arousal to interfere with the achievement of their intended goal (e.g., nourishing their child). They can use preemptive strategies when they notice their level of emotional arousal begin to increase. However, once emotional intensity increases, the use of strategies that are more cognitive (e.g., rationalization) may be less effective than more visceral strategies that change the experience of the body (e.g., hot shower, deep breathing). If parents were to go with the behavioral urges associated with their emotional experience, they may meet their goal, but ineffectively (e.g., nourishing their child with heightened expressed emotion). Rather, they must "actively cope" by inhibiting their action urge in the service of a more adaptive manner in which to achieve the goal.

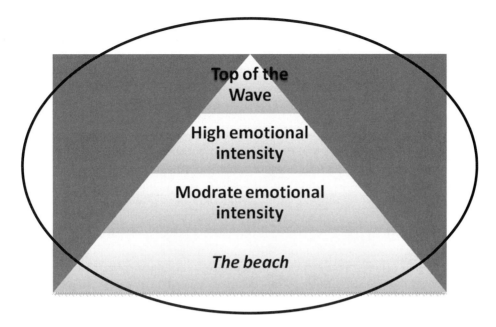

FIGURE 19.2. After the goal has been achieved, the message communicated by the emotion is considered as resulting in enhanced self-knowledge, self-trust (via "self-parenting" construct) and future learning. In Phase 3, parents guide their children in the use of emotion regulatory strategies and to reflect on the motivational salience of their emotional experience.

Imagine a father exhausted after a day of work. He arrives home angry because of situations at work and is concerned about the financial well-being of his family because, in part, of the expensive health care costs of his child's eating disorder. He sits down to dinner and his son with AN is struggling to finish his meal and refuses his parents' requests to increase his intake. The father's anger progresses to rage. He is poised to try to force his child to eat as that is the seemingly shortest path to head off the danger his malnutrition is signaling. If his partner were to try to "reason with him" about his son's struggles, the father may not have access to reasoning skills for such strategies to benefit him. Rather, if his partner were to suggest a strategy that targeted the somatic concomitants of emotional arousal, that may be more effective. For instance, the partner could suggest: "We're all tense right now. Let's go sit on the porch for a few moments, take some deep breaths, and start this meal over." The family members could then regain a sense of calm and reapproach the situation that challenged them.

Once parents are adept at identifying their own emotional intensity and gently guiding their emotional experience in the service of goal-directed actions, they are directly helping their children achieve these same skills via their example. Furthermore, parents learn to gently guide their children in the use of emotion regulatory strategies, much as they would hug a toddler having an emotional outburst to help him calm down.

A child with an eating disorder is extremely agitated, shouting, "I hate myself, I hate myself! I am so fat and you are making me fat!" while scratching her skin and sobbing. The parent knows her child is "on the wave" and thus any verbal strategy would be ineffective. Rather, the parent focuses on the child's bodily experiences and wants to soothe her child via somatosensory stimulation. The parent gives the child a strong hug—which the child initially pushes away from, but the parent persists—symbolically helping the child fight the disorder, and gently rocks the child as the child continues to sob and then to collapse, reminiscent of the parent's experience of temper tantrums of the child as a toddler.

Finally, parents help their children learn about how eating disorder symptoms facilitate emotional avoidance. To paraphrase, "When the eating disorder is loud, emotions are strong." Thus, rather than focusing on symptoms and getting lost in content related to eating disorder pathology, parents first recognize the emotion–eating disorder symptom connection and join with their child (rather than merely telling their child what to do), guiding her or him in the use of strategies to help the child reengage in goal-directed action ("We're both upset; let's go sit on the porch, get some fresh air, and clear our heads"). Later, after the emotional intensity of the moment has passed and illness management has proceeded, there is an opportunity for the parent to make the symptom–emotion link for the child. "Your eating disorder was really giving you are hard time today. Did something happen that you would like to talk about?" By making affective experience something that can be observed and labeled, we attempt to take away the fear of emotions in both the parents themselves and as they observe affective intensity in their child (see Figure 19.2).

Core Skill: Self-Awareness ("Responsive Self-Parenting")

Emotions are not just something to be endured, however. Rather, affective experience provides vital information about the motivational state of an individual at the moment. According to some theorists, the physiological reactivity (e.g., pounding heart), urge for action, and mood-congruent cognition that accompany emotional experience signal basic motivational drives (e.g., to approach, to avoid) (Bradley & Lang, 2007). Failing to acknowledge such a state is to avoid an opportunity to broaden self-knowledge. Ideally, there is a back-and-forth "dance with oneself": an individual explores internal experiences, deciphering, integrating, or responding to the motivated states of emotional experience; the body responds with pain, pleasure, satiety. These transactions serve as critical content for the formation of self-knowledge ("I learn when this experience happens, I feel this way in my body and I interpret that to mean this."). Thus, after parents and their child "surf" the wave, they are instructed to investigate the situations that led to the intensified affect (Figure 19.2) so that the experience can be used to learn more about themselves (their needs, preferences, etc). Emotions are framed as a curiosity, a useful tool by which individuals can become fully connected and not afraid of their internal experiences. Via the back-and-forth trial and error learning of deciphering and attuning to emotional experience, an individual becomes self-aware and attuned: a potential antithesis to the physiological muting of the starvation of AN.

Core Skill: Mindful Elaboration of Experience ("Process versus Outcome")

The extreme striving for achievement (or "outcome focus") of individuals with eating disorders may prevent flexible responding and optimal learning. The "process versus outcome" philosophy that guides GPT was designed to helped parents strike a balance between using high performance standards to choose their direction, but to be mindful enough of unfolding present moment experiences that they learn from each step along the path, and become flexible enough to choose a "side road" if new learning highlights the more optimal nature of this new route. This framework was designed to serve as an antithesis to the relentless drive of those with AN, in which basic needs are sacrificed in the service of rigid performance standards (Zucker, Herzog, Moskovich, Merwin, & Linn, 2011). By role-modeling the value of trial and error learning, the intention is to address anhedonia and perfectionism in both parents and child (Slade & Owens, 1998; Zucker et al., 2011).

For many with AN, self-worth is defined concretely on the basis of performance parameters ("I am worthy because I achieved such and so"). Such an unrealistic belief system was reasoned to make the engagement in activities negatively reinforced. In other words, a focus on outcomes diminishes the pleasure of ongoing mastery. Instead, activities are undertaken to avoid guilt, not to achieve pleasure. Such a biased focus on outcomes makes the experience of activities less rewarding, both because they are not being fully attended to in the moment and because there is a looming potential threat of failure (Owens & Slade, 2008). Instead, we shift the focus to the value of learning. Inasmuch as the most optimal learning happens when mistakes are made, mistakes become something to look "forward" to: opportunities for new learning. Thus, mistakes also are curiosities, chances to expand one's skill of observation to all that is unfolding in the present moment so that optimal learning can unfold. Learning replaces achievement as the compass that guides the path. As learning is never done, the endless path is intended to become an exciting adventure, not the hopelessness of perfectionism indicative that no effort is ever enough.

Core Skill: Self-Care

When parents perform the behavior they wish to see their child perform, they potently communicate the importance of that behavior. "Do as I say, not as I do" does not work well for adolescents, whose increasingly maturing cognitive capacities enhance their abilities to critically reason and thus judge the authenticity of parental requests. For an adolescent, adults symbolize what they will experience in the future. Given the mixed motivations for treatment in those with AN, powerful motivators are required for them to be willing to forgo their symptoms and face the challenges of adolescent maturation and, eventually, adulthood. Role-modeling by parents is a powerful vehicle to influence changes in behavior irrespective of the child's motivation for treatment.

Unfortunately, achievement-striving parents often role-model self-neglect. Although parents can readily recognize the dangerous effects of the relentless striving characteristic of their child on her or his health, they may be less aware of the chronic impact of sleep deprivation, skipped meals, lack of balance between leisure and work, et cetera, on their own mental health and, ultimately, productivity. To address this neglect, in GPT, parents set a weekly self-care goal, a deliberate, planned activity they engage in as a symbolic kind gesture toward themselves that has no intended purpose but the enjoyment of that moment in time. Children observe this change in the behavior of parents in relation to their own well-being and the greater balance they are achieving between leisure and work, and perhaps the thought of becoming an adult is then not as scary.

> For his self-care homework, an overworked father made a pact to come home in time for dinner 3 nights per week to join the family and to not read e-mail on Sundays.

Logistics of GPT

The parent skills group meets weekly in approximately 90-minute sessions for 20 weeks. There are entry points for new group members every 4 weeks, when the core skill of the emotional wave is reviewed. Parents design a personalized homework assignment each week in which they focus on four key areas:

1. An unhealthy symptom in their child and a related behavioral management plan to address that symptom (e.g., not eating enough food; plan: monitor breakfast and have child come home for lunch).
2. A healthy coping strategy that will be increased in the child (e.g., expression of negative emotions; plan: when parents notice eating disorder symptoms are loud, ask child if anything is wrong—don't just focus on symptoms).
3. A healthy coping strategy that parents will work on role-modeling (e.g., parent being dishonest about feelings for fear of upsetting her or his child; plan: parent will role model greater honesty about feelings).
4. Self-care (e.g., parents not spending enough time together; plan: parents will go on a date).

The group begins with the review of homework, with an emphasis on what did not go well and what was learned. New material is taught and new homework is assigned. Despite high acceptability ratings (Zucker, Marcus, & Bulik, 2006), the evidence base for this treatment remains limited.

Health Communication to Lessen Caregiver Burden

Images and messages influence behavior. In the field of health communication, there are examples of messaging campaigns that have had profound effects on public behavior (e.g., smoking) (Cunningham, Faulkner, Selby, & Cordingley, 2006; Grandpre, Alvaro, Burgoon, Miller, & Hall, 2003; Invernizzi, Falomir-Pichastor, Munoz-Rojas, & Mugny, 2003). This field offers innovative techniques and tools that may be usefully leveraged to influence parent behavior. Patel, Shafer, Zucker, and Bulik (Patel, Shafer, Zucker, & Bulik, 2011) investigated barriers for parents in obtaining needed services and explored ways to better communicate to them to facilitate their help-seeking behavior. Specifically, these investigators were interested in influencing parents' willingness to take better care of themselves.

Lack of knowledge is a critical barrier to self-care behavior in parents. Parents are often unaware that they may face many barriers to participating in self-care activities (Haigh & Treasure, 2002). There has been little research on what may motivate or dissuade a parent of a child with an eating disorder from participating in self-care behaviors, and as to what messages may help parents change behavior in an environment that blames parents of children with eating disorders because of the stigma associated with the disease. To guide the development of health messages for parents, work was influenced by the tenets of the transactional model of stress and coping (TMSC) and the transtheoretical model (TTM) (Glanz & Schwartz, 2008; Prochaska, Redding, & Evers, 2008). These models describe the dynamic and recursive process of behavior change: how from one moment to the next, an individual may deny the very presence of a problem, but then passionately commit to radical shifts in behavior that may alter the disease course. The key message of these models is that strategies to influence behavior must match the motivational state of the individual. Otherwise, communication is both invalidating of the patient's present moment experience and inevitably ineffective. In focus groups with parents of a child with an eating disorder, Patel and colleagues explored motivators and barriers to engage in their own self-care. These authors further tested five sample message campaigns compiled on the basis of reviews of extant research and consultation with providers of eating disorder services.

Results indicated that messages from health care providers can have a powerful impact on parent behavior. Parents identified lack of time and their need for permission from health care professionals to take time for themselves as the main barriers to self-care. The main motivator for parents to engage in coping behaviors was awareness of a connection between self-care and their child's health outcomes. Two health message print campaigns were well received: (1) in one poster, a mother in her 50s spoke about the importance of parents taking a lead in destigmatizing eating disorders and the need for self-care, and (2) in a second poster, a family was seen hugging, with the child with the eating disorder speaking about the importance of her father getting support. The tagline "Caring for yourself is caring for your child" was strongly endorsed. Suggestions for changes in the elements of messages were directly related to the barriers and motivators that were expressed. For example, self-care resources should be more prominent because parents saw time as a barrier and needed to access information quickly. Inherent in these messages were several theory-driven elements. For example, raising awareness of the problem and appealing to emotion are important components of the theory of change model. Theory-based elements in the ads were seen as important. For example, the importance of the perceived controllability of stress is an important element in the TMSC model. Parents appreciated validation of their appraisal of their controllability of stress in the ad copy. The processes of change (TTM) the ads embodied, including social liberation, self-liberation, consciousness raising, helping relationships, self- and environmental reevaluation, and dramatic relief, were also seen as important by parents. Thus, messages for parents of children with eating disorders should include theory-based message elements explicitly based on the barriers and motivators to engaging in self-care behaviors.

Conclusion

The value of a participant approach in which parents are a crucial part of the treatment team is increasingly being acknowledged. A variety of service models have been developed to assist parents in their role and minimize their burden, but the evidence base is limited. Given the importance of their role in the treatment team, as well as the importance of fostering caregivers' mental health, there is an imperative need to more formally investigate services that may reduce burden, protect the mental health of the family, and, potentially, help sustain treatment gains.

Although all of these approaches are united in their mission to help parents, the diversity of both content and format and the lack of systematic study precludes a determination of the most efficacious method to support parents. Furthermore, the impact of these approaches on parents' mental health has not been a direct focus. Nonetheless, these, these program descriptions offer important starting points to spur more focused research.

References

Berkman, N. D., Bulik, C. M., Brownley, K. A., Lohr, K. N., Sedway, J. A., Rooks, A., et al. (2006). Management of eating disorders. *Evidence Report/Technology Assessment, 135*, 1–166.

Bradley, M. M., & Lang, P. J. (2007). Emotion and motivation. In J. T. Cacioppo, L. G. Tassinary, & G. G. Berntson (Eds.), *Handbook of psychophysiology* (pp. 581–607). New York: Cambridge University Press.

Brosch, T., Pourtois, G., & Sander, D. (2010). The perception and categorisation of emotional stimuli: A review. *Cognition and Emotion, 24*(3), 377–400.

Bulik, C. M., Sullivan, P. F., Tozzi, F., Furberg, H., Lichtenstein, P., & Pedersen, N. L. (2006). Prevalence, heritability, and prospective risk factors for anorexia nervosa. *Archives of General Psychiatry, 63(3)*, 305–312.

Butzlaff, R. L., & Hooley, J. M. (1998). Expressed emotion and psychiatric relapse: A meta-analysis. *Archives of General Psychiatry, 55*(6), 547–552.

Cunningham, J. A., Faulkner, G., Selby, P., & Cordingley, J. (2006). Motivating smoking reductions by framing health information as safer smoking tips. *Addictive Behaviors, 31*(8), 1465–1468.

Dare, C., & Eisler, I. (2000). A multi-family group day treatment programme for adolescent eating disorder. *European Eating Disorders Review, 8*(1), 4–18.

de la Rie, S. M., Noordenbos, G., & van Furth, E. F. (2005). Quality of life and eating disorders. *Quality of Life Research, 14*(6), 1511–1522.

de la Rie, S. M., Van Furth, E. F., De Koning, A., Noordenbos, G., & Donker, M. C. (2005). The quality of life of family caregivers of eating disorder patients. *Eating Disorders, 13*(4), 345–351.

Eisler, I., Dare, C., Hodes, M., Russell, G. F. M., Dodge, E., & Le Grange, D. (2000). Family therapy for adolescent anorexia nervosa: The results of a controlled comparison of two family interventions. *Journal of Child Psychology and Psychiatry, 41*(6), 727–736.

Eisler, I., Simic, M., Russell, G. F., & Dare, C. (2007). A randomised controlled treatment trial of two forms of family therapy in adolescent anorexia nervosa: A five-year follow-up. *Journal of Child Psychology and Psychiatry, 48*(6), 552–560.

Garner, D., Rockert, W., Olmsted, M., Johnson, C., & Coscina, D. (1985). Psychoeducational principles in the treatment of bulimia and anorexia nervosa. In D. M. Garner & P. E. Garfinkel (Eds.), *Handbook of psychotherapy for anorexia nervosa and bulimia* (pp. 513–572). New York: Guilford Press.

Geist, R., Heinmaa, M., Stephens, D., Davis, R., & Katzman, D. K. (2000). Comparison of family therapy and family group psychoeducation in adolescents with anorexia nervosa. *Canadian Journal of Psychiatry, 45*(2), 173–178.

Glanz, K., & Schwartz, M. D. (2008). Stress, coping, and health behavior. In K. Glanz, B. K. Rimer, & K. Viswanath (Eds.), *Health behavior and health education* (4th ed., pp. 211–236). San Francisco: Jossey-Bass.

Grandpre, J., Alvaro, E. M., Burgoon, M., Miller, C. H., & Hall, J. R. (2003). Adolescent reactance and anti-smoking campaigns: A theoretical approach. *Health Communication, 15*(3), 349–366.

Greenberg, L. S., & Paivio, S. C. (2003). *Working with emotions in psychotherapy*. New York: Guilford Press.

Haigh, R., & Treasure, J. (2002). Investigating the needs of carers in the area of eating disorders: Development of the Carers' Needs Assessment Measure (CaNAM). *Euorpean Eating Disorder Review, 11*(2), 125–141.

Holliday, J., Wall, E., Treasure, J., & Weinman,

J. (2005). Perceptions of illness in individuals with anorexia nervosa: A comparison with lay men and women. *International Journal of Eating Disorders, 37*(1), 50–56.

Holtkamp, K., Herpertz-Dahlmann, B., Vloet, T., & Hagenah, U. (2005). Group Psychoeducation for parents of adolescents with eating disorders: The Aachen Program. *Eating Disorders: The Journal of Treatment and Prevention, 13*(4), 381–390.

Invernizzi, F., Falomir-Pichastor, J. M., Munoz-Rojas, D., & Mugny, G. (2003). Social influence in personally relevant contexts: The respect attributed to the source as a factor increasing smokers' intention to quit smoking. *Journal of Applied Social Psychology, 33*(9), 1818–1836.

Kaskutas, L. A. (2009). Alcoholics Anonymous effectiveness: Faith meets science. *Journal of Addictive Diseases, 28*(2), 145–157.

Kaskutas, L. A., Subbaraman, M. S., Witbrodt, J., & Zemore, S. E. (2009). Effectiveness of Making Alcoholics Anonymous Easier: A group format 12-step facilitation approach. *Journal of Substance Abuse Treatment, 37*(3), 228–239.

Kaye, W. H., Lilenfeld, L. R., Plotnicov, K., Merikangas, K. R., Nagy, L., Strober, M., et al. (1996). Bulimia nervosa and substance dependence: Association and family transmission. *Alcoholism—Clinical and Experimental Research, 20*(5), 878–881.

Keys, A. (1950). *The biology of human starvation.* Minneapolis: University of Minnesota Press.

Leichner, P., Hall, D., & Calderon, R. (2005). Meal support training for friends and families of patients with eating disorders. *Eating Disorders: The Journal of Treatment and Prevention, 13*(4), 407–411.

Lewinsohn, P. M., Sullivan, J. M., & Grosscup, S. J. (1980). Changing reinforcing events: An approach to the treatment of depression. *Psychotherapy: Theory, Research and Practice, 17*(3), 322–334.

Lilenfeld, L. R., Kaye, W. H., Greeno, C. G., Merikangas, K. R., Plotnicov, K., Pollice, C., et al. (1998). A controlled family study of anorexia nervosa and bulimia nervosa: Psychiatric disorders in first-degree relatives and effects of proband comorbidity.

Archives of General Psychiatry, 55(7), 603–610.

Linehan, M. M. (1993). *Cognitive-behavioral treatment of borderline personality disorder.* New York: Guilford Press.

Lock, J., Agras, W. S., Bryson, S., & Kraemer, H. C. (2005). A comparison of short- and long-term family therapy for adolescent anorexia nervosa. *Journal of the American Academy of Child and Adolescent Psychiatry, 44*(7), 632–639.

Lock, J., & Le Grange, D. (2005). Family-based treatment of eating disorders. *International Journal of Eating Disorders, 37,* S64–S67.

O'Hara, S. K., & Smith, K. C. (2007). Presentation of eating disorders in the news media: What are the implications for patient diagnosis and treatment? *Patient Education and Counseling, 68*(1), 43–51.

Owens, R. G., & Slade, P. D. (2008). So perfect it's positively harmful?: Reflections on the adaptiveness and maladaptiveness of positive and negative perfectionism. *Behavior Modification, 32*(6), 928–937.

Pasold, T. L., Boateng, B. A., & Portilla, M. G. (2010). The use of an outpatient treatment group for children and adolescents with eating disorders. *Eating Disorders, 18,* 318–332.

Patel, S. J., Shafer, A., Zucker, N. L., & Bulik, C. M. (2011). Caring for yourself is caring for your child: Helping parents of children with eating disorders receive health care for themselves. In M. Brann (Ed.), *Contemporary case studies in health communication: Theoretical and applied approaches* (pp. 149–165). Dubuque, IA: Kendall Hunt.

Pearce, J. M. S. (2004). Richard Morton: Origins of anorexia nervosa. *European Neurology, 52*(4), 191–192.

Prochaska, J. O., Redding, C. A., & Evers, K. E. (2008). The transtheoretical model and stages of change In K. Glanz, B. K. Rimer, & K. Viswanath (Eds.), *Health behavior and health education* (4th ed., pp. 97–122). San Francisco: Jossey-Bass.

Propper, C., & Moore, G. A. (2006). The influence of parenting on infant emotionality: A multi-level psychobiological perspective. *Developmental Review, 26*(4), 427–460.

Rainville, P., Bechara, A., Naqvi, N., & Damasio, A. R. (2006). Basic emotions are associated with distinct patterns of cardiorespiratory activity. *International Journal of Psychophysiology, 61*(1), 5–18.

Ruggiero, G. M., Bertelli, S., Boccalari, L., Centorame, F., Ditucci, A., La Mela, C., et al. (2008). The influence of stress on the relationship between cognitive variables and measures of eating disorders (in healthy female university students): A quasi-experimental study. *Eating and Weight Disorders: Studies on Anorexia Bulimia and Obesity, 13*(3), 142–148.

Schmidt, U., & Treasure, J. (2006). Anorexia nervosa: Valued and visible. A cognitive-interpersonal maintenance model and its implications for research and practice. *British Journal of Clinical Psychology, 45,* 343–366.

Siegel, M., Brisman, J., & Weinshel, M. (1989). *Surviving an eating disorders: Strategies for families and friends.* New York: Harper-Collins.

Slade, P. D., & Owens, R. G. (1998). A dual process model of perfectionism based on reinforcement theory. *Behavior Modification, 22*(3), 372–390.

Stein, D., Lilenfeld, L. R., Plotnicov, K., Pollice, C., Rao, R., Strober, M., et al. (1999). Familial aggregation of eating disorders: Results from a controlled family study of bulimia nervosa. *International Journal of Eating Disorders, 26*(2), 211–215.

Szmukler, G. I., Eisler, I., Russell, G., & Dare, C. (1985). Anorexia nervosa, parental "expressed emotion" and dropping out of treatment. *British Journal of Psychiatry, 147,* 265–271.

Treasure, J., Murphy, T., Szmukler, T., Todd, G., Gavan, K., & Joyce, J. (2001). The experience of caregiving for severe mental illness: A comparison between anorexia nervosa and psychosis. *Social Psychiatry and Psychiatric Epidemiology, 36*(7), 343–347.

Uehara, T., Kawashima, Y., Goto, M., Tasaki, S., & Someya, T. (2001). Psychoeducation for the families of patients with eating disorders and changes in expressed emotion: A preliminary study. *Comprehensive Psychiatry, 42*(2), 132–138.

van Furth, E. F., Van Strien, D. C., Martina, L. M., van Son, M. J., Hendrickx, J. J., & van Engeland, H. (1996). Expressed emotion and the prediction of outcome in adolescent eating disorders. *International Journal of Eating Disorders, 20*(1), 19–31.

Vaughn, C. E., & Leff, J. (1976). The measurement of expressed emotion in the families of psychiatric patients. *British Journal of Social and Clinical Psychology, 15,* 157–165.

Whitney, J., Murray, J., Gavan, K., Todd, G., Whitaker, W., & Treasure, J. (2005). Experience of caring for someone with anorexia nervosa: Qualitative study. *British Journal of Psychiatry, 187,* 444–449.

Wildes, J. E., Ringham, R. M., & Marcus, M. D. (2010). Emotion avoidance in patients with anorexia nervosa: Initial test of a functional model. *International Journal of Eating Disorders, 43*(5), 398–404.

Wilson, G. T., & Schlam, T. R. (2004). The transtheoretical model and motivational interviewing in the treatment of eating and weight disorders. *Clinical Psychology Review, 24*(3), 361–378.

Zachar, P. (2010). Defending the validity of pragmatism in the classification of emotion. *Emotion Review, 2*(2), 113–116.

Zucker, N., Losh, M., Bulik, C., LaBar, K., Piven, J., & Pelphrey, K. (2007). Anorexia nervosa and autism spectrum disorders: Guided inquiry into social cognitive endophenotypes. *Psychological Bulletin, 133,* 976–1006.

Zucker, N. L., Herzog, D., Moskovich, A., Merwin, R., & Linn, T. (2011). Incorporating dispositional traits into the treatment of anorexia nervosa. In R. A. H. Adan & W. H. Kaye (Eds.), *Behavioral neurobiology of eating disorders* (pp. 289–314). Berlin: Springer-Verlag.

Zucker, N. L., Marcus, M. D., & Bulik, C. (2006). A group parent training program: A novel approach for eating disorder management. *Eating and Weight Disorders: Studies on Anorexia, Bulimia and Obesity, 11,* 78–82.

CHAPTER 20

Treatments Targeting Aberrant Eating Patterns in Overweight Youth

Kerri N. Boutelle
Marian Tanofsky-Kraff

With the current high rates of pediatric obesity (Ogden, Carroll, Curtin, Lamb, & Flegal, 2010), there is an urgent need to better understand the etiology and treatment of overeating in children. Approximately one-third of children in the United States are either overweight or obese, defined as equal to or above the 85th body mass index (BMI, kg/m²) percentile for age and sex (Ogden et al., 2010). Although behavioral treatments for overweight youth typically include recommendations to decrease overeating, very few treatments to date have specifically targeted aberrant overeating patterns. Aberrant overeating patterns in youth refer to a range of eating behaviors that involve a lack of restraint in food intake, which include binge and loss-of-control (LOC) eating, emotional eating, eating in secret, and eating in the absence of hunger (EAH). Such behaviors have been associated with adverse physical and psychological outcomes (Shomaker, Tanofsky-Kraff, & Yanovski, 2011). Therefore, targeting aberrant eating patterns may provide a point of intervention for excessive weight gain and exacerbated disordered eating in youth (Tanofsky-Kraff, Wilfley, et al., 2007). In this chapter, we first define the types of aberrant eating patterns identified in the literature. A summary of the cross-sectional relationships and the longitudinal impact that aberrant eating patterns have on the physical and psychological well-being of children follow. Finally, we discuss novel treatments currently in development to address these eating behaviors.

A question that often arises in regard to targeting overeating patterns in youth is, Why focus specifically on eating patterns rather than energy intake and physical activity? First, it is well established that overweight and obesity result from an energy imbalance in which intake exceeds expenditure. Today children are exposed to large portions of palatable, inexpensive, and energy-dense foods, which is thought to increase the likelihood of excess intake and ultimately to contribute to excess weight gain in youth (Hill & Peters, 1998). Second, studies of behavioral weight loss in preteens show that these programs are limited in ability to impact the symptoms of disordered eating (Epstein, Paluch, Saelens, Ernst, & Wilfley, 2001). In addition, there is an emerging body of literature suggesting that there are potential compensatory responses to increased exercise that result in increased intake (Church, Earnest, Skinner, & Blair, 2007; King et al., 2007;

Sonneville & Gortmaker, 2008). A 2-year longitudinal study of 538 adolescents found that when adolescents initiate an exercise program, they end up eating, on average, 100 more calories more than they burn (Sonneville & Gortmaker, 2008). Finally, there may be a practical reason for targeting overeating in youth: it may be easier to skip a candy bar than to have the child play outside for an hour to burn the calories consumed. However, this possibility warrants empirical testing. For these reasons, a new field is emerging that focuses specifically on intervening in aberrant eating behaviors in youth.

What Are Aberrant Eating Patterns That Promote Overweight in Youth?

"Aberrant eating patterns" refers to eating for reasons not motivated by biological hunger (Shomaker, Tanofsky-Kraff, & Yanovski, in press). Specifically, the aberrant eating patterns described in this chapter include binge eating, LOC eating, EAH, eating in secret, and emotional eating.

Binge Eating

According to DSM-IV-TR, binge eating is defined as the consumption of an objectively large amount of food while experiencing a sense of loss of control over eating (American Psychiatric Association, 2000). Binge eating is relatively common among youth (Glasofer et al., 2007; Lamerz et al., 2005; Tanofsky-Kraff et al., 2004), with prevalence estimates ranging from 2 to 40% depending on the age and characteristics (e.g., community vs. weight loss treatment seeking) of the sample studied.

Cross-sectional data point to a relationship between the presence of binge-eating episodes and overweight or obesity in childhood. For instance, among young children (6 years of age), parental reports of binge eating were correlated with the children's overweight status (Lamerz et al., 2005). In a large survey-based study of boys and girls (9–14 years), children's self-report of binge eating in the past month were associated with higher body weight (Field et al., 1999). A consistent relationship between binge eating and body weight has also been found among older children. In a school-based sample, overweight adolescents were more likely to report binge eating than their normal weight peers (Neumark-Sztainer et al., 1997). Similar findings have been reported in other adolescent community samples using survey methods (Ackard, Neumark-Sztainer, Story, & Perry, 2003; Field, Colditz, & Peterson, 1997). Children and adolescents with binge eating can also be distinguished by increased psychopathology (e.g., depressive symptoms and disordered eating attitudes) as compared with their counterparts without binge eating (e.g., Goossens, Braet, & Decaluwe, 2007; Goossens, Soenens, & Braet, 2009; Tanofsky-Kraff, 2008).

Binge-eating behaviors have been shown to predict weight gain in a number of longitudinal pediatric studies. Among adolescent girls in a community sample, binge eating was associated with elevated weight gain (Stice, Cameron, Killen, Hayward, & Taylor, 1999) and obesity onset (Stice, Presnell, & Spangler, 2002) over a 4-year period. In a large community cohort of youth 9–14 years of age, boys, but not girls, who self-reported binge eating in a survey gained significantly more weight as compared with those who reported no binge eating (Field et al., 2003). Among 6- to 12-year-old children at heightened risk for adult obesity by virtue of their own overweight status or parental overweight, self-reported binge-eating episodes predicted greater gains in body fat mass approximately 4 years later (Tanofsky-Kraff et al., 2006). The literature on the psychological outcomes of children and adolescents who report binge eating is surprisingly sparse. There are prospective data suggesting that binge eating is predictive of increases in depressive symptoms in a community sample of adolescents (Presnell, Stice, Seidel, & Madeley, 2009). However, the authors also found that depressive symptoms were predictive of eating pathology, suggesting that depressive and binge-eating symptomatology may contribute reciprocally over time.

LOC Eating

LOC eating refers to a child's perception of eating without the ability to stop. LOC eating can occur with or without episodes of overeating, thus encompassing binge-eating episodes. The notion that the experience of LOC is the more relevant component of a binge episode is often adopted in child studies. This is likely due to the difficulty involved in making a size criterion determination for children of different ages because physically developing boys and girls have vastly varying energy needs. For example, the consumption of an entire large pizza by a child or adolescent of any age would likely be considered *unambiguously* large. In contrast, the amount of five slices of pizza eaten by a 16-year-old boy might be less clear and thus deemed an *ambiguously* large amount of food. The consumption of this food, even if accompanied by a sense of loss of control over eating, might not be classified as an objective binge-eating episode. Furthermore, in younger children, the amount of food consumed in an eating episode may be limited by parental controls, masking how much a child might have eaten given the opportunity.

The emerging data on LOC eating suggest that its prevalence ranges from 4 to 45%, with higher estimates among overweight youth (vs. nonoverweight), adolescents (vs. preadolescents), and when assessed via questionnaire (vs. semistructured interview) (Tanofsky-Kraff, 2008). Youth with LOC—both those reporting objective and subjective episodes—are more likely to be heavier and/or to have greater fat mass than youth with no LOC episodes (Shomaker et al., 2010; Tanofsky-Kraff, Goossens, et al., 2007). Children and adolescents with LOC eating, whether assessed by questionnaire or interview, also exhibit greater psychological symptoms and disordered eating cognitions and behaviors (Goossens et al., 2007; Morgan et al., 2002; Tanofsky-Kraff et al., 2004, 2008; Tanofsky-Kraff, Theim, et al., 2007), as well as dysfunctional emotion regulation strategies (Czaja, Rief, & Hilbert, 2009), as compared with their counterparts without LOC. Notably, there are prospective data showing that children who report LOC eating gain more weight over time than their peers without such episodes (Tanofsky-Kraff et al., 2009).

Eating in Secret or Hiding Food

Eating in secret, a behavior that is often clinically reported, is included in the diagnostic features of binge-eating disorder. However, very little is known about the prevalence rates of eating in secret among overweight and obese youth. Like many of these behaviors, it may overlap with binge eating and LOC eating and/or EAH. One of the few studies specifically including an independent report of eating in secret showed that in a sample of young women who were dieting (ages 16–24), eating in secret was one of the predictive behaviors identifying those who will develop an eating disorder (Fairburn, Cooper, Doll, & Davies, 2005). In a study of 108 overweight adolescents, one-third of those sampled endorsed eating in secret in the last month (Knatz et al., 2011). Adolescents who eat in secret have higher levels of depression (Knatz et al., 2011). In another study, 23% of adolescent girls reported eating alone (Vervaet & Van Heeringen, 2000). More data are required to understand the relationship between eating in secret and more exacerbated disordered eating and excessive weight gain in youth.

Eating in the Absence of Hunger

EAH is a behavioral measure of overeating, which was initially described in a longitudinal study of preschool children and their parents (Fisher & Birch, 1999). In this study, girls were assessed for EAH before they entered kindergarten (age 5 years) and again 2 years later. Girls were fed a standard lunch, after which hunger ratings were obtained to ensure that the girls were full. Next, participants were allowed to play with toys and were offered access to a variety of palatable snack foods. Intake of snack foods was measured and girls were divided into high- and low-intake groups using a median split based on calories consumed. Sixty-eight percent of girls in the high-intake group at age 5 years were also in the high intake group at age 7 years. Notably, girls in the high-intake group at 5 and 7 years of age were 4.6 times more likely to be overweight than girls who were low on EAH. Fisher and Birch (2002) suggested that EAH represents a stable phenotypic behavior in young girls that is equivalent to disinhibited eating in adults. A number of subsequent studies have examined EAH in overweight children and have demonstrated that children who are overweight or at higher risk of becoming overweight eat significantly more than normal-weight/lower-risk children in the EAH paradigm (Faith et al., 2006; Fisher & Birch, 2002; Fisher et al., 2007; Francis & Birch, 2005; Moens & Braet, 2007; Shunk & Birch, 2004). In contrast to binge and LOC eating, EAH can occur with or without a cognitive understanding by the child of how much the child ate, and can occur with or without distress by the child (Shomaker et al., in press).

Emotional Eating

Emotional eating is defined as "eating in response to a range of negative emotions such as anxiety, depression, anger, and loneliness to cope with negative affect" (Faith, Allison, & Geliebter, 1997). Emotional eating may be relatively common in overweight youth. A study of 55 overweight children (5–13 years of age) seeking weight loss treatment found that 63% endorsed the question, "Do you ever eat because you feel bad, sad, bored, or because of any other mood?" (Shapiro et al., 2007). Emotional eating, like EAH, has been shown to be significantly associated with LOC eating (Tanofsky-Kraff, Theim, et al., 2007). In adolescents, emotional eating is correlated with constructs of disturbed eating and symptoms of depression and anxiety (Van Strien, Engels, Van Leeuwe, & Snoek, 2005). Some (Braet & Van Strien, 1997), but not all (Snoek, Van Strien, Janssens, & Engels, 2007; Tanofsky-Kraff, Theim, et al., 2007) studies have found emotional eating to be associated with overweight among youth and predictive of overeating in cross-sectional structural models (Van Strien et al., 2005). However, longitudinal prospective data are needed to determine if there is, indeed, a predictive relationship between emotional eating and excessive weight gain.

In summary, binge eating, LOC eating, eating in secret, EAH, and emotional eating are aberrant eating patterns that may be associated with adverse physical and psychological outcomes. In general, aberrant overeating patterns in youth have not been considered as targets for treatment in children. The standard approach to obesity in children has been behavioral weight loss, which aims to reduce overall caloric intake as part of a comprehensive program that includes behavioral skills (stimulus control, removing all triggering foods from the home, increasing cues to do physical activity), parenting skills, and increasing physical activity (Epstein, Myers, Raynor, & Saelens, 1998). Notably, the majority of published studies of behavioral weight loss have excluded children who endorse symptoms of an eating disorder. Considering the high prevalence of aberrant eating patterns among overweight youth, it is important to develop programs specifically targeting these behaviors to promote weight loss, prevent further weight gain, and possibly prevent the development of a full-syndrome eating disorder.

Treatment Programs Targeting Aberrant Eating Patterns

In recent years, there has been a burgeoning effort to develop programs designed to target aberrant eating among youth. Although preliminary in nature, new interventions offer optimism for future development and dissemination. Each of these treatment programs is described below.

Interventions Targeting Overeating in Preschoolers

The first study specifically targeting overeating in youth was published in 2000. Susan Johnson provided 6 weeks of age-appropriate training to identify internal cues of hunger and satiety to 25 preschoolers (Johnson, 2000). The intervention was held once per week in school. The first day of the intervention included a skit with themes of hunger, eating to fullness, and signals associated with overeating. In addition, the children were taught the meaning of the terms "mouth" (where you chew food), "esophagus" (where food goes when you swallow), and "stomach" (where swallowed food goes). The following week, the children watched *Winnie the Pooh and the Honey Jar* and afterward discussed hunger, overeating, and the results of chronic overeating. During week 3, doll play was used to identify internal cues of hunger and satiety. Androgynous dolls with a mouth, esophagus, and a place for a stomach on the exterior of the doll abdomen were used. In addition, several sets of stomachs were made from nylon material and filled with salt to varying degrees to represent (1) an empty stomach that was hungry, (2) a stomach that was a little full, and (3) a stomach that was very full. These stomachs could be attached to the dolls with Velcro strips. Following these visits, each child was seen before and after snack time 1 day per week over the course of a 4-week period. Children were asked to compare the three doll stomachs to their own stomachs and report whether they were hungry, a little full, or very full. This activity was repeated throughout the day with the children.

The outcome measure was a compensation index, which was created by providing children either a high-energy or a low-energy preload drink and then measuring food intake at lunch. The children also completed a compensation evaluation with the other drink (high- or low-energy) at a second evaluation. At baseline, these children showed little evidence of compensation for the difference in energy in the two drinks and exhibited a large deviation from the ideal compensation for caloric intake preload. After 6 weeks of the intervention, children improved their compensation index and the deviation from the ideal compensation decreased significantly. These exciting findings suggest that children respond to age-appropriate training that focuses on responding to internal cues of hunger and satiety, and that these changes translate into responsiveness in eating (Johnson, 2000).

Interventions Targeting EAH

The Regulation of Cues Intervention

In the late 1960s, Schachter formulated the "externality theory of obesity" (Schachter, 1971; Schachter & Rodin, 1974). This theory states that both obese rats and human beings are more reactive to external cues (time, presence and quality of food, situational effects, etc.) and less sensitive to internal hunger and satiety signals than their lean counterparts. When considering the treatment of children who eat in the absence of hunger, the two main tenets of Schachter's theory, increased sensitivity to food cues and decreased sensitivity to internal cues, could be useful for identifying treatments that may reduce a child's overeating when not biologically hungry. Theoretically, sensitivity to external food cues may be understood in terms of Pavlovian conditioning. The conditioning model of binge eating (Jansen, 1994, 1998) suggests that through Pavlovian conditioning, cues such as the sight, smell, and taste of food, as well as rituals for eating, environment where eating occurs, and affective states and food-related cognitions, can elicit physiological responses that are experienced as craving. Food intake may, in terms of Pavlovian conditioning, be considered an unconditioned stimulus, whereas its metabolic responses are unconditioned responses. Cues that signal food intake, such as sight, smell, and taste of food, may start to act as conditioned stimuli that can trigger cue reactivity or conditioned responses. In principle, the association between urges to eat and external cues should be amenable to extinction through systematic exposure (Wardle, 1990).

Treatments that target decreased sensitivity to external cues and increased sensitivity to internal cues could logically be applied to the treatment of overweight children. Treatments that reduce sensitivity to external cues, including cue reactivity and sensitivity training and exposure with response prevention, have been found to decrease cue reactivity in the usage of alcohol (Drummond & Glautier, 1994; Monti & Rohsenow, 1999), drugs (Childress et al., 1993; Franken, de Haan, van der Meer, Haffmans, & Hendriks, 1999), nicotine (Havermans, Debaere, Smulders, Wiers, & Jansen, 2003; Niaura et al., 1999), and purging behavior (Bulik, Sullivan, Carter, McIntosh, & Joyce, 1998; Carter, Bulik, McIntosh, & Joyce, 2002; Toro et al., 2003). These programs attempt to decrease sensitivity to external cues by extinguishing the relationship between the conditioned stimulus and the unconditioned stimulus in the presence of the triggering cues. In terms of treatment for overeating, these programs could theoretically train the individual to decrease his or her reactivity when faced with potential binge-type (e.g., highly palatable) foods, thus decreasing the urge to overeat.

A treatment that increases sensitivity to internal cues in overweight adults is appetite awareness training (Craighead & Allen, 1995). The focus of this treatment is to train participants to regulate their eating by responding to hunger and appetite. One of the main tenets of this approach is that focusing on food may lead to feelings of deprivation, thoughts about food, and a cycle of overeating. This treatment does not prescribe a diet, and participants are taught to recognize and respond to hunger signals from their bodies.

The fundamental aim of appetite awareness training is to learn to use the body's internal signals to decide when and how much to eat. This program has been shown to decrease the frequency of binge eating in adults (Craighead & Allen, 1995), and has demonstrated preliminary efficacy in a 6-session children's appetite awareness training (CAAT) program. In a pilot study of 45 8- to 12-year-old children randomized to CAAT or a delayed wait-list control (Bloom, Sharpe, Heriot, Zucker, & Craighead, 2005), results indicated that, on average, CAAT children lost a modest, but significantly greater amount of weight (419 grams), whereas the wait-list children gained weight (1.12 kg).

The regulation of cues program (ROC) was developed by the first author (K. N. B.) and Nancy Zucker, with the assistance of Carol Peterson. This treatment specifically focuses on training overweight children who are high in EAH to become more sensitive to hunger and satiety cues, and to reduce sensitivity to external cues to eat. ROC targets EAH in overweight children and is currently under development in two phases. The first phase evaluates cue responsivity training and children's appetite awareness training in overweight boys and girls (8–12 years) who are high in EAH (>10% daily caloric intake needs). The second phase evaluates a combined treatment program against a comparison group.

In the early developmental stages of this endeavor, we evaluated the potential efficacy of an 8-week cue-exposure treatment program (Volcravo) and CAAT program on EAH in 36 obese children who had high EAH. Both Volcravo and CAAT included experiential training in parent–child groups. Assessments were conducted at baseline, posttreatment, 6 months posttreatment, and 12 months posttreatment. Results showed that both Volcravo and CAAT significantly reduced subjective bulimic episodes (LOC) and objective bulimic episodes (LOC and overeating) on the Eating Disorders Examination for children, and effects were maintained at 12 months posttreatment (Boutelle, Zucker, Rydell, Cafri, et al., 2009; Boutelle, Zucker, Rydell, Peterson, & Harnack, 2009). In addition, Volcravo resulted in significant decreases in EAH posttreatment whereas the CAAT program showed no impact on EAH. No significant impact was seen on children's body mass index (BMI) with either treatment. We found that both treatments were acceptable to children and parents; however, participants had difficulties understanding craving in Volcravo without some training in the concept of hunger. On the basis of these results, we developed the combined 14-visit program (ROC).

The ROC treatment focuses on training overweight children who are high on EAH and their parents to be more sensitive to their hunger and satiety cues, and to learn to resist overeating when exposed to eating cues when not hungry. This is accomplished by providing psychoeducation about hunger and satiety and Pavlovian conditioning, self-monitoring of hunger and cravings, experiential learning, parent training, and child and parent skill building to resist food cues. ROC is conducted in separate parent and child groups (approximately 10 parent/child pairs), with parent/child pairs coming back together for experiential learning in each group meeting. The parent and child groups cover similar information, but the child group is taught in a more age-appropriate manner (for children 8–12) and the parent groups also include behavioral parent training. The first five group visits focus on learning to monitor hunger and parallels what was developed for appetite awareness training (Craighead & Allen, 1995) in adults, and the next seven visits include learning to habituate and extinguish responses to food cues.

In this program hunger is monitored on a scale of 1 to 5. Children and parents are taught to monitor hunger and eat when they are at 2 or 3, and stop when they are at 4.

Participants are encouraged to avoid the ends of the hunger meter as getting too low on the hunger meter can result in overeating because of physiological hunger and not stopping until 5 can result in being overstuffed. To emphasize this skill, parents and children bring a meal to the first five sessions, and every session is initiated by eating their dinner and monitoring their hunger at the beginning, middle, and end of the meal. Learning about and becoming more sensitive to hunger feelings is a crucial component of ROC.

The next seven visits focus on cue–exposure treatment, which includes craving monitoring. Craving is described to families as the urge to eat when they are not physically hungry. This urge to eat includes "liking" something and "wanting" something in the absence of physical hunger. During this phase of the program parents and children continue to monitor hunger, but they also begin monitoring cravings and complete "exposures" (which are described below) in the groups and at home. Parents and children are taught about the impossibility of avoiding overeating cues in today's society, and how they can learn to reduce their cravings over time. Exposures are based on cue-exposure treatment (Monti & Rohsenow, 1999) for addictions, and we have adapted them for food cues. An exposure session consists of children and parents who hold the food and rate their cravings, smell the food and rate their cravings, take two bites of the food and rate their cravings, and continue to look at the food while rating their cravings every 30 seconds. Participants continue to rate their cravings on a scale from 1 to 5 (highest) until their cravings are at less than 2, at which point they discard the food. Families identify a list of six highly craved foods and bring in one food each week.

Parents are taught behavioral parent management skills in the parenting group without the children. These skills include daily meetings, positive parenting skills, self-monitoring, modeling behaviors for the ROC program, active listening and empathy, planning ahead for high-risk situations, and a motivation system. In addition, parents are educated on stimulus control in the home to increase the chances that the child will maintain healthy eating at home. Each parent/child pair is assigned to have a ROC meeting every day to discuss their progress in the program. In addition, parent/child pairs create a motivation system in which the child earns points by complying with the recommendations in the ROC program, which may be exchanged for motivators (e.g., sleepovers, being queen of the family for a day, special privileges, weekend away with Mom or Dad) at a future date.

As part of the ROC program, parents and children are taught about nine "tricky hungers," which frame a discussion for each group. These tricky hungers include ignoring fullness, getting too hungry, feeding your feelings, eating too fast, eating food because it's there, responding to media, who cares response, eating for entertainment, eating because other people are eating, and food rules. In the groups, children and parents are taught methods to manage tricky hungers (or coping skills), which include delaying tactics, activity substitution, relaxation, mindful eating, media awareness, empathy, cost–benefit analyses, distraction, assertiveness, self-motivational statements, and moderate thinking.

Notably, unlike traditional behavioral weight-loss programs, the ROC program does not require high levels of physical activity or dietary restriction. However, physical activity is mentioned as a method for reducing cravings and managing tricky hungers.

We recruited 44 8- to 12-year-old children who were high in EAH at baseline (>10% daily caloric needs) and randomized them to either the ROC program or a comparison group. Children and parents in the ROC program attended 4 months of parent and child separate groups, with *in vivo* experiences conducted with parent/child pairs. Only post-treatment data were available at the time of this writing. The treatment was acceptable to both parents and children, and families liked the combination of monitoring hungers as well as cravings. Preliminary analysis suggests that the children in ROC decreased their BMI at posttreatment as compared with those in the comparison group, but the change only approached significance. Interestingly, children's self-efficacy for eating in a healthy manner when down, stressed, or bored improved in the ROC group as compared with the comparison group.

Case Example

Sarah was an-11 year-old obese girl who attended treatment with her father, Scott. Scott and Sarah attended all eight sessions of the Volcravo (cue reactivity) program. Sarah showed an extreme sensitivity to food cues, and she and her father openly discussed her difficulties in resisting food cues. Sarah would come home from school and immediately ask about a snack, and then about dinner. She constantly requested food because she was "always" hungry. In the child group, Sarah had no trouble understanding the concepts taught in the program. However, she struggled at the beginning to implement those con-cepts. During the first few exposures, Sarah made comments about how difficult it was to "ride out" her cravings. She would ask for "just one more bite" or say "This is a waste of good food" or "We went out of our way to get this. I should eat it all. " As she became more skilled at riding out the craving wave, Sarah voiced fewer and fewer frustrations. She seemed to really benefit from using deep breathing exercises and distraction, and especially puzzlers, to help her ride out the craving wave. She would, however, humor-ously comment on her father's difficulty to ride the wave. Scott was very much aware of himself as a role model and could empathize with Sarah's struggles with oversensitivity to food cues. In the parent group, Scott reported using very specific and immediate positive feedback, reported practicing "catching Sarah practicing her Volcravo coping skills," and also used humor to avert the black-and-white thinking. Scott talked in the group about wanting to work with Sarah on concepts for the program without triggering concerns about her body. They worked well together as a team and were consistent in parent–child meetings. By the end of the program, the father and daughter were skilled at riding the craving wave, both in and out of session.

Interventions That Focus on LOC Eating

Interpersonal Psychotherapy

Given that LOC, with or without reported overeating, predicts excessive weight gain (Stice et al., 1999; Tanofsky-Kraff et al., 2006, 2009), reducing such behaviors may be an important weight maintenance intervention in youth who are still growing. Studies testing the efficacy of various psychotherapies for the treatment of binge-eating disorder (BED) in overweight adults have reported reductions in binge-eating episodes (Tanofsky-Kraff, Wilfley, et al., 2007). Abstinence rates across studies ranged from 33 to 77% at final assessment (Tanofsky-Kraff, Wilfley, et al., 2007). Results indicate that those who cease to binge eat tend to maintain their body weights during and following treatment. In approximately 50% of adult studies that used therapy, participants who remained abstinent from binge eating lost modest amounts of weight by the time of their last assessment (Tanofsky-Kraff, Wilfley, et al., 2007). Because many adults with BED report not having been overweight prior to binge eating on a regular basis (Fairburn, Cooper, Doll, Norman, & O'Connor, 2000; Mussell et al., 1995), decreasing LOC eating episodes may reduce the likelihood of excessive weight gain and prevent the onset of obesity. To date, there is a dearth of treatment research in adolescents with binge or LOC eating. Indeed, only one study provides preliminary evidence that reducing binge episodes may impact body weight in youth (Jones et al., 2008).

A number of psychotherapeutic interventions are effective in the treatment of BED in adults (Tanofsky-Kraff, Wilfley, et al., 2007). Unlike other approaches, interpersonal psychotherapy (IPT) targets negative affect by addressing social interactions that are related to mood. Interpersonal relationships and social functioning are of vital importance to adolescents (Mufson, Dorta, Moreau, & Weissman, 2004) and thus motivate them to engage more fully in a prevention program. IPT is acceptable to adolescents with depression (Moreau, Mufson, Weissman, & Klerman, 1991) and those at risk for depression (Young, Mufson, & Davies, 2006). IPT is effective in decreasing negative affect and improving interpersonal and social functioning in such youth (Mufson, Dorta, Wickramaratne, et al., 2004; Rossello & Bernal, 1999). In regard to BED, IPT is based on the assumption that binge eating occurs in response to poor social functioning, such as isolation and rejection, and consequent negative moods (Wilfley, Pike, & Striegel-Moore, 1997). Indeed, adults with BED often suffer from social impairment and poor relationships (Crow, Agras, Halmi, Mitchell, & Kraemer, 2002; Johnson, Spitzer, & Williams, 2001). Furthermore, based on the self-reports of 8- to 17-year-olds, negative affect mediated the cross-sectional relationship between social problems/interpersonal sensitivity and LOC episodes by use of structural equation modeling (Elliott et al., 2010). IPT focuses on improving the interpersonal difficulties and conflicts and social deficits (Klerman, Weissman, Rounsaville, & Chevron, 1984) that may perpetuate LOC and emotional eating (Wilfley, Frank, Welch, Spurrell, & Rounsaville, 1998). IPT is effective in decreasing binge episodes and inducing weight stability in overweight adults with BED (Wilfley et al., 1993, 2002; Wilson, Wilfley, Agras, & Bryson, 2010).

IPT may be particularly appropriate for adolescents at high risk for adult obesity (Tanofsky-Kraff, Wilfley, et al., 2007). Overweight youth report frequent teasing, social isolation, and generally compromised interpersonal functioning (Hayden-Wade et al., 2005; Pearce, Boergers, & Prinstein, 2002; Strauss & Pollack, 2003). As compared with adolescents with healthy weights, heavier teens are often teased about their appearance, stigmatized, and socially rejected (Strauss & Pollack, 2003). Overweight adolescents may be more likely to experience poorer social functioning and negative feelings about themselves regarding their body shape and weight (Fallon et al., 2005; Schwimmer, Burwinkle, & Varni, 2003; Striegel-Moore, Silberstein, & Rodin, 1986). Because adolescents often use peer relationships as a crucial measure of self-evaluation (Mufson, Dorta, Moreau, et al., 2004), the chance of improving relationships may motivate teens to participate in IPT groups. IPT directly targets social difficulties and negative moods. Because prospective studies in youth have found depressive symptoms to predict weight gain and obesity onset (Anderson, Cohen, Naumova, & Must, 2006; Goodman & Whitaker, 2002; Pine, Goldstein, Wolk, & Weissman, 2001; Stice, Presnell, Shaw, & Rohde, 2005), the proven efficacy of IPT in decreasing depressive symptoms may serve to decrease an additional risk factor for inappropriate weight gain. Finally, IPT improves social support, which has been demonstrated to increase weight loss and assist with weight maintenance in overweight adults (Wing & Jeffery, 1999) and children (Wilfley et al., 2007).

IPT for the Prevention of Excessive Weight Gain

IPT for the prevention of excessive weight gain (IPT-WG; Tanofsky-Kraff, Wilfley, et al., 2007), developed by the second author (M. T.-K.), expands upon Young and colleagues' (2006) manual addressing the prevention of depression, with modifications based on an adaptation of group IPT for BED by Wilfley, MacKenzie, Welch, Ayres, and Weissman (2000). IPT-WG is similar to the original IPT (Weissman, Markowitz, & Klerman, 2000) in that it initially involves an "interpersonal inventory" (Mufson, Dorta, Moreau, et al., 2004) so that therapists can learn about the patient's relationships and the context in which LOC episodes are manifested, as well as set goals for the program. The manifestation of the patient's symptoms is then conceptualized in one of four problem areas: (1) interpersonal deficits, (2) interpersonal role disputes, (3) role transitions, and (4) grief. *Interpersonal deficits* apply to those patients who are either socially isolated or are involved in chronically unfulfilling relationships. For patients in this problem area, unsatisfying relationships and/or inadequate social support are frequently the results of poor social skills. *Interpersonal role disputes* refers to conflicts with a significant other (e.g., a parent, other family member, or peer) that emerge from differences in expectations about the relationship. *Role transitions* include difficulties associated with a change in life status (e.g., changes in schools, graduation, moving, parental divorce). The problem area of *grief* is identified when the onset of the patient's symptoms is associated with either the recent or past loss of a person or a relationship. Making use of this framework for defining one or more interpersonal problem areas, IPT focuses on identifying and changing the maladaptive interpersonal context in which the eating problem has developed and been maintained. The group program is delivered in three phases: initial (providing the rationale for IPT, developing rapport among group members); middle (the work phase during which members share personal relationship experiences and role-play new ways of communication); and termination (preparing for saying good-bye and planning future work on goals). The following considerations are specific to IPT-WG.

TARGETED POPULATION

IPT-WG includes adolescents endorsing LOC eating with or without elevated mood symptoms. Furthermore, targeted teens have a BMI between the 75th and 97th percentiles for age and sex (Ogden et al., 2002). Although the current criterion for youth at risk for overweight is a BMI ≥ 85th percentile (Ogden et al., 2006), a prospective study found that for children between the 75th and 84th percentiles, 35% became overweight and 36% became obese in adulthood (Freedman, Khan, Dietz, Srinivasan, & Berenson, 2001). Moreover, Field, Cook, and Gillman (2005) found that youth (8–15 years) between the 75th and 84th BMI percentiles were 20 times more likely to become overweight 8–15 years later, as compared with those below the 50th percentile. Only adolescents up to the 97th percentile in BMI are targeted because individuals with more severe overweight are at greater risk for obesity-related health comorbidities (Weiss et al., 2004) and thus may require more intensive weight-loss treatment.

INTERVENTION TARGET

Broadly, the focus of IPT-WG involves linking difficult relationships and negative affect to LOC eating. The pretreatment session focuses on reviewing the teen's current body weight and eating patterns that place him or her at high risk for excessive weight gain and adult obesity. Psychoeducation on the relationship between adult obesity and impaired health, and psychological and social functioning is discussed. During the interpersonal inventory and throughout the group sessions, participants are encouraged to link their moods and interactions to their eating patterns.

ADDITIONAL SPECIFIC MODIFICATIONS

Length of Intervention. IPT-WG involves 12 weeks of group meetings and one pregroup session during which the interpersonal inventory is conducted. There are also two individual meetings, one at midtreatment (in or near Session 6) and one at posttreatment (1–2 weeks following the final session of the group). A brief (15- to 30-minute) individual midtreatment meeting is scheduled with the therapists for each group member to review the progress made on his or her individual goals, to identify/clarify any work that remains for the second half of the program, and to assess the participant's experience in the group to date. This meeting is an opportunity for the teen to voice any potential concerns with other group members that the participant might otherwise feel uncomfortable addressing in the group. Therapists can brainstorm with the member to generate other ways to understand the discomfort with other group participants and how, if appropriate, concerns might be addressed within the group milieu. Therapists also encourage the member to understand such concerns in a broader context within IPT-WG so that the participant may better understand his or her own contribution to the discomfort. Therapists and the member may then reformulate the goal(s) to work on this problem. In some cases, a member may have accomplished a goal set prior to entering the group. In this case, the goal may be refined, based on progress, or a new goal can be set. At posttreatment there is a brief (15-minute) individual meeting of the therapists and each group member to review the participant's progress and the work that should be continued in the future.

Therapists. We recommend that two therapists lead the group sessions so that productive communication may be modeled. In addition, one therapist may assist in role-playing, particularly at times when group members are reserved, while the second therapist participates in coaching along with other group members.

Group Sessions. Following discussions of interpersonal events, participants are frequently asked if they have noticed changes in their eating. Although clear links between relationships, mood, and eating are made, the group sessions focus largely on interpersonal communication and building skills to improve relationships. Finally, toward the end of each session, leaders check in with participants who have been more reserved to gain their perspective on the discussions throughout the session.

A particularly useful aspect of Young and Mufson's IPT prevention of depression program (Young et al., 2006) is the inclusion of six flash cards showing specific IPT skills that participants are encouraged to reference while working on interpersonal interactions during group sessions. These skills are "Strike while the iron is cold," "Use I statements," "Be specific," "Put yourself in their shoes," "Have some solutions in mind," and "Don't give up" (Young et al., 2006). For the purposes of IPT-WG, we have added a seventh flash card that includes the skill, "What you don't say speaks volumes," to help group members realize how their facial expressions, body language, and tone can impact interpersonal interactions.

- *Initial phase*: IPT-WG differs minimally from Young and Mufson's adaptation (Young et al., 2006). However, following the opening introductions and activities of the first session, IPT-WG participants share their own goals for the group. Psychoeducation does not focus on levels of depressive symptom severity, but rather on obesity, eating disturbances, and related behaviors such as chronic dieting and LOC or emotional eating. The group is provided with case examples that illustrate a young adult with BED, a teenager with uncomplicated obesity, and an adolescent at high risk for adult obesity by virtue of a current BMI percentile above average and LOC eating behaviors. The last example is designed to reflect characteristics of teens participating in the group. During this stage, members role-play fictional conflicts, most of which are common to teens (e.g., arguing with a parent about curfew). By the end of this phase, participants are encouraged to link their own interpersonal conflicts to their eating. For example, a member might discuss a personal tendency to avoid arguments by walking away and then, in turn, overeating and feeling unable to stop.
- *Middle phase*: During this phase, participants are encouraged to discuss interpersonal conflicts that occurred over the week and then analyze them during the group session. Members are asked to practice role-playing how a conversation might progress using new skills. Group leaders assign specific tasks for participants to try at home.
- *Termination phase*: In addition to acknowledging the difficulty in ending the group, the therapists focus on the work accomplished and assure members of their achievements and abilities to continue to make improvements in their relationships and eating patterns. Plans for future work and warning signs, signaling a need to seek additional help, are discussed.

As described by Mufson and colleagues, members use the IPT group sessions to discuss problems they are having with family and friends and to learn whether or not their situations differs from those of other adolescents (Mufson, Gallagher, Dorta, & Young, 2004). Overweight adolescents and those at risk for overweight can identify with one another regarding body shape and weight and eating concerns, as well as problems more specific to teenagers such as peer pressure. Group members then generate potential solutions to problems and practice role-playing by utilizing their newly learned skills within the group before attempting new forms of communication in their outside relationships (Young et al., 2006). Ultimately, by finding ways to improve interactions with parents and peers and subsequently developing more satisfying relationships, teens who are overweight and at risk for overweight can improve their self-esteem and mood while reducing their reliance on disturbed eating patterns to cope with negative interactions and emotions. In turn, we hypothesize that such individuals will be less likely to gain excessive weight attributable to LOC eating.

CASE EXAMPLE

The following case example briefly illustrates the presentation of a patient at intake. We have additionally outlined the conceptualization as well as the agreed-upon goals.

Presentation. Nancy is a 14-year-old female with a BMI between the 85th and 90th percentiles for her age and sex. At intake, she reported engaging in three episodes of LOC eating during the month prior to intake. Although she was unable to link her LOC eating episodes to a specific interaction or trigger, she reported feeling "numbed out" while eating and guilt following such episodes. Nancy described intense distress concerning her body weight and shape, as well as her eating habits both during and outside episodes of LOC. She indicated that she spent a considerable number of days during the past month dieting because of the fear that she might gain more weight or become fat. She reported that she looks "ugly." In addition, Nancy endorsed eating in response to feeling excited and reported that she eats when she is not hungry, if she feels tired, or if the food around her looks, tastes, or smells very good. Nancy did not appear to suffer from any diagnosable psychiatric disturbance, but reported some symptoms of depression and anxiety. Her general self-esteem was normative, but her self-esteem related to her body was quite low.

Nancy reported a great deal of conflict with her family, particularly with her mother whom she described as hurtful and mean. Her mother, a slender and successful professional, frequently criticized Nancy, both privately and publicly, about her body weight. They often argued about Nancy's grades and, according to Nancy, she was excluded from a family vacation as the result of one poor grade. Furthermore, her mother does not allow her certain privileges that her friends are granted, such as staying out late on weekend nights. She reported that she and her mother cannot "talk" but only "yell." Fights typically resulted in Nancy's "giving up" for fear that she might lose additional privileges. Thus, she expended a great deal of energy in holding in her frustration. Although she reported satisfaction with her social life, during her pretreatment meeting it became evident that she often did not share her feelings with other girls whom she described as her best friends. Furthermore, Nancy often refrained from sharing differences of opinions with her friends for fear that they might "turn on her." She reported feeling irritable much of the time.

Conceptualization. Nancy and her mother had difficulty in negotiating their relationship and Nancy's role as an adolescent trying, unsuccessfully, to assert independence (role dispute). Furthermore, Nancy had difficulty in telling her mother that criticisms, particularly about her body weight, were hurtful and unacceptable to her. Nancy also suffered from interpersonal deficits. She lacked the capacity to state her desires, feelings, and opinions with her friends because of a fear of being disliked and rejected. With her mother, she was unable to communicate her feelings without becoming frustrated and, therefore, often opted to avoid discussion. To deal with her negative feelings, she avoided communication and turned to food.

Goals. The therapists and Nancy agreed on the following therapy goals: First, Nancy would more directly express to her mother how her comments about Nancy's weight make her feel. Moreover, she agreed to work on expressing these feelings more consistently, calmly, and without fear that she might lose privileges. Second, Nancy would work to begin sharing her feelings more in order to reduce her irritability and prevent her frustration from building up and thus lessen the likelihood of her turning to food.

In Table 20.1 we illustrate the courses of treatment for three additional cases (Tanofsky-Kraff, Wilfley, et al., 2007). In a pilot study testing IPT-WG as compared with

TABLE 20.1. IPT-WG Sample Case Conceptualizations and Courses of Treatment

LOC eating precipitant(s)	Interpersonal functioning	Problem area	Goal	Initial phase	Middle phase	Termination phase
Case 1						
Sadness, stress, and worry	Repeated heated arguments with mother	Role dispute	Gain perspective to decrease frustration and remain calm when communicating with mother	Sharing feelings of frustration with mother; in group role-play of discussions with mother	Discuss resistance to speaking with mother; with group encouragement, begin productive dialogues with mother	Emphasis on improved communication skills; discussion of transferring use of skills to other close interpersonal relationships; gaining other outside supports
Case 2						
Avoiding conflict and negative affect	Does not express negative feelings or discomfort with conflict in multiple relationships	Interpersonal deficits	Become more comfortable with conflict and work on expressing feelings	Discuss discomfort about interactions involving conflict	Practice sharing feelings via role-playing; encouraged to communicate feelings with less tense relationship	Emphasis on improved communication skills; focus on future generalizing of skills to several situations
Case 3						
Boredom and frustration	Expresses emotions/needs to family (especially parents) in nonproductive manner	Role dispute	Use more constructive communication to express self	Communication analysis and in group role play of poor interactions	Continued role-playing specific situations and trying out discussions with siblings	Emphasis on improved communication skills; focus on future sharing of deeper personal conflicts with parents

Note. From Tanofsky-Kraff, Wilfley, et al. (2007). Copyright 2007 by Marian Tanofsky-Kraff. Reprinted by permission.

a standard health education program (Bravender, 2005), IPT-WG was shown to be both feasible and acceptable to adolescent girls (Tanofsky-Kraff et al., 2009). Moreover, more girls in IPT than in health education experienced weight stabilization or weight loss, as compared with weight gain, at the last measured observation. An adequately powered controlled trial is currently under way to determine the effectiveness of IPT-WG for the prevention of excess weight gain.

Summary

In conclusion, binge eating, LOC eating, EAH, eating in secret, and emotional eating are aberrant eating patterns that have traditionally not been considered as treatment targets in youth with eating and weight-related problems. Although further research is required for a complete understanding of the correlates and outcomes of such behaviors, there are data to support the possibility that these patterns can overlap and predict adverse outcomes. Considering the high prevalence of pediatric obesity and the generally poor long-term maintenance of traditional weight loss treatment programs, targeting aberrant eating patterns may offer a novel approach to reducing the current rates of obesity. Moreover, such approaches may have the added benefit of simultaneously preventing the development of full-syndrome eating disorders.

References

Ackard, D. M., Neumark-Sztainer, D., Story, M., & Perry, C. (2003). Overeating among adolescents: Prevalence and associations with weight-related characteristics and psychological health. *Pediatrics, 111*, 67–74.

American Psychiatric Association. (2000). *Diagnostic and statistical manual of mental disorders* (4th ed., text rev.). Washington, DC: American Psychiatric Association.

Anderson, S. E., Cohen, P., Naumova, E. N., & Must, A. (2006). Association of depression and anxiety disorders with weight change in a prospective community-based study of children followed up into adulthood. *Archives of Pediatrics and Adolescent Medicine, 160*(3), 285–291.

Bloom, T., Sharpe, L., Heriot, S., Zucker, N., & Craighead, L. (2005, June). *Children's appetite-awareness training (CAAT): A cognitive-behavioural intervention in the treatment of childhood obesity.* Paper presented at the WHO Expert Meeting on Childhood Obesity, Kobe, Japan.

Boutelle, K. N., Zucker, N., Rydell, S., Cafri, G., Peterson, C., & Harnack, L. (2009). *Changes in restraint and binge eating in treatments for childhood overeating: The effect of focusing on external and internal cues.* Paper presented at the Eating Disorders Research Society, New York.

Boutelle, K. N., Zucker, N., Rydell, S., Peterson, C., & Harnack, L. (2009). *VOLCRAVO: An exposure-based intervention to address food cravings and eating in the absence of hunger in children.* Paper presented at the Association of Behavioral and Cognitive Therapies, Washington, DC.

Braet, C., & Van Strien, T. (1997). Assessment of emotional, externally induced and restrained eating behaviour in nine- to twelve-year-old obese and non-obese children. *Behavior Research and Therapy, 35*(9), 863–873.

Bravender, T. (2005). *Health, education, and youth in Durham: HEY-Durham curricular guide* (2nd ed.). Durham, NC: Duke University.

Bulik, C. M., Sullivan, P. F., Carter, F. A., McIntosh, V. V., & Joyce, P. R. (1998). The role of exposure with response prevention in the cognitive-behavioural therapy for bulimia nervosa. *Psychological Medicine, 28*(3), 611–623.

Carter, F. A., Bulik, C. M., McIntosh, V. V., & Joyce, P. R. (2002). Cue reactivity as a predictor of outcome with bulimia nervosa. *International Journal of Eating Disorders, 31*(3), 240–250.

Childress, A. R., Hole, A. V., Ehrman, R. N., Robbins, S. J., McLellan, A. T., & O'Brien, C. P. (1993). Cue reactivity and cue reactivity interventions in drug dependence. *NIDA Research Monograph, 137*, 73–95.

Church, T. S., Earnest, C. P., Skinner, J. S., & Blair, S. N. (2007). Effects of different doses of physical activity on cardiorespiratory fitness among sedentary, overweight or obese postmenopausal women with elevated blood pressure: A randomized controlled trial. *Journal of the American Medical Association, 297*(19), 2081–2091.

Craighead, L. W., & Allen, H. N. (1995). Appetite awareness training: A cognitive-behavioral intervention for binge-eating. *Cognitive and Behavioral Practice, 2*(2), 249–270.

Crow, S. J., Agras, W. S., Halmi, K., Mitchell, J. E., & Kraemer, H. C. (2002). Full syndromal versus subthreshold anorexia nervosa, bulimia nervosa, and binge eating disorder: A multicenter study. *International Journal of Eating Disorders, 32*(3), 309–318.

Czaja, J., Rief, W., & Hilbert, A. (2009). Emotion regulation and binge eating in children. *International Journal of Eating Disorders, 42*(4), 356–362.

Drummond, D. C., & Glautier, S. (1994). A controlled trial of cue exposure treatment in alcohol dependence. *Journal of Consulting and Clinical Psychology, 62*(4), 809–817.

Elliott, C. A., Tanofsky-Kraff, M., Shomaker, L. B., Columbo, K. M., Wolkoff, L. E., Ranzenhofer, L. M., et al. (2010). An examination of the interpersonal model of loss of control eating in children and adolescents. *Behavior Research and Therapy, 48*(5), 424–428.

Epstein, L. H., Myers, M. D., Raynor, H. A., & Saelens, B. E. (1998). Treatment of pediatric obesity. *Pediatrics, 101*(3, Pt. 2), 554–570.

Epstein, L. H., Paluch, R. A., Saelens, B. E., Ernst, M. M., & Wilfley, D. E. (2001). Changes in eating disorder symptoms with pediatric obesity treatment. *Journal of Pediatrics, 139*(1), 58–65.

Fairburn, C. G., Cooper, Z., Doll, H. A., & Davies, B. A. (2005). Identifying dieters who will develop an eating disorder: A prospective, population-based study. *American Journal of Psychiatry, 162*(12), 2249–2255.

Fairburn, C. G., Cooper, Z., Doll, H. A., Norman, P., & O'Connor, M. (2000). The natural course of bulimia nervosa and binge eating disorder in young women. *Archives of General Psychiatry, 57*(7), 659–665.

Faith, M. S., Allison, D. B., & Geliebter, A. (1997). Emotional eating and obesity: Theoretical considerations and practical recommendations. In S. Dalton (Ed.), *Obesity and weight control: The health professional's guide to understanding and treatment* (pp. 439–465). Gaithersburg, MD: Aspen.

Faith, M. S., Berkowitz, R. I., Stallings, V. A., Kerns, J., Storey, M., & Stunkard, A. J. (2006). Eating in the absence of hunger: A genetic marker for childhood obesity in prepubertal boys? *Obesity, 14*(1), 131–138.

Fallon, E. M., Tanofsky-Kraff, M., Norman, A. C., McDuffie, J. R., Taylor, E. D., Cohen, M. L., et al. (2005). Health-related quality of life in overweight and nonoverweight black and white adolescents. *Journal of Pediatrics, 147*(4), 443–450.

Field, A. E., Austin, S. B., Taylor, C. B., Malspeis, S., Rosner, B., Rockett, H. R., et al. (2003). Relation between dieting and weight change among preadolescents and adolescents. *Pediatrics, 112*, 900–906.

Field, A. E., Camargo, C. A., Jr., Taylor, C. B., Berkey, C. S., Frazier, A. L., Gillman, M. W., et al. (1999). Overweight, weight concerns, and bulimic behaviors among girls and boys. *Journal of the American Academy of Child and Adolescent Psychiatry, 38*, 754–760.

Field, A. E., Colditz, G. A., & Peterson, K. E. (1997). Racial differences in bulimic behaviors among high school females. *Annals of the New York Academy of Sciences, 817*, 359–360.

Field, A. E., Cook, N. R., & Gillman, M. W.

(2005). Weight status in childhood as a predictor of becoming overweight or hypertensive in early adulthood. *Obesity Research, 13*(1), 163–169.

Fisher, J. O., & Birch, L. L. (1999). Restricting access to foods and children's eating. *Appetite, 32*(3), 405–419.

Fisher, J. O., & Birch, L. L. (2002). Eating in the absence of hunger and overweight in girls from 5 to 7 years of age. *American Journal of Clinical Nutrition, 76*(1), 226–231.

Fisher, J. O., Cai, G., Jaramillo, S. J., Cole, S. A., Comuzzie, A. G., & Butte, N. F. (2007). Heritability of hyperphagic eating behavior and appetite-related hormones among Hispanic children. *Obesity, 15*(6), 1484–1495.

Francis, L. A., & Birch, L. L. (2005). Maternal influences on daughters' restrained eating behavior. *Health Psychology, 24*(6), 548–554.

Franken, I. H., de Haan, H. A., van der Meer, C. W., Haffmans, P. M., & Hendriks, V. M. (1999). Cue reactivity and effects of cue exposure in abstinent posttreatment drug users. *Journal of Substance Abuse Treatment, 16*(1), 81–85.

Freedman, D. S., Khan, L. K., Dietz, W. H., Srinivasan, S. R., & Berenson, G. S. (2001). Relationship of childhood obesity to coronary heart disease risk factors in adulthood: The Bogalusa heart study. *Pediatrics, 108*(3), 712–718.

Glasofer, D. R., Tanofsky-Kraff, M., Eddy, K. T., Yanovski, S. Z., Theim, K. R., Mirch, M. C., et al. (2007). Binge eating in overweight treatment-seeking adolescents. *Journal of Pediatric Psychology, 32*(1), 95–105.

Goodman, E., & Whitaker, R. C. (2002). A prospective study of the role of depression in the development and persistence of adolescent obesity. *Pediatrics, 110*(3), 497–504.

Goossens, L., Braet, C., & Decaluwe, V. (2007). Loss of control over eating in obese youngsters. *Behavior Research and Therapy, 45*(1), 1–9.

Goossens, L., Soenens, B., & Braet, C. (2009). Prevalence and characteristics of binge eating in an adolescent community sample. *Journal of Clinical Child and Adolescent Psychology, 38*(3), 342–353.

Havermans, R. C., Debaere, S., Smulders, F. T.,

Wiers, R. W., & Jansen, A. T. (2003). Effect of cue exposure, urge to smoke, and nicotine deprivation on cognitive performance in smokers. *Psychology of Addictive Behaviors, 17*(4), 336–339.

Hayden-Wade, H. A., Stein, R. I., Ghaderi, A., Saelens, B. E., Zabinski, M. F., & Wilfley, D. E. (2005). Prevalence, characteristics, and correlates of teasing experiences among overweight children vs. non-overweight peers. *Obesity Research, 13*(8), 1381–1392.

Hill, J. O., & Peters, J. C. (1998). Environmental contributions to the obesity epidemic. *Science, 280*, 1371–1374.

Jansen, A. (1994). The learned nature of binge eating. In C. Legg & D. A. Booth (Eds.), *Appetite, neural and behavioral bases* (pp. 193–211). Oxford, UK: Oxford University Press.

Jansen, A. (1998). A learning model of binge eating: Cue reactivity and cue exposure. *Behavior Research and Therapy, 36*(3), 257–272.

Johnson, J. G., Spitzer, R. L., & Williams, J. B. (2001). Health problems, impairment and illnesses associated with bulimia nervosa and binge eating disorder among primary care and obstetric gynaecology patients. *Psychological Medicine, 31*(8), 1455–1466.

Johnson, S. L. (2000). Improving preschoolers' self-regulation of energy intake. *Pediatrics, 106*(6), 1429–1435.

Jones, M., Luce, K. H., Osborne, M. I., Taylor, K., Cunning, D., Doyle, A. C., et al. (2008). Randomized, controlled trial of an Internet-facilitated intervention for reducing binge eating and overweight in adolescents. *Pediatrics, 121*(3), 453–462.

King, N. A., Caudwell, P., Hopkins, M., Byrne, N. M., Colley, R., Hills, A. P., et al. (2007). Metabolic and behavioral compensatory responses to exercise interventions: Barriers to weight loss. *Obesity, 15*(6), 1373–1383.

Klerman, G. L., Weissman, M. M., Rounsaville, B. J., & Chevron, E. S. (1984). *Interpersonal psychotherapy of depression.* New York: Basic Books.

Knatz, S., Manginot, T., Story, M., Neumark-Sztainer, D., & Boutelle, K. (2011). Prevalence rates and psychological predictors of secretive eating in overweight and obese adolescents. *Childhood Obesity, 7*(1), 30–35.

Lamerz, A., Kuepper-Nybelen, J., Bruning, N., Wehle, C., Trost-Brinkhues, G., Brenner, H., et al. (2005). Prevalence of obesity, binge eating, and night eating in a cross-sectional field survey of 6-year-old children and their parents in a German urban population. *Journal of Child Psychology and Psychiatry and Allied Disciplines, 46*(4), 385–393.

Moens, E., & Braet, C. (2007). Predictors of disinhibited eating in children with and without overweight. *Behavior Research and Therapy, 45*(6), 1357–1368.

Monti, P. M., & Rohsenow, D. J. (1999). Coping-skills training and cue-exposure therapy in the treatment of alcoholism. *Alcohol Research Health, 23*(2), 107–115.

Moreau, D., Mufson, L., Weissman, M. M., & Klerman, G. L. (1991). Interpersonal psychotherapy for adolescent depression: Description of modification and preliminary application. *Journal of the American Academy of Child and Adolescent Psychiatry, 30*(4), 642–651.

Morgan, C., Yanovski, S., Nguyen, T., McDuffie, J., Sebring, N., Jorge, M., et al. (2002). Loss of control over eating, adiposity, and psychopathology in overweight children. *International Journal of Eating Disorders, 31*(4), 430–441.

Mufson, L., Dorta, K. P., Moreau, D., & Weissman, M. M. (2004). *Interpersonal psychotherapy for depressed adolescents* (2nd ed.). New York: Guilford Press.

Mufson, L., Dorta, K. P., Wickramaratne, P., Nomura, Y., Olfson, M., & Weissman, M. M. (2004). A randomized effectiveness trial of interpersonal psychotherapy for depressed adolescents. *Archives of General Psychiatry, 61*(6), 577–584.

Mufson, L., Gallagher, T., Dorta, K. P., & Young, J. F. (2004). A group adaptation of interpersonal psychotherapy for depressed adolescents. *American Journal of Psychotherapy, 58*(2), 220–237.

Mussell, M. P., Mitchell, J. E., Weller, C. L., Raymond, N. C., Crow, S. J., & Crosby, R. D. (1995). Onset of binge eating, dieting, obesity, and mood disorders among subjects seeking treatment for binge eating disorder. *International Journal of Eating Disorders, 17*(4), 395–401.

Neumark-Sztainer, D., Story, M., French, S. A., Hannan, P. J., Resnick, M. D., & Blum, R. W. (1997). Psychosocial concerns and health-compromising behaviors among overweight and nonoverweight adolescents. *Obesity Research, 5,* 237–249.

Niaura, R., Abrams, D. B., Shadel, W. G., Rohsenow, D. J., Monti, P. M., & Sirota, A. D. (1999). Cue exposure treatment for smoking relapse prevention: A controlled clinical trial. *Addiction, 94*(5), 685–695.

Ogden, C. L., Carroll, M. D., Curtin, L. R., Lamb, M. M., & Flegal, K. M. (2010). Prevalence of high body mass index in US children and adolescents, 2007–2008. *Journal of the American Medical Association, 303*(3), 242–249.

Ogden, C. L., Carroll, M. D., Curtin, L. R., McDowell, M. A., Tabak, C. J., & Flegal, K. M. (2006). Prevalence of overweight and obesity in the United States, 1999–2004. *Journal of the American Medical Association, 295*(13), 1549–1555.

Ogden, C. L., Kuczmarski, R. J., Flegal, K. M., Mei, Z., Guo, S., Wei, R., et al. (2002). Centers for Disease Control and Prevention 2000 growth charts for the United States: Improvements to the 1977 National Center for Health Statistics version. *Pediatrics, 109*(1), 45–60.

Pearce, M. J., Boergers, J., & Prinstein, M. J. (2002). Adolescent obesity, overt and relational peer victimization, and romantic relationships. *Obesity Research, 10*(5), 386–393.

Pine, D. S., Goldstein, R. B., Wolk, S., & Weissman, M. M. (2001). The association between childhood depression and adulthood body mass index. *Pediatrics, 107*(5), 1049–1056.

Presnell, K., Stice, E., Seidel, A., & Madeley, M. C. (2009). Depression and eating pathology: Prospective reciprocal relations in adolescents. *Clinical Psychology and Psychotherapy, 16*(4), 357–365.

Rossello, J., & Bernal, G. (1999). The efficacy of cognitive-behavioral and interpersonal treatments for depression in Puerto Rican adolescents. *Journal of Consulting and Clinical Psychology, 67*(5), 734–745.

Schachter, S. (1971). Some extraordinary facts about obese humans and rats. *American Psychologist, 26*, 129–144.

Schachter, S., & Rodin, J. (1974). *Obese humans and rats.* Washington, DC: Erlbaum/Halsted.

Schwimmer, J. B., Burwinkle, T. M., & Varni, J. W. (2003). Health-related quality of life of severely obese children and adolescents. *Journal of the American Medical Association, 289*(14), 1813–1819.

Shapiro, J. R., Woolson, S. L., Hamer, R. M., Kalarchian, M. A., Marcus, M. D., & Bulik, C. M. (2007). Evaluating binge eating disorder in children: Development of the Children's Binge Eating Disorder Scale (C-BEDS). *International Journal of Eating Disorders, 40*(1), 82–89.

Shomaker, L. B., Tanofsky-Kraff, M., Elliott, C., Wolkoff, L. E., Columbo, K. M., Ranzenhofer, L. M., et al. (2010). Salience of loss of control for pediatric binge episodes: Does size really matter? *International Journal of Eating Disorders, 43*(8), 707–716.

Shomaker, L. B., Tanofsky-Kraff, M., & Yanovski, J. A. (in press). Disinhibited eating and body weight in youth. In V. R. Preedy, R. R. Watson, & C. R. Watson (Eds.), *International handbook of behavior, food and nutrition.* New York: Springer.

Shunk, J. A., & Birch, L. L. (2004). Girls at risk for overweight at age 5 are at risk for dietary restraint, disinhibited overeating, weight concerns, and greater weight gain from 5 to 9 years. *Journal of the American Dietetic Association, 104*(7), 1120–1126.

Snoek, H. M., Van Strien, T., Janssens, J. M., & Engels, R. C. (2007). Emotional, external, restrained eating and overweight in Dutch adolescents. *Scandanavian Journal of Psychology, 48*(1), 23–32.

Sonneville, K. R., & Gortmaker, S. L. (2008). Total energy intake, adolescent discretionary behaviors and the energy gap. *International Journal of Obesity, 32*(Suppl. 6), S19–S27.

Stice, E., Cameron, R. P., Killen, J. D., Hayward, C., & Taylor, C. B. (1999). Naturalistic weight-reduction efforts prospectively predict growth in relative weight and onset of obesity among female adolescents. *Journal of Consulting and Clinical Psychology, 67*(6), 967–974.

Stice, E., Presnell, K., Shaw, H., & Rohde, P. (2005). Psychological and behavioral risk factors for obesity onset in adolescent girls: A prospective study. *Journal of Consulting and Clinical Psychology, 73*(2), 195–202.

Stice, E., Presnell, K., & Spangler, D. (2002). Risk factors for binge eating onset in adolescent girls: A 2-year prospective investigation. *Health Psychology, 21*(2), 131–138.

Strauss, R. S., & Pollack, H. A. (2003). Social marginalization of overweight children. *Archives of Pediatrics and Adolescent Medicine, 157*(8), 746–752.

Striegel-Moore, R. H., Silberstein, L. R., & Rodin, J. (1986). Toward an understanding of risk factors for bulimia. *American Psychologist, 41*(3), 246–263.

Tanofsky-Kraff, M. (2008). Binge eating among children and adolescents. In E. Jelalian & R. Steele (Eds.), *Handbook of child and adolescent obesity* (pp. 41–57). New York: Springer.

Tanofsky-Kraff, M., Cohen, M. L., Yanovski, S. Z., Cox, C., Theim, K. R., Keil, M., et al. (2006). A prospective study of psychological predictors of body fat gain among children at high risk for adult obesity. *Pediatrics, 117*(4), 1203–1209.

Tanofsky-Kraff, M., Goossens, L., Eddy, K. T., Ringham, R., Goldschmidt, A., Yanovski, S. Z., et al. (2007). A multisite investigation of binge eating behaviors in children and adolescents. *Journal of Consultation and Clinical Psychology, 75*(6), 901–913.

Tanofsky-Kraff, M., Theim, K. R., Yanovski, S. Z., Bassett, A. M., Burns, N. P., Ranzenhofer, L. M., et al. (2007). Validation of the emotional eating scale adapted for use in children and adolescents (EES-C). *International Journal of Eating Disorders, 40*(3), 232–240.

Tanofsky-Kraff, M., Wilfley, D. E., Young, J. F., Mufson, L., Yanovski, S. Z., Glasofer, D. R., et al. (2007). Preventing excessive weight gain in adolescents: Interpersonal psychotherapy for binge eating. *Obesity, 15*(6), 1345–1355.

Tanofsky-Kraff, M., Yanovski, S. Z., Schvey, N. A., Olsen, C. H., Gustafson, J., & Yanovski, J. A. (2009). A prospective study of loss of control eating for body weight gain in children at high risk for adult obesity. *International Journal of Eating Disorders, 42*(1), 26–30.

Tanofsky-Kraff, M., Yanovski, S. Z., Wilfley, D. E., Marmarosh, C., Morgan, C. M., & Yanovski, J. A. (2004). Eating disordered behaviors, body fat, and psychopathology in overweight and normal weight children. *Journal of Consulting and Clinical Psychology, 72*, 53–61.

Toro, J., Cervera, M., Feliu, M. H., Garriga, N., Jou, M., Martinez, E., et al. (2003). Cue exposure in the treatment of resistant bulimia nervosa. *International Journal of Eating Disorders, 34*(2), 227–234.

Van Strien, T., Engels, R. C., Van Leeuwe, J., & Snoek, H. M. (2005). The Stice model of overeating: Tests in clinical and non-clinical samples. *Appetite, 45*(3), 205–213.

Vervaet, M., & Van Heeringen, C. (2000). Eating style and weight concerns in young females. *Eating Disorders, 8*(3), 233–240

Wardle, J. (1990). Conditioning processes and cue exposure in the modification of excessive eating. *Addictive Behaviors, 15*(4), 387–393.

Weiss, R., Dziura, J., Burgert, T. S., Tamborlane, W. V., Taksali, S. E., Yeckel, C. W., et al. (2004). Obesity and the metabolic syndrome in children and adolescents. *New England Journal of Medicine, 350*(23), 2362–2374.

Weissman, M. M., Markowitz, J., & Klerman, G. L. (2000). *Comprehensive guide to interpersonal psychotherapy.* New York: Basic Behavioral Science Books.

Wilfley, D. E., Agras, W. S., Telch, C. F., Rossiter, E. M., Schneider, J. A., Cole, A. G., et al. (1993). Group cognitive-behavioral therapy and group interpersonal psychotherapy for the nonpurging bulimic individual: A controlled comparison. *Journal of Consulting and Clinical Psychology, 61*(2), 296–305.

Wilfley, D. E., Frank, M. A., Welch, R. R., Spurrell, E. B., & Rounsaville, B. J. (1998). Adapting interpersonal psychotherapy to a group format (IPT-G) for binge eating disorder: Toward a model for adapting empirically supported treatments. *Psychotherapy Research, 8*, 379–391.

Wilfley, D. E., MacKenzie, K. R., Welch, R. R., Ayres, V. E., & Weissman, M. M. (2000). *Interpersonal psychotherapy for group.* New York: Basic Books.

Wilfley, D. E., Pike, K. M., & Striegel-Moore, R. H. (1997). Toward an integrated model of risk for binge eating disorder. *Journal of Gender, Culture, and Health, 2*, 1–3.

Wilfley, D. E., Stein, R. I., Saelens, B. E., Mockus, D. S., Matt, G. E., Hayden-Wade, H. A., et al. (2007). Efficacy of maintenance treatment approaches for childhood overweight: A randomized controlled trial. *Journal of the American Medical Association, 298*(14), 1661–1673.

Wilfley, D. E., Welch, R. R., Stein, R. I., Spurrell, E. B., Cohen, L. R., Saelens, B. E., et al. (2002). A randomized comparison of group cognitive-behavioral therapy and group interpersonal psychotherapy for the treatment of overweight individuals with binge-eating disorder. *Archives of General Psychiatry, 59*(8), 713–721.

Wilson, G. T., Wilfley, D. E., Agras, W. S., & Bryson, S. W. (2010). Psychological treatments of binge eating disorder. *Archives of General Psychiatry, 67*(1), 94–101.

Wing, R. R., & Jeffery, R. W. (1999). Benefits of recruiting participants with friends and increasing social support for weight loss and maintenance. *Journal of Consulting and Clinical Psychology, 67*(1), 132–138.

Young, J. F., Mufson, L., & Davies, M. (2006). Efficacy of interpersonal psychotherapy—adolescent skills training: An indicated preventive intervention for depression. *Journal of Child Psychology and Psychiatry, 47*(12), 1254–1262.

CHAPTER 21

Pharmacotherapy for Eating Disorders in Children and Adolescents

Jennifer Couturier
Wendy Spettigue

Although the use of medications to treat children and adolescents suffering from eating disorders is common in clinical practice, there is actually little empirical support for the use of medication in this population. This chapter reviews the literature on pharmacotherapy for children and adolescents with eating disorders, first focusing on anorexia nervosa (AN), then on bulimia nervosa (BN), followed by a short comment on eating disorder not otherwise specified (EDNOS), including binge-eating disorder (BED). The literature was reviewed by searching the PubMed database for all articles on medication use in the child and adolescent population using the terms "medication," "antipsychotic," "antidepressant," "pharmacotherapy," "child," "adolescent," "eating disorders," "anorexia nervosa," "bulimia nervosa," and "binge-eating disorder." Because of the paucity of literature in the child and adolescent area, some studies on pharmacotherapy for adults with eating disorders are discussed, as well as some recent research findings presented at conferences.

Pharmacotherapy for AN

In general, treatment guidelines suggest that medication should not be used as the primary treatment for children and adolescents with AN (American Psychiatric Association, 2006; National Institute for Clinical Excellence, 2004). These guidelines suggest that family-based psychological treatments that focus on renourishment of the affected child should be the first-line treatment for children and adolescents with AN, and that medication should be used only to treat comorbid conditions. However, caution should be used in treating depressive or obsessive–compulsive symptoms, especially those associated with low body weight, as these symptoms often resolve with weight gain (Meehan, Loeb, Roberto, & Attia, 2006). In these situations, a good longitudinal history is important in determining whether the comorbid symptoms preceded the onset of the eating disorder, in which case treatment of these comorbidities is indicated once the patient has been renourished. There is currently little evidence that medication is effective for patients in the starved state, although the atypical antipsychotics may be useful, particularly in agitated patients.

Antipsychotics

Atypical antipsychotics are being increasingly used for the treatment of AN in both adults and youth. They have known calming properties, and their side effects of sedation and weight gain, which can be problematic for other populations, are of potential benefit for patients who need to gain weight. Additional symptom targets for the atypical agents include body image distortion, obsessiveness, and anxiety. Therefore, although the exact mechanism by which these medications work in AN are unknown, they appear to have some usefulness in terms of both weight gain and cognition. The literature on the use of atypical antipsychotics in adolescent AN is mostly limited to case reports; thus, some additional results from recent conference proceedings, and some studies involving adults, are discussed here.

After clozapine, olanzapine is the atypical antipsychotic associated with the most weight gain (Sussman, 2001; Taylor & McAskill, 2000). (Clozapine should be avoided in this population because of serious side effects of significant postural hypotension and agranulocytosis.) Dennis, Le Grange, and Bremer (2006) used olanzapine at a dose of 5 mg daily in five adolescent females with AN and found an increase in body mass index (BMI), reduction of body concerns, and improvements in sleep and anxiety concerning food and weight. Another case series, involving four patients ages 10–12 years, used olanzapine at a dose of 2.5 mg daily to treat children and adolescents with AN at low body weights (Boachie, Goldfield, & Spettigue, 2003). The authors reported improvements in compliance and weight gain, as well as decreases in agitation. Mehler and colleagues (2001) also reported on five female patients ages 12–17 years on a dose range of 5 mg–12.5 mg per day of olanzapine. They found improvements in body image distortion and rigidity. La Via, Gray, and Kaye (2000) described two females with AN who experienced reduction of inner tension and "paranoid ideas" with the use of 10 mg daily of olanzapine. One of these patients was a 16-year-old. There is also a case report of a 15-year-old treated with 10 mg of olanzapine daily who experienced an increase in BMI, along with a reduction of obsessive–compulsive symptoms, exercising, and anorexic cognitions (Ercan, Copkunol, Cykoethlu, & Varan, 2003). There is an additional case report of using olanzapine to treat a 17-year-old girl with AN and comorbid pervasive developmental disorder not otherwise specified at dose of 5 mg daily (Tateno, Teshirogi, Kamasaki, & Saito, 2008). The authors reported weight restoration and improvements in eating behavior within 5 months of initiating treatment.

In terms of treatment with other atypical antipsychotics, even fewer studies exist. Quetiapine has been used in three subjects ages 11–15 years with severe AN (lengthy hospitalization, use of nasogastric tubes, and BMI 12.3 to 13.9) (Mehler-Wex, Romanos, Kirchheiner, & Schulze, 2008). Two of these patients were treated with quetiapine, 100 mg twice daily, and one with 250 mg twice daily. The authors reported improvements in body image disturbance, weight phobia, and "paranoid ideas." Initial fatigue and constipation were side effects. As part of a larger study that also involved adults, Powers, Bannon, Eubanks, and McCormick (2007) reported on an open-label study of quetiapine. There were six adolescents ages 14–18 years in this study. The dose of quetiapine ranged from 150 mg daily to 300 mg daily. Improvements in anxiety and depression were noted.

There have also been two cases of adolescents described in which risperidone (1.5 mg daily) was added to antidepressant treatment, with improvements in anxiety and weight gain (Newman-Toker, 2000). In addition, there is one case report describing a 12-year-old girl with autism and AN who benefited from treatment with risperidone at a dose of 0.5 mg twice daily (Fisman, Steele, Short, Byrne, & Lavallee, 1996). However, a recent double-blind, placebo-controlled trial of risperidone involving 41 subjects ages 12–21 years found no significant differences between groups other than in drive for thinness (Hagman et al., 2009). The dose of risperidone in this study was started at 0.5 mg daily and tapered up by 0.5 mg per week to a maximum of 4 mg daily based on tolerability. The authors concluded that their results do not support the use of risperidone in the weight restoration phase of treatment for young patients with AN.

The safety of the atypical agents is yet to be determined, although they are thought to be safer than the typical agents. There are two studies providing details on adverse events in children and adolescents. Norris and colleagues (in press) completed a retrospective chart review that compared 43 adolescents with AN treated with olanzapine (mean age 14.4 years) with 43 matched control subjects. The authors described those patients treated with olanzapine as having greater illness severity and higher rates of comorbidity, as compared with those not treated with olanzapine. Inpatients treated with olanzapine had longer lengths of stay and higher BMIs at discharge than those in the control group, but there was no difference between groups in the rate of weekly weight gain. The authors reported adverse events in 56% of patients, the most common being sedation. Abnormal lipid profiles were reported in 29% of those youth who were tested. Olanzapine was discontinued in one patient after experiencing significant elevations in liver function tests (alanine aminotransferase increased from 101 to 457, aspartate aminotransferase increased from 61 to 297). Another patient experienced extrapyramidal side effects, which occurred at a low dosage (1.25 mg), and a further 11 patients (24%) stopped the medication secondary to other undesirable side effects, including perceived excess weight gain, increased hunger, subjective change in personality, increased agitation, nausea, vomiting, elevated prolactin, hypotension, eye twitching, and decreased motivation/energy. The most commonly cited reasons for termination of olanzapine were improvements in patients' psychological status or weight restoration (50%), refusal to continue taking medication (20%), and undesirable side effects (19%). Interestingly, 36% of patients restarted the olanzapine after initial discontinuation, most commonly because of increased psychological distress or significant weight loss.

The second study examined olanzapine and risperidone safety and tolerability in 25 adolescents with AN as compared with 25 control subjects who were not treated with these medications (Steinegger, Pinhas, Boachie, & Katzman, 2007). No laboratory or clinical side effects were identified in the majority of patients. Several patients decided to discontinue the medication (13% of those taking risperidone and 22% of those taking olanzapine). There were no differences in outcomes in terms of menstrual status, BMI, total admissions, or final disposition; however, discharge from the program was significantly faster in those treated with these medications.

In adult patients with AN, a recent randomized controlled trial has provided more support for the potential benefit of olanzapine. Bissada, Tasca, Barber, and Bradwejn (2008) randomized 34 women within a day treatment program to receive either olanzapine or placebo. The dose was started at 2.5 mg daily and then slowly titrated up to a maximum of 10 mg daily. The average daily dose was 6.61 mg. As compared with the placebo group, those taking olanzapine experienced a greater rate of weight gain and a decrease in obsessive symptoms. Brambilla and colleagues (2007) also found that in 30 patients with AN, those with the binge–purge type experienced improvements in BMI, depression, and "direct aggressiveness" when 2.5 mg–5 mg daily of olanzapine was used in combination with cognitive-behavioral therapy. One additional randomized trial compared eight patients treated with olanzapine (10 mg average dose) with seven patients given chlorpromazine (50 mg average dose) (Mondraty et al., 2005). This study demonstrated that although the group treated with olanzapine experienced significantly less rumination, no difference in weight gain was seen between the groups. There have also been several open trials of olanzapine showing various degrees of benefit for adults with AN (Barbarich, McConaha, Gaskill, et al., 2004; Malina et al., 2003; Powers, Santana, & Bannon, 2002), as well as open trials with quetiapine in adult populations (Bosanac et al., 2007; Powers et al., 2007). It should be noted that the atypical antipsychotic ziprasidone is not recommended because of the risk of QTc prolongation. (For more on the topic of atypical antipsychotics and QTc prolongation in AN, see Ritchie and Norris, 2009).

Typical antipsychotics have also been studied in adults with AN, beginning with a trial of chlorpromazine in 1960 (Dally & Sargant, 1960). Although patients gained weight, many experienced seizures and increased purging. Pimozide (Vandereycken & Pierloot, 1982) and sulpiride (Vandereycken, 1984) have also been studied in comparison with placebo, although with no significant benefit. It is thought that the risks such as seizures, cardiac conduction problems, and QTc prolongation outweigh any possible benefit with the typical antipsychotics.

Antidepressants

Antidepressants were first considered as possible treatments for AN in adults because the illness was associated with high rates of comorbid depression, and it was speculated that both disorders might have a common pathogenesis (Pollice, Kaye, Greeno, & Weltzin, 1997). However, results from earlier trials of antidepressants for the treatment of low-weight adults with AN were disappointing. This likely explains the lack of systematic research on antidepressant treatment for AN in youth. There is one retrospective study that compared 19 adolescent patients with AN taking selective serotonin reuptake inhibitors (SSRIs) with 13 patients with AN not treated with SSRIs (Holtkamp et al., 2005). The authors found that there were no differences between these groups, in terms of BMI, eating disorder psychopathology, or depressive and obsessive–compulsive symptoms, after evaluating patients on admission, discharge, and 1-year follow-up. The SSRIs involved in this study included fluoxetine (*n* = 7, mean dose 35 mg once daily), fluvoxamine (*n* = 8, mean dose 120 mg once daily), and sertraline (*n* = 4, mean dose 100 mg once daily). There is one other case-control study examining fluoxetine as an adjunct to intensive multidisciplinary inpatient treatment (Strober, Pataki, Freeman, & DeAntonio, 1999). No beneficial effect was found in global clinical severity of eating behavior or weight phobia. In terms of non-SSRI antidepressant treatment, there is one case report on the use of mirtazapine in a 16-year-old female hospitalized for AN and depression (Jaafar, Daud, Rahman, & Baharudin, 2007). The authors found positive results and suggested that further study of this medication is needed.

As previously mentioned, the studies of antidepressants for the treatment of adults with AN have been discouraging. Fluoxetine showed no benefit as compared with placebo in hospitalized patients (Attia, Haiman, Walsh, & Flater, 1998), even with the addition of tryptophan, which was used in an effort to increase serotonin substrate (Barbarich, McConaha, Halmi, et al., 2004). Furthermore, the studies on antidepressants to prevent relapse in adult patients with AN have shown mixed results. A study by Kaye and colleagues (2001) reported an increased time to relapse with fluoxetine treatment as compared with placebo in 35 patients who were weight restored; however, results must be interpreted with caution, given the high dropout rate: in the fluoxetine group, 10/16 (63%) completed the study, and in the placebo group only 3/19 (16%) completed the study. A more recent well-designed large randomized controlled trial comparing fluoxetine with placebo was less encouraging. The study involved 93 adults with AN whose weight had been restored in an inpatient or day treatment program. Patients in both groups were followed for 1 year and received outpatient cognitive-behavioral therapy. The results showed no significant difference in the time to relapse between the medication and control groups (Walsh et al., 2006). However, attrition rates in this study were also over 50%, making definitive conclusions problematic.

Historically, the tricyclic antidepressants (amitriptyline, clomipramine) have been studied in controlled trials with no benefit observed in terms of weight gain in hospitalized patients (Biederman et al., 1985; Halmi, Eckert, LaDu, & Cohen, 1986; Lacey & Crisp, 1980). These medications also had significant side effects, including prolongation of the QTc interval as well as constipation.

Despite these discouraging findings, some clinicians believe that children and adolescents may be more responsive than adults to SSRIs, possibly because these patients have typically had a shorter duration of illness and because parents might be more likely to ensure compliance with medication use. However, given the paucity of evidence and recent concerns about the safety of SSRIs in adolescents and children in terms of suicidal ideation, it is prudent to advise caution in using this class of medications for children and adolescents with AN (Lock, Walker, Rickert, & Katzman, 2005).

Other Medications

In addition to the antipsychotics and antidepressants used to treat AN, other medications have also been examined in randomized trials but have not proved efficacious and/ or have demonstrated detrimental side effects. Lithium showed some benefit in weight gain in a small placebo-controlled trial in adults but has significant side effects (Gross et al., 1981). Zinc has shown inconclusive results in three double-blind placebo-controlled trials, one of which involved children and adolescents (Birmingham, Goldner, & Bakan, 1994; Katz et al., 1987; Lask, Fosson, Rolfe, & Thomas, 1993). Cyproheptadine, which has appetite-enhancing effects, produced no significant benefit in weight gain in adults with AN (Goldberg, Halmi, Eckert, Casper, & Davis, 1979; Halmi et al., 1986). The prokinetic agent cisapride, once commonly used to treat gastric distress, has since been removed from the market because of QTc prolongation and cardiac arrhymias (Stacher et al., 1993; Szmukler, Young, Miller, Lichtenstein, & Binns, 1995). There have also been some small open trials of naloxone (Moore, Mills, & Forster, 1981) and naltrexone (Marrazzi, Bacon, Kinzie, & Luby, 1995) showing some benefits; however, no larger trials exist. Tetrahydrocannabinol was also compared with diazepam in an effort to increase appetite, but no benefit was found (Gross et al., 1983). Finally, estrogen has been studied in an effort to treat osteopenia and osteoporosis in AN. However, a recent meta-analysis failed to demonstrate clear efficacy in increasing bone-mineral density (Sim et al., 2010). In fact, estrogen may have negative psychological effects, as it artificially induces a menstrual cycle, thereby enhancing the denial associated with AN. Because of inconclusive results and risk of harm, estrogen is not recommended in this population (Sim et al., 2010).

Pharmacotherapy for BN

Treatment guidelines suggest that cognitive-behavioral therapy specifically adapted for BN should be offered as a first-line treatment, with fluoxetine added as adjunctive treatment for both adults and adolescents with BN (National Institute for Clinical Excellence, 2004). Patients should be informed that the long-term effects of treatment with fluoxetine are unknown. In terms of pharmacotherapy, antidepressants, particularly SSRIs, currently have the greatest evidence base for the treatment of BN, although the antidepressant bupropion is contraindicated because of the risk of seizures.

Antidepressants

Tricyclic antidepressants were first studied for the treatment of adults with BN because of the observation that depression was a common comorbidity, and that mood was related to binge eating and purging. It was hypothesized that improvement in mood might help patients to better control these symptoms (Mitchell, Agras, & Wonderlich, 2007). Early trials of imipramine and amitriptyline showed significant improvement in those taking the medications as compared with placebo, which was believed to be due to the antidepressant properties of these medications (Mitchell & Groat, 1984; Pope, Hudson, Jonas, & Yurgelun-Todd, 1983). This led to trials of monoamine oxidase inhibitors, SSRIs and other antidepressants in adults with BN, with similarly positive results. Further trials made clear that the antidepressants are effective for reducing binge-eating and purging symptoms even in nondepressed patients.

Although literature on medication use in adults with BN is abundant, only one pharmacotherapy study specific to adolescents with BN could be found. This was an open trial of fluoxetine in 10 adolescents ages 12–18 years (Kotler, Devlin, Davies, & Walsh, 2003). These adolescents received 8 weeks of fluoxetine at a daily dose of 60 mg along with supportive psychotherapy. The dose was titrated upwards as follows: 20 mg daily for 3 days, then 40 mg daily for 3 days, then up to 60 mg daily. The frequencies of binge episodes decreased significantly from an average of 4.1 to 0 episodes per week, and weekly purges decreased from 6.4 to 0.4 episodes. Seventy percent of patients were rated as improved or much improved on the clinical global impressions-improvement scale. No significant side effects were noted, and there were no dropouts due to adverse effects from the medication. Whether patients maintained these benefits over the long term is unknown.

In contrast to the single medication trial for adolescents with BN, there have been many studies confirming the effectiveness of SSRIs, particularly fluoxetine, for adults with BN. In fact, fluoxetine has received approval from the FDA for this patient population. It has been shown to be effective in reducing symptoms of binge eating and purging when used at a dose of 60 mg daily in several double-blind trials (Beumont et al., 1997; Fluoxetine Bulimia Nervosa Collaborative Study Group, 1992; Goldstein, Wilson,

Thompson, Potvin, & Rampey, 1995). The multisite BN collaborative trial was 8 weeks in duration, involving 387 women, in which 60 mg of fluoxetine was compared with 20 mg and with placebo. A 67% reduction in frequency of binge eating and 56% reduction in frequency of purging were observed in the 60 mg group, which were clearly superior to results in the 20 mg and placebo groups (Fluoxetine Bulimia Nervosa Collaborative Study Group, 1992). In a long-term follow-up study over a 1-year period, those who had responded to fluoxetine acutely at a dose of 60 mg daily were treated with a maintenance dose of 60 mg daily (Romano, Halmi, Sarkar, Koke, & Lee, 2002). Compared to those acute responders who were switched to a placebo, those who remained on a maintenance dose of 60 mg of fluoxetine experienced a significantly increased time to relapse, leading investigators to conclude that fluoxetine should be continued for a period of at least 1 year.

A Cochrane Review concluded that fluoxetine is the most systematically studied antidepressant agent and that its better side effect profile makes it superior to other drugs in treating BN. The reviewers suggested that fluoxetine should be the first-line agent for BN and that a daily dose of 60 mg is more effective than a dose of 20 mg (Bacaltchuk & Hay, 2003). Eight weeks appears to be an appropriate period to determine effectiveness. Other authors have indicated that treatment with fluoxetine decreases binge frequency by an average of 56%, as compared with 11% in placebo treatment (Jimerson, Herzog, & Brotman, 1993). Decreases in purging frequencies are similar. The effect of fluoxetine in treating BN does not appear to be related to the presence of a comorbid depression, as those with depression and those without depression fare equally well (Goldstein, Wilson, Ascroft, & al-Banna, 1999).

In terms of other SSRIs, sertraline has also been shown to be effective for adults with BN. Milano, Petrella, Sabatino, and Capasso (2004) completed a small randomized controlled trial involving 20 female outpatients at a mean dose of 100 mg daily. Individuals taking sertraline had significantly decreased frequencies of binge–purge episodes as compared with those taking a placebo. Fichter, Kruger, Rief, Holland, and Dohne (1996) found that fluvoxamine at a mean dose of 182 mg daily prevented relapse at a significantly higher rate as compared with placebo in a study of 117 adolescent and adult females with BN.

There have also been randomized controlled studies on non-SSRI antidepressants demonstrating effectiveness, as compared with placebo, including trazodone (Pope, Keck, McElroy, & Hudson, 1989) and desipramine (Walsh, Hadigan, Devlin, Gladis, & Roose, 1991). Because of the side effect profile of the tricyclic antidepressants, including cardiac complications associated with the electrolyte abnormalities seen in BN, and risks of death in overdose, SSRIs are a much preferred option, and the tricyclic antidepressants should generally be avoided. Monoamine oxidase inhibitors such as brofaromine have also been studied (Kennedy et al., 1993), but because of the risk of a hypertensive crisis during a binge episode, are not recommended.

Other Medications

With respect to other classes of medications, the anticonvulsant and mood stabilizer topiramate has also demonstrated effectiveness in a randomized controlled study of adults with BN (Hedges et al., 2003; Hoopes et al., 2003). This study randomized 68 subjects ages 16–50 years to treatment with topiramate (mean dose of 100 mg daily) or placebo over 10 weeks. Rates of abstinence from binge–purge episodes were 23% in the medication group as compared with 6% in the placebo group. Body dissatisfaction and drive for thinness were also significantly improved in the medication group. However, subjects experienced a 1.8-kg weight loss, so caution must be used in patients who are at average or below average weight. Side effects included word finding difficulties, somnolence, dizziness, and paresthesias. Ondansetron, a potent antiemetic drug, has also shown greater efficacy than placebo in a small randomized controlled trial involving 26 adult females with BN (Faris et al., 2000). However, because of its high cost it is not usually a feasible option.

Pharmacotherapy for EDNOS

Children and adolescents are often seen with a diagnosis of EDNOS, leaving clinicians uncertain of which course of treatment to take. Guidelines suggest that these individuals should be treated with the protocol for the disorder that most closely resembles their symptomatology (National Institute for Clinical Excellence, 2004). Therefore, if dietary restriction is most prominent, a protocol for AN may be considered, whereas if binge eating or purging is the main problem, a protocol for BN may be most appropriate. In general, atypical antipsychotics can be considered for low-weight, agitated patients who are struggling with the process of weight gain and renourishment, whereas fluoxetine is the first choice for young patients close to or above ideal weight who have symptoms of binge eating or purging, or comorbid affective or anxiety disorders.

For BED, no medication trials involving children and adolescents could be found. There are some clinical trials of pharmacotherapy for adults with BED, which are discussed here. For adults and adolescents with BED, psychological treatments adapted for BED, such as cognitive-behavioral therapy, dialectical behavior therapy, and interpersonal therapy, are suggested first-line treatments, with SSRIs as adjunctive treatments (National Institute for Clinical Excellence, 2004). A recent meta-analysis indicated that for adults with BED, psychotherapy (mainly cognitive-behavioral therapy) and structured self-help demonstrated the highest rates of abstinence from binge eating, followed by combination treatments and pharmacotherapy alone (Vocks et al., 2010). This meta-analysis concluded that pharmacotherapy has a moderately positive effect on binge eating and depressive symptoms; however, cognitions surrounding eating and body weight and shape were not affected. These results were similar to the conclusions found in another recent meta-analysis by Reas and Grilo (2008).

The SSRIs that have been studied in randomized controlled trials for adults with BED include fluoxetine, fluvoxamine, sertraline, citalopram, and escitalopram (see Brownley, Berkman, Sedway, Lohr, & Bulik, 2007, for a systematic review; see also Guerdjikova et al., 2008). Doses are generally in the upper range, as in the treatment protocols for BN. One trial compared fluoxetine (mean dose 71.3 mg daily) with placebo in 60 adults with BED and found significantly decreased weekly binge frequency (Arnold et al., 2002). Similar results were seen for fluvoxamine (dose range 50–300 mg daily) as compared with placebo in 85 adults with BED (Hudson et al., 1998). However, in a second trial involving fluvoxamine, no differences were found (Pearlstein et al., 2003). Sertraline (mean dose 187 mg daily) (McElroy et al., 2000), and citalopram (40–60 mg daily) (McElroy, Hudson, et al., 2003) have also shown some positive effects on binge eating as compared with placebo. In addition, in a 12-week double-blind placebo-controlled trial of escitalopram for BED, Guerdjikova and colleagues (2008) concluded that escitalopram was efficacious in reducing weight and the global severity of illness, but not obsessive–compulsive symptoms; no definitive conclusions could be drawn about the medication's effect in decreasing symptoms of bingeing.

Anticonvulsants such as topiramate (McElroy, Arnold, et al., 2003; McElroy, Hudson, et al., 2007), zonisamide (McElroy, Kotwal, et al., 2006), and lamotrigine (Guerdjikova et al., 2009) have also been studied in randomized controlled trials for BED with some benefit; however, there can be significant side effects such as memory impairment and Stevens–Johnson syndrome. Weight loss drugs, such as sibutramine (Appolinario et al., 2003; Wilfley et al., 2008) and orlistat (Grilo, Masheb, & Salant, 2005), have also shown some benefit for binge eating, but have unpleasant side effects such as dry mouth, constipation, oily stools, and flatulence. Because of the absence of studies in the pediatric population, as well as the risk of significant side effects, these medications are not recommended for children and adolescents with BED. Alternatively, atomoxetine has shown some promising results in terms of decreasing binge episodes as compared with placebo in adults with BED (McElroy, Guerdjikova, et al., 2007). Although it has not been studied in children and adolescents with BED, this medication has been used and studied in children and adolescents with attention-deficit/hyperactivity disorder (ADHD), potentially making it a more acceptable option. Thus, for children and adolescents with BED, psychological interventions should be attempted first, with SSRIs and possibly atomoxetine as medication adjuncts.

Some eating disturbances in children are distinct from AN, BN, and EDNOS, as weight and shape concerns are not present. Some of these include selective eating, food avoidance emotional disorder, food phobias, functional dysphagia, and food refusal (Nicholls & Bryant-Waugh, 2009). First-line treatment for all of these disorders is non-pharmacological, ranging from parent education, through behavioral interventions, to psychotherapy. There is very little literature on the use of psychopharmacological treatment for these disorders. There is one case series of three children treated successfully with low-dose SSRIs for severe "choking phobias" (Banerjee, Bhandari, & Rosenberg, 2005). Food phobias and selective eating may be more common in children with pervasive developmental disorders, another comorbid condition with eating disorders in the pediatric population. As mentioned earlier, there are two case reports of atypical antipsychotics used successfully to treat young patients with comorbid AN and pervasive developmental disorder (Fisman et al., 1996; Tateno et al., 2008), suggesting that perhaps the atypical antipsychotics may be of benefit in this population. In clinical practice, symptom targets for medication use in cases where there is an atypical eating disturbance are often anxiety and agitation, hence the potential benefit of the SSRIs and atypical antipsychotics. However, further study is needed in this population of children in order to better understand these presentations and potential treatments.

Clinical Implications

There are several complicating factors in attempting to use medications in a clinical setting with children and adolescents with eating disorders. First, pharmacological studies on a younger population are notoriously challenging. This means that clinicians have few studies on which to base clinical decisions. At the same time, although parents are likely to be compliant in bringing their child to appointments, they may be hesitant to put their child on medication, especially when evidence regarding efficacy and safety is lacking. In addition, eating disorders have medical complications that must be considered in prescribing medication. In AN, medications should be started at the lowest possible dose to minimize side effects (i.e., olanzapine 1.25 or 2.5 mg daily, given at bedtime; quetiapine 25 or 50 mg daily, given at bedtime; or risperidone 0.25 mg daily) and tapered up gradually. Although there is a lack of evidence to support target doses, clinical use suggests targets of 2.5 to 7.5 mg daily of olanzapine, 0.5 to 1.0 mg daily of risperidone, or 50 to 150 mg daily of quetiapine. Issues of postural hypotension must be monitored when starting an atypical agent. Baseline bloodwork should be done, and liver function tests and fasting glucose, prolactin, and lipids monitored regularly. Drugs such as the atypical antipsychotics, especially risperidone, can raise prolactin levels, thereby interfering with the menstrual cycle. Electrocardiograms (EKGs) should be monitored in order to detect possible QTc prolongation. In addition, eating disorder symptoms such as nausea and constipation can be exacerbated by many psychotropic medications, including SSRIs and atypical antipsychotics, possibly interfering with the goal of increased food intake. Doses of SSRIs in the higher range are generally recommended in treating BN and BED, making the discussion and monitoring of side effects even more critical, particularly the risk of increased suicidal ideation in youth.

Many psychological symptoms of starvation resolve with weight restoration alone. A careful history should be obtained to ascertain whether depressive or obsessive–compulsive symptoms began prior to weight loss or are severe enough to warrant treatment. In these situations, guidelines for the comorbid condition should be followed, and medication should be started only after the patient has been almost fully weight restored. All possible methods to restore weight using nutrition should be attempted prior to adding medication. If patients have been started on a medication such as an atypical antipsychotic at a low weight, tapering of that medication is warranted once patients are weight restored. In practice, many clinicians prefer to use atypical antipsychotics such as olanzapine to help very agitated, low-weight patients reach a healthy weight and then taper off these medications and start an SSRI such as fluoxetine to treat comorbid anxiety or depression once the patients are at or close to ideal body weight. Generally, weight restoration above 85% of ideal body weight should be targeted prior to starting a patient on an SSRI, given that below this weight, SSRIs are likely not effective. In fact, SSRIs have been shown not to be effective for treating depression (without an eating disorder) when patients exhibit dietary restriction, likely due to a lack of serotonin substrate (Delgado et al., 1999).

Finally, patients with eating disorders commonly have comorbid psychiatric conditions. There is significant crossover among these disorders, and they co-occur with high rates of mood and anxiety disorders (including generalized anxiety disorder, social phobia, obsessive–compulsive disorder, panic disorder, major depressive disorder, and adjustment disorders), as well as other less common comorbidities. For example, consider a patient with BN with comorbid bipolar disorder. Lithium could be dangerous because of the rapid shifts in fluid and electrolyte levels that occur with purging. Valproic acid and lithium can lead to weight gain, which can hinder compliance. Lamotrigine is an option, but there is a risk of Stevens–Johnson syndrome, and evidence in this population is lacking. Topiramate has been studied only in adults and older adolescents and has significant side effects, but is perhaps one option to consider in this complex clinical picture in an older adolescent.

Another fairly common comorbidity is ADHD in combination with BN. In this case, stimulants are likely to cause appetite suppression, which can then worsen the symptoms of dietary restriction, when normalization of eating throughout the day is critical to recovery from BN. Moreover, the risk of abuse of stimulants for this appetite suppression effect is substantial. Perhaps atomoxetine might have less effect on appetite as compared with other stimulants, although this is debatable. A delay in treatment with stimulants until symptoms of BN are better under control is a possible option in this scenario.

Substance abuse is another common complicating comorbidity in eating disorders, especially with BN. Ideally, dual care designed to address both disorders concurrently is recommended (Harrop & Marlatt, 2010). Some psychotherapies, including cognitive-behavioral therapy and dialectical behavior therapy, can be adapted to treat both disorders (Sysko & Hildebrandt, 2009). There is no literature on the treatment of comorbid substance abuse and eating disorders in youth, and only one report of a psychopharmacological trial of naltrexone with cognitive-behavioral therapy for the treatment of alcohol-dependent women with eating disorders, showing no benefit from the use of naltrexone (O'Malley et al., 2007).

Summary and Future Directions

In conclusion, evidence-based pharmacological treatment for children and adolescents with eating disorders is not yet possible because of the limited number of studies available. On the basis of studies in adults and some case reports in adolescents, it appears that olanzapine and other atypical antipsychotics may be helpful for AN at low body weights to help with eating-related anxiety and weight gain. The atypical antipyschotic ziprasidone and the typical antipsychotics are not recommended because of the risk of prolongation of the QTc interval. It remains uncertain whether SSRIs are helpful in preventing relapse in AN, though the current evidence is not encouraging. Generally, medications for AN should be reserved for treating comorbid conditions such as obsessive–compulsive disorder, other anxiety disorders, and depression, only if the comorbid presentation warrants pharmacological treatment, and only once the patient has been weight restored.

For children and adolescents with BN the first-line pharmacological option is fluoxetine, given the large evidence base for this drug with the adult population and the small open trial involving adolescents with BN. For treatment of BN, studies suggest that SSRIs such as fluoxetine are effective in reducing the symptoms of binge eating and purging and should be continued for 8 months to 1 year to prevent relapse. It must be kept in mind that cognitive-behavioral therapy modified for BN is still the first-line treatment before a trial of medication, although this treatment modality may not be available to all clinicians and patients. Often, in clinical practice, an SSRI is started in combination with cognitive-behavioral therapy. Tricyclic antidepressants and monoamine oxidase inhibitors are not recommended in the treatment of eating disorders because of serious adverse effects, and buproprion is contraindicated because of the risk of seizures.

In treating children and adolescents with EDNOS, it is best to follow treatment recommendations for the disorder that the symptoms most closely resemble. For example, treatment for dietary restriction may follow treatment guidelines for AN, whereas binge-eating or purging behavior may compel a clinician to follow guidelines for BN. There are no studies of youth with BED; however, SSRIs are likely the safest option.

Further medication trials are needed in order to delineate which, if any, pharmacological treatments are safe and efficacious for treating children and adolescents with eating disorders. Given the pressing need for these trials and the costs and challenges associated with such studies in children and adolescents, collaboration between sites and increased funding for multisite trials are strongly recommended.

References

American Psychiatric Association. (2006). Treatment of patients with eating disorders (3rd ed.). *American Journal of Psychiatry, 163*(7, Suppl.), 4–54.

Appolinario, J. C., Bacaltchuk, J., Sichieri, R., Claudino, A. M., Godoy-Matos, A., Morgan, C., et al. (2003). A randomized, double-blind, placebo-controlled study of sibutramine in the treatment of binge-eating disorder. *Archives of General Psychiatry, 60*(11), 1109–1116.

Arnold, L. M., McElroy, S. L., Hudson, J. I., Welge, J. A., Bennett, A. J., & Keck, P. E. (2002). A placebo-controlled, randomized trial of fluoxetine in the treatment of binge-eating disorder. *Journal of Clinical Psychiatry, 63*(11), 1028–1033.

Attia, E., Haiman, C., Walsh, B. T., & Flater, S. R. (1998). Does fluoxetine augment the inpatient treatment of anorexia nervosa? *American Journal of Psychiatry, 155*(4), 548–551.

Bacaltchuk, J., & Hay, P. P. J. (2003). Antidepressants versus placebo for people with bulimia nervosa. *Cochrane Database System Reviews*, Issue 4 (Article No. CD003391), DOI: 10.1002/14651858.CD003391.

Banerjee, S. P., Bhandari, R. P., & Rosenberg, D. R. (2005). Use of low-dose selective serotonin reuptake inhibitors for severe, refractory choking phobia in childhood. *Journal of Developmental and Behavioral Pediatrics, 26*(2), 123–127.

Barbarich, N. C., McConaha, C. W., Gaskill, J., La Via, M., Frank, G. K., Achenbach, S., et al. (2004). An open trial of olanzapine in anorexia nervosa. *Journal of Clinical Psychiatry, 65*(11), 1480–1482.

Barbarich, N. C., McConaha, C. W., Halmi, K. A., Gendall, K., Sunday, S. R., Gaskill, J., et al. (2004). Use of nutritional supplements to increase the efficacy of fluoxetine in the treatment of anorexia nervosa. *International Journal of Eating Disorders, 35*(1), 10–15.

Beumont, P. J., Russell, J. D., Touyz, S. W., Buckley, C., Lowinger, K., Talbot, P., et al. (1997). Intensive nutritional counselling in bulimia nervosa: A role for supplementation with fluoxetine? *Australian and New Zealand Journal of Psychiatry, 31*(4), 514–524.

Biederman, J., Herzog, D. B., Rivinus, T. M., Harper, G. P., Ferber, R. A., Rosenbaum, J. F., et al. (1985). Amitriptyline in the treatment of anorexia nervosa: A double-blind, placebo-controlled study. *Journal of Clinical Psychopharmacology, 5*(1), 10–16.

Birmingham, C. L., Goldner, E. M., & Bakan, R. (1994). Controlled trial of zinc supplementation in anorexia nervosa. *International Journal of Eating Disorders, 15*(3), 251–255.

Bissada, H., Tasca, G. A., Barber, A. M., & Bradwejn, J. (2008). Olanzapine in the treatment of low body weight and obsessive thinking in women with anorexia nervosa: A randomized, double-blind, placebo-controlled trial. *American Journal of Psychiatry, 165*(10), 1281–1288.

Boachie, A., Goldfield, G. S., & Spettigue, W. (2003). Olanzapine use as an adjunctive treatment for hospitalized children with anorexia nervosa: Case reports. *International Journal of Eating Disorders, 33*(1), 98–103.

Bosanac, P., Kurlender, S., Norman, T., Hallam, K., Wesnes, K., Manktelow, T., et al.

(2007). An open-label study of quetiapine in anorexia nervosa. *Human Psychopharmacology, 22*(4), 223–230.

Brambilla, F., Garcia, C. S., Fassino, S., Daga, G. A., Favaro, A., Santonastaso, P., et al. (2007). Olanzapine therapy in anorexia nervosa: Psychobiological effects. *International Clinical Psychopharmacology, 22*(4), 197–204.

Brownley, K. A., Berkman, N. D., Sedway, J. A., Lohr, K. N., & Bulik, C. M. (2007). Binge eating disorder treatment: A systematic review of randomized controlled trials. *International Journal of Eating Disorders, 40*(4), 337–348.

Dally, P. J., & Sargant, W. (1960). A new treatment of anorexia nervosa. *British Medical Journal, 5188*, 1770–1773.

Delgado, P. L., Miller, H. L., Salomon, R. M., Licinio, J., Krystal, J. H., Moreno, F. A., et al. (1999). Tryptophan-depletion challenge in depressed patients treated with desipramine or fluoxetine: Implications for the role of serotonin in the mechanism of antidepressant action. *Biological Psychiatry, 46*(2), 212–220.

Dennis, K., Le Grange, D., & Bremer, J. (2006). Olanzapine use in adolescent anorexia nervosa. *Eating and Weight Disorders, 11*(2), e53–e56.

Ercan, E. S., Copkunol, H., Cykoethlu, S., & Varan, A. (2003). Olanzapine treatment of an adolescent girl with anorexia nervosa. *Human Psychopharmacology, 18*(5), 401–403.

Faris, P. L., Kim, S. W., Meller, W. H., Goodale, R. L., Oakman, S. A., Hofbauer, R. D., et al. (2000). Effect of decreasing afferent vagal activity with ondansetron on symptoms of bulimia nervosa: A randomised, double-blind trial. *Lancet, 355*, 792–797.

Fichter, M. M., Kruger, R., Rief, W., Holland, R., & Dohne, J. (1996). Fluvoxamine in prevention of relapse in bulimia nervosa: Effects on eating-specific psychopathology. *Journal of Clinical Psychopharmacology, 16*(1), 9–18.

Fisman, S., Steele, M., Short, J., Byrne, T., & Lavallee, C. (1996). Case study: Anorexia nervosa and autistic disorder in an adolescent girl. *Journal of the American Academy of Child and Adolescent Psychiatry, 35*(7), 937–940.

Fluoxetine Bulimia Nervosa Collaborative Study Group. (1992). Fluoxetine in the treatment of bulimia nervosa. A multicenter, placebo-controlled, double-blind trial. *Archives of General Psychiatry, 49*(2), 139–147.

Goldberg, S. C., Halmi, K. A., Eckert, E. D., Casper, R. C., & Davis, J. M. (1979). Cyproheptadine in anorexia nervosa. *British Journal of Psychiatry, 134*, 67–70.

Goldstein, D. J., Wilson, M. G., Ascroft, R. C., & al-Banna, M. (1999). Effectiveness of fluoxetine therapy in bulimia nervosa regardless of comorbid depression. *International Journal of Eating Disorders, 25*(1), 19–27.

Goldstein, D. J., Wilson, M. G., Thompson, V. L., Potvin, J. H., & Rampey, A. H., Jr. (1995). Long-term fluoxetine treatment of bulimia nervosa. Fluoxetine Bulimia Nervosa Research Group. *British Journal of Psychiatry, 166*(5), 660–666.

Grilo, C. M., Masheb, R. M., & Salant, S. L. (2005). Cognitive behavioral therapy guided self-help and orlistat for the treatment of binge eating disorder: A randomized, double-blind, placebo-controlled trial. *Biological Psychiatry, 57*(10), 1193–1201.

Gross, H., Ebert, M. H., Faden, V. B., Goldberg, S. C., Kaye, W. H., Caine, E. D., et al. (1983). A double-blind trial of delta 9-tetrahydrocannabinol in primary anorexia nervosa. *Journal of Clinical Psychopharmacology, 3*(3), 165–171.

Gross, H., Ebert, M. H., Faden, V. B., Goldberg, S. C., Nee, L. E., & Kaye, W. H. (1981). A double-blind controlled trial of lithium carbonate in primary anorexia nervosa. *Journal of Clinical Psychopharmacology, 1*(6), 376–381.

Guerdjikova, A. I., McElroy, S. L., Kotwal, R., Welge, J. A., Nelson, E., Lake, K., et al. (2008). High-dose escitalopram in the treatment of binge-eating disorder with obesity: A placebo-controlled monotherapy trial. *Human Psychopharmacology, 23*(1), 1–11.

Guerdjikova, A. I., McElroy, S. L., Welge, J. A., Nelson, E., Keck, P. E., & Hudson, J. I. (2009). Lamotrigine in the treatment of binge-eating disorder with obesity: A randomized, placebo-controlled monotherapy trial. *International Clinical Psychopharmacology, 24*(3), 150–158.

Hagman, J., Gralla, J., Sigel, E., Dodge, M., Ellert, S., Gardner, R., et al. (2009). *A double-blind, placebo controlled study of risperidone for anorexia nervosa.* Paper presented at the American Academy of Child and Adolescent Psychiatry, Honolulu, Hawaii.

Halmi, K. A., Eckert, E., LaDu, T. J., & Cohen, J. (1986). Anorexia nervosa: Treatment efficacy of cyproheptadine and amitriptyline. *Archives of General Psychiatry, 43*(2), 177–181.

Harrop, E. N., & Marlatt, G. A. (2010). The comorbidity of substance use disorders and eating disorders in women: Prevalence, etiology, and treatment. *Addictive Behaviors, 35*(5), 392–398.

Hedges, D. W., Reimherr, F. W., Hoopes, S. P., Rosenthal, N. R., Kamin, M., Karim, R., et al. (2003). Treatment of bulimia nervosa with topiramate in a randomized, double-blind, placebo-controlled trial: Part 2. Improvement in psychiatric measures. *Journal of Clinical Psychiatry, 64*(12), 1449–1454.

Holtkamp, K., Konrad, K., Kaiser, N., Ploenes, Y., Heussen, N., Grzella, I., et al. (2005). A retrospective study of SSRI treatment in adolescent anorexia nervosa: Insufficient evidence for efficacy. *Journal of Psychiatric Research, 39*(3), 303–310.

Hoopes, S. P., Reimherr, F. W., Hedges, D. W., Rosenthal, N. R., Kamin, M., Karim, R., et al. (2003). Treatment of bulimia nervosa with topiramate in a randomized, double-blind, placebo-controlled trial: Part 1. Improvement in binge and purge measures. *Journal of Clinical Psychiatry, 64*(11), 1335–1341.

Hudson, J. I., McElroy, S. L., Raymond, N. C., Crow, S., Keck, P. E., Jr., Carter, W. P., et al. (1998). Fluvoxamine in the treatment of binge-eating disorder: A multicenter placebo-controlled, double-blind trial. *American Journal of Psychiatry, 155*(12), 1756–1762.

Jaafar, N. R., Daud, T. I., Rahman, F. N., & Baharudin, A. (2007). Mirtazapine for anorexia nervosa with depression. *Australian and New Zealand Journal of Psychiatry, 41*(9), 768–769.

Jimerson, D. C., Herzog, D. B., & Brotman, A. W. (1993). Pharmacologic approaches in the treatment of eating disorders. *Harvard Review of Psychiatry, 1*(2), 82–93.

Katz, R. L., Keen, C. L., Litt, I. F., Hurley, L. S., Kellams-Harrison, K. M., & Glader, L. J. (1987). Zinc deficiency in anorexia nervosa. *Journal of Adolescent Health Care, 8*(5), 400–406.

Kaye, W. H., Nagata, T., Weltzin, T. E., Hsu, L. K., Sokol, M. S., McConaha, C., et al. (2001). Double-blind placebo-controlled administration of fluoxetine in restricting- and restricting-purging-type anorexia nervosa. *Biological Psychiatry, 49*(7), 644–652.

Kennedy, S. H., Goldbloom, D. S., Ralevski, E., Davis, C., D'Souza, J. D., & Lofchy, J. (1993). Is there a role for selective monoamine oxidase inhibitor therapy in bulimia nervosa?: A placebo-controlled trial of brofaromine. *Journal of Clinical Psychopharmacology, 13*(6), 415–422.

Kotler, L. A., Devlin, M. J., Davies, M., & Walsh, B. T. (2003). An open trial of fluoxetine for adolescents with bulimia nervosa. *Journal of Child and Adolescent Psychopharmacology, 13*(3), 329–335.

Lacey, J. H., & Crisp, A. H. (1980). Hunger, food intake and weight: The impact of clomipramine on a refeeding anorexia nervosa population. *Postgraduate Medical Journal, 56*(Suppl. 1), 79–85.

Lask, B., Fosson, A., Rolfe, U., & Thomas, S. (1993). Zinc deficiency and childhood-onset anorexia nervosa. *Journal of Clinical Psychiatry, 54*(2), 63–66.

La Via, M. C., Gray, N., & Kaye, W. H. (2000). Case reports of olanzapine treatment of anorexia nervosa. *International Journal of Eating Disorders, 27*(3), 363–366.

Lock, J., Walker, L. R., Rickert, V. I., & Katzman, D. K. (2005). Suicidality in adolescents being treated with antidepressant medications and the black box label: Position paper of the Society for Adolescent Medicine. *Journal of Adolescent Health, 36*(1), 92–93.

Malina, A., Gaskill, J., McConaha, C., Frank, G. K., LaVia, M., Scholar, L., et al. (2003).

Olanzapine treatment of anorexia nervosa: A retrospective study. *International Journal of Eating Disorders, 33*(2), 234–237.

Marrazzi, M. A., Bacon, J. P., Kinzie, J., & Luby, E. D. (1995). Naltrexone use in the treatment of anorexia nervosa and bulimia nervosa. *International Clinical Psychopharmacology, 10*(3), 163–172.

McElroy, S. L., Arnold, L. M., Shapira, N. A., Keck, P. E., Jr., Rosenthal, N. R., Karim, M. R., et al. (2003). Topiramate in the treatment of binge eating disorder associated with obesity: A randomized, placebo-controlled trial. *American Journal of Psychiatry, 160*(2), 255–261.

McElroy, S. L., Casuto, L. S., Nelson, E. B., Lake, K. A., Soutullo, C. A., Keck, P. E., Jr., et al. (2000). Placebo-controlled trial of sertraline in the treatment of binge eating disorder. *American Journal of Psychiatry, 157*(6), 1004–1006.

McElroy, S. L., Guerdjikova, A., Kotwal, R., Welge, J. A., Nelson, E. B., Lake, K. A., et al. (2007). Atomoxetine in the treatment of binge-eating disorder: A randomized placebo-controlled trial. *Journal of Clinical Psychiatry, 68*(3), 390–398.

McElroy, S. L., Hudson, J. I., Capece, J. A., Beyers, K., Fisher, A. C., & Rosenthal, N. R. (2007). Topiramate for the treatment of binge eating disorder associated with obesity: A placebo-controlled study. *Biological Psychiatry, 61*(9), 1039–1048.

McElroy, S. L., Hudson, J. I., Malhotra, S., Welge, J. A., Nelson, E. B., & Keck, P. E., Jr. (2003). Citalopram in the treatment of binge-eating disorder: A placebo-controlled trial. *Journal of Clinical Psychiatry, 64*(7), 807–813.

McElroy, S. L., Kotwal, R., Guerdjikova, A. I., Welge, J. A., Nelson, E. B., Lake, K. A., et al. (2006). Zonisamide in the treatment of binge eating disorder with obesity: A randomized controlled trial. *Journal of Clinical Psychiatry, 67*(12), 1897–1906.

Meehan, K. G., Loeb, K. L., Roberto, C. A., & Attia, E. (2006). Mood change during weight restoration in patients with anorexia nervosa. *International Journal of Eating Disorders, 39*(7), 587–589.

Mehler, C., Wewetzer, C., Schulze, U., Warnke, A., Theisen, F., & Dittmann, R. W. (2001). Olanzapine in children and adolescents with chronic anorexia nervosa. A study of five cases. *European Child and Adolescent Psychiatry, 10*(2), 151–157.

Mehler-Wex, C., Romanos, M., Kirchheiner, J., & Schulze, U. M. E. (2008). Atypical antipsychotics in severe anorexia nervosa in children and adolescents: Review and case reports. *European Eating Disorders Review, 16*(2), 101–108.

Milano, W., Petrella, C., Sabatino, C., & Capasso, A. (2004). Treatment of bulimia nervosa with sertraline: A randomized controlled trial. *Advances in Therapy, 21*(4), 232–237.

Mitchell, J. E., Agras, S., & Wonderlich, S. (2007). Treatment of bulimia nervosa: Where are we and where are we going? *International Journal of Eating Disorders, 40*(2), 95–101.

Mitchell, J. E., & Groat, R. (1984). A placebo-controlled, double-blind trial of amitriptyline in bulimia. *Journal of Clinical Psychopharmacology, 4*(4), 186–193.

Mondraty, N., Birmingham, C. L., Touyz, S., Sundakov, V., Chapman, L., & Beumont, P. (2005). Randomized controlled trial of olanzapine in the treatment of cognitions in anorexia nervosa. *Australas Psychiatry, 13*(1), 72–75.

Moore, R., Mills, I. H., & Forster, A. (1981). Naloxone in the treatment of anorexia nervosa: Effect on weight gain and lipolysis. *Journal of the Royal Society of Medicine, 74*(2), 129–131.

National Institute for Clinical Excellence. (2004). *Eating disorders: Core interventions in the treatment and management of anorexia nervosa, bulimia nervosa and related eating disorders.* London: Author.

Newman-Toker, J. (2000). Risperidone in anorexia nervosa. *Journal of the American Academy of Child and Adolescent Psychiatry, 39*(8), 941–942.

Nicholls, D., & Bryant-Waugh, R. (2009). Eating disorders of infancy and childhood: Definition, symptomatology, epidemiology, and comorbidity. *Child and Adolescent Psychiatric Clinics of North America, 18*(1), 17–30.

Norris, M. L., Spettigue, W., Buchholz, A., Henderson, K. Maras, D., & Gomez, R. (in press). Olanzapine use for the adjunctive treatment of adolescents with anorexia nervosa. *Journal of Child and Adolescent Psychopharmacology.*

O'Malley, S. S., Sinha, R., Grilo, C. M., Capone, C., Farren, C. K., McKee, S. A., et al. (2007). Naltrexone and cognitive behavioral coping skills therapy for the treatment of alcohol drinking and eating disorder features in alcohol-dependent women: A randomized controlled trial. *Alcoholism: Clinical and Experimental Research, 31*(4), 625–634.

Pearlstein, T., Spurell, E., Hohlstein, L. A., Gurney, V., Read, J., Fuchs, C., et al. (2003). A double-blind, placebo-controlled trial of fluvoxamine in binge eating disorder: A high placebo response. *Archives of Women's Mental Health, 6*(2), 147–151.

Pollice, C., Kaye, W. H., Greeno, C. G., & Weltzin, T. E. (1997). Relationship of depression, anxiety, and obsessionality to state of illness in anorexia nervosa. *International Journal of Eating Disorders, 21*(4), 367–376.

Pope, H. G., Jr., Hudson, J. I., Jonas, J. M., & Yurgelun-Todd, D. (1983). Bulimia treated with imipramine: A placebo-controlled, double-blind study. *American Journal of Psychiatry, 140*(5), 554–558.

Pope, H. G., Jr., Keck, P. E., Jr., McElroy, S. L., & Hudson, J. I. (1989). A placebo-controlled study of trazodone in bulimia nervosa. *Journal of Clinical Psychopharmacology, 9*(4), 254–259.

Powers, P. S., Bannon, Y., Eubanks, R., & McCormick, T. (2007). Quetiapine in anorexia nervosa patients: An open label outpatient pilot study. *International Journal of Eating Disorders, 40*(1), 21–26.

Powers, P. S., Santana, C. A., & Bannon, Y. S. (2002). Olanzapine in the treatment of anorexia nervosa: An open label trial. *International Journal of Eating Disorders, 32*(2), 146–154.

Reas, D. L., & Grilo, C. M. (2008). Review and meta-analysis of pharmacotherapy for binge-eating disorder. *Obesity, 16*(9), 2024–2038.

Ritchie, B., & Norris, M. L. (2009). QTc prolongation associated with atypical antipsychotic use in the treatment of adolescent-onset anorexia nervosa. *Journal of the Canadian Academy of Child and Adolescent Psychiatry, 18*(1), 60–63.

Romano, S. J., Halmi, K. A., Sarkar, N. P., Koke, S. C., & Lee, J. S. (2002). A placebo-controlled study of fluoxetine in continued treatment of bulimia nervosa after successful acute fluoxetine treatment. *American Journal of Psychiatry, 159*(1), 96–102.

Sim, L. A., McGovern, L., Elamin, M. B., Swiglo, B. A., Erwin, P. J., & Montori, V. M. (2010). Effect on bone health of estrogen preparations in premenopausal women with anorexia nervosa: A systematic review and meta-analyses. *International Journal of Eating Disorders, 43*(3), 218–225.

Stacher, G., Abatzi-Wenzel, T. A., Wiesnagrotzki, S., Bergmann, H., Schneider, C., & Gaupmann, G. (1993). Gastric emptying, body weight and symptoms in primary anorexia nervosa. Long-term effects of cisapride. *British Journal of Psychiatry, 162*, 398–402.

Steinegger, C., Pinhas, L., Boachie, A., & Katzman, D. (2007). *The safety and tolerability of atypical antipsychotics in the treatment of adolescents with anorexia nervosa.* Paper presented at the International Conference on Eating Disorders, Baltimore.

Strober, M., Pataki, C., Freeman, R., & DeAntonio, M. (1999). No effect of adjunctive fluoxetine on eating behavior or weight phobia during the inpatient treatment of anorexia nervosa: An historical case-control study. *Journal of Child and Adolescent Psychopharmacology, 9*(3), 195–201.

Sussman, N. (2001). Review of atypical antipsychotics and weight gain. *Journal of Clinical Psychiatry, 62*(Suppl. 23), 5–12.

Sysko, R., & Hildebrandt, T. (2009). Cognitive-behavioural therapy for individuals with bulimia nervosa and a co-occurring substance use disorder. *European Eating Disorders Review, 17*(2), 89–100.

Szmukler, G. I., Young, G. P., Miller, G., Lichtenstein, M., & Binns, D. S. (1995). A controlled trial of cisapride in anorexia nervosa. *International Journal of Eating Disorders, 17*(4), 347–357.

Tateno, M., Teshirogi, H., Kamasaki, H., & Saito, T. (2008). Successful olanzapine treatment of anorexia nervosa in a girl with pervasive developmental disorder not otherwise specified. *Psychiatry and Clinical Neurosciences, 62*(6), 752.

Taylor, D. M., & McAskill, R. (2000). Atypical antipsychotics and weight gain: A systematic review. *Acta Psychiatrica Scandinavica, 101*(6), 416–432.

Vandereycken, W. (1984). Neuroleptics in the short-term treatment of anorexia nervosa: A double-blind placebo-controlled study with sulpiride. *British Journal of Psychiatry, 144,* 288–292.

Vandereycken, W., & Pierloot, R. (1982). Pimozide combined with behavior therapy in the short-term treatment of anorexia nervosa. A double-blind placebo-controlled cross-over study. *Acta Psychiatrica Scandinavica, 66*(6), 445–450.

Vocks, S., Tuschen-Caffier, B., Pietrowsky, R., Rustenbach, S. J., Kersting, A., & Herpertz, S. (2010). Meta-analysis of the effectiveness of psychological and pharmacological treatments for binge eating disorder. *International Journal of Eating Disorders, 43*(3), 205–217.

Walsh, B. T., Hadigan, C. M., Devlin, M. J., Gladis, M., & Roose, S. P. (1991). Long-term outcome of antidepressant treatment for bulimia nervosa. *American Journal of Psychiatry, 148*(9), 1206–1212.

Walsh, B. T., Kaplan, A. S., Attia, E., Olmsted, M., Parides, M., Carter, J. C., et al. (2006). Fluoxetine after weight restoration in anorexia nervosa: A randomized controlled trial. *Journal of the American Medical Association, 295*(22), 2605–2612.

Wilfley, D. E., Crow, S. J., Hudson, J. I., Mitchell, J. E., Berkowitz, R. I., Blakesley, V., et al. (2008). Efficacy of sibutramine for the treatment of binge eating disorder: A randomized multicenter placebo-controlled double-blind study. *American Journal of Psychiatry, 165*(1), 51–58.

■ PART VI ■
PREVENTION

CHAPTER 22

Prevention of Eating Disorders in Children and Adolescents

Dianne Neumark-Sztainer

E ating disorder prevention involves the reduction or elimination of important, modifiable risk factors for eating disorders and the promotion of factors that are protective against eating disorders. Eating disorder prevention can be done at the individual, family, group, institutional, community, or societal level. Eating disorder prevention can be done with individuals at risk for eating disorders (e.g., adolescent girls) and their caretakers (e.g., parents, teachers, or health care providers). It can be done within one-to-one conversations (e.g., between parents and their children) or within group settings (e.g., classrooms). Policies aimed at eating disorder prevention can be put in place at the institutional or community level, such as within schools, youth activities, community centers, fitness centers, and clinics. Eating disorder prevention can also be done at the societal level, in order to implement cultural shifts in factors that can increase risk for eating disorders (e.g., media images). In fact, in order for eating disorder prevention to be most effective, it probably needs to be occurring at all of these different levels.

This chapter provides an overview of key risk and protective factors that can be addressed within interventions aimed at eating disorder prevention in children and adolescents. Examples of interventions that can be implemented within school and other community-based settings are provided. Ideas for parents and health care providers interested in promoting a positive body image and healthy eating practices among children and adolescents are presented. The importance of addressing risk factors at the societal level is also discussed. Given the high prevalence of obesity among young people and the current attention and funds being directed toward the prevention of obesity, ideas for integrating interventions aimed at the prevention of obesity and eating disorders are described.

Risk and Protective Factors to Be Addressed in Preventing Eating Disorders

Interventions aimed at preventing eating disorders deal with risk and protective factors for eating disorders, rather than with eating disorders per se. Risk and protective factors include variables that have been found to be associated with eating disorders or disordered eating behaviors, such as extreme weight control behaviors or binge eating. Clinical reports of commonalities seen among individuals with eating disorders can provide important insight into patterns worthy of further research. Cross-sectional associations inform us about the association between two variables at the same point in time, longitudinal associations provide information about temporality (i.e., which came first), and intervention studies can inform us about whether the manipulation of one variable can lead to changes in another variable. Thus, risk and protective factors identified in longitudinal studies carry more weight than those identified in cross-sectional studies, and the strongest evidence comes from intervention studies.

Key factors identified as risk factors for either eating disorders or disordered eating behaviors include body dissatisfaction, weight concerns, internalization of the thin ideal, dieting behaviors, media influences, peer teasing, and unhealthy weight control behaviors (Levine & Smolak, 2006, p.101) These factors are commonly addressed within prevention programs, given their strong associations with eating disorders or disordered eating, their suitability for addressing within school-based interventions, and their potential amenability. Furthermore, there is value in preventing these outcomes above and beyond their direct association with eating disorders. Young people who feel better about their bodies may be more likely to engage in healthier behaviors, such as becoming involved in physical activity and eating more fruits and vegetables, and thus have better mental and physical health outcomes (Neumark-Sztainer, Levine, et al., 2006; van den Berg & Neumark-Sztainer, 2007). Furthermore, shifts in social norms, such as a decrease in discussions about feeling fat or diets, offer the potential for a positive "herd" effect, meaning that individuals who are not participating in a particular program may also benefit—that is, be less likely to have body dissatisfaction or engage in unhealthy dieting behaviors and thus be at lower risk for eating disorders.

It is noteworthy that there are additional risk factors for eating disorders that are also important to take into account in the development and implementation of interventions aimed at preventing eating disorders. For example, sexual abuse has been identified as a risk factor for eating disorders and disordered eating behaviors (Neumark-Sztainer, Story, Hannan, Beuhring, & Resnick, 2000; Wonderlich et al., 2000). Given the sensitivity and complexity of sexual abuse, it is often not addressed within school-based eating disorder prevention programs. However, it is certainly a factor worthy of exploration within clinical settings. Other risk factors that also need to be taken into account in the planning of eating disorder prevention interventions include nonmodifiable risk factors. These are risk factors that can be used to target high-risk populations with interventions. For example, girls are at higher risk than boys for eating disorders, and thus prevention programs often specifically target girls or are designed to meet the needs of girls even if offered within mixed-gender groups (e.g., classrooms).

It is also important to think about protective factors that can be addressed within prevention interventions. Protective factors work to decrease the effects of risk factors and operate in the presence of risk (Bernat & Resnick, 2006; Resnick, 2000). Children and adolescents live within a social environment that bombards them with mixed messages regarding food and weight. For example, the environment simultaneously encourages the pursuit of an extremely thin body and the consumption of large portions of high-calorie fast food. Thus, protective factors may help young people mitigate the effects of living in such a society. For instance, more frequent family meals have been found to be cross-sectionally and longitudinally protective against extreme weight control behaviors in adolescent girls (Neumark-Sztainer, Eisenberg, Fulkerson, Story, & Larson, 2008; Neumark-Sztainer, Wall, Story, & Fulkerson, 2004). Family meals have also been found to be protective for other outcomes; more frequent family meals are associated with better dietary intake, higher levels of psychosocial well-being, academic success, and lower levels of substance use (Neumark-Sztainer, Larson, Fulkerson, Eisenberg, & Story, 2010). Thus, encouraging families to eat together more frequently may be effective in decreasing the risk for eating disorders and is also likely to have other beneficial outcomes. The potential for multiple benefits is important for parents who may not be concerned about the prevention of eating disorders in their children, but may be concerned about their children's academic success or risk for substance use. Similarly, the enhancement of media literacy skills has the potential to protect children from being negatively influenced by media images portraying dangerously thin models and promoting quick-fix diets (Levine & Smolak, 2006, pp. 306–344). In addition, media literacy skills can help children in dealing with other potentially harmful messages such as advertisements for alcohol or fast foods. Programs aimed at improving self-esteem in young people have the potential to protect children from an array of harmful outcomes and to promote overall well-being, in addition to decreasing risk for eating disorders (O'Dea, 2004). Time-strapped schools may be reluctant to implement programs that work only toward the prevention of eating disorders, but may be more likely to implement programs that have the potential to protect children from a variety of harmful outcomes.

Given the high prevalence of overweight young people, and the emphasis on obesity prevention, it seems important to identify risk and protective factors that have relevance for obesity, in addition to eating disorders/disordered eating, in young people. The identification of shared risk and protective factors can guide interventions that work toward the prevention of both eating disorders and obesity. In an analysis of data from Project EAT-I and II, a 5-year longitudinal study of eating- and weight-related issues in 2,500 adolescent girls and boys, a number of shared risk and protective factors for overweight status and disordered eating behaviors were identified that are suitable for addressing within interventions (Neumark-Sztainer et al., 2007). Family members teasing a person about his or her weight, personal weight concerns, and dieting/unhealthy weight control behaviors were found to strongly and consistently predict overweight status, binge eating, and extreme weight control behaviors 5 years later. Family meals, regular meal patterns, and reading magazine articles about dieting and weight loss were also associated with weight-related outcomes, although there were differences in the strength and consistency of associations across outcomes and genders. Thus, programs that target these risk and protective factors may be effective in preventing both eating disorders and obesity in young people.

School- and Community-Based Interventions with Children and Adolescents

The majority of interventions implemented with children and adolescents have been done within schools. Interventions have been implemented within elementary schools, middle schools, high schools, and colleges/universities. There have also been a few interventions implemented within community groups, such as the Girl Scouts, Free to be Me, and Full of Ourselves, but these have been the exception, rather than the rule (Neumark-Sztainer, Sherwood, Coller, & Hannan, 2000; Sjostrom & Steiner-Adair, 2005; Steiner-Adair et al., 2002). Schools are excellent places for interventions inasmuch as they offer venues for easily reaching children from diverse backgrounds who might have less accessibility to clinic or community programs. A number of reviews have been conducted on the effectiveness of eating disorder prevention interventions, most of which have been implemented within school or community settings (Holt & Ricciardelli, 2008; Levine & Smolak, 2006, pp. 179–223; Neumark-Sztainer, Levine, et al., 2006; Pratt & Woolfenden, 2002; Stice, Shaw, & Marti, 2007). Overall, the findings suggest that interventions have shown modest success in decreasing risk factors and increasing protective factors for eating disorders and that further work is needed to improve the effectiveness of such interventions. Given that much has been written about school-based interventions for young people, the different types of approaches commonly used, and the effectiveness of these interventions, this chapter focuses on other areas for prevention. Thus, the discussion of school-based interventions is limited to a discussion on the value of investing in training school staff, the importance of comprehensive school-based interventions, and the need to develop mechanisms for the dissemination of programs developed and evaluated within research frameworks.

The majority of interventions conducted within schools focus on the students. However, given that teachers have daily contact with young people, it can be very important to target teachers with interventions aimed at preventing eating disorders among students (Piran, 2004). Furthermore, this can be a more time-efficient use of eating disorder specialists and other health care professionals who are often invited to come into schools to do some type of prevention work, such as talking with students in their health classes. One strategy is to train teachers to properly implement an eating disorder prevention curriculum. Another equally and potentially more valuable intervention is to work with educators in changing the way they think about and treat their own bodies and how they discuss topics related to dieting, body satisfaction, eating, and physical activity with their students. It is important to increase teachers' awareness about the importance of avoiding discussions about their own dieting behaviors with their students, as well as comments to the students about their need to lose weight. It may be particularly important to work with teachers who deal with health-related topics, such as physical education teachers, health teachers, and coaches. Weighting for You! is an example of a short (90-minute) training program aimed at helping high school faculty and staff increase their (1) awareness of their own weight-related attitudes and beliefs, (2) knowledge about weight-related disorders, and (3) skills in providing support to students at risk for, or experiencing, a weight-related problem (Toledo & Neumark-Sztainer, 1999). McVey and colleagues evaluated their Web-based prevention program, Student Body, in a controlled study design with 78 elementary schoolteachers and 89 local public health practitioners who provide support to schools (McVey, Gusella, Tweed, & Ferrari, 2009). The program was found to enhance participants' awareness about how weight bias can be present in their teaching practices and how this can trigger students' body image concerns. The website is an excellent resource for educators and public health practitioners (McVey et al., 2006). In Australia, the Victorian State Government, along with philanthropic organizations, has provided funding to train teachers in the delivery of the program BodyThink, aimed at improving body image and self-esteem in children (ages 11–14) (Paxton, in press; Richardson, Paxton, & Thomson, 2009). The Butterfly Foundation conducts half-day training programs for teachers and other community professionals interested in implementing the program (Richardson et al., 2009). Given the amount of time teachers spend with young people, the suitability of the school environment for learning, and the ability of schools to reach out to a captive audience of young people, more work is needed in the implementation and evaluation of interventions that specifically target teachers.

A positive trend within the literature on school-based interventions aimed at eating disorder prevention is an increased focus on the school as a whole, rather than solely on the implementation of educational programs within the classroom. The idea of a school-based comprehensive program has been described in the literature (Neumark-Sztainer, 1996; O'Dea & Maloney, 2000), and there have been efforts to implement more comprehensive interventions within school settings. Piran (1998, 1999) did her pioneering work in eating disorder prevention within a residential ballet school, using a whole-school approach based on a highly participatory model and feminist principles. Piran's intervention did not involve a class curriculum but rather focused on changing the school environment and culture to promote healthier eating and more positive body images. Although the evaluation design did not allow for a control school, the approach appeared to be successful with girls achieving significant improvements in body image, disordered eating behaviors, and eating disorder risk. Furthermore, Piran's work set the stage for thinking about school-based prevention of eating disorders in a holistic manner. Another example of a whole-school prevention approach is the V.I.K. (Very Important Kids) program, which was aimed at changing an elementary school's culture in regard to teasing behaviors, including weight-based teasing (Haines, Neumark-Sztainer, Perry, Hannan, & Levine, 2006). The program was informed by an in-depth formative assessment with students, parents, school staff, and a V.I.K advisory board comprising various members of the school community (Haines, Neumark-Sztainer, & Thiel, 2007). The V.I.K. program included activities at the individual level (e.g., an after-school program and the development of a theater production based on the children's experiences with artists from Illusion Theater), the school environmental level (e.g., a half-day training for teachers, a no-teasing school campaign, and a book focusing on teasing to be read by all students), and the family level (e.g., family nights, V.I.K. booths at parent–teacher conferences, and a theater production by the children for families at the Illusion Theater in downtown Minneapolis). Program evaluation indicated that V.I.K. was successful in decreasing teasing in the school that received the intervention, as compared with a control school, although further evaluation in a larger study is needed. McVey and her colleagues have also implemented and evaluated an impressive comprehensive school-based intervention, Healthy Schools–Healthy Kids (McVey, Tweed, & Blackmore, 2007). Activities included school staff training, parent education, in-class curriculum, peer support groups, a play production, posters and videos, and public service announcements for the entire school. The findings suggested that there were some positive changes regarding the internalization of media ideals and disordered eating behaviors, particularly among the high-risk students. Important steps for the future of comprehensive school-based interventions include involvement of the school food service and the physical education department, integration of efforts aimed at preventing a broad spectrum of weight-related problems in youth, strong evaluation designs, and mechanisms for the dissemination of such complex models of intervention.

A major challenge to be addressed is how best to disseminate school and community-based programs that have been developed and evaluated within a research framework.

Research grants provide funding for the development and evaluation of eating disorder interventions, and for staff time during this process, but typically very minimal, if any, funding is provided for the dissemination of programs for wider use. It is imperative to find ways to realistically link researchers who have designed and evaluated eating disorder prevention programs to schools and community organizations interested in disseminating cutting-edge interventions. The use of technology has the potential to help in dissemination, as intervention materials can easily be placed on websites. For example, our research team placed all of the intervention materials for New Moves, a school-based program aimed at preventing weight-related problems in adolescent girls, on a website in order to more widely disseminate the program materials (Neumark-Sztainer, 2009a; Neumark-Sztainer, Flattum, Story, Feldman, & Petrich, 2008; Neumark-Sztainer et al., 2010). However, in order to properly implement interventions, particularly comprehensive school-based interventions, it will not be enough to provide intervention materials. Rather, there is a need for tailoring programs to meet the needs of specific populations, training staff, dealing with school logistics, and optimally, conducting some type of ongoing evaluation.

Working with Parents of Children and Adolescents

Parents of children and adolescents often struggle with how best to address eating- and weight-related issues with their children. Many parents question how they can help their children have a healthy dietary intake, a healthy body weight, and a positive self-image. In working with parents, a balance may be needed between helping parents recognize the important role they play in shaping their children's eating behaviors, physical activity patterns, and body image, and reducing feelings of blame if problems do develop. It can be useful to share a version of the social-ecological model with parents, in which the layers of influence on children's weight-related outcomes are shown in concentric circles around the child (see Figure 22.1). More proximal layers of influence (e.g., familial) are shown closer to the child, and more distal levels (e.g., societal) are farther away (Bronfenbrenner, 1986; Neumark-Sztainer, 2005). Layers of influence include children's individual characteristics (e.g., genetic dispositions), family influences (e.g., weight-related discussions at home), peer influences (e.g., peer dieting), school factors (e.g., bullying policies), community factors (e.g., presence of fast food restaurants), and societal factors (e.g., media messages). The diagram clearly shows that although parents can play a very important role in influencing their children, there are many other influences, and even if parents do everything "right," children may develop weight-related problems. The role of parents can be viewed as a "filter" of negative messages and a "reinforcer" of positive messages from these different outer layers of influence. For example, parents can filter out negative media messages about the importance of a perfect body by limiting the use of magazines with messages of this type that come into the home. Furthermore, parents can avoid reinforcing these harmful messages by refraining from talking about their own body dissatisfaction. Instead, parents can look for positive societal messages to reinforce, such as by pointing out successful family members who have made important contributions because of their careers.

Parents of adolescents face particular challenges. Their role changes as children become more independent. On the basis of research findings examining associations

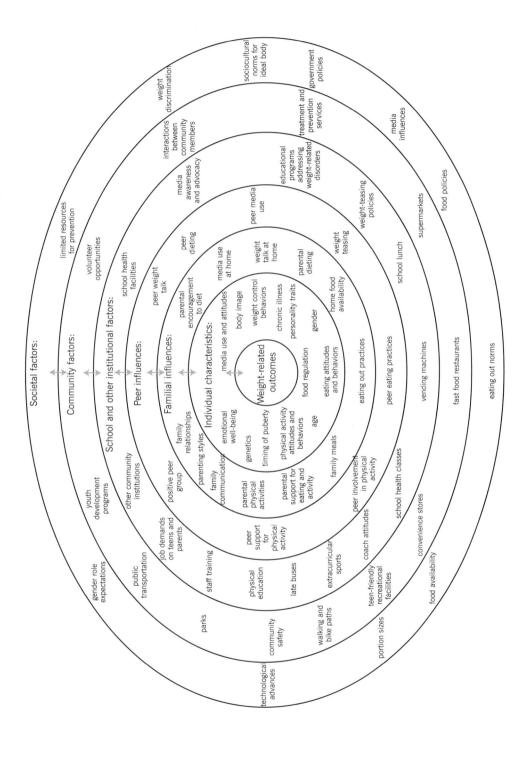

FIGURE 22.1. Factors of relevance to weight-related outcomes to be addressed within prevention interventions: An ecological perspective. From Neumark-Sztainer (2005). Copyright 2005 by Dianne Neumark-Sztainer. Adapted with permission from The Guilford Press.

between familial factors and adolescent outcomes, four "cornerstones" for parents were developed to guide parents in helping their children develop healthy body weights and positive body images (Neumark-Sztainer, 2005). An underlying aim of these cornerstones, listed in Figure 22.2, is to guide parents to *talk less* about weight-related topics and *do more* to help their children feel better about themselves and make it easier for their children to engage in healthy eating and physical activity behaviors.

Although the potential value of working with parents in the prevention of eating disorders is widely recognized, the vast majority of eating disorder prevention interventions have had minimal parental components. In large part, this is due to logistical difficulties in reaching parents through school-based interventions. Efforts to reach parents that our research team has used within interventions have included parent postcards, talks for parents, parent–child events, theater productions by children for parents, and books for parents. An important future step is considering how best to reach out to parents.

One area of promise includes parent-to-parent outreach. Within the eating disorder world, parents of children who have had eating disorders are becoming more visible and speaking out about their experiences and what they have learned from them. Parents of children who have had eating disorders can play a crucial role in helping other parents in recognizing early signs of potential problems and can provide suggestions and support. They also can assist in the prevention of risk factors and in the promotion of protective factors against eating disorders. The National Eating Disorders Association (NEDA) in the United States is developing the NEDA Navigator Program as a way to catalyze the

---

1. **Model healthy behaviors for your children.**
   - Avoid dieting, or at least unhealthy dieting behaviors.
   - Avoid making weight-related comments as much as possible.
   - Engage in regular physical activity that you enjoy.
   - Model healthy (but not perfect) eating patterns and food choices.

2. **Provide an environment that makes it easy for your children to make healthy choices.**
   - Make healthy food choices readily available.
   - Establish family meal norms that work for your family.
   - Make physical activity the norm in your family and limit TV watching.
   - Support your teen's efforts to get involved in physical activity.

3. **Focus less on weight; instead focus on behaviors and overall health.**
   - Encourage your teen to adopt healthy behaviors without focusing on weight loss.
   - Help your teen develop an identity that goes beyond physical appearance.
   - Establish a no-tolerance policy for weight teasing in your home.

4. **Provide a supportive environment with lots of talking and even more listening.**
   - Be there to listen and provide support when your teen discusses weight concerns.
   - When your teen talks about fat, find out what's really going on.
   - Keep the lines of communication open, no matter what.
   - Provide unconditional love, not based on weight, and let your child know it.

FIGURE 22.2. The four cornerstones for parents for promoting a healthy weight and positive body image in their teenage children. From Neumark-Sztainer (2005). Copyright 2005 by Dianne Neumark-Sztainer. Reprinted with permission from The Guilford Press.

experience and wisdom gained by parents (and friends, family members, and others) to help other parents and loved ones in need of support and information about navigating the world of eating disorders (National Eating Disorders Association, 2009).

Another area that shows promise includes ongoing conversations between children's health care providers (e.g., pediatricians) and parents. Parents tend to trust their children's health care providers, and hearing about the importance of working to prevent weight-related problems from such a valued source can be important. Suggestions for health care providers are included in the following section.

The Role of Health Care Providers

Pediatricians and other primary health care providers working with children and adolescents have an important role to play in the prevention of eating disorders through their work with children and adolescents and with their parents. Health care providers are often concerned about the high prevalence of obesity among their patients, thus it seems wise to incorporate messages of relevance to a broad spectrum of weight-related problems into such discussions. Health care providers need to become aware of the importance of having a positive body image and avoiding unhealthy weight control practices, for the prevention of both obesity and eating disorders.

The spectrum of weight-related problems shown in Figure 22.3 may be a useful tool for health care providers to use with young people and their parents. This spectrum shows five dimensions of weight-related problems, including weight control practices, physical activity behaviors, body image, eating behaviors, and weight status. It further shows that a child can range from healthy to problematic for each dimension. The aim is to keep to

	Healthy ⟶ ⟶ ⟶			Problematic
Weight control practices:	Healthy eating	Dieting	Unhealthy weight control behaviors	Anorexia or bulimia nervosa
Physical activity behaviors:	Regular physical activity	Minimal or excessive activity	Lack of, or obsessive, physical activity	"Anorexia athletica"
Body image:	Body appreciation	Mild body dissatisfaction	Moderate body dissatisfaction	Severe body dissatisfaction
Eating behaviors:	Regular eating patterns	Erratic eating behaviors	Binge eating	Binge-eating disorder
Weight status:	Healthy body weight	Mildly overweight or underweight	Overweight or underweight	Severe overweight or underweight

FIGURE 22.3. The spectrum of weight-related problems in adolescents. From Neumark-Sztainer (2005). Copyright 2005 by Dianne Neumark-Sztainer. Adapted with permission from The Guilford Press.

the healthy side on each dimension, but to recognize that different children may have different patterns. For example, an overweight child who avoids unhealthy weight control behaviors will need different guidance than an overweight child with a high level of body dissatisfaction who goes from diet to diet. This spectrum can also be a helpful tool to use in discussing early prevention and identification of emerging problems.

Five recommendations for health care providers to help prevent both obesity and eating disorders emerged from a review of research findings from Project EAT, in conjunction with other relevant studies. These recommendations are included in Figure 22.4 and have been previously described (Neumark-Sztainer, 2009b). Two important caveats need to be taken into account in regard to these recommendations. First of all, given that the recommendations emerged from a study focusing on adolescents, they are written with adolescents in mind and may be most appropriate for this age group. That said, most of the recommendations (e.g., have more regular and enjoyable family meals) appear similarly appropriate for younger children. Second, although these are research-based recommendations, the feasibility and effectiveness of their implementation in preventing eating disorders and other weight-related problems have not yet been empirically evaluated.

The first recommendation emphasizes the importance of discouraging dieting and, instead, supporting positive eating and physical activity behaviors that can be implemented on an ongoing basis. Because dieting may mean different things to different people, health care providers should inquire about the use of weight control behaviors and, if they are being used, what exactly is being done. It may be helpful to let young people know that "going on a diet" has actually been found to lead to weight gain, rather than weight loss, over time (Field et al., 2003; Neumark-Sztainer, Wall, et al., 2006; Stice, Cameron, Killen, Hayward, & Taylor, 1999).

Promoting a positive body image is the focus of the second recommendation for health care providers working with children and adolescents. Although questions remain to be answered about the association between body image and the use of health-promoting and health-compromising behaviors, existing research suggests that body dissatisfaction does not predict greater use of healthy weight management behaviors, such as physical activ-

---

1. Inform young people that dieting, and particularly unhealthy weight control behaviors, may be counterproductive. Instead encourage positive eating and physical activity behaviors that can be maintained on a regular basis.

2. Do not use body dissatisfaction as a motivator for change. Instead, help young people care for their bodies so that they will want to nurture them through healthy eating, physical activity, and positive self-talk.

3. Encourage families to have regular, and enjoyable, family meals and to provide a home environment in which the healthy choices are the easy choices.

4. Encourage families to avoid weight talk: talk less about weight and do more to help children and adolescents achieve a weight that is healthy for them.

5. Assume overweight children and adolescents have experienced weight mistreatment and address this with youth and their families.

FIGURE 22.4. Preventing obesity and eating disorders in adolescents: Five recommendations for health care providers. From Neumark-Sztainer (2009b). Copyright 2009 by Elsevier. Reprinted by permission.

ity or fruit and vegetable intake (Neumark-Sztainer, Paxton, Hannan, Haines, & Story, 2006). Furthermore, a study of overweight adolescent girls found that body dissatisfaction predicts weight gain over time, even after adjusting for body mass index (BMI) at baseline (van den Berg & Neumark-Sztainer, 2007). Thus, health care providers should do all they can to help young people feel better about their bodies so that they will nurture them through healthy eating, physical activity, and positive self-talk.

The third recommendation involves the encouragement of more frequent and enjoyable family meals and the provision of a home environment that makes it easy for children to engage in healthier behaviors. As discussed earlier, family meals have been found to be protective against extreme weight control behaviors in adolescent girls, even after a 5-year follow-up period and after statistical adjustments for potential confounders such as family weight concerns and discussions (Neumark-Sztainer, Eisenberg, et al., 2008; Neumark-Sztainer et al., 2004).

The fourth recommendation is to encourage families to talk less about weight and do more to facilitate healthy eating and physical activity. Parental recognition of weight talk by family members and efforts to curb these discussions are crucial. It may be useful to let parents know that the most important behaviors to change in regard to weight talk may be the easiest to implement. For example, although not entirely clear-cut, research suggests that weight-related comments made directly to a child, such as teasing about weight and encouragement to diet, may be more harmful than indirect factors, such as observing a parent dieting or having a parent who has a high level of body dissatisfaction (Dixon, Adair, & O'Connor, 1996; Fulkerson et al., 2002; Keel, Heatherton, Hamden, & Hornig, 1997; Keery, Eisenberg, Boutelle, Neumark-Sztainer, & Story, 2006). Furthermore, it will probably be easier for parents to stop making weight-related comments in front of their children than for parents to stop thinking about their own body image concerns.

Finally, the fifth recommendation is to assume that young people have experienced mistreatment in regard to their weight and to address this issue. Given the high prevalence of teasing about weight and its associations with disordered eating behaviors, children need to know that this type of behavior is unacceptable and need the skills to cope with teasing directed at them or their peers (Hayden-Wade et al., 2005; Neumark-Sztainer, Story, & Faibisch, 1998; Neumark-Sztainer et al., 2007; Puhl & Latner, 2007). Discussing weight-related teasing with patients may be beyond the realm of comfort for many health care providers, yet it does need to be acknowledged and discussed with youth who have been teased about their weight. Medical providers can involve the use of mental health care providers when necessary, such as when there appears to be a serious problem, and when such services are available. Many young people who have been the victims of weight-teasing may feel as though they deserved it or that it was meant to be funny, and need to hear that neither is true or acceptable.

The role of health care providers in treating eating disorders among children and adolescents is well accepted, and different models are presented throughout this book. The role of health care providers in the prevention of eating disorders has been less well studied, and less is known about successful models. The five recommendations described here provide a starting point for discussions with young people and their families. Further work is needed to determine strategies for addressing these recommendations within clinical settings and the effectiveness of the various approaches.

Changing Societal Norms

If we are to see significant decreases in the prevalence of weight-related problems, including disordered eating behaviors and eating disorders, changes are needed at the societal level (Austin, 2000, 2001; Irving, 1999; Levine, 2010; Levine & Murnen, 2009; Paxton, in press). There is a need to change the culture of a society in which risk factors for eating disorders (e.g., body dissatisfaction and dieting) are allowed, and even encouraged, to thrive. Although living in such a society does not lead to the onset of eating disorders in all exposed to it, dangerous societal norms can increase the risk in vulnerable individuals. By significantly modifying social norms regarding body image and dieting behaviors, we have the potential to see not only a decrease in the prevalence of eating disorders, but also an improvement in the quality of life among people who are unhappy with their bodies and engage in unhealthy eating and dieting behaviors. Somewhat ironically, as discussed below, we may also expect see a decrease in the prevalence of obesity.

Working toward changes at the broader societal level can seem overwhelming in terms of the implementation of interventions and the assessment of their impact. Indeed, it can be very difficult to evaluate the effects of interventions operating at this level. In spite of the challenges, we are witnessing incremental and important changes at the societal level.

For example, making a change within the advertising world can seem like a hopeless venture, but we are seeing some positive changes. Although not without its flaws, the Dove Campaign for Real Beauty shines as an example of how women can be reached through the promotion of "real women," who may differ from the typical ideals seen in advertising in regard to body shape and size, age, hair color, or skin (Unilever, 2009). Across Europe, people are speaking out against the portrayal of extremely thin models, and their messages are being heard with responses coming from magazines and government. Within the United States, the National Eating Disorders Association operates a media watchdog program to encourage responsible media messages regarding body image issues (National Eating Disorders Association, 2010a). The Media Watchdog program was created to improve media messages about size, weight, and beauty. The program brings students, educators, health professionals, parents, eating disorders sufferers, and concerned consumers together to encourage companies and advertisers to send healthy media messages regarding body size and shape.

In Australia, serious steps are being taken "to develop a strategic national approach to negative body image in a coordinated, targeted, and effective way" (Australian Government, 2009). The Eating Disorder Coalition (*www.eatingdisorderscoalition.org*), composed of parents and professionals concerned about eating disorders, are lobbying in Washington, D.C., for legislative change, including the FREED Act (Federal Response to Eliminate Eating Disorders). The American Psychological Association (APA) has adopted an important policy statement regarding the prevention of eating disorders and obesity (Smith & APA Public Interest Government Relations Office, 2008a, 2008b). The Tri Delta sorority's steps toward ending "fat talk" (or at least avoiding it for 1 week) have received an abundance of attention in the media (Chadwick, 2009) and the movie it put together for Fat Talk Free Week has received many hits on youtube.com (TriDeltaEO, 2008). These efforts, and many others, offer the promise of hope for meaningful change within our society. Many of these endeavors were spearheaded by small groups of con-

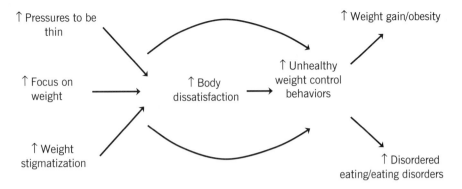

FIGURE 22.5. The current situation.

cerned individuals, demonstrating the importance of the actions of each one of us and the potential for making a difference.

By taking advantage of the current interest in working toward the prevention of obesity at a societal and environmental level, we may also be able to take strides in decreasing risk factors for eating disorders. Figure 22.5 shows the current situation regarding weight-related pressures within our society. Westernized societies focus heavily on weight, which leads to high levels of body dissatisfaction and the use of unhealthy weight control practices, which are associated with the onset of disordered eating/eating disorders and with weight gain/obesity. The situation is further compounded by easy access to calorie-rich foods and many opportunities to be sedentary. Figure 22.6 shows a proposed alternate route that offers more support for healthy eating and physical activity with less emphasis on weight per se. This alternate situation may be less likely to lead to body dissatisfaction and the use of unhealthy weight control practices and more likely to lead to healthier eating and physical activity patterns, which, in turn should lead to lower prevalences of eating disorders and obesity. Important aims for the prevention of eating disorders are to make changes within the home, school, workplace, neighborhood, and broader societal environments that place less emphasis on weight but provide more support for healthy eating and physical activity.

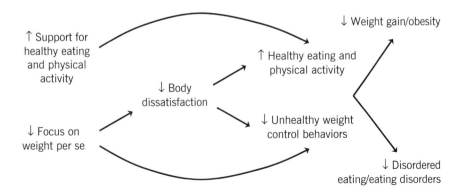

FIGURE 22.6. An alternate route.

Summary and Future Directions

In reviewing the work that has been done in the field of eating disorder prevention to date, it is important to keep in mind that this is a relatively new field. In preparing an article that discussed the field of eating disorder prevention and the next steps to be taken in moving forward, we found more than 50 articles in the scientific literature describing evaluations of eating disorder prevention programs during the decade 1994–2005 and noted that only six evaluated programs were published prior to that period (Neumark-Sztainer, Levine, et al., 2006). Since 2005, the research within the field of eating disorder prevention has continued to flourish as its importance becomes more widely recognized (Berger, Sowa, Bormann, Brix, & Strauss, 2008; Holt & Ricciardelli, 2008; Levine & Smolak, 2006, pp. 179–223; Neumark-Sztainer, Levine, et al., 2006; Pratt & Woolfenden, 2002; Stice et al., 2007). Although a great deal has been learned during this period, clearly much work remains.

The majority of peer-reviewed, evaluated interventions aimed at preventing eating disorders have been conducted within school settings, and many have been primarily classroom-based programs. Although the school is an excellent place to reach out to large numbers of children and adolescents, we need to move beyond the strategy of using classroom curricula to more comprehensive school-based programs. This is not to say that the development and implementation of appropriate classroom curricula should stop, but rather that these programs are unlikely to be successful in leading to significant and long-term changes on their own. That said, it is important to note that the implementation and evaluation of comprehensive school-based interventions are challenging and costly. In 1996 I published an article describing a framework for implementing a comprehensive school-based program to prevent a broad spectrum of weight-related problems, but have yet to implement and evaluate such a comprehensive program to assess its feasibility, effectiveness, and potential for dissemination (Neumark-Sztainer, 1996). Within the field of obesity prevention, there has been a move toward the implementation of comprehensive school-based programs that include significant changes in the school environment to promote healthier eating and physical activity behaviors (Story, Nanney, & Schwartz, 2009). Within the eating disorder prevention field, we also need to employ such comprehensive models or link up with the obesity prevention efforts to ensure that interventions are appropriate for different weight-related problems.

We also need to work toward the wider implementation and evaluation of eating disorder prevention interventions outside the school setting. Here, too, we can expect to see numerous obstacles. For example, modifications within health systems to train health care providers in eating disorders, and to allow adequate time for addressing risk and protective factors for eating disorders with children and their families, will require efforts and creativity at different levels. Changing norms regarding the acceptability of extremely thin images of women in magazines often seems nearly impossible. And discussing the importance of eating disorders in the wake of public health concern about the high prevalence of obesity in young people can seem futile, and practically irrelevant, at times. Yet changes within these, and other, arenas are happening. The passion and dedication of professionals and parents in preventing eating disorders accounts for much of the success to date and offers promise for overcoming these and other obstacles. For example, Michael Levine serves as a wealth of inspiration and information to those interested in this field and maintains a listing of eating disorder prevention work (Levine & Smolak, 2006, 2007, 2009). Contact him at *levine@kenyon.edu*. The website for the National Eating Disorders Association includes many resources to help in the prevention and early identification of eating disorders (National Eating Disorders Association, 2010b). The work done by Carolyn Becker and her team in changing social norms regarding fat talk and other eating disorder risk factors within college sororities offers a light at the end of a dark tunnel (Becker, Ciao, & Smith, 2008; Becker, Smith, & Ciao, 2005; Becker, Stice, Shaw, & Woda, 2009). Who would have thought that sororities would be taking such a leading role in this important work? Groups such as the Eating Disorder Coalition, the National Eating Disorders Association, and the Academy for Eating Disorders are working toward, and leading to, change in national policies regarding eating disorders within the United States. In Australia, numerous efforts are being implemented to change local and national policies of relevance to eating disorder prevention. Parents of children who have suffered from eating disorders, who were once shunned and silenced, have been active in taking a major role in accomplishing these changes. Finally, people from all walks of life seem to be rethinking how they talk about weight and dieting. Although the focus on a "strong body" and "healthy eating" may, at times, be body dissatisfaction and dieting in disguise, at least there is recognition of a new way to talk about our bodies and how we eat. It is exciting to look back at all that has occurred within the field of eating disorder prevention over the past two decades. It is even better to look forward and get involved in efforts aimed at the promotion of healthy body image and the prevention of disordered eating behaviors and eating disorders in young people.

References

Austin, S. B. (2000). Prevention research and eating disorders: Theory and new directions. *Psychological Medicine, 30*(6), 1249–1262.

Austin, S. B. (2001). Population-based prevention of eating disorders: An application of the Rose Prevention Model. *Preventive Medicine, 32*, 268–283.

Australian Government. (2009). Body image. Retrieved January 26, 2010, from *www.youth.gov.au/bodyimage.html*.

Becker, C. B., Ciao, A. C., & Smith, L. M. (2008). Moving from efficacy to effectiveness in eating disorders prevention: The Sorority Body Image Program. *Cognitive and Behavioral Practice, 15*(1), 18–27.

Becker, C. B., Smith, L. M., & Ciao, A. C. (2005). Reducing eating disorder risk factors in sorority members: A randomized trial. *Behavior Therapy, 36*, 245–253.

Becker, C. B., Stice, E., Shaw, H., & Woda, S. (2009). Use of empirically supported interventions for psychopathology: Can the participatory approach move us beyond the research-to-practice gap? *Behaviour Research and Therapy, 47*(4), 265–274.

Berger, U., Sowa, M., Bormann, B., Brix, C., & Strauss, B. (2008). Primary prevention of eating disorders: Characteristics of effective programmes and how to bring them to broader dissemination. *European Eating Disorders Review, 16*(3), 173–183.

Bernat, D. H., & Resnick, M. D. (2006). Healthy youth development: Science and strategies. *Journal of Public Health Management and Practice, 12*(Suppl. 6), S10–S16.

Bronfenbrenner, M. (1986). Ecology of the family as a context for human development: Research perspectives. *Developmental Psychology, 22*, 723–742.

Chadwick, D. (2009). You'd be so pretty if … *Psychology Today*. Retrieved from *www.*

psychologytoday.com/blog/youd-be-so-pretty-if/200910/what-we-dont-say-out-loud-the-internal-dialogue.

Dixon, R., Adair, V., & O'Connor, S. (1996). Parental influences of the dieting beliefs and behaviors of adolescent females in New Zealand. *Journal of Adolescent Health, 19,* 303–307.

Field, A. E., Austin, S. B., Taylor, C. B., Malspeis, S., Rosner, B., Rockett, H. R., et al. (2003). Relation between dieting and weight change among preadolescents and adolescents. *Pediatrics, 112*(4), 900–906.

Fulkerson, J. A., McGuire, M. T., Neumark-Sztainer, D., Story, M., French, S. A., & Perry, C. L. (2002). Weight-related attitudes and behaviors of adolescent boys and girls who are encouraged to diet by their mothers. *International Journal of Obesity, 26,* 1579–1587.

Haines, J., Neumark-Sztainer, D., Perry, C. L., Hannan, P. J., & Levine, M. P. (2006). V.I.K. (Very Important Kids): A school-based program designed to reduce teasing and unhealthy weight-control behaviors. *Health Education Research, 21,* 884–895.

Haines, J., Neumark-Sztainer, D., & Thiel, L. (2007). Addressing weight-related issues in an elementary school: What do students, parents, and school staff recommend? *Eating Disorders, 15*(1), 5–21.

Hayden-Wade, H. A., Stein, R. I., Ghaderi, A., Saelens, B. E., Zabinski, M. F., & Wilfley, D. E. (2005). Prevalence, characteristics, and correlates of teasing experiences among overweight children vs. non-overweight peers. *Obesity Research, 13*(8), 1381–1392.

Holt, K. E., & Ricciardelli, L. A. (2008). Weight concerns among elementary school children: A review of prevention programs. *Body Image, 5*(3), 233–243.

Irving, L. M. (1999). A bolder model of prevention: Science, practice, and activism. In N. Piran, M. Levine, & C. Steiner-Adair (Eds.), *Preventing eating disorders: A handbook of interventions and special challenges* (pp. 63–83). Philadelphia: Brunner/Mazel.

Keel, P. K., Heatherton, T. F., Hamden, J. L., & Hornig, C. D. (1997). Mothers, fathers, and

daughters: Dieting and disordered eating. *Eating Disorders, 5*(3), 216–228.

Keery, H., Eisenberg, M. E., Boutelle, K., Neumark-Sztainer, D., & Story, M. (2006). Relationships between maternal and adolescent weight-related behaviors and concerns: The role of perception. *Journal of Psychosomatic Research, 61,* 105–111.

Levine, M. (2010). Combating the negative impact of mass media. *Eating Disorders Review, 20*(6), 1–4.

Levine, M. P., & Murnen, S. K. (2009). "Everybody knows that mass media are/are not [pick one] a cause of eating disorders": A critical review of evidence for a causal link between media, negative body image, and disordered eating in females. *Journal of Social and Clinical Psychology, 28*(1), 9–42.

Levine, M. P., & Smolak, L. (2006). *The prevention of eating problems and eating disorders: Theory, research, and practice.* Mahwah, NJ: Erlbaum.

Levine, M. P., & Smolak, L. (2007). Prevention of negative body image, disordered eating, and eating disorders: An update. In S. Wonderlich, J. Mitchell, M. de Zwaan, & H. Steiger (Eds.), *Eating disorders review* (Vol. 18, Part 3, pp. 1–13). Oxford, UK: Radcliffe.

Levine, M. P., & Smolak, L. (2009). Prevention of negative body image and disordered eating in children and adolescents: Recent developments and promising directions. In L. Smolak & J. K. Thompson (Eds.), *Body image, eating disorders, and obesity in youth* (2nd ed., pp. 215–239). Washington, DC: American Psychological Association.

McVey, G., Gusella, J., Tweed, S., & Ferrari, M. (2009). A controlled evaluation of web-based training for teachers and public health practitioners on the prevention of eating disorders. *Eating Disorders, 17*(1), 1–26.

McVey, G., Gussella, J., Tweed, S., Ferrari, M., Roussel, J., & Colpitts, L. (2006). The student body: Promoting health at any size. Retrieved January 26, 2010, from *www.aboutkidshealth.ca/thestudentbody.*

McVey, G., Tweed, S., & Blackmore, E. (2007). Healthy Schools–Healthy Kids: A controlled evaluation of a comprehensive universal eating disorder program. *Body Image, 4*(2), 115–226.

National Eating Disorders Association. (2009). *NEDA outlook: Newsletter of the National Eating Disorders Association, 23.* Seattle, WA: Author. Retrieved from *www.nationaleatingdisorders.org/uploads/file/in-the-news/NEDA%20Outlook_Nov2009.pdf.*

National Eating Disorders Association. (2010a). Media watchdog. Seattle, WA: Author. Retrieved January 29, 2010, from *www.nationaleatingdisorders.org/programs-events/media-watchdog.php.*

National Eating Disorders Association. (2010b). NEDA. Seattle, WA: Author. Retrieved January 26, 2010, from *www.nationaleatingdisorders.org.*

Neumark-Sztainer, D. (1996). School-based programs for preventing eating disturbances. *Journal of School Health, 66*(2), 64–71.

Neumark-Sztainer, D. (2005). *"I'm, like, SO fat!": Helping your teen make healthy choices about eating and exercise in a weight-obsessed world.* New York: Guilford Press.

Neumark-Sztainer, D. (2009a). *New moves online.* Retrieved January 26, 2010, from *www.newmovesonline.com.*

Neumark-Sztainer, D. (2009b). Preventing obesity and eating disorders in adolescents: What can health care providers do? *Journal of Adolescent Health, 44*(3), 206–213.

Neumark-Sztainer, D., Eisenberg, M. E., Fulkerson, J. A., Story, M., & Larson, N. I. (2008). Family meals and disordered eating in adolescents: Longitudinal findings from Project EAT. *Archives of Pediatrics and Adolescent Medicine, 162,* 17–22.

Neumark-Sztainer, D., Flattum, C. F., Story, M., Feldman, S., & Petrich, C. A. (2008). Dietary approaches to healthy weight management for adolescents: The New Moves model. *Adolescent Medicine: State of the Art Reviews, 19*(3), 421–430.

Neumark-Sztainer, D., Friend, S. E., Flattum, C. F., Hannan, P. J., Story, M., Bauer, K. W., et al. (2010). New moves: Preventing weight-related problems in adolescent girls: A group-randomized study. *American Journal of Preventive Medicine, 39*(5), 421–432.

Neumark-Sztainer, D., Larson, N. I., Fulkerson, J. A., Eisenberg, M. E., & Story, M. (2010). Family meals and adolescents: What have we learned from Project EAT (Eating Among Teens). *Public Health Nutrition, 13,* 1113–1121.

Neumark-Sztainer, D., Levine, M. P., Paxton, S. J., Smolak, L., Piran, N., & Wertheim, E. H. (2006). Prevention of body dissatisfaction and disordered eating: What next? *Eating Disorders, 14*(4), 265–285.

Neumark-Sztainer, D., Paxton, S. J., Hannan, P. J., Haines, J., & Story, M. (2006). Does body satisfaction matter?: Five-year longitudinal associations between body satisfaction and health behaviors in adolescent females and males. *Journal of Adolescent Health, 39,* 244–251.

Neumark-Sztainer, D., Sherwood, N. E., Coller, T., & Hannan, P. J. (2000). Primary prevention of disordered eating among preadolescent girls: Feasibility and short-term impact of a community based intervention. *Journal of the American Dietetic Association, 100*(12), 1466–1473.

Neumark-Sztainer, D., Story, M., & Faibisch, L. (1998). Perceived stigmatization among overweight African American and Caucasian adolescent girls. *Journal of Adolescent Health, 23*(5), 264–270.

Neumark-Sztainer, D., Story, M., Hannan, P. J., Beuhring, T., & Resnick, M. D. (2000). Disordered eating among adolescents: Associations with sexual/physical abuse and other familial/psychosocial factors. *International Journal of Eating Disorders, 28*(3), 249–258.

Neumark-Sztainer, D., Wall, M., Guo, J., Story, M., Haines, J., & Eisenberg, M. (2006). Obesity, disordered eating, and eating disorders in a longitudinal study of adolescents: How do dieters fare five years later? *Journal of the American Dietetic Association, 106,* 559–568.

Neumark-Sztainer, D., Wall, M., Haines, J., Story, M., Sherwood, N. E., & van den Berg, P. (2007). Shared risk and protective factors for overweight and disordered eating in adolescents. *American Journal of Preventive Medicine, 33,* 359–369.

Neumark-Sztainer, D., Wall, M., Story, M., & Fulkerson, J. A. (2004). Are family meal patterns associated with disordered eating behaviors among adolescents? *Journal of Adolescent Health, 35*(5), 350–359.

O'Dea, J., & Maloney, D. (2000). Preventing eating and body image problems in children and adolescents using the Health Promoting Schools Framework. *Journal of School Health, 70*(1), 18–21.

O'Dea, J. A. (2004). Evidence for a self-esteem approach in the prevention of body image and eating problems among children and adolescents. *Eating Disorders, 12*(3), 225–239.

Paxton, S. (in press). Public health interventions for body dissatisfaction and eating disorders: Learning from Victoria. In G. McVey, M. Levine, N. Piran, & B. Ferguson (Eds.), *Prevention of eating-related disorders: Collaborative research, advocacy and policy change.* Waterloo, ON, Canada: Wilfred Laurier University Press.

Piran, N. (1998). A participatory approach to the prevention of eating disorders in a school. In W. Vandereycken & G. Noordenbos (Eds.), *The prevention of eating disorders* (pp. 173–186). New York: New York University Press.

Piran, N. (1999). Eating disorders: A trial of prevention in a high-risk school setting. *Journal of Primary Prevention, 20,* 75–90.

Piran, N. (2004). Teachers: On "being" (rather than "doing") prevention. *Eating Disorders: Journal of Treatment and Prevention, 12,* 1–9.

Pratt, B. M., & Woolfenden, S. R. (2002). Interventions for preventing eating disorders in children and adolescents. *Cochrane Database Systematic Reviews,* Issue 2 (Article No. CD002891), DOI: 10.1002/14651858. CD002891.

Puhl, R. M., & Latner, J. D. (2007). Stigma, obesity, and the health of the nation's children. *Psychological Bulletin, 133,* 557–580.

Resnick, M. D. (2000). Protective factors, resiliency and healthy youth development. *Adolescent Medicine: State of the Art Reviews, 11*(1), 157–165.

Richardson, S. M., Paxton, S. J., & Thomson, J. S. (2009). Is BodyThink an efficacious body image and self-esteem program?: A controlled evaluation with adolescents. *Body Image, 6*(2), 75–82.

Sjostrom, L. A., & Steiner-Adair, C. (2005). Full of ourselves: A wellness program to advance girl power, health and leadership: An eating disorders prevention program that works. *Journal of Nutrition Education and Behavior, 37*(Suppl. 2), S141–S144.

Smith, J., & APA Public Interest Government Relations Office. (2008a). Recommendations to prevent youth obesity and disordered eating. Retrieved February 16, 2009, from *www.apa.org/about/gr/pi.advocacy/2008/obesity.pdf.*

Smith, J., & APA Public Interest Government Relations Office. (2008b). Shared risk factors for youth obesity and disordered eating. Retrieved February 19, 2009, from *www.apa.org/about/gr/pi/advocacy/2008/shared-risk.pdf.*

Steiner-Adair, C., Sjostrom, L., Franio, D. L., Pai, S., Tucker, R., Becker, A. E., et al. (2002). Primary prevention of risk factors for eating disorders in adolescent girls: Learning from practice. *International Journal of Eating Disorders, 32,* 401–411.

Stice, E., Cameron, R. P., Killen, J. D., Hayward, C., & Taylor, C. B. (1999). Naturalistic weight-reduction efforts prospectively predict growth in relative weight and onset of obesity among female adolescents. *Journal of Consulting and Clinical Psychology, 67*(6), 967–974.

Stice, E., Shaw, H., & Marti, C. N. (2007). A meta-analytic review of eating disorder prevention programs: Encouraging findings. *Annual Review of Clinical Psychology, 3,* 207–231.

Story, M., Nanney, M. S., & Schwartz, M. B. (2009). Schools and obesity prevention: Creating school environments and policies to promote healthy eating and physical activity. *Milbank Quarterly, 87*(1), 71–100.

Toledo, T., & Neumark-Sztainer, D. (1999). Weighting for you! Training for high school faculty and staff in the prevention and detection of weight-related disorders among adolescents. *Journal of Nutrition Education, 31*(5), 283A.

TriDeltaEO (Producer). (2008, January 29). Tri Delta—Fat Talk Free Week. Video retrieved from *www.youtube.com/watch?v=RKPaxD61lwo.*

Unilever. (2009). Dove Campaign for Real Beauty. Retrieved January 29, 2010, from *www.dove.us/#/cfrb/.*

van den Berg, P., & Neumark-Sztainer, D. (2007). Fat 'n happy 5 years later: Is it bad for overweight girls to like their bodies? *Journal of Adolescent Health, 41,* 415–417.

Wonderlich, S. A., Crosby, R. D., Mitchell, J. E., Roberts, J. A., Haseltine, B., DeMuth, G., et al. (2000). Relationship of childhood sexual abuse and eating disturbance in children. *Journal of the American Academy of Child and Adolescent Psychiatry, 39*(10), 1277–1283.

CHAPTER 23

Innovative Approaches to Prevention and Intervention

The Internet

Angela Celio Doyle
Roslyn Binford Hopf
Debra L. Franko

The use of the Internet has grown exponentially over the past two decades and now reaches the vast majority of people in developed nations. There is great potential for the Internet as a platform to provide psychological interventions, including programs to prevent and treat eating and weight disorders. In a recent population-based study, more than 43% of adolescent females reported body disparagement, disordered eating, or full-syndrome eating disorders (Ackard, Fulkerson, & Neumark-Sztainer, 2007), and a growing number of males are affected by disordered eating as well (Muise, Stein, & Arbess, 2003). It is widely recognized that rates of obesity are also climbing rapidly, such that almost one in six adolescents are now considered overweight (Hedley et al., 2004) and higher rates of eating disorder symptoms are found among heavier adolescents (Neumark-Sztainer, Story, Hannan, Perry, & Irving, 2002). Many individuals are reluctant to seek help for negative body image or eating disorder symptoms because of shame or embarrassment and, even if help is desired, cost may be an impediment to receiving traditional services. Innovative approaches to the prevention and treatment of eating disorders are required in order to reach more individuals, particularly in geographical areas without adequate access to professionals with expertise in eating disorders. The Internet provides an innovative medium that may facilitate prevention and intervention efforts. A growing number of studies have reported on the efficacy of Internet programs in such endeavors.

Advantages of the Internet in the Prevention and Treatment of Eating Disorders

Adolescents and young adults are the group at highest risk for the development of eating disorders (Striegel-Moore & Bulik, 2007). They also represent a complex target group for a number of developmental reasons, including their drive for autonomy, tendency to focus on the present, experimenting/risk-taking behaviors, variable attention spans, busy schedules, identity issues, and being highly attuned to the latest brands, fads, and celebrities (Arnett, 2007). Children and adolescents spend an average of 5½ hours a day using media, which is more time than that spent doing anything else other than sleeping (Henry J. Kaiser Family Foundation, 2004). Adolescents use the Internet more than any other age group. In a recent study by the Pew Internet and American Life Project (Jones & Fox, 2009), results indicated that 93% of youth ages 12–17 are online and their primary activities are watching videos (57%), engaging in social networking (65%), making purchases (38%), and seeking health information (28%). In a Kaiser Family Foundation report (Rideout, 2010), as cited in a recent *Pediatrics* article by Strasburger, Jordan, and Donnerstein (2010), 8- to 18-year-olds spend on average 90 minutes per day on the Internet. In 2009 children under 12 years old constituted nearly 16 million, or 9.5%, of active online users, and time spent online by this group has increased 63% in the last 5 years, from nearly 7 hours in May 2004 to more than 11 hours online in May 2009, according to Nielsen Online (2009). Given the ubiquitous nature of online behavior in the lives of young people, utilizing the Internet for prevention and intervention efforts is an optimal strategy for reaching this group.

Internet-based programs are accessible to large groups, cost-effective, and much less labor intensive than face-to-face interventions. Moreover, multimedia technology has several distinct benefits over traditional formats (Budman, 2000). Internet-based programs can provide a multisensory experience, which conveys information more vividly and memorably than single-medium presentations. Individuals are more naturally "literate" in learning via visual images and have to do less decoding than when presented with text (Seeck, Schomer, Mainwaring, & Ives, 1995). The multimedia approach encourages active participation in the experience by allowing the user to physically interact with the content. Finally, Internet-based programs provide flexible delivery and can be tailored to suit a wide range of learning styles and needs.

The specific merits of Internet-based programs for eating disorder prevention and treatment include (1) anonymity, (2) varying models of care, (3) program reach, and (4) technological benefits provided by current Internet capabilities. Each is addressed here in turn.

Online intervention delivery can assist in overcoming obstacles unique to body image and eating disorders (Paxton & Franko, 2010). The first advantage of Internet-based programs is that users can obtain information, participate in chat groups with others, and interact anonymously. For people at risk for or struggling with eating disorders, this may be a distinct advantage because of the shame, secrecy, and embarrassment often experienced. In particular, high levels of shame associated with disordered eating symptomatology have been found to be related to a reluctance to seek help (Hepworth & Paxton, 2007). Skarderud (2003) suggests that the anonymity associated with an Internet-delivered intervention can assist in overcoming this hurdle to seeking treatment. The Internet offers a way to learn more about eating disorders, and potentially even receive help, without risk of disclosure.

However, this advantage can also become a disadvantage in the context of Internet-based treatment if, unbeknownst to his or her therapist, an individual deteriorates in a dangerous way and does not inform the therapist. It is critical to thoroughly assess Internet-based treatment participants to ensure suitability for the particular program and to determine the likelihood of risky behaviors, an issue that is addressed later in the chapter.

The continuum of care model is widely used in both intervention and prevention efforts for eating disorders (Wilson, Grilo, & Vitousek, 2007). In the universal prevention sphere, the Internet can reach large numbers of young people with the provision of psychoeducational programs, which are often carried out with the use of school-based approaches (Cousineau et al., 2010; Franko et al., 2008; O'Dea & Abraham, 2000). A more selective prevention endeavor, in which the targeted group has been determined to be at risk of developing an eating disorder, has also has been carried out with multimedia programs (e.g., Franko et al., 2005; Taylor et al., 2006). Even within a universal prevention program, algorithms can be programmed through self-report quizzes that guide participants who report higher levels of symptomatology to more tailored prevention topics, thereby simultaneously providing universal and targeted prevention (Luce et al., 2005). The Internet offers the possibility of providing treatment at a lower level of intensity than one-on-one in-person therapy as a first-line approach. Treatment protocols that provide online counseling from a therapist and a self-help manual have been found to be efficacious, and positive findings have recently been reported (Fernández-Aranda et al., 2009; Pretorius et al., 2009). Particularly in locations where there are waiting lists for treatment, providing an online option offers a reasonable response to those seeking care.

A significant advantage of Internet-based programs is the ability to reach large numbers of people regardless of time of day or geographic location. Internet-based technologies can be used as a means of extending access to those in need of an intervention who, by virtue of location do not have access to care. Technological approaches attempt to overcome the practical difficulties of receiving in-person intervention, such as geographic centralization of specialist services, and can reduce costs to the participants (Heinicke, Paxton, McLean, & Wertheim, 2007; Myers, Swan-Kremeier, Wonderlich, Lancaster, & Mitchell, 2004). In addition, computer-based technologies are being used as a means of providing support groups for individuals with eating disorders. Analogous to face-to-face support groups, chat room support groups have been established in which registered participants may log into a chat room and discuss issues in an unstructured way in the presence of a facilitator (Brooke, Pethick, & Greenwood, 2007; Darcy & Dooley, 2007). Evidence from a study involving a chat room support group suggested that almost 80% of participants preferred the chat room conversations to face-to-face conversations (Zabinski, Wilfley, et al., 2001).

Finally, Internet-based prevention and treatment programs have a number of advantages that relate to the availability and sophistication of the available technology. Current software allows for ease in changing or updating Web-based content, as well as the ability to program algorithms that release content based on user characteristics or responses. Moreover, users can be provided with instant feedback, based on individual input and on the algorithms that guide the program. Online multimedia applications increasingly allow not only for targeting information to groups, but for tailoring of personal health information, which can offer advantages over standard text- or video-based education materials and may approximate counseling information provided by a therapist. Indeed, with a new generation of Internet-based programs, messages can be both *targeted* to a group (e.g., to females or to adolescents who are at risk because of membership in a given group, i.e., gymnasts) and *tailored* to current eating and lifestyle habits (e.g., provision of unique combinations of messaging to the adolescent who skips breakfast or relies on protein shakes for a meal). In addition, usage can be tracked in terms of time of day, hours of usage, and movement on the website to better understand the user's interaction with the program. Finally, several platforms allow for self-monitoring of eating behaviors, cognitions, and emotions, which is altogether more user-friendly than traditional paper-based formats.

Recent Research

Research has begun to examine whether the Internet and other related technological media such as chat rooms and SMS (i.e., instant messaging) are helpful in disseminating prevention and intervention programming for eating disorders and overweight in children and adolescents.

Technology in the Delivery of Weight-Related Psychoeducation

Two studies have evaluated the feasibility and acceptance of an interactive program in delivering psychoeducational information regarding puberty, self-esteem, body image and other related topics to young adolescents.

Cousineau, Franko, Green, Watt, and Rancourt (2006) examined the feasibility of an interactive computer program called *Body Morph* in providing information about puberty to 34 sixth- and seventh-grade girls ($N = 17$) and boys ($N = 17$). In the program, an animated teenager introduces students to an interactive book titled *Body Morph*, which presents physiological information about hormones, growth spurts, secondary sex characteristics, and normal body changes/weight gain. Skills training material is focused on challenging peer pressure and examining the cultural norms of the ideal body image as a determinant of self-esteem. Girls and boys read material specific to their genders via a "frequently asked questions" bulletin board that addresses common concerns regarding puberty in boys (e.g., "Some of my buddies have deeper voices and I still sound like I'm 8. Why?") and girls (e.g., "Why am I gaining weight while my girlfriends are still skinny?").

Students significantly improved their knowledge about puberty after participating in *Body Morph*. In particular, an association between an increase in knowledge of puberty and less internalization of the male sociocultural ideal was found in boys. Participants reported being very satisfied with the program. As pointed out by the authors, this approach allows for information about puberty to be presented in a confidential manner. Indeed, the provision of information related to puberty or other sensitive topics may prove less embarrassing to students if the material is presented online, versus face-to-face, and adolescents may learn more as a result.

Using an interactive Internet-based prevention program called *Trouble on the Tightrope: In Search of Skateboard Sam*, Cousineau and colleagues (2010) randomized 190 young adolescents (mean age = 11.7; $n = 108$ girls, $n = 82$ boys) to either the *Skateboard Sam* intervention or a control group in which students viewed science-based websites. The *Skateboard Sam* program presented information about puberty, self-esteem, body image, nutrition, physical activity, and peer relations via games, quizzes, and videos in which animated teenagers described their pubertal challenges. Those who completed the program increased their knowledge about puberty relative to controls. Weight-related body esteem and self-esteem were moderated by pubertal status (i.e., scores on these measures were more improved for those adolescents in the intervention group who had already begun puberty), indicating that education about these topics was particularly salient for those who were going through the process. Improvements in self-esteem were observed in girls who participated in *Skateboard Sam*; however, decreases in self-worth and self-esteem were observed for boys in the intervention condition. Findings from both of these programs offer evidence for the feasibility and effectiveness of providing health education through the Internet.

Technology in the Delivery of Targeted Prevention for Eating Disorders

My Body, My Life: Body Image Program for Adolescent Girls

Using a synchronous (real-time) online group format, Heinicke and colleagues (2007) evaluated the effects of administering an Internet-based intervention called *My Body, My Life: Body Image Program for Adolescent Girls* to adolescent girls (N = 73, range = 12–18, mean age = 14.4) who self-identified as having body image or eating problems. Participants were randomly assigned to the intervention group (*n* = 36) or a delayed treatment control group (*n* = 37). Groups of four to eight girls met with a therapist online for 90 minutes for 6 weeks. Sessions were primarily used to talk about eating concerns and body image, as well as to learn strategies to improve these issues. A discussion board was also offered to allow participants an opportunity to stay in contact with the other group members in the interim periods between chats.

My Body, My Life is based on a cognitive-behavioral approach and focuses on improving body image, eating issues, motivation for change, and unhealthy eating patterns. The program content includes a description of the rationale for normalizing eating, self-monitoring, and a context for examining relationships between low self-esteem, depression, interpersonal relationships, and body dissatisfaction. Social pressures, social comparison, teasing, and fat talk are also discussed. Additional components of the program include cognitive restructuring (e.g., challenging irrational beliefs and negative thoughts about one's body) and learning strategies to prevent relapse. Each week, participants were asked to read the psychoeducational information and complete the intervention activities, which corresponded to each session, detailed in a self-help manual. The group chat for the week was based on this material.

Body dissatisfaction, disordered eating, and depressive symptomatology were significantly improved at the end of the intervention. Moreover, these improvements were maintained at 2- and 6-month follow-up. Intervention participants showed significant improvements over control participants on most measures of eating pathology, as well as depressive symptoms. Qualitative data provide further support for the online intervention. Most participants reported feeling comfortable using the Internet, with only 15% reporting that they would have rather met face-to-face. Although group members never met in person, they encouraged and supported each other and reported feeling reassured that others experienced similar feelings of body image–related distress. These findings suggest that synchronous online chat room technology can successfully deliver group therapy for female adolescents at risk of developing an eating disorder.

ES[S]PRIT

ES[S]PRIT is an Internet-based prevention and early intervention program for university students who are at risk of developing an eating disorder (Bauer, Moessner, Wolf, Haug, & Kordy, 2009). The program utilizes a stepped-care approach by offering support based on the participants' degree of impairment. Progressively more intensive components are offered as symptom intensity increases, starting with psychoeducation, then symptom monitoring, supportive feedback, peer support (i.e., moderated Internet forum), and, finally, professional online counseling (i.e., individual chat session with a clinician). If a participant develops significant eating disorder symptoms, a referral to the university counseling center is made for face-to-face treatment.

In order to match the intensity of support to the needs of each participant, a monitoring/automated feedback program continuously tracks the symptoms and impairment of each participant during the study. After a participant completes the monitoring assessment, the program determines whether the pattern of change has (1) improved, (2) deteriorated, or remained either (3) functional or (4) dysfunctional since the last monitoring assessment. Then a feedback message is selected by chance from a pool of 10–15 statements corresponding to this specific pattern of change and is sent to the participant through the program. These feedback messages provide support as well as advice on how participants can improve their eating behavior and attitudes about shape and weight. An e-mail is automatically sent to the online counselor if a participant's functioning significantly deteriorates.

This program was piloted with a sample of college women ($N = 44$, mean age = 31, $SD = 12.7$). Findings indicate that *ES[S]PRIT* is a technically feasible program that may assist in the earlier referral of individuals to more intensive interventions such as face-to-face therapy. In addition, 83% of the scheduled monitoring assessments were completed, which suggests good compliance with the monitoring component of the program (Bauer et al., 2009).

The feasibility and acceptability of this program for younger adolescents (range = 13–16 years) is currently being tested in an ongoing study. The program content was adapted to a younger group by using more teenage-appropriate language. Preliminary findings indicate that 88% of participants ($N = 178$) were "overall satisfied" with the *YoungES[S]PRIT* program (Lindenberg, Bauer, Moessner, & Kordy, 2010).

Student Bodies

Student Bodies is an 8–10 week, Internet-based multimedia program that uses a self-help cognitive-behavioral approach to decrease weight and shape concerns and unhealthy weight regulation behaviors (e.g., extreme dietary restriction, excessive exercise). The program content includes (1) psychoeducational readings on body image, media influences, nutrition, dieting, physical activity, and eating disorders; (2) cognitive-behavioral exercises; (3) the use of an online body image journal to record thoughts, feelings and events that trigger body dissatisfaction; and (4) an electronic discussion board (asynchronous) or chat room group (synchronous) that is either moderated or unmoderated.

The efficacy of this online intervention has been extensively tested for college-age students at high risk of developing eating disorders (Celio et al., 2000; Low et al., 2006; Winzelberg et al., 1998, 2000; Zabinski, Celio, Jacobs, Manwaring, & Wilfley, 2003;

Zabinski, Pung, et al., 2001; Zabinski, Wilfley, Calfas, Winzelberg, & Taylor, 2004). Overall, significant improvements have been found on measures of eating disorder attitudes and behaviors (reductions in body image dissatisfaction, problematic eating disorder behaviors, and shape and weight concerns) for those in the *Student Bodies* program as compared with control participants, with effect sizes of 0.30 to 0.67. Furthermore, participation in *Student Bodies* was associated with a lower likelihood of eating disorder diagnosis among college-age women who reported engaging in compensatory behaviors and were at a higher weight at baseline assessment (Taylor et al., 2006).

Given the success of this online intervention in college-age students, the effectiveness of *Student Bodies* was tested in a younger population. Within a high school sample, Abascal, Bruning Brown, Winzelberg, Dev, and Taylor (2004) investigated whether *Student Bodies* was effective when students were allocated into separate groups based on degree of risk and motivation so as to provide a more supportive environment among similarly thinking and feeling peers. Degree of risk of developing an eating disorder (low/high) and level of motivation to improve their body images (low/high) were determined prior to beginning the intervention. Seventy-eight girls (13–16 years) were randomized to (1) a higher-risk and more highly motivated group, (2) a lower-risk or less motivated group, or (3) a combined group.

Although eating disorder attitudes and behaviors significantly improved in all of the groups (effect sizes = 0.49–0.75), participants in the higher-risk, more highly motivated group experienced significantly more positive interactions (e.g., made positive comments about others, about their own progress or about the program) and made significantly fewer negative comments about the program in the online group discussion, as compared with the higher-risk and more highly motivated participants in the combined group. This appears to suggest that girls found the group to be more supportive when the other group members were similar to them in terms of risk and level of motivation.

Luce and colleagues (2005) evaluated the feasibility of screening for eating disorders and overweight within *Student Bodies* and giving individualized feedback about the degree of risk of developing an eating disorder and/or obesity among female high school students ($N = 174$) in 10th grade. Students were assessed online. The algorithm identified 111 "no-risk," 36 "eating disorder risk," 16 "overweight risk," and 5 "both risks." Fifty-six percent of the "eating disorder risk" and 50% of the "overweight risk" groups decided to participate in the recommended targeted intervention once they received feedback on their risks. Shape and weight concerns were significantly lessened in all groups.

In another randomized, controlled evaluation of *Student Bodies* with high school girls, a supplemental online program for the students' parents was evaluated (Bruning Brown, Winzelberg, Abascal, & Taylor, 2004). The unstructured parent program was available for use during 4 weeks of the 8-week intervention period for the high school participants. It provided psychoeducational materials focused on accepting variations in weight and shape; discouraging critical comments and teasing related to eating, weight, and shape; and identifying disordered eating habits or attitudes. Exercises were provided to assist parents in determining if they were contributing to unhealthy attitudes toward weight, shape, and/or eating, and guidance was given to help parents improve their communication about these issues with their adolescent. A discussion board was also provided for parents to discuss topics and interact anonymously. Eleven of 22 *Student Bodies* participants' parents used the supplemental program and, among the 11 parents using the program, a high degree of use and satisfaction was reported. Pre–post analyses indicated improvements on parent measures of critical attitudes regarding weight/shape toward others in the intervention group, as compared with the waiting-list control group. There were no differences in students' outcomes on measures of eating disorder attitudes and behaviors, based on parental use of the supplemental program.

Technology in the Delivery of Treatment for Eating Disorders

As in the adult literature, in which only one Internet-based treatment program for eating disorders has published results (Fernández-Aranda et al., 2009), only one program for adolescents has been studied to date. Pretorius and colleagues (2009) examined the feasibility, acceptance, and effectiveness of a multimedia Internet-based cognitive-behavioral therapy (CBT) intervention for bulimia nervosa (BN) symptomatology in adolescents (N = 101, mean age = 18) with BN or eating disorder not otherwise specified (EDNOS). Adolescents were randomly assigned to either the intervention condition, which included (1) the *Overcoming Bulimia Online* program (Williams, Aubin, Cottrell, & Harkin, 1998), (2) separate moderated electronic message boards for participants and parents, and (3) weekly e-mail support from a CBT-experienced therapist or a control condition.

Results included significant reductions in objective binge eating, purging, dietary restraint, and concerns about shape, weight and eating; these improvements were maintained at 6-month follow-up. Participant perspectives of the intervention program were positive. In addition to evaluating the program as accessible, convenient, and confidential, many participants reported that this program gave them the needed knowledge and confidence to seek professional help or to confide in a parent or other authority figure (e.g., teacher) about their eating disorder. Therefore, it appears that this program might be helpful as a first step in providing treatment for adolescents with BN.

Technology in the Delivery of Weight Management Programs

The use of modern communication technologies in the delivery of weight management programs to address pediatric and adolescent obesity and overweight, as well as co-occurring binge eating and body image disparagement, has recently been studied.

Student Bodies 2

A recent randomized controlled trial (RCT) evaluated an Internet-based program that simultaneously addressed weight loss and eating disorder attitudes and behaviors in adolescents (Celio Doyle et al., 2008). Eighty overweight adolescents were randomized to either *Student Bodies 2* (SB2; n = 40) or usual care (UC; n = 40). Members of the UC group received basic information on nutrition and physical activity but were not given specific instructions on behavior modification.

SB2 utilizes a cognitive-behavioral approach and was specifically designed to help overweight adolescent girls and boys lose weight and improve body image. The 16-week intervention included education about healthy nutritional choices (e.g., portion control), physical activity, behavior modification for managing weight, and cognitive activities to improve body image (e.g., cognitive restructuring). Participants were asked to keep an online body image diary to record triggers for body dissatisfaction. The first 8 weeks of the program focused on weight loss, and the latter 8 weeks targeted improving body image. Adolescents were expected to record their daily food intake, amount of physical activity obtained, and their weight via an online journal. Once a week, *SB2* participants received an e-mail newsletter that included personalized feedback about their eating, exercise, weight, and other targeted activities. In addition, groups of 8–13 adolescents at a time participated in an asynchronous, moderated discussion group that provided a forum to seek support, build relationships, and problem solve. Parents were also sent a monthly newsletter through the mail to encourage them to create a positive and constructive home environment that would enable their child to achieve his or her goals.

Body mass index (BMI) *z*-scores were reduced in the *SB2* group as compared with the UC group from baseline to postintervention. However, this difference was not maintained at 4-month follow-up because of weight loss in the UC participants from postintervention to follow-up. *SB2* participants reported using healthy eating-related (e.g., monitoring caloric intake) and physical activity-related (implementing problem-solving skills to increase physical activity) weight loss skills more frequently than UC participants postintervention and at 4-month follow-up. As discussed earlier, use of these healthy lifestyle changes could be equated with weight loss or weight maintenance in the future. Finally, this delivery approach was acceptable to patients, as satisfaction ratings of the program were quite high.

SB2-BED

Jones and colleagues (2008) conducted a randomized controlled trial (RCT) evaluating a modified version of *SB2* that concurrently targeted binge eating and weight maintenance in adolescents. One hundred five male and female high school students at risk for overweight were randomized to *SB2-BED* (*Student Bodies 2–Binge Eating Disorder*; *n* = 52) or a wait-list control (*n* = 53). Significant decreases in BMI, binge-eating episodes, and shape/weight concerns were found among adolescents who participated in the *SB2-BED* intervention. Individuals in the *SB2-BED* group who reported episodes of objective overeating or binge eating prior to beginning the intervention were found to have significantly greater weight loss at follow-up assessment, in comparison with the control group.

The findings of both of these controlled studies indicate that the Internet-delivered intervention *SB2* is moderately effective in short-term weight loss and weight maintenance and is very effective in reduction of binge eating and promotion of healthy eating-related and physical activity-related weight loss skills. These investigations also provide support for programs that manage weight and reduce eating disorder attitudes and behaviors simultaneously.

Internet-Based Behavioral Weight Management Program for African American Adolescent Girls and Their Parents

An interactive Internet-based behavioral weight management program was compared with an educational control group, consisting of static websites and face-to-face sessions, in a sample of African American girls (*N* = 57; 11–15 years) who were overweight and had at least one overweight biological parent (Williamson et al., 2005). Overweight parents (*N* = 57) also participated in the study. After 6 months of participation in the study, adolescents in the Internet program decreased their mean body fat more than controls, and parents in the Internet program reduced their mean body weight more than controls. Unfortunately, this weight loss was regained over the next 18 months, resulting in no between-group differences at 2-year follow-up (Williamson et al., 2006). The authors posited that this lack of weight loss maintenance was related to decreased use of the web-site over the course of the follow-up period.

Text Messaging Program for Weight Control

A novel approach that could be applied in the treatment of overweight children was recently described by Shapiro and colleagues (2008). Specifically, the feasibility and acceptance of using short message service (SMS, or text messaging) for self-monitoring healthy behaviors as an intervention for weight control in children was tested. Fifty-eight children (5–13 years) and their parents were randomized to a monitor condition via SMS ($n = 18$), a monitor condition via paper diary ($n = 18$), or a control condition that did not include monitoring ($n = 22$), for 8 weeks.

All children and their parents participated in three in-person, 90-minute, weekly group education sessions that targeted three behaviors: (1) increasing physical activity (5,000 steps daily); (2) decreasing screen time (< 1 hour total screen time per day of tele-vision, video games, computers, etc.); and (3) reducing sugar-sweetened beverage (SSB) consumption. Participants in the SMS group were provided with a mobile phone and were requested to send two text messages (one SMS from the parent and one SMS from the child) with responses to the following questions: (1) "What was the number on your pedometer today?" (2) "How many SSBs did you drink today?" (3) "How many min-utes of screen time did you have today?" Participants using the paper diaries recorded this information on a self-monitoring form. SMS participants received an immediate, automated text message, which provided feedback employing an algorithm based on the following information: (1) how many goals were met and (2) any improvement or dete-rioration from the previous day. For instance, if the participant met his or her behavioral goals for physical activity and screen time but did not meet the goal for SSB, the par-ticipant would receive the following text message: "Wow, you met your step and screen time goals—Congratulations! What happened to beverages?" Families in the "paper diary" condition received delayed verbal feedback at the in-person meetings. Members of the control group participated in the intervention sessions but were not instructed to self-monitor. Children who self-monitored via SMS technology had somewhat lower attrition rates (28%) as compared with 61% and 50% in the paper diary and control groups, respectively. Moreover, adherence to self-monitoring was significantly greater in the SMS group (43%) than the paper diary group (19%). It appears that children prefer a program that incorporates a technological device (i.e., SMS) rather than a traditional self-monitoring program, suggesting that SMS is a viable and effective alternative for self-monitoring healthy behaviors in children.

In summary, a small but growing body of research literature supports the efficacy of modern communication technologies in the delivery of psychoeducational prevention and intervention approaches to children and adolescents at risk of and presenting with eating disorders and/or overweight. These programs appear to be helpful in engendering attitudinal and behavioral changes and are well liked by participants.

Risk Management and Areas for Development

Concerns about Internet-delivered prevention and treatment include maintaining confidentiality, crisis management, and technical difficulties that lead to frustration and reduced compliance by participants (Zabinski, Celio, Wilfley, & Taylor, 2003). It is critical that investigators be conscious of risk management procedures while using this mode of delivery. Risks include a breach of confidentiality through a variety of means, whether intentional or unintentional (e.g., hackers), the worsening of participants' psychological symptoms and the presence of more serious psychological problems that cannot be addressed in a timely or sufficiently aggressive manner via the Internet. Risk management procedures should include password protection, an automated time out of the program after a certain duration of no activity, and the avoidance of using protected health information online, at a minimum. To protect participants who are at high risk of developing an eating disorder and for those who are receiving treatment online, it is important to clearly state the purpose of the program (e.g., does the program constitute treatment?) and the limits of availability of any moderators, counselors, or other administrative personnel involved in the program. Obtaining phone numbers and other contact information from family members to use in case of an emergency, such as an indication of suicidality by the adolescent in an online self-monitoring form, is very important. Furthermore, it is also prudent to identify local clinical care and to provide participants and their families with this information to use in case of emergency. With good risk management, the benefits of Internet and other technology-delivered programs likely outweigh the risks.

Several areas of Internet-based programs have gone relatively unexamined and are worthy of additional attention in research studies. First, most Internet programs that have been developed primarily target the individual child or adolescent, to the exclusion of parents or family. However, there have been a small number of studies to date that have included a parallel or supplemental program focused on parents (e.g., Bruning Brown et al., 2004; Pretorius et al., 2009; Shapiro et al., 2008; Williamson et al., 2005). The role of parents as a resource in treatment has been recognized (Le Grange, Lock, Loeb, & Nicholls, 2010), and Internet programs that capitalize on this resource may enhance outcomes, especially in regard to adherence. For example, Pretorius and colleagues (2009) found that participants completed a median of only three of eight online sessions. Thus, perhaps parental intervention can assist in increasing adherence to Internet-based programs. Second, alternative Internet-based technologies beyond text-driven psychoeducation and asynchronous discussion boards have been only minimally studied. Real-time chat rooms or instant messaging may encourage greater use of online programs because of these technologies being more relevant and modern. Other Internet-based technologies are used very frequently by adolescents (e.g., social networking sites), but have not yet been studied as media for eating disorder prevention or treatment. A recent Pew Internet report by Lenhart, Purcell, Smith, and Zickuhr (2010) shows that in 2009, 14% of adolescents were blogging, 73% of online adolescents were using social networking sites (e.g., Facebook, MySpace), and 8% were using Twitter. As of 2009, 75% of adolescents and 58% of 12-year olds had cell phones and more than a quarter of youth used cell phones to access the Internet wirelessly. As the use of these technologies increases, employing SMS as well as Internet-based applications available through cell phones appears to be a promising direction.

A challenge faced in developing programs using innovative technology is evident in the changing patterns of use by children and adolescents. For instance, the rate of cell phone ownership by adolescents has almost doubled since 2004, but the percentage of adolescents who blog online was reduced by half over a period of 3 years (28% in 2006 to 14% in 2009). This quickly shifting landscape of technology and user preferences makes it extremely difficult to quickly identify a form of technology, adapt a prevention program or intervention specifically for that mode of delivery, obtain funding for the research, and execute a study to evaluate outcomes. To complicate matters further, once an innovative approach has been shown to be efficacious, because of the extremely fast pace of technological advances, the original program may quickly appear outdated and unappealing to users. These efforts are particularly hampered by the relatively limited research funding in academic settings. In comparison, private companies are better able to keep up with technological advances, but their programs may or may not be driven by research findings.

Future Directions

The Internet and related technological devices have become central aspects of our day-to-day functioning and social interactions. Research on the role of the Internet in the prevention and treatment of eating disorders in children and adolescents suggests that the use of technology holds great promise for our abilities to address these problems through innovative, cost-effective, and appealing means. Keeping up with technology and user preferences, particularly in a group that is rapidly taking up new technology, remains a significant challenge. Collaboration with other investigators working with technology and improving connections with technology-based private industry may help to improve our ability to "stay current," as well as to disseminate these programs widely, once there is evidence of their effectiveness.

References

Abascal, L., Bruning Brown, J. B., Winzelberg, A. J., Dev, P., & Taylor, C. B. (2004). Combining universal and targeted prevention for school-based eating disorder programs. *International Journal of Eating Disorders, 35*, 1–5.

Ackard, D. M., Fulkerson, J. A., & Neumark-Sztainer, D. (2007). Prevalence and utility of DSM-IV eating disorder diagnostic criteria among youth. *International Journal of Eating Disorders, 40*, 409–417.

Arnett, J. J. (2007). *Adolescence and emerging adulthood: A cultural approach.* Upper Saddle River, NJ: Prentice Hall.

Bauer, S., Moessner, M., Wolf, M., Haug, S., & Kordy, H. (2009). ES[S]PRIT: An Internet-based programme for the prevention and early intervention of eating disorders in college students, *British Journal of Guidance and Counselling, 37*, 327–336.

Brooke, L., Pethick, L., & Greenwood, K. (2007, August). *Internet-based support for people with an eating disorder.* Paper presented at the Australian and New Zealand Academy of Eating Disorders Conference, Melbourne, Australia.

Bruning Brown, J., Winzelberg, A. J., Abascal, L. B., & Taylor, C. B. (2004). An evaluation of an Internet-delivered eating disorder prevention program for adolescents and their parents. *Journal of Adolescent Health, 35,* 290–296.

Budman, S. H. (2000). Behavioral health care dot-com and beyond: Computer-mediated communications in mental health and substance abuse treatment. *American Psychologist, 55,* 1290–1300.

Celio, A. A., Winzelberg, A. J., Wilfley, D. E., Springer, E. A., Dev, P., & Taylor, C. B. (2000). Reducing risk factors for eating disorders: Comparison of an Internet and a classroom-delivered psychoeducational program. *Journal of Consulting and Clinical Psychology, 68,* 650–657.

Celio Doyle, A., Goldschmidt, A., Huang, C., Winzelberg, A. J., Taylor, C. B., & Wilfley, D. E. (2008). Reduction of overweight and eating disorder symptoms via the Internet in adolescents: A randomized controlled trial. *Journal of Adolescent Health, 43,* 172–179.

Cousineau, T. M., Franko, D. L., Green, T. C., Watt, M., & Rancourt, D. (2006). Body Morph: Feasibility testing of an interactive CD-ROM to teach young adolescents about puberty. *Journal of Youth and Adolescence, 35,* 1015–1021.

Cousineau, T. M., Franko, D. L., Trant, M., Rancourt, D., Ainscough, J., Chaudhuri, A., et al. (2010). Teaching adolescents about changing bodies: Randomized controlled trial of an Internet puberty education and body dissatisfaction prevention program. *Body Image, 74*(4), 296–300.

Darcy, A. M., & Dooley, B. (2007). A clinical profile of participants in an online support group. *European Eating Disorders Review, 15,* 185–195.

Fernández-Aranda, F., Nunez, A., Martinez, C., Krug, I., Cappozzo, M., Carrard, I., et al. (2009). Internet-based cognitive-behavioral therapy for bulimia nervosa: A controlled study. *Cyberpsychological Behavior, 12,* 37–41.

Franko, D. L., Cousineau, T. M., Trant, M., Green, T. C., Rancourt, D., Thompson, D., et al. (2008). Motivation, self-efficacy, physical activity, and nutrition in college students: Randomized controlled trial of an Internet-based education program. *Preventive Medicine, 47,* 369–377.

Franko, D. L., Mintz, L. B., Villapiano, M., Green, T. C., Mainelli, D., Folensbee, L., et al. (2005). Food, mood, and attitude: Reducing risk for eating disorders in college women. *Health Psychology, 24,* 567–578.

Hedley, A. A., Ogden, C. L., Johnson, C. L., Carroll, M. D., Curtin, L. R., & Flegal, K. M. (2004). Prevalence of overweight and obesity among US children, adolescents, and adults, 1999–2002. *Journal of the American Medical Association, 291,* 2847–2850.

Heinicke, B. E., Paxton, S. J., McLean, S. A., & Wertheim, E. H. (2007). Internet-delivered targeted group intervention for body dissatisfaction and disordered eating in adolescent girls: A randomized controlled trial. *Journal of Abnormal Child Psychology, 35,* 379–391.

Henry J. Kaiser Family Foundation. (2004). The role of the media in childhood obesity. *Issue Brief,* 1–12. Retrieved February 20, 2009, from *www.kff.org/entmedia/7030.cfm.*

Hepworth, N., & Paxton, S. J. (2007). Pathways to help-seeking in bulimia nervosa and binge eating problems: A concept mapping approach. *International Journal of Eating Disorders, 40,* 493–504.

Jones, M., Luce, K. H., Osborne, M. I., Taylor, K., Cunning, D., Celio Doyle, A., et al. (2008). Randomized, controlled trial of an Internet-facilitated intervention for reducing binge eating and overweight in adolescents. *Pediatrics, 121,* 453–462.

Jones, S., & Fox, S. (2009). Generations online in 2009. Washington, DC: Pew Research Center. Available at *www.pewinternet.org/~/media//Files/Reports/2009/PIP_Generations_2009.pdf.*

Le Grange, D., Lock, J., Loeb, K., & Nicholls, D. (2010). Academy for Eating Disorders position paper: The role of the family in eating disorders. *International Journal of Eating Disorders, 43,* 1–5.

Lenhart, A., Purcell, K., Smith, A., & Zickuhr, K. (2010). Social media and young adults. Washington, DC: Pew Research Center. Available at *pewinternet.org/~/media//Files/Reports/2010/PIP_Social_Media_and_Young_Adults_Report.pdf.*

Lindenberg, K., Bauer, S., Moessner, M., &

Kordy, H. (2010, February). *Individual-isierte Essstörungsprävention bei Schül-erInnen [Individualized eating disorder prevention for students]*. Paper presented at 2. Kongress der Deutschen Gesellschaft fuer Essstoerungen (DGESS) [2nd Annual Congress of the German Society for Eating Disorders], Aachen, Germany.

Low, K. G., Charanasomboon, S., Lesser, J., Reinhalter, K., Martin, R., Jones, H., et al. (2006). Effectiveness of a computer-based interactive eating disorders prevention program at long-term follow-up. *Eating Disorders, 14*(1), 17–30.

Luce, K. H., Osborne, M. I., Winzelberg, A. J., Das, S., Abascal, L. B., Celio, A. A., et al. (2005). Application of an algorithm-driven protocol to simultaneously provide universal and targeted prevention programs. *International Journal of Eating Disorders, 37*, 220–226.

Muise, A. M., Stein, D. G., & Arbess, G. (2003). Eating disorders in adolescent boys: A review of the adolescent and young adult literature. *Journal of Adolescent Health, 33*, 427–435.

Myers, T. C., Swan-Kremeier, L., Wonderlich, S., Lancaster, K., & Mitchell, J. E. (2004). The use of alternative delivery systems and new technologies in the treatment of patients with eating disorders. *International Journal of Eating Disorders, 36*, 123–143.

Neumark-Sztainer, D. M., Story, M., Hannan, P. J., Perry, C. L., & Irving, L. M. (2002). Weight-related concerns and behaviors among overweight and nonoverweight adolescents: Implications for preventing weight-related disorders. *Archives of Pediatrics and Adolescent Medicine, 156*, 171–178.

Nielsen Online. (2009). *en-us.nielsen.com/main/news/news_releases/2009/july/Nielsen_Online_Data_Quick_Take_Kids_Online*. Accessed March 12, 2010.

O'Dea, J. A., & Abraham, S. (2000). Improving the body image, eating attitudes and behaviors of young male and female adolescents: A new educational approach which focuses on self-esteem. *International Journal of Eating Disorders, 28*, 43–57.

Paxton, S. J., & Franko, D. L. (2010). Body image and eating disorders. In M. A. Cuc-

ciare & K. R. Weingardt (Eds.), *Using technology to support evidence-based behavioral health practices: A clinician's guide* (pp. 151–168). New York: Taylor & Francis.

Pretorius, N., Arcelus, J., Beecham, J., Dawson, H., Doherty, F., Eisler, I., et al. (2009). Cognitive-behavioural therapy for adolescents with bulimic symptomatology: The acceptability and effectiveness of Internet-based delivery. *Behavior Research and Therapy, 47*, 729–736.

Rideout, V. (2010). *Generation M2: Media in the lives of 8- to 18-year-olds*. Menlo Park, CA: Kaiser Family Foundation.

Seeck, M., Schomer, D., Mainwaring, N., & Ives, J. (1995). Selectively distributed processing of visual object recognition in the temporal and frontal lobes of the human brain. *Annals of Neurology, 37*, 538–545.

Shapiro, J. R., Bauer, S., Hamer, R. M., Kordy, H., Ward, D., & Bulik, C. M. (2008). Use of text messaging for monitoring sugar-sweetened beverages, physical activity, and screen time in children: A pilot study. *Journal of Nutrition Education, 40*, 385–391.

Skarderud, F. (2003). Sh@me in cyberspace. Relationships without faces: The e-media and eating disorders. *European Eating Disorders Review, 11*, 155–169.

Strasburger, V. C., Jordan, A. B., & Donnerstein, E. (2010). Health effects of media on children and adolescents. *Pediatrics, 125*, 756–767.

Striegel-Moore, R. H., & Bulik, C. M. (2007). Risk factors for eating disorders. *American Psychologist, 62*, 181–198.

Taylor, C. B., Bryson, S., Luce, K. H., Cunning, D., Doyle, A., Abascal, L. B., et al. (2006). Prevention of eating disorders in at-risk college-age women. *Archives of General Psychiatry, 63*, 881–888.

Williams, C. J., Aubin, S. D., Cottrell, D., & Harkin, P. J. R. (1998). *Overcoming bulimia: A self-help package*. Leeds, UK: University of Leeds.

Williamson, D. A., Martin, P. D., White, M. A., Newton, R., Walden, H., York-Crowe, E., et al. (2005). Efficacy of an Internet-based behavioral weight loss program for overweight adolescent African-American girls. *Eating and Weight Disorders, 10,* 193–203.

Williamson, D. A., Walden, H. M., White, M. A., York-Crowe, E., Newton, R. L., Alfonso, A., et al. (2006). Two-year Internet-based randomized controlled trial for weight loss in African-American girls. *Obesity, 114,* 1231–1243.

Wilson, G. T., Grilo, C. M., & Vitousek, K. M. (2007). Psychological treatment of eating disorders. *American Psychologist, 62,* 199–216.

Winzelberg, A. J., Eppstein, D., Eldredge, K. L., Wilfley, D. E., Dasmashapatra, R., Dev, P., et al. (2000). Effectiveness of an Internet-based program for reducing risk factors for eating disorders. *Journal of Consulting and Clinical Psychology, 68,* 346–350.

Winzelberg, A. J., Taylor, C. B., Sharpe, T. M., Eldredge, K. L., Dev, P., & Constantinou, P. S. (1998). Evaluation of a computer-mediated eating disorder intervention program. *International Journal of Eating Disorders, 24,* 339–349.

Zabinski, M. F., Celio, A., Wilfley, D. E., & Taylor, C. B. (2003). Prevention of eating disorders and obesity via the Internet. *Cognitive Behaviour Therapy, 32,* 137–150.

Zabinski, M. F., Celio, A. A., Jacobs, J., Manwaring, J., & Wilfley, D. E. (2003). Internet-based prevention of eating disorders. *European Eating Disorders Review, 11,* 183–197.

Zabinski, M. F., Pung, M. A., Wilfley, D. E., Eppstein, D. L., Winzelberg, A. J., Celio, A., et al. (2001). Reducing risk factors for eating disorders: Targeting at-risk women with a computerized psychoeducational program. *International Journal of Eating Disorders, 29,* 401–408.

Zabinski, M. F., Wilfley, D. E., Calfas, K. J., Winzelberg, A. J., & Taylor, C. B. (2004). An interactive psychoeducational intervention for women at risk of developing an eating disorder. *Journal of Consulting and Clinical Psychology, 72,* 914–919.

Zabinski, M. F., Wilfley, D. E., Pung, M. A., Winzelberg, A. J., Eldredge, K., & Taylor, C. B. (2001). An interactive Internet-based intervention for women at risk of eating disorders: A pilot study. *International Journal of Eating Disorders, 30,* 129–137.

PART VII

THE ROLE OF PARENTS

■ CHAPTER 24 ■

A Parent's Perspective on Family Treatment

Harriet Brown

From the moment our daughter was diagnosed with anorexia—and, truly, even before the diagnosis—my husband and I found ourselves in a kind of alternate universe. Everything we'd known about our daughter for 14 years had been turned upside down. The calm, poised, funny young woman we knew had become a gaunt, unrecognizable, anxiety-wracked creature who seemed possessed by a force we instinctively loathed. The close relationship we had enjoyed since she was born was suddenly fraught with a level of terror and rage and insanity we'd never seen before. Our daughter had disappeared, and what made her disappearance so frightening to us was that she was still right there in front of us. If she had run away or gone missing, we would have known what to do: call the police, mount a search, pull in friends and family to help. But faced with this strange persona who spoke with her mouth and looked out of her eyes and yet was profoundly, viscerally different, we became disoriented and fearful.

Everything we read, everyone we talked to, suggested that this was how things would be for years to come. That our daughter as we knew her had vanished, maybe for good, certainly for a long time. We felt lost. We *were* lost, and worse, we felt helpless, and that was the most disorienting thing of all. Because like most parents, we were used to supporting our child. We knew how to read her moods. We bandaged her scrapes. We nursed her through the flu. We knew how to feed her, mind and soul as well as body. We knew what made her eyes light up and her delighted laugh ring out across the kitchen.

At least, we *had* known. Now we were locked in a kind of mortal combat with someone we could not and did not want to understand.

When we stumbled upon family-based treatment (FBT), my husband and I knew immediately that we wanted to try it. Much later, I wondered why. What about FBT spoke to us? What made it seem like the right approach? As a journalist, I'd done my homework and knew that outcomes with FBT looked promising. But our decision to try FBT wasn't intellectual; it was made with our hearts, not our heads.

I've since come to understand that what grabbed us was the notion that we could *do* something to help our daughter. That we didn't have to sit at the table and watch her refuse to eat. We didn't have to hear her shriek and watch her starve and say nothing, or harangue her and feel ineffectual. We could take action. This was an immensely appealing idea, long before we had the foggiest notion of what exactly we might be doing.

That sense of being able to create change, to make a difference, is what led my husband and me toward FBT, despite the fact that we had no real FBT therapist. We had no program to back us up. We had only a handful of articles and reports from other parents and the willingness of our pediatrician and therapist to try it our way.

And somehow, that was enough. Despite our stumbles and insecurities (Is this really what we're supposed to be doing? *How* are we supposed to do it?), despite the relentless nature of parenting a child with anorexia, despite our own despair and the criticisms of others who didn't understand what we were doing (especially family members, who repeatedly "voiced concern" that we weren't taking care of our daughter properly), we made it through. Our daughter ate (a miracle in itself, in those early days). And over the course of a year or so, she came back to us, and to herself.

*   *   *

Parenting a child with an eating disorder is hard. Actually, that bland statement doesn't convey even a fraction of the stress families go through. Caring for a child in the grip of anorexia, bulimia, or another eating disorder is one of the most rigorous, confounding, and painful experiences any family can go through, comparable to the stress of caring for someone with psychosis (Treasure et al., 2001).

Historically, parents have been sidelined in the recovery process, relegated to watching their child suffer, feeling shame, guilt, and confusion. Fortunately, FBT has helped change the culture around parent involvement in eating disorders treatment. The last decade or so of studies clearly show that parents often represent an adolescent's best chance of recovery from an eating disorder. What the studies don't show—yet—is that FBT is good for parents as well as kids because it gives parents a unique and vital role in the work of helping a child recover.

Which isn't to say that this work is easy. On the contrary: Most parents say FBT is by far the most challenging experience they've ever gone through. We plan meals, calculate calories, shop and cook endlessly. We sit at the table for hours each day as one meal or snack blends into the next. We absorb the tears, the rage, and the terror of our child and the rest of the family. We learn to face down the eating disorder, to stand with our children as they battle the delusions and compulsions that make eating disorders so hard to rout.

But despite the hardships, many parents feel grateful to have a role, to be able to do something to help. Traditional eating disorders treatment, which often includes "parentectomies," can wind up fracturing family relationships. But most families who come through the FBT recovery process say they're stronger, more empowered, and ultimately more bonded because of what they have been through together.

I'll never forget a conversation one mom described to me, years after her daughter had recovered. She was remembering, with her teenage son, who was a few years younger than his sister, how difficult family meals had been during refeeding. And her son told her that the hardest part of his sister's illness wasn't those conflict-ridden meals; it was watching her starve, before the family took on refeeding. Even for a 12-year-old who was mostly an observer, the idea of taking action was preferable to sitting by helplessly.

That, to me, is the most beautiful thing about FBT. The fact that it works? That's pretty great, too. But that's really the icing on the cake. So to speak.

*   *   *

One of the toughest aspects of FBT (or any eating disorders treatment) is that it doesn't follow the trajectory we expect: Kid gets sick. Parent takes kid to doctor. Treatment commences. Kid starts to feel better. Kid recovers. End of story.

With eating disorders, the storyline goes more like this: Parents slowly realize something is wrong with kid. Kid insists he or she feels fine. Parents take kid to doctor. Treatment commences. Kid starts to feel much, *much* worse. Family life goes out the window. Months of conflict ensue, with kid insisting he or she is fine, not sick at all. Eventually, if everyone's lucky, kid recovers. Maybe end of story, or maybe just the first act in a long, drawn-out play.

Treatment makes kids feel worse, not better. It brings out the eating-disordered personality, which often resembles an *Exorcist*-type demon that shocks and horrifies parents. Parents begin to question themselves: *Things weren't so bad before we started trying to get her to eat. Are we making it worse? Maybe she really doesn't need all that food. Maybe she's different from other kids. Maybe she's not really sick. Maybe all this food really is killing her, just as she says.*

Parents, like sufferers, fall prey to the cognitive distortions of the eating disorder.

You see the problem? Every family struggles with this, no matter how dedicated and knowledgeable they are. Not only that, we struggle with it over and over. We will need support from an FBT therapist on this count through the entire recovery process.

The fact that treatment also goes against the grain of the conventional wisdom about food—eat as little as possible, avoid fat, exercise like crazy—doesn't help, either. Some parents have to get past their own issues with food, even if they don't think they have any, to help their child. The more knowledge we have about how refeeding works and why all this food is necessary, the better.

*   *   *

One of the most important things a therapist does is prepare a family for what might happen during recovery. Several times during our daughter's recovery, my husband and I were told by professionals, "I've never seen behaviors like these. Your daughter is very sick—too sick to stay home with you." We had to read Ancel Keys's Minnesota Starvation Experiment to understand that anxiety, depression, rage, withdrawal, and self-harm typically *intensify* once a child begins eating and gaining weight. Parents who think their child's behaviors and reactions are extreme or frightening are more apt to give up on FBT. But if they know what to expect, they're more likely to hang in there during the worst of the behaviors. If parents know, for instance, that many eating-disordered patients report that they "hear voices," they won't panic if their child mentions the voice in her head. If they know that many teens with eating disorders exhibit a kind of alternate personality during recovery, they won't be as shocked if and when it surfaces.

Parents also need to know when behaviors and symptoms are out of the ordinary. Sobbing, screaming, and throwing things fall within the range of "normal" behaviors during refeeding; jumping out of a car, persistent head banging, and other serious attempts at self-injury might signal the need for a higher level of care. Parents need guidance about when and how to keep a child safe.

No matter how much parents wish the therapist could just tell them what to do and exactly how to do it, the process doesn't work that way. And that's OK. A child struggling with an eating disorder needs to know on a profound level that someone is bigger than the disorder. That someone can stand beside the child 24/7, can talk back to the voice in her head, can override the self-destructive compulsions that drive the child toward starvation. And that someone can never be the therapist because the therapist sees the family for only an hour each week. Families are the ones at the table six times a day. Families are the ones who rock a sobbing child after each meal, who dream up distractions, who insist in the face of rage and sometimes violence on the full complement of calories.

In that sense, the role of the family in FBT is no different from the role of the family in life: We're the ultimate support system. The buck stops with us. As much as we may plead with therapists to tell us what to do, damn it, we know that we know our child better than anyone else. Better than the therapist or the psychiatrist or the experts who write about eating disorders. That is both our handicap and our greatest strength.

Parents can and must lead the way in their child's recovery. But we can't do it alone. We can't do it without the guidance, support, encouragement, and information therapists bring us. We can't do it without hope—the hope that our child really can and will recover fully from the eating disorder. Because one thing we may not even realize ourselves is that we're scared. Terrified, actually. The kind of fear that makes your teeth chatter, that wakes you at 3:00 A.M., that makes you question your entire vision of the universe. It's easy to get lost in that fear. Just as our child must trust us to be bigger than the eating disorder, we must trust that the therapist can see the path ahead, the way through the terror. We need to believe that we're on a path, even if it's a winding, indirect one, even if it takes us places we really don't want to go. We need the kind of hope that keeps us moving forward even through the dark times.

Nor can we do this without information—about neurobiology, metabolism, all the whys and wherefores of what our child is going through. It helps us to have the therapist's respect, too, to know that just as we believe in our child's ability to recover, the therapist believes in our ability to do what's needed, even if we screw up (and we will, we will), even if we get stuck in denial at first, even if we sometimes weep and gnash our teeth at the unfairness and horror of it all.

At the end of the session, when we wipe our eyes and pick ourselves up off the therapist's chairs, part of what helps us walk out the door is knowing there's someone who understands, who can guide us and empathize with us, who can cheer and encourage and support our family through the long nightmare of recovery. And for that, we are truly, deeply grateful.

Reference

Treasure, J., Murphy, T., Szmukler, G., Todd, G., Gavin, K., & Joyce, K. (2001). The experience of caregiving for severe mental illness: A comparison between anorexia nervosa and psychosis. *Social Psychiatry and Psychiatric Epidemiology, 36*(7), 343–347.

CONCLUDING COMMENTS

■ CHAPTER 25 ■

Where Are We Going from Here?

James Lock

This book is one of the first to focus in a comprehensive way on eating disorders in children and adolescents. It is, in this sense, already initiating new directions in the area of eating disorders simply by gathering together the information in this volume. In a way, given the age of onset of most eating disorder symptoms and disorders, it is surprising that this book should be so late in coming (Hoek & van Hoeken, 2003; Lucas, Beard, & O'Fallon, 1991; van Son et al., 2006). Many reports have focused on adults with eating disorders, so perhaps the most important contribution this book can make is to focus attention on the need to grow the clinical and research literature in the area of child and adolescent eating disorders. However, the expert authors in this volume have provided additional, more specific, suggestions for how we might proceed in order to make progress in understanding and treating eating disorders in younger populations. This chapter is an opportunity to summarize, examine, and extend some of the suggestions these authors have made for future directions for clinical and research work with younger populations (Lock, 2010).

Next Steps in Understanding the Biological Basis of Eating Disorders

In the first part of this volume ("Etiology and Neurobiology"), the authors of the included chapters stress the promise and importance of genetic and neurobiological factors in understanding the etiology and possible application to clinical problems and treatment. Strober and Peris (Chapter 4) suggest that gene–family environment interaction deserves further research in order to better understand how gene expression and family interactions may affect the development or maintenance of eating disorders (Strober, 2007; Strober, Freeman, Lampert, Diamond, & Kaye, 2000; Strober & Humphrey, 1987; Strober, Morrell, Burroughs, Salkin, & Jacobs, 1985; Woodside et al., 2002). Racine, Root, Klump, and Bulik (Chapter 3, this volume) especially note that current data highlight the relative influence of genes and environment on eating disorders as differing across the lifespan and that, somewhat surprisingly, genetic factors are more important *after* puberty (Klump, Keel, Sisk, & Burt, 2010). According to these authors, this could mean that early onset (prepubertal) eating disorders might have a different etiology than those that develop postpubertally. Another possibility however, is that early onset of a disorder may represent greater penetrance of genetic factors leading to early onset, a view supported by some literature that finds very early onset eating disorders have a poorer prognosis (Bryant-Waugh, Knibbs, Fosson, Kaminski, & Lask, 1988; Walford & McCune, 1991). However, the interaction between genes and pubertal development, especially as it may relate to hormonal changes during this period, is a key area for further exploration. For example, a recent study of digit ratio in males with eating disorders, suggests that the degree of in uterine brain exposure to testosterone may contribute to variations in risk of developing an eating disorder (Smith, Hawkeswood, & Joiner, 2010). Those having higher levels of exposure (leading to lower digit ratios and higher masculinization of the brain) reported lower drive for thinness. This study may help explain why a genetic vulnerability could be mediated by hormones leading to different expression by gender and partially explain why eating disorders occur more frequently in females.

In line with this thinking, in Chapter 2, this volume, on the neurobiology of eating disorders, Kaye suggests that the rise in estrogen levels associated with puberty in females likely affects the serotonin system or levels of neuropeptides that influence feeding, emotionality, and other behaviors (Rubinow, Schmidt, & Roca, 1998). In addition, a recent meta-analytic study of a more than 2,000 participants from eight independent case–control association studies examining the serotonin transporter gene found that anorexia nervosa (AN) was significantly associated with the s allele and s carrier genotype (Lee & Lin, 2010). These results suggest that genetic variance of the serotonin transporter gene promoter contributed to the susceptibility of AN. These studies emphasize the importance of examining the relationship between gene expression, hormones, and neurotransmitters in the context of brain development and eating disorders.

Examination of the neurobiological nature of eating disorders is still at a relatively early stage. Recent studies have focused on cognitive processes as possible endophenotypes of eating disorders, in particular problems in cognitive flexibility (set shifting) and global thinking (weak central coherence) (Holliday, Tchanturia, Landau, & Collier, 2005; Lopez, Tchanturia, Stahl, Booth, et al., 2008; Lopez, Tchanturia, Stahl, & Treasure, 2008; Roberts, Tchanturia, Stahl, Southgate, & Treasure, 2005). Preliminary studies have found evidence that a thinking style characterized as relatively rigid and unduly focused on detail is found in adults with AN. There is a single study by Zastrow and colleagues (2009) that found evidence that decreased activation in the anterior cingulate and striatum is associated with impaired cognitive-behavioral flexibility in adults with AN. Other studies suggest that cognitive inhibition may play an important role in both AN and bulimia nervosa (BN), albeit by different mechanisms (Marsh, Maia, & Peterson, 2009; Marsh, Steinglass, et al., 2009). In AN, overinhibition may support obsessive thinking and anxiety, whereas disinhibition, a common behavioral characteristic in patients with BN, may increase the risk in subjects with BN. In support of this view, a recent study found that patients who binge eat or purge regardless of primary diagnosis demonstrated increased activation in the right dorsolateral prefrontal cortex, an executive control region, suggesting inefficient or possibly compensatory activation (i.e., recruitment of additional brain regions and/or discrepant brain activation patterns, leading to improved cognitive ability) (Lock, Garrett, Beenhaker, & Reiss, 2011). Although studies of cognitive style and the search for neural correlates for these processes are still preliminary, future research in these areas may help to increase our understanding of fundamental disease processes in the thinking of patients with eating disorders and, in turn, suggest novel ways to intervene through cognitive remediation (Baldock & Tchanturia, 2007; Tchanturia, Davies, & Campbell, 2007) or medications.

Of course, there are many other promising avenues for research in understanding the neurobiological underpinnings of eating disorders, including studies that relate eating disorder psychopathology to that of related disorders, such as anxiety disorders, obsessive–compulsive disorders, and depression (Anderluch, Tchanturia, Rabe-Hesketh, & Treasure, 2003; Godart, Flament, Perdereau, & Jeammet, 2002; Holtkamp, Muller, Heussen, Remschmidt, & Herperz-Dahlmann, 2005; Le Grange & Lock, 2002, 2007; Le Grange, Loeb, Orman, & Jellar, 2004; Wagner et al., 2006). Because some behavioral and psychological traits associated with these other disorders predate as well as often continue during and after an eating disorder, studies of the biological basis of these other disorders may likely shed light on the etiology of eating disorders as well (Kaye, Fudge, & Paulus, 2009).

Next Steps in Improving Our Understanding of the Epidemiology and Course of Eating Disorders in Youth

As noted by Norris, Bondy, and Pinhas (Chapter 5, this volume), there are significant gaps in our understanding of the epidemiology of eating disorders. These authors identify a number of key research areas that need further attention even before we try to undertake large-scale and expensive population-based studies. To begin with, there is a need for a clear classification rubric for eating disorders in children and adolescents that is developmentally sensitive, a problem discussed more specifically in later paragraphs (Workgroup & Adolescents, 2007). Without progress in the area of classification it will be impossible to elucidate accurate rates of eating disorders in youth. The particular problem of the high apparent rate of eating disorder not otherwise specified (EDNOS) is highlighted, as this category is currently not only the biggest, but also the most imprecise diagnostic group (Fairburn & Bohn, 2005; Peebles, Hardy, Wilson, & Lock, 2010; Turner & Bryant-Waugh, 2004). Recent work by Peebles and colleagues, for example, applied a set of broadened criteria for AN and BN to a large data set and found that EDNOS could be reduced from 60 to 15% by recategorizing adolescents as having AN and BN by allowing weight thresholds and frequency of binge eating and purging behaviors to be more flexible (Peebles et al., 2010). This study also found that within the broader groups with AN and BN, medical problems were similar, though medical problems of the groups with AN and BN themselves continued to differ. Another study found few clinical differences between full threshold and subthreshold diagnostic groups in adolescents with BN (Le Grange et al., 2006). Further studies are needed to examine these kinds of criteria changes used in classification.

There is also a dearth of epidemiological information on eating disorders in early childhood, in part because no uniform classification for many of these disorders is available (Bryant-Waugh & Lask, 1995; Nicholls, Chater, & Lask, 2000). At the other end of the spectrum, problems of deciding who no longer has an eating disorder (remission and/or recovery) are also contentious and require further study and clinical and research consensus (Couturier & Lock, 2006b, 2006c). Work in this area has begun, but current studies illustrate how severe the problem is by documenting that recovery can range from 3% to 96% in the same population, depending on the definitions used. Progress on these classification and definitional issues must be achieved in advance of large-scale epidemiological studies, but there is, nonetheless, a need for population-based incidence, prevalence, and outcome studies that are powered appropriately with adequate sample sizes in order for there to be statistically significant, generalizable, and interpretable results that can inform policy decisions.

Progress in understanding the course and outcome remains limited, though Steinhausen's heroic work over many decades has helped considerably (Steinhausen, 2002, 2009; Steinhausen, Rauss-Mason, & Seidel, 1991, 1993; Steinhausen & Weber, 2009). Data related to course and outcome are limited by some of the same definitional problems in regard to recovery and classification discussed earlier. Another area of particular interest for future research relevant to younger patients is that of mitigating factors affecting course. Although data suggest that patients with early-adolescence onset may have better prognoses, patients with prepubertal onset tend to fare worse (Bryant-Waugh et al., 1988; Lask & Bryant-Waugh, 1992). Furthermore, comorbid psychiatric disorders are common both premorbidly and after an acute episode of AN is resolved (Herzog, Keller, Sacks, Yeh, & Lavori, 1992; Wentz, Gillberg, Gillberg, & Rastam, 2001; Zipfel, Lowe, Deter, & Herzog, 2000). There is some evidence that response to treatment is moderated by these comorbid obsessive and compulsive features in AN. A study comparing doses of family-based treatment (FBT) found that those with high levels of obsessive–compulsive disorder (OCD) features did better with more treatment (Lock, Agras, Bryson, & Kraemer, 2005). A number of studies suggest that a longer duration of the disorder predicts poorer outcome (Eisler et al., 1997; Russell, Szmukler, Dare, & Eisler, 1987). What is unclear is why this is so. Is the group that has persistent AN simply more ill at baseline, or was treatment failure the cause of the development of a more chronic course? As Steinhausen notes, there is limited knowledge about how interventions affect the course of the illness, and the scarcity of controlled intervention studies with a sufficient duration of follow-up is a major obstacle in the field of outcome research in AN, even though several studies of FBT for AN suggest durable effects of treatment (Eisler et al., 1997; Eisler, Simic, Russell, & Dare, 2007; Lock, Couturier, & Agras, 2006; Lock, Couturier, Bryson, & Agras, 2006). In addition, better understanding of the continuity and discontinuity of AN and the factors influencing this process need further study. "Crossover" rates between AN and BN, of 10 to 30%, support the notion that there is substantial instability in diagnostic classification (Eddy et al., 2008). This may relate to duration of illness, age, or other factors. Studies examining these aspects of the course of eating disorders in youth are needed.

Most of the problems described for adolescent AN are pertinent to adolescent BN as well, but there are even fewer studies of adolescent samples with BN and longer-term course is largely unknown for BN (Le Grange, Crosby, Rathouz, & Leventhal, 2007; Schmidt et al., 2007). A recent long-term follow-up study of late adolescent-onset BN (mean age 20 plus or minus 2 years) found that 75% of patients were in remission at 20-year follow-up, but 4.5% continued to have a clinically significant eating disorder (Keel, Graemer, Joiner, & Haedt, 2010). In addition, as with AN, the long-term effects of treatment of BN are largely unknown, as no longer-term follow-up of a sample of adolescents treated in a randomized controlled trial (RCT) is yet available.

Next Steps in Improving Diagnosis and Classification of Child and Adolescent Eating Disorders

With the development of the *Diagnostic and Statistical Manual of Mental Disorders* (5th ed.) (DSM-5) well under way, there may be progress in improving the classification of child and adolescent eating disorders. Bryant-Waugh and Nicholls (Chapter 7, this volume) suggest that the next most important step in improving diagnosis and classification of eating problems in younger children is to develop a consensus on clinical diagnostic groups and collect clinical data that allow examination of the utility of various formulations (Workgroup & Adolescents, 2007). Field trials using definitions for some of these disorders are part of the DSM-5 work plan. Retrieving data from these field trials is a good next step in understanding how best to classify these relatively rare disorders.

Turning to the classification of adolescent "classic" eating disorders (e.g., AN, BN, and EDNOS), Eddy, Herzog, and Zucker (Chapter 8, this volume) suggest that longitudinal studies of adolescence-onset eating disorders are needed to answer questions about the specific criteria needed for diagnosis (e.g., weight thresholds, body image distortion, behavioral frequency or duration, certain cognitive requirements, etc.). They also suggest that other types of empirical approaches to the study of classification, such as taxometric analyses, may be useful in addressing whether the relationship between different eating disorder diagnostic groups (or empirically derived classes) is truly discontinuous and qualitative (taxonic) versus continuous and quantitative (dimensional).

Classification of eating disorders in males remains a problem, with limited data available to help in understanding gender-specific aspects of eating disorders. An example is the clinical presentation of muscle dysphoria, sometimes called "reverse anorexia," wherein males are preoccupied by the need for an increasingly lean and muscular physique. Because overexercising is the main behavioral symptom of muscle dysphoria, some have argued that it is not an eating disorder. However, muscle dysphoria shares many behavioral and cognitive features with AN. In a recent review, Murray, Reiger, Touyz, and Garcia (2010) argue that muscle dysmorphia should likely be considered an eating disorder, specifically highlighting the effects of gender behaviors, beliefs, and stereotypes contributing to the symptom profile. In particular, the authors note the use of anabolic steroids as a means of achieving the desired body type, a strategy not typically employed by women with eating disorders. A better understanding of how boys and men present, should be classified, and are treated in the context of eating, shape, and weight concerns remains an important area for future research (Darcy, Celio Doyle, Lock, Doyle, & Le Grange, in press; Lock, 2008).

Next Steps in Developing Appropriate Assessment Approaches in Child and Adolescent Eating Disorders

Katzman and Findlay (Chapter 9, this volume) point out the importance of early detection of eating disorders to prevent a range of medical problems associated with malnutrition and binge eating and purging. The authors' review identifies many important areas where information is lacking. A key area where there is little systematic guidance concerns what constitutes a medical emergency for adolescents with eating disorders (Fisher et al., 1995). Current decisions about medical hospitalization are based on consensus opinion and are best fitted to medical instability related to malnutrition. However, a recent report suggests that degree of weight loss (rather than absolute weight), rate of weight loss, and phosphorus levels are better predictors of severe medical problems than bradycardia, hypothermia, or orthostasis, which are the principle reasons for medical hospitalization of patients with eating disorders in the United States at this time (Lock & Peebles, 2010). Another key area relates to determining the role of weight restoration in AN. Some authors have suggested that menstrual return is a sufficient marker for healthy weight (at least in females); however, a recent study suggests that for bone health, higher weight and greater weight change are needed for bone health restoration (Olmos et al., 2010). Because costs of hospitalization drive the overall high costs of treatment for eating disorders, it is critical to better understand the medical basis for these decisions (Agras, 2001; Crow & Nyman, 2004; Lock, Couturier, & Agras, 2008; Striegel-Moore, Leslie, Petrill, Garvin, & Rosenheck, 2000). In addition, to make sure that our treatments have appropriate medical goals that can ensure that adolescents recover their full physical health, it is important to set weight restoration goals at the appropriate levels. Conducting studies that provide clear evidence supporting the medical necessity for hospitalization and for recovery is a crucial next step in improving our understanding of eating disorders in youth.

Similarly, assessments specific to younger patients are needed to assist in diagnosis. As Loeb, Brown, and Goldstein (Chapter 10, this volume) point out, there are a number of challenges to developing such measures. They propose that using parents as informants may minimize error, but note that parent reports may be less reliable for secretive disorders such as BN (Couturier & Lock, 2006a; Couturier, Lock, Forsberg, Vanderheyden, & Lee, 2007). At this point, studies are under way to determine how instruments such as the Eating Disorder Examination (EDE), incorporating parental report, can be used. Determining when and how best to incorporate these parental reports is another important area for research. With the developing awareness of eating disorders in young males, it is important to better understand how well the EDE works with boys. Current data suggest that the EDE is generally useful, though there may be ways to improve it by incorporating male-specific types of concerns (leanness, muscularity, etc.; Darcy, Celio Doyle, et al., in press).

Next Steps in Better Understanding Treatment and Prevention of Eating Disorders in Youth

Little systematic evidence is available that documents the usefulness of intensive interventions in adolescent eating disorders. In fact, the evidence that is available suggests that for most adolescents, hospital care is not better than general community care (Crisp et al., 1991; Gowers et al., 2007; Gowers, Weetman, Shore, Hussain, & Elvins, 2000). Nonetheless, as Tantillo and Kreipe (Chapter 11, this volume) as well as many clinicians attest, there is a subgroup of young patients who likely need and benefit from such care. Identifying for whom and under what circumstances such care is beneficial is a critical next step in treatment research. A current study of the Westmead group in Sydney, Australia, promises to provide systematic evidence about how best to combine hospital care with FBT. These researchers randomized 82 subjects to short hospitalization plus FBT versus longer hospitalization (weight restoration and longer psychological treatment) plus FBT. These authors have already found that FBT reduces relapse to hospitalization (Wallis, Rhodes, Kohn, & Madden, 2007). Such studies may help inform health care systems on how best to utilize limited hospital resources as well as help keep patients at home with families and in their communities. Nonetheless, for some patients who have no parents or whose parents cannot or will not help them, professional care, including intensive treatments in hospitals, day programs, and residential treatment centers, may be needed. Studies on how best to identify these patients, what kinds of intensive treatments are most effective, and how to transition care into less restrictive settings are needed.

Outpatient treatment for adolescent AN remains understudied, with fewer than 500 adolescents systematically studied in RCTs (Le Grange & Lock, 2005; Lock et al., 2010). Few studies compare active treatments, and although FBT has a greater evidence base than other approaches, it is not particularly helpful for 15 to 20% of adolescents with AN. Studies that examine augmentation strategies for standard FBT constitute one promising area of research, including the use of FBT in the context of additional professional support to families in hospitals, day programs, or other residential programs. Such treatment augmentation is clinically already under way in a variety of programs, but how useful these strategies may be remains an open question. In addition, studies that explore matching patients to FBT (moderators) as well as studies that examine how FBT works (mediation) are needed (Kraemer, Frank, & Kupfer, 2006; Lock, Couturier, et al., 2006). These types of studies require larger samples and likely require complex multisite designs if they are to be successful. A particular augmentation strategy that is currently being studied is a multifamily group (MFG) format, as described by Eisler (2005; see Fairbairn, Simic, and Eisler, Chapter 13, this volume). Data are currently being analyzed that compare standard FBT to FBT plus MFG. Results from this study—which should be forthcoming soon—may help determine how best to use MFGs in clinical practice as well as identify the next steps for research of this approach. Other approaches that support families in a group format deserve research and clinical attention. Groups have the potential for being highly efficient and cost-effective, while also providing interfamily support. Fortunately, data are also being analyzed in a pilot comparison of family education groups with FBT by Zucker, Marcus, and Bulik (2006).

Turning to individual treatment approaches for adolescent AN, there remains a great deal of work to do. At this point, developmentally tailored treatments such as adolescent-focused therapy (AFT) are useful (Lock, Le Grange, Agras, Moye, Bryson, & Jo, 2010; Robin et al., 1999), but other possible individual approaches, such as cognitive-behavioral therapy (CBT) and interpersonal therapy (IPT) in particular, have scarcely been examined (McIntosh et al., 2005). Pilot studies would be an appropriate first step. As suggested by Loeb, Craigen, Goldstein, Lock, and Le Grange (Chapter 18, this volume), studies that provide evidence for effectiveness for early intervention are also needed. A study examining a version of FBT for subsyndromal AN is under way at Mount Sinai Hospital.

Treatment for adolescent BN is even less studied than treatment for adolescent AN, with fewer than 200 subjects studied in RCTs (Le Grange, Crosby, Rathouz, & Leventhal, 2007; Schmidt et al., 2007). Data from the two studies examining FBT suggest it is useful, but whether it is better than another active treatment (e.g., CBT) remains unclear (Lock, 2005). A multisite study is under way comparing FBT with CBT and supportive psychotherapy (SPT). This study is a reasonable next step in treatment studies for adolescent BN, but there is a need to examine other treatments such as IPT and medications for BN in this younger age group. As Campbell and Schmidt (Chapter 16, this volume) point out, evidence suggests that CBT is useful when adapted to address the developmental needs of this age group. Studies that incorporate families in CBT in a developmentally appropriate way are a reasonable alternative, given findings suggesting that FBT is useful for adolescent BN. Studies examining early intervention to prevent more chronic and less responsive forms of BN are needed for the adolescent age group. Moderators and mediators of FBT for BN are unexamined and could shed light on which treatment works best for whom and how treatments work (Le Grange, Crosby, & Lock, 2008; Lock, Le Grange, & Crosby, 2008). As noted by Moye, Fitzpatrick, and Hoste (Chapter 14, this volume), psychological treatment in the form of SFT is also useful for adolescent BN, though it may work more slowly than FBT (Le Grange, Crosby, Rathouz, & Leventhal, 2007). SPT may be more acceptable to adolescents in some cases than FBT or CBT, as some adolescents resist involving their parents and resent the homework and relatively narrow focus of CBT (Fairburn, 1981; Fairburn, Cooper, & Shafran, 2002, 2008). SPT may be especially attractive to older adolescents interested in a more introspective therapy. Future studies of SPT may examine some of these factors as moderators of treatment response.

Interventions to address overeating and obesity are being studied, as Boutelle and Tanofsky-Kraff (Chapter 20, this volume) have pointed out. Given the prevalence of pediatric obesity and ineffectiveness of weight loss treatment programs, novel approaches that target aberrant eating patterns may provide a way forward in this challenging area. Group and individual IPT and family interventions may be useful, and further study is needed (Rieger et al., 2010; Tanofsky-Kraff et al., 2007; Wilfley et al., 2002). New studies examining the possibility of an FBT-type intervention for adolescent obesity are being conducted by Loeb and Le Grange. Though these studies are preliminary in nature, the findings suggesting that parents can be helpful in other eating problems in children are encouraging.

The use of Internet-based interventions may also present an opportunity for treating child and adolescent eating disorders, given that this age group is comfortable with this form of communication and the early indications that it may be useful (Luce et al., 2008; Peebles et al., submitted). Because the Internet and other related devices are increasingly important in our lives, and especially in adolescents' lives, it is important to find ways to use them to address eating-related problems. For example, a recent study found that text messaging might be useful in improving self-monitoring in adults with BN, with 87% adherent to self-monitoring (Shapiro et al., 2010). As self-monitoring is particularly challenging for adolescents, the use of this type of reminder might improve feasibility and acceptability of this crucial element of CBT for this younger age group as well. Studies examining these possibilities are important avenues for treatment development. In addition, the use of Web-based programs for prevention of eating disorders is now known to be effective in college-age students. The use of Web-based prevention and early intervention for AN remains an important area of study. Jacobi and colleagues at the Technical University of Dresden are piloting a study doing just that by employing an FBT psychoeducational model for parents of adolescents at risk for AN.

As noted by Couturier and Spettigue (Chapter 21, this volume), evidence-based pharmacological treatment for children and adolescents with eating disorders is not yet possible because of the limited number of studies available (Couturier & Lock, 2007). These authors correctly note that RCTs examining medication are needed. However, prior to this, there is a lack of compelling preliminary data suggesting the feasibility, acceptability, and likely efficacy of particular compounds (Halmi, 2008). To date, few such preliminary studies suggest that further study of particular compounds is warranted (Boachie, Goldfield, & Spettigue, 2003; Kotler, Devlin, Davies, & Walsh, 2003; Norris, Spettigue, Buchholz, Henderson, & Obeid, 2010). However, more clinical case series data are needed in large samples as there may well be a subgroup of patients who may respond differentially to medications. Again, given the pressing need for these trials and the costs and challenges associated with such studies in children and adolescents, multi-site studies will ultimately be needed.

Prevention of eating disorders remains an important but difficult goal. We know many of the risks and protective factors, particularly for binge eating and obesity (Jacobi, Hayward, de Zwaan, Kraemer, & Agras, 2004), but interventions with younger populations remain understudied (Taylor et al., 2006). Conducting school-based programs is an important and likely useful strategy for younger patients (McVey, Davis, Tweed, & Shaw, 2004), but early identification and intervention by pediatricians and family members are also needed (Peebles, Wilson, & Lock, 2006). The development and study of prevention in this age group is an important area for future research.

Next Steps for Parent and Patient Involvement

Unlike many other psychiatric disorders at this point, eating disorders have a relatively underdeveloped network of patient and family advocates for prevention. The reasons for this are complex, but it is likely due, to a large extent, to the long history of blaming parents for causing these disorders and the associated parental shame and guilt that have prevented potential advocates from speaking out (Bruch, 1973; Gull, 1874; Silverman, 1997). Like parents of children with mental retardation, schizophrenia, bipolar disorder, and autism, parents of children with eating disorders are finally being let off the hook, which is helping to empower them to take action (Eisler, 2005; Le Grange, Lock, Loeb, & Nicholls, 2010). As compared with other psychiatric disorders of similar incidence and prevalence and severity, and despite being a stated research priority area for the National Institutes of Mental Health (NIMH), research funding for eating disorders is not getting its fair share of the pie (Agras et al., 2004). Furthermore, insurance companies have selectively disallowed treatment for eating disorders (Crow & Nyman, 2004; Silber, 1994; Striegel-Moore et al., 2000). As Harriet Brown (Chapter 24, this volume) illustrates, family involvement is beginning to increase as families learn more about the biological basis of these disorders and about their important role in helping their children recover. In the last several years, two Web-based parent organizations have been founded (*Maudsleyparents.org* and *FEAST.org*), both designed to facilitate parents' learning about how they can help their children, to promote awareness about eating disorders, and to advocate for changes in legislative and research agendas that encourage fair access and coverage for treatment of children with eating disorders. Several important additions to the literature are now available for parents, including an educational handbook (Lock & Le Grange, 2005), a parent-authored book about experiences of treatment and recovery (Alexander & Le Grange, 2009), and a book to support professional and carers (Treasure, Schmidt, & Macdonald, 2009), focused on how to better understand their children and themselves when dealing with serious eating disorders in their families.

Professionals joining together with patients and families to promote awareness, encourage treatment, promote research, and decrease stigma is a crucial step forward in the field. For too long professionals and parents and patients have been on different sides, but this is changing (Le Grange et al., 2010). As professionals, we need to learn how better to involve patients and families and encourage their participation and feedback in what we do (Darcy et al., 2010; Krautter & Lock, 2004; Le Grange & Gelman, 1998). Parents can also support one another, and this may well increase their abilities to take on the challenge of eating disorders (Rhodes, Baillee, Brown, & Madden, 2008; Rhodes, Madden, & Brown, 2009). Making these relationships work is the next key step in moving forward in advocacy, research, and access to appropriate treatments.

References

Agras, W. S. (2001). The consequences and costs of the eating disorders. *Psychiatric Clinics of North America, 24,* 371–381.

Agras, W. S., Brandt, H., Bulik, C. M., Dolan-Sewell, R., Fairburn, C. G., Halmi, C. A., et al. (2004). Report of the National Institutes of Health workshop on overcoming barriers to treatment research in anorexia nervosa. *International Journal of Eating Disorders, 35,* 509–521.

Alexander, J., & Le Grange, D. (2009). *My kid is back: Empowering parents to beat anorexia nervosa.* Carlton, Victoria, Australia: Melbourne University.

Anderluch, M., Tchanturia, K., Rabe-Hesketh, S., & Treasure, J. L. (2003). Childhood obsessive–compulsive personality traits in adult women with eating disorders: Defining a broader eating disorder phenotype. *American Journal of Psychiatry, 160,* 242–247.

Baldock, E., & Tchantaria, K. (2007). Translating laboratory research into practice: Foundations, functions, and future of cognitive remediation therapy for anorexia nervosa. *Therapy, 4,* 1–8.

Boachie, A., Goldfield, G., & Spettigue, W. (2003). Olanzapine use as an adjunctive treatment for hospitalized children with anorexia nerovsa: Case reports. *International Journal of Eating Disorders, 33,* 98–103.

Bruch, H. (1973). *Eating disorders: Obesity, anorexia nervosa, and the person within.* New York: Basic Books.

Bryant-Waugh, R., Knibbs, J., Fosson, A.,

Kaminski, Z., & Lask, B. (1988). Long-term follow-up of patients with early onset anorexia nervosa. *Archives of Diseases of Childhood, 63,* 5–9.

Bryant-Waugh, R., & Lask, B. (1995). Eating disorders in children. *Journal of Child Psychology and Psychiatry, 36,* 191–202.

Couturier, J., & Lock, J. (2006a). Denial and minimization in adolescent anorexia nervosa. *International Journal of Eating Disorders, 39,* 175–183.

Couturier, J., & Lock, J. (2006b). What constitutes remission in adolescent anorexia nervosa: A review of various conceptualizations and a quantitative analysis. *International Journal of Eating Disorders, 39,* 175–183.

Couturier, J., & Lock, J. (2006c). What is recovery in adolescent anorexia nervosa? *International Journal of Eating Disorders, 39,* 550–555.

Couturier, J., & Lock, J. (2007). Review of medication use for children and adolescents with eating disorders. *Journal of the Canadian Academy of Child and Adolescent Psychiatry, 16,* 173–176.

Couturier, J., Lock, J., Forsberg, S., Vanderheyden, D., & Lee, H. Y. (2007). The addition of a parent and clinician component to the eating disorder examination for children and adolescents. *International Journal of Eating Disorders, 40,* 472–475.

Crisp, A. H., Norton, K., Gowers, S., Halek, C., Bowyer, C., Yeldham, D., et al. (1991). A controlled study of the effect of therapies aimed at adolescent and family psychopathology in anorexia nervosa. *British Journal of Psychiatry, 159,* 325–333.

Crow, S., & Nyman, J. (2004). The cost-effectiveness of anorexia nervosa treatment. *International Journal of Eating Disorders, 35,* 155–160.

Darcy, A., Celio Doyle, A., Lock, J., Doyle, P., & Le Grange, D. (in press). The Eating Disorder Examination in adolescent males: How does it compare to adolescent females? *International Journal of Eating Disorders.*

Darcy, A., Katz, S., Fitzpatrick, K., Forsberg, S., Ultzinger, L., & Lock, J. (2010). All better … How former patients define recovery and engage in treatment. *European Eating Disorders Review, 18,* 260–270.

Eddy, K., Dorer, D., Franko, D., Tahilani, K., Thompson-Brenner, H., & Herzog, D. B. (2008). Diagnostic crossover in anorexia nervosa and bulimia nervosa: Implications for DSM 5. *American Journal of Psychiatry, 165,* 245–250.

Eisler, I. (2005). The empirical and theoretical base of family therapy and multiple family day therapy for adolescent anorexia nervosa. *Journal of Family Therapy, 27,* 104–131.

Eisler, I., Dare, C., Russell, G. F. M., Szmukler, G. I., Le Grange, D., & Dodge, E. (1997). Family and individual therapy in anorexia nervosa: A five-year follow-up. *Archives of General Psychiatry, 54,* 1025–1030.

Eisler, I., Simic, M., Russell, G., & Dare, C. (2007). A randomized controlled treatment trial of two forms of family therapy in adolescent anorexia nervosa: A five-year follow-up. *Journal of Child Psychology and Psychiatry, 48,* 552–560.

Fairburn, C. (1981). A cognitive behavioural approach to the treatment of bulimia. *Psychological Medicine, 11*(4), 707–711.

Fairburn, C., & Bohn, K. (2005). Eating disorder NOS (EDNOS): An example of the troublesome eating disorder not otherwise specified (NOS) category in DSM-IV. *Behavior Research and Therapy, 43,* 691–701.

Fairburn, C. G., Cooper, Z., & Shafran, R. (2002). Cognitive behaviour therapy for eating disorders: A "transdiagnostic" theory and treatment. *Behavior Research and Therapy, 41,* 509–528.

Fairburn, C. G., Cooper, Z., & Shafran, R. (2008). Enhanced cognitive behavioral therapy for eating disorders ("CBT-E"): An overview. In C. G. Fairburn (Ed.), *Cognitive behavior therapy and eating disorders* (pp. 23–34). New York: Guilford Press.

Fisher, M., Golden, N., Katzman, D., Kreipe, R., Rees, J., Schebendach, J., et al. (1995). Eating disorders in adolescents: A background paper. *Journal of Adolescent Health, 16,* 420–437.

Godart, N., Flament, M., Perdereau, F., & Jeammet, P. (2002). Comorbidity between eating disorders and anxiety disorders: A review. *International Journal of Eating Disorders, 32,* 253–270.

Gowers, S., Clark, A., Roberts, C., Griffiths, A., Edwards, V., Bryan, C., et al. (2007). Clinical effectiveness of treatments for anorexia nervosa in adolescents. *British Journal of Psychiatry, 191,* 427–435.

Gowers, S., Weetman, J., Shore, R., Hussain, F., & Elvins, R. (2000). The impact of hospitalisation on the outcome of adolescent anorexia nervosa. *British Journal of Psychiatry, 45,* 138–141.

Gull, W. (1874). Anorexia nervosa (apepsia hysterica, anorexia hysterica). *Transactions of the Clinical Society of London, 7,* 222–228.

Halmi, C. A. (2008). The perplexities of conducting randomized, double-blind, placebo-controlled treatment trials in anorexia nervosa patients. *American Journal of Psychiatry, 165,* 1227–1228.

Herzog, D. B., Keller, M. B., Sacks, N. R., Yeh, C. J., & Lavori, P. W. (1992). Psychiatric comorbidity in treatment-seeking anorexics and bulimics. *Journal of the American Academy of Child and Adolescent Psychiatry, 31*(5), 810–818.

Hoek, H. W., & van Hoeken, D. (2003). Review of prevalence and incidence of eating disorders. *International Journal of Eating Disorders, 34,* 383–396.

Holliday, J., Tchanturia, K., Landau, S., & Collier, D. (2005). Is impaired set-shifting an endophenotype of anorexia nervosa? *American Journal of Psychiatry, 162,* 2269–2275.

Holtkamp, K., Muller, B., Heussen, N., Remschmidt, H., & Herperz-Dahlmann, B.

(2005). Depression, anxiety, and obsessionality in long-term recovered patients with adolescent-onset anorexia nervosa. *European Child and Adolescent Psychiatry, 14,* 106–110.

Jacobi, C., Hayward, C., de Zwaan, M., Kraemer, H., & Agras, W. (2004). Coming to terms with risk factors for eating disorders: Application of risk terminology and suggestions for a general taxonomy. *Psychological Bulletin, 130,* 19–65.

Kaye, W., Fudge, J., & Paulus, M. (2009). New insights into symptoms and neurocircuit function in anorexia nervosa. *Nature Reviews/Neuroscience, 10,* 573–584.

Keel, P., Graemer, J., Joiner, T., & Haedt, A. (2010). Twenty-year follow-up of bulimia nervosa and related eating disorders not otherwise specified. *International Journal of Eating Disorders, 43,* 491–497.

Klump, K. L., Keel, P. K., Sisk, C., & Burt, S. A. (2010). Preliminary evidence that estradiol moderates genetic influences on disordered eating attitudes and behaviors during puberty. *Psychological Medicine, 40,* 1745–1753.

Kotler, L., Devlin, B., Davies, M., & Walsh, B. T. (2003). An open trial of fluoextine in adolescents with bulimia nervosa. *Journal of Child and Adolescent Psychopharmacology, 13,* 329–325.

Kraemer, H., Frank, E., & Kupfer, D. (2006). Moderators of treatment outcomes: Clinical, Research, and Policy importance. *Journal of the American Medical Association, 296,* 1286–1289.

Krautter, T., & Lock, J. (2004). Is manualized family-based treatment for adolescent anorexia nervosa acceptable to patients?: Patient satisfaction at end of treatment. *Journal of Family Therapy, 26,* 65–81.

Lask, B., & Bryant-Waugh, R. (1992). Early-onset anorexia nervosa and related eating disorders. *Journal of Child Psychology and Psychiatry, 33,* 281–300.

Lee, Y., & Lin, P.-Y. (2010). Association between serotonin transporter gene polymorphism and eating disorders: A meta-analytic study. *International Journal of Eating Disorders, 43,* 498–504.

Le Grange, D., Binford, R., Peterson, C., Crow, S., Crosby, R., Klein, M., et al. (2006). DSM-IV threshold versus sub-threshold bulimia nervosa. *International Journal of Eating Disorders, 39,* 462–467.

Le Grange, D., Crosby, R., & Lock, J. (2008). Predictors and moderators of outcome in family-based treatment for adolescent bulimia nervosa. *Journal of the American Academy of Child and Adolescent Psychiatry, 47,* 464–470.

Le Grange, D., Crosby, R., Rathouz, P., & Leventhal, B. (2007). A randomized controlled comparison of family-based treatment and supportive psychotherapy for adolescent bulimia nervosa. *Archives of General Psychiatry, 64,* 1049–1056.

Le Grange, D., & Gelman, T. (1998). The patient's perspective of treatment in eating disorders: A preliminary study. *South African Journal of Psychology, 28,* 182–186.

Le Grange, D., & Lock, J. (2002, August). Bulimia nervosa in adolescents: Treatment, eating pathology, and comorbidity. *South African Psychiatry Review,* 19–22.

Le Grange, D., & Lock, J. (2005). The dearth of psychological treatment studies for anorexia nervosa. *International Journal of Eating Disorders, 37,* 79–81.

Le Grange, D., & Lock, J. (2007). *Treating bulimia in adolescents: A family-based approach.* New York: Guilford Press.

Le Grange, D., Lock, J., Loeb, K., & Nicholls, D. (2010). The role of the family in eating disorders: An Academy of Eating Disorders position paper. *International Journal of Eating Disorders, 43,* 1–5.

Le Grange, D., Loeb, K. L., Orman, S., & Jellar, C. (2004). Bulimia nervosa: A disorder in evolution? *Archives of Pediatrics and Adolescent Medicine, 158,* 478–482.

Lock, J. (2005). Adjusting cognitive behavioral therapy for adolescent bulimia nervosa: Results of a case series. *American Journal of Psychotherapy, 59,* 267–281.

Lock, J. (2008). Fitting square pegs into round holes: Males with eating disorders. *Journal of Adolescent Health, 44,* 99–100.

Lock, J. (2010). Controversies and advances in child and adolescent eating disorders. In W.

S. Agras (Ed.), *Oxford handbook of eating disorders* (pp. 51–74). Oxford, UK: Oxford University Press.

Lock, J., Agras, W. S., Bryson, S., & Kraemer, H. (2005). A comparison of short- and long-term family therapy for adolescent anorexia nervosa. *Journal of the American Academy of Child and Adolescent Psychiatry, 44,* 632–639.

Lock, J., Couturier, J., & Agras, W. S. (2006). Comparison of long-term outcomes in adolescents with anorexia nervosa treated with family therapy. *American Journal of Child and Adolescent Psychiatry, 45,* 666–672.

Lock, J., Couturier, J., & Agras, W. S. (2008). Costs of remission and recovery using family therapy for adolescent anorexia nervosa: A descriptive study. *Eating Disorders, 16,* 322–330.

Lock, J., Couturier, J., Bryson, S., & Agras, W. S. (2006). Predictors of dropout and remission in family therapy for adolescent anorexia nervosa in a randomized clinical trial. *International Journal of Eating Disorders, 39,* 639–647.

Lock, J., Garrett, A., Beenhaker, J., & Reiss, A. (2011). Aberrant brain activation during a response inhibition task in adolescent eating disorder subtypes. *American Journal of Psychiatry, 168,* 55–64.

Lock, J., & Le Grange, D. (2005). *Help your teenager beat an eating disorder.* New York: Guilford Press.

Lock, J., Le Grange, D., Agras, W. S., Moye, A., Bryson, S., & Jo, B. (2010). Randomized clinical trial comparing family-based treatment to adolescent focused individual therapy for adolescents with anorexia nervosa. *Archives of General Psychiatry, 67,* 1025–1032.

Lock, J., Le Grange, D., & Crosby, R. (2008). Exploring possible mechanisms of change in family based treatment for bulimia nervosa. *Journal of Family Therapy, 30,* 260–271.

Lock, J., & Peebles, R. (2010). *Predictors of serious medical complications in adolescent females hospitalized for eating disorders.* Paper presented at the Academy of Eating Disorders, Saltzburg, Austria.

Lopez, C., Tchanturia, K., Stahl, D., Booth, R., Holliday, J., & Treasure, J. (2008). An examination of the concept of central coherence in women with anorexia nervosa. *International Journal of Eating Disorders, 41,* 143–152.

Lopez, C., Tchanturia, K., Stahl, D., & Treasure, J. (2008). Central coherence in women with bulimia nervosa. *International Journal of Eating Disorders, 41,* 340–354.

Lucas, A. R., Beard, C. M., & O'Fallon, W. M. (1991). 50-year trends in the incidence of anorexia nervosa in Rochester, Minn.: A population-based study. *American Journal of Psychiatry, 148,* 917–929.

Luce, J., Osborne, M., Taylor, K., Cunning, D., Doyle, A., Wilfley, D., et al. (2008). Randomized, controlled trial of an Internet-facilitated intervention for reducing binge eating and overweight in adolescents. *Pediatrics, 121,* 453–462.

Marsh, R., Maia, T., & Peterson, B. (2009). Functional disturbances within frontostriatal circuits across multiple childhood psychopathologies. *American Journal of Psychiatry, 166,* 664–674.

Marsh, R., Steinglass, J., Gerber, A., O'Leary, G., Wang, Z., Murphy, D., et al. (2009). Deficient activity in the neural systems that mediate self-regulatory control in bulimia nervosa. *Archives of General Psychiatry, 66,* 51–63.

McIntosh, V. W., Jordan, J., Carter, F. A., Luty, S. E., McKenzie, J. M., Bulik, C. M., et al. (2005). Three psychotherapies for anorexia nervosa: A randomized, controlled trial. *American Journal of Psychiatry, 162,* 741–747.

McVey, G., Davis, R., Tweed, S., & Shaw, B. (2004). Evaluation of a school-based program designed to improve body image satisfaction, global self-esteem, and eating attitudes and behaviors: A replication study. *International Journal of Eating Disorders, 36,* 1–11.

Murray, S., Reiger, E., Touyz, S., & Garcia, Y. (2010). Muscle dysphoria and the DSM-5 cunundrum: Where does it belong? A review paper. *International Journal of Eating Disorders, 43,* 481–491.

Nicholls, D., Chater, R., & Lask, B. (2000).

Children into DSM don't go: A comparison of classification systems for eating disorders in childhood and adolescence. *International Journal of Eating Disorders, 28*, 317–324.

Norris, R., Spettigue, W., Buchholz, A., Henderson, K., & Obeid, N. (2010). Factors influencing research drug trials in adolescents with anorexia nervosa. *Eating Disorders, 18*, 210–217.

Olmos, J., Valero, C., del Barrio, A., Amado, J., Hernandez, J., Menedez-Arango, J., et al. (2010). Time course of bone loss in patients with anorexia nervosa. *International Journal of Eating Disorders, 43*, 537–542.

Peebles, R., Hardy, K., Wilson, J., & Lock, J. D. (2010). Eating disorders not otherwise specified: Are diagnostic criteria for eating disorders markers of medical severity? *Pediatrics, 125*, 1193–1201.

Peebles, R., Wilson, J., Borzehowski, D., Hardy, K., Lock, J., Mann, J., et al. *Disordered eating in a digital age: Eating behaviors, health and quality of life in users of websites with pro-eating disorder content.* Manuscript submitted for publication.

Peebles, R., Wilson, J., & Lock, J. (2006). How do children and adolescents with eating disorders differ at presentation? *Journal of Adolescent Health, 39*, 800–805.

Rhodes, P., Baillee, A., Brown, J., & Madden, S. (2008). Can parent-to-parent consultation improve the effectiveness of the Maudsley model of family-based treatment for anorexia nervosa? A randomized control trial. *Journal of Family Therapy, 30*, 96–198.

Rhodes, P., Madden, S., & Brown, J. (2009). Parent-to-parent consultation in the Maudsley model of family-based treatment of anorexia nervosa: A qualitative study. *Journal of Marital and Family Therapy, 35*, 181–192.

Rieger, E., Van Buren, D., Bishop, M., Tanofsky-Kraff, M., Welch, R., & Wilfley, D. (2010). An eating disorder-specific model of interpersonal therapy (IPT-ED): Causal pathways and treatment implications. *Clinical Psychology Review, 30*, 400–410.

Roberts, M., Tchanturia, K., Stahl, D., Southgate, L., & Treasure, J. (2005). A systematic review and meta-analysis of set-shifting

ability in eating disorders. *Psychological Medicine, 37*, 1075–1084.

Robin, A., Siegal, P., Moye, A., Gilroy, M., Dennis, A., & Sikand, A. (1999). A controlled comparison of family versus individual therapy for adolescents with anorexia nervosa. *Journal of the American Academy of Child and Adolescent Psychiatry, 38*(12), 1482–1489.

Rubinow, D. R., Schmidt, P. J., & Roca, C. A. (1998). Estrogen–serotonin interactions: Implications for affective regulation. *Biological Psychiatry, 44*, 839–850.

Russell, G. F., Szmukler, G. I., Dare, C., & Eisler, I. (1987). An evaluation of family therapy in anorexia nervosa and bulimia nervosa. *Archives of General Psychiatry, 44*(12), 1047–1056.

Schmidt, U., Lee, S., Beecham, J., Perkins, S., Treasure, J. L., Yi, I., et al. (2007). A randomized controlled trial of family therapy and cognitive behavior therapy guided self-care for adolescents with bulimia nervosa and related conditions. *American Journal of Psychiatry, 164*, 591–598.

Shapiro, J., Bauer, S., Andrews, E., Pitesky, E., Bulik-Sullivan, B., Hamer, R., et al. (2010). Mobile therapy: Use of text-messaging in the treatment of bulimia nervosa. *International Journal of Eating Disorders, 43*, 513–519.

Silber, T. (1994). Eating disorders and health insurance. *Archives of Pediatrics and Adolescent Medicine, 148*, 785–788.

Silverman, J. (1997). Charcot's comments on the therapeutic role of isolation in the treatment of anorexia nervosa. *International Journal of Eating Disorders, 21*, 295–298.

Smith, A., Hawkeswood, B., & Joiner, T. (2010). The measure of a man: Associations between digit ratio and disordered eating in males. *International Journal of Eating Disorders, 43*, 543–548.

Steinhausen, H. (2002). The outcome of anorexia nervosa in the 20th century. *American Journal of Psychiatry, 159*, 1284–1293.

Steinhausen, H. (2009). Outcome of eating disorders. *Child and Adolescent Psychiatric Clinics of North America, 18*, 225–242.

Steinhausen, H., Rauss-Mason, C., & Seidel,

R. (1991). Follow-up studies of anorexia nervosa: A review of four decades of outcome research. *Psychological Medicine, 21,* 447–454.

Steinhausen, H., Rauss-Mason, C., & Seidel, R. (1993). Short-term and intermediate term outcome in adolescent eating disorders. *Acta Psychiatrica Scandinavica, 88,* 169–173.

Steinhausen, H., & Weber, S. (2009). The outcome of bulimia nervosa: Findings from one-quarter century of research. *American Journal of Psychiatry, 166,* 1331–1341.

Striegel-Moore, R., Leslie, D., Petrill, S. A., Garvin, V., & Rosenheck, R. A. (2000). One-year use and cost of inpatient and outpatient services among female and male patients with an eating disorder: Evidence from a national database of health insurance claims. *International Journal of Eating Disorders, 27,* 381–389.

Strober, M. (2007). The association of anxiety disorders and obsessive compulsive personality disorder with anorexia nervosa: Evidence from a family study with discussion of nosological and neurodevelopmental implications. *International Journal of Eating Disorders, 40,* S46–S51.

Strober, M., Freeman, A., Lampert, C., Diamond, J., & Kaye, W. H. (2000). Controlled family study of anorexia nervosa and bulimia nervosa: Evidence of shared liability and transmission of partial syndromes. *American Journal of Psychiatry, 157,* 393–401.

Strober, M., & Humphrey, L. (1987). Family contributions to the etiology and course of anorexia nervosa and bulimia nervosa. *Journal of Consulting Clinical Psychology, 55,* 654–659.

Strober, M., Morrell, W., Burroughs, J., Salkin, B., & Jacobs, C. (1985). A controlled family study of anorexia nervosa. *Journal of Psychiatric Research, 19,* 239–246.

Tanofsky-Kraff, M., Wilfley, D., Young, J., Mufson, L., Yanovski, S. Z., Glasofer, D., et al. (2007). Preventing excessive weight gain in adolescents: Interpersonal psychotherapy for binge eating. *Obesity, 15,* 1345–12355.

Taylor, C. B., Bryson, S., Luce, K. H., Cunning, D., Celio Doyle, A., Abascal, L. B., et al. (2006). Prevention of eating disorders in at-risk college-age women. *Archives of General Psychiatry, 63,* 881–888.

Tchanturia, K., Davies, H., & Campbell, I. (2007). Cognitive remediation for patients with anorexia nervosa: Preliminary findings. *Annals of General Psychiatry, 14,* 1–6.

Treasure, J., Schmidt, U., & Macdonald, P. (2009). *The clinician's guide to collaborative caring in eating disorders: The new Maudsley method.* New York: Routledge.

Turner, H., & Bryant-Waugh, R. (2004). Eating disorder not otherwise specified (EDNOS): Profiles of clients presenting at a community eating disorder service. *European Eating Disorders Review, 12,* 18–26.

van Son, G., van Hoeken, D., Aad, I., Bartelds, A., van Furth, E., & Hoek, H. (2006). Time trends in the incidence of eating disorders: A primary care study in the Netherlands. *International Journal of Eating Disorders, 39,* 565–569.

Wagner, A., Barbarich-Marstellar, N., Frank, G., Bailer, U., Wonderlich, S., Crosby, R., et al. (2006). Personality traits after recovery from eating disorders: Do subtypes differ? *International Journal of Eating Disorders, 39,* 276–284.

Walford, G., & McCune, N. (1991). Long-term outcome in early onset anorexia nervosa. *British Journal of Psychiatry, 159,* 383–389.

Wallis, A., Rhodes, P., Kohn, M., & Madden, S. (2007). Five years of family based treatment for anorexia nervosa: The Maudsley model at the Children's Hospital at Westmead. *International Journal of Adolescent Medicine and Health, 19,* 277–283.

Wentz, E., Gillberg, C., Gillberg, I. C., & Rastam, M. (2001). Ten-year follow-up of adolescent-onset anorexia nervosa: Psychiatric disorders and overall functioning scales. *Journal of Child Psychology and Psychiatry, 42,* 613–622.

Wilfley, D., Welch, R., Stein, R., Spurrell, E., Cohen, L., Saelens, B., et al. (2002). A randomized clinical comparison of group cognitive behavioral therapy and group interpersonal therapy for the treatment of overweight individuals with binge-eating disorder. *Archives of General Psychiatry, 59,* 713–721.

Woodside, B., Bulik, C. M., Halmi, C. A., Fichter, M., Kaplan, A. S., Berrettini, W., et al. (2002). Personality, perfectionism, and attitudes toward eating in parents of individuals with eating disorders. *International Journal of Eating Disorders, 31,* 290–299.

Workgroup for the Classification of Child and Adolescent Eating Disorders. (2007). Classification of child and adolescent eating disturbances. *International Journal of Eating Disorders, 40,* S117–S122.

Zastrow, A., Kaiser, S., Stippich, C., Walther, S., Herzog, W., Tchanturia, K., et al. (2009). Neural correlates of impaired cognitive-behavioral flexibility in anorexia nervosa. *American Journal of Psychiatry, 166,* 608–616.

Zipfel, S., Lowe, B., Deter, H. C., & Herzog, W. (2000). Long-term prognosis in anorexia nervosa: Lessons from a 21-year follow-up study. *Lancet, 355,* 721–722.

Zucker, N. L., Marcus, M. D., & Bulik, C. (2006). A group parent training program: A novel approach for eating disorder management. *Eating and Weight Disorders: Studies on Anorexia, Bulimia and Obesity, 11,* 78–82.

Author Index

Subject Index

Page numbers followed by *f* indicate figure, *t* indicate table